Neuroscience for the Study of Communicative Disorders

Second Edition

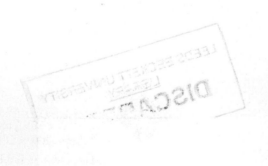

Neuroscience for the Study of Communicative Disorders

Second Edition

Subhash C. Bhatnagar, PhD

Speech Pathology and Audiology Department
Marquette University
Milwaukee, Wisconsin

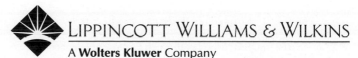

LIPPINCOTT WILLIAMS & WILKINS
A **Wolters Kluwer** Company

Philadelphia • Baltimore • New York • London
Buenos Aires • Hong Kong • Sydney • Tokyo

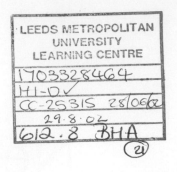

Editor: Timothy L. Julet
Managing Editor: Linda S. Napora
Marketing Manager: Christen DeMarco
Production Editor: Paula C. Williams
Compositor: Maryland Composition, Inc.
Printer: Courier

351 West Camden Street
Baltimore, Maryland 21201-2436 USA

530 Walnut Street
Philadelphia, Pennsylvania 19106-3621 USA

Printed in the United States of America

Library of Congress Cataloging-in-Publication Data

Bhatnagar, Subhash Chandra.
  Neuroscience for the study of communicative disorders / Subhash C. Bhatnagar.–2nd ed.
    p. ; cm.
  Includes bibliographical references and index.
  ISBN 0-7817-2346-9
  1. Communicative disorders–Pathophysiology. 2. Neurosciences. I. Title.
  [DNLM: 1. Central Nervous System–anatomy & histology. 2. Central Nervous System–physiology. 3. Communication Disorders–physiopathology. WL 300 B575n 2001]
  RC243 .B53 2001
  612.8–dc21

                                                                    2001038869

The publishers have made every effort to trace the copyright holders for borrowed material. If they have inadvertently overlooked any, they will be pleased to make the necessary arrangements at the first opportunity.

To purchase additional copies of this book call our customer service department at **(800) 638-3030** or fax orders to **(301) 824-7390.** International customers should call **(301) 714-2324.**

Visit Lippincott Williams & Wilkins on the Internet: **http://www.lww.com.** Lippincott Williams & Wilkins customer service representatives are available from 8:30 am to 6:00 pm, EST, Monday through Friday, for telephone access.

01 02 03
1 2 3 4 5 6 7 8 9 10

In memory of
My father, Shri. Chiranji L. Bhatnagar who
nurtured and inspired me
and
My friend, Orlando J. Andy
for his encouragement and support

Foreword

I am honored to be asked to write the Foreword for *Neuroscience for the Study of Communicative Disorders*. This Second Edition has been updated, as well as expanded and enhanced to meet the book's primary goal of making neuroscience reachable to students of human behavior, many of whom have limited backgrounds in science.

The essence of the text, with its commitment to enhancing the learning process remains untouched. This Second Edition builds upon the success of the first edition and has the same approach: sensitivity to student needs and ways to meet those needs. The Second Edition benefits from the use of color enhancement, the presentation of additional case studies, the development of a set of systematic rules for localizing brain damage, and more informative, extensive, and explicit tables and figures, glossary terms, medical abbreviations, and so forth.

Students of communication and its disorders will quickly feel at home with this book. It highlights issues in neuroscience that are basic to the study of communicative disorders and deals with those issues from the perspective of the communication disorders student. Guidance is provided by the learning objectives and the carefully crafted review questions. The book teaches problem-solving skills, an absolute necessity for any student of the neurosciences who is interested in keeping up with this complex and ever-evolving field.

I believe that as this book becomes the standard for teaching neuroscience to students of communicative disorders, the quality of their understanding will escalate. I am also confident that working clinicians and professionals in medically related fields will be well served in relying on this text as a reference that provides the essentials while avoiding oversimplification of neuroscience. *Neuroscience for the Study of Communicative Disorders* is a balanced and focused text that provides readers at all levels with an opportunity to learn the basics of neuroscience.

Audrey L. Holland, PhD
Regents' Professor
Department of Speech and Hearing Sciences
University of Arizona
Tucson, Arizona

_____ Preface to the Second Edition

We believed that neuroscience could be simplified and presented in such a way so that its learning poses a challenge for students and allows them to engage in clinical application of neurological concepts. In the first edition of _Neuroscience for the Study of Communicative Disorders_, we made efforts to avoid excessive details, while at the same time maintaining a sense of the complexity of the material. We used concise descriptions, along with extensive illustrations of structures and neuronal pathways, to explain the anatomy and physiology of the brain and to promote an analytic approach to brain function. This discussion, along with the visual approach to neuroscience, proved to be challenging to students. The encouraging feedback from many colleagues and students reinforced our belief that this was an effective method of teaching neuroscience.

This same belief, which has helped our colleagues and benefited students in the field of communicative disorders, has guided the revision of the book. In this _Second Edition_, efforts have been made to improve further the visual presentation of neuroscience, to reduce excessive detail, to increase the simplicity of presentation and, most importantly, to stimulate an analytic approach to neuroscience. Problem-solving skills have been enhanced by the inclusion of rules for lesion localizing, enabling students to relate functions with structures. Through the incorporation of case studies and lesion localizing rules, the learning of neuroscience becomes more interactive and enjoyable. The highlights of the revised text are:

- _Use of color to identify and demarcate structures and pathways of interest;_
- _Updated discussion of neurodiagnostic images and common neurological concepts, and techniques and treatment;_
- _Discussion of respiratory physiology;_
- _Review of physiology of consciousness;_
- _Inclusion of lesion localization rules for promoting reasoning and analytic approach;_
- _Presentation of user-friendly case studies to promote problem-solving skills;_
- _35 summary tables to consolidate learning;_
- _35 additional illustrations to help with the visual learning of neurostructures;_
- _180 medical abbreviations and 140 Greek/Latin lexical roots to simplify the learning of medical terms;_
- _More than 200 definitions in the glossary to facilitate learning;_
- _Additional review questions to allow students to assess their knowledge._

Instructors are encouraged to reorganize the order and control the quantity of material presented. The bulleted outlines can help instructors to reorder and reprioritize the book content to suit their teaching needs.

Preface to the First Edition

Neuroscience for the Study of Communicative Disorders is primarily a textbook for a semester-long graduate level course in neuroscience for students in communicative disorders and sciences; many of these students have only a limited background in biology, chemistry, physiology, and physics. The book can also be used by working clinicians and by professionals in other medically associated fields. The purpose of the book is to describe the basics of neuroscience. We have made every effort to present facts of neuroscience and eliminate excessive details. *By eliminating the encyclopedic details of anatomy and physiology, we have provided the essentials while avoiding the oversimplification of neuroscience.* We have used concise though simplified descriptions along with extensive illustrations of structures and neuronal connections to explain the anatomy and physiology of the brain. This will enable readers to relate functions with structures in both the central and peripheral nervous systems. With this simple approach, students in communicative disorders will not feel overwhelmed by neurological complexity but will be challenged as they learn neuroscience.

Why Neuroscience?

Communicative disorders and neuroscience are two closely related disciplines. One basic concern of neuroscience that relates to the study of speech-language pathologies is the cortical representation of linguistic, congitive, gestural, and mnemonic (memory) faculties unique to the human brain. This association underscores why students in communicative disorders need a background in neuroscience. Knowledge of the nervous system helps students to understand the functional organization of the brain and will help them grasp the genesis, nature, and scope of neurogenic communicative breakdown. This also enables students to understand brain abnormalities and neurological illnesses, appreciate the physiology of treatment efficacy or limitations, follow neurolinguistic research, and relate their knowledge to the broader application of the profession.

Organization

The 20 chapters are arranged in a sequence that facilitates learning. Chapter 1 deals with the rationale for studying neuroscience and introduces technical terms, functional classifications, and principles that govern brain functions. Chapters 2–6 focus on the neuroanatomical knowledge needed for understanding the functional organization of the brain. These include the gross external and internal neuroanatomical structures, basic neuronal principles underlying impulse generation and transmission, subcortical structures and their functions, and embryological concepts. Chapters 7–10 focus on anatomy and physiology of sensory systems that include somatic sensation (pain, temperature, touch), vision, hearing, and equilibrium. Chapters 11–14 deal with the various levels of organization important in motor functions, including speech production. Cranial nerve functions have been examined in depth in Chapter 15 because of their importance in sensorimotor functions, motor speech processes, special sensations, and swallowing. Chapter 16 covers the anatomy and physiology of the axial brain, which includes the autonomic nervous system, limbic system, hypothalamus, and reticular formation. These systems are essential to survival and involve more complex neural mechanisms that are only indirectly related to the primary concern of professionals in communicative disorders. We have deliberately cut the scope of these topics, retaining discussions of essential concepts only to help students appreciate their importance. Chapter 17 and 18 provide a basic understanding of the circulation of cerebrovascular and cerebrospinal fluid systems and their pathologies. Higher mental functions that are significant to students and professionals in communicative disorders and sciences are discussed in Chapter 19. A more detailed discussion of aphasia, dementia, dysarthria, and apraxia can be found in numerous excellent texts. Chapter 20 includes a basic description of clinical and diagnostic techniques needed in medical and research settings. Diagnostic methods include brain imaging techniques, cerebral dominance determining tests such as dichotic listening and sodium amytal infusion, and brain electrical activity mapping. Additional issues relevant to the clinical setting include evoked potentials, nerve conduction, neurosurgical procedures used for cortical and subcortical ablations, genetic patterns of inheritance, and specific neurological disorders such as seizures, encephalopathies, myopathies, peripheral neuropathies, and cerebral infections.

This book incorporates the following practical teaching concepts:

- Learning objectives are listed before each chapter to assist students in identifying the scope of knowledge they will gain;
- Important technical terms are italicized in the text;
- Extensive illustrations that are clear and well-labeled have been used to facilitate the visual learning of complex anatomical details (illustrations are further supplemented by charts and tables that summarize crucial inforamtion);
- Clinical discussions are often used to nurture analytical reasoning and problem solving ability;
- Case studies in most chapters provide an opportunity to examine the clinical application of the information;
- Summaries at the end of each chapter help readers check the information covered;
- Technical terms are listed at the end of each chapter; readers should check whether they understand the terms before continuing to the next chapter (most technical terms are defined in the Glossary);
- Review questions at the end of each chapter serve to consolidate the learning; those who can answer the questions can begin to think in terms of applying the knowledge to clinical settings and problem solving;
- Appendices contain explanations of common medical abbreviations, prefixes, suffixes, and Greek and Latin lexical roots; a substantial Glossary of technical terms is also provided.

Teaching Neuroscience

Despite its admitted complexity, the human nervous system is organized logically along principles and systems; its complexity can be overcome by a systematic approach to learning. Colleagues who teach neuroscience are advised to use the following time-tested approaches:

Promote orientation to visual learning. Repeated visual orientation to gross and internal structures of the brain in relation to their functions is needed for overcoming anatomical and physiological complexities. Chapters 2 and 3 provide the anatomical background needed for understanding the functional organization of the brain.

Foster functional learning. Relate each structure to its functional relevance. For example, how does the pathology of a structure at a specific brain level relate to a pattern of sensorimotor deficit, and would it affect the body parts ipsilateral or contralateral to the lesion? Examining such questions will nurture a grasp of the organization of the brain.

Avoid short cuts. To understand functions of the nervous system, it is essential to study neuroanatomy. Strategies or priorities that stress only the functions will actually restrict the understanding of neuroscience needed to comprehend its applications to brain and behavior.

Subhash C. Bhatnagar, PhD
Orlando J. Andy, MD

Acknowledgments

I am indebted to the following who have helped me in the second edition of the book:

One of my teachers—who preferred to remain anonymous—for reading a large part of the book and giving me most valuable suggestions for improving the anatomical and clinical details.

Dr. Robin L. Curtis from the Department of Cell Biology, Neurobiology, and Anatomy at the Medical College of Wisconsin for his valuable comments on chapters related to sensory motor systems.

Dr. Duane E. Haines from the Department of Anatomy at the University of Mississippi Medical Center, Jackson for his support throughout this work and for allowing us to use the serial brain dissections from his Brain Atlas.

Dr. Arnold E. Aronson from the Department of Neurology, Mayo Medical School for many clinical ideas and his comments on the chapter related to cranial nerves.

Dr. Howard Kirshner from the Department of Neurology, Vanderbilt College of Medicine for his comments on some case studies and for providing me with PET images.

Dr. Varun K. Saxena from the Center for Neurological Disorders Milwaukee for many discussions, and for his comments on clinical issues related to the vascular accidents.

Dr. Leighten Mark from the Department of Neuroradiology at the Medical College of Wisconsin for providing me with MR and CT images and commenting on my discussion of neuroradiology.

Dr. Edward W. Korabic from Marquette University and Dr. Tom White from SUNY/Buffalo for their comments on the auditory system.

Dr. Donald A. Neuman from Marquette University for reviewing the respiratory physiology section in the chapter on axial brain.

Dr. Patricia A. Marquardt for her assistance in reviewing Greek and Latin details in the glossary.

Dr. Arun V. Parikh, a consulting psychiatrist, for assistance in reviewing neurobehavioral problems.

Dr. Waleed S. Najeeb from Mepoint Sleep Disorder Center in Milwaukee, for comments on the disorders of consciousness.

Nick Schroeder for assistance with artwork.

I am also grateful to many of my colleagues and students, who have used the book over the years and have provided me with numerous suggestions. In particular, I thank Dr. Brooke Hallowell from the Ohio State University at Athens, who has been the most enthusiastic about this book and who has given me invaluable suggestions for revision. Over the years, many of my students at Marquette University have helped me with the revision. In particular, I acknowledge the assistance of Allyson Goetschel, Cara Koch, Clare Burgess, Kay Eason, and Jill Stukenberg.

Last, but not least, I thank my wife Priti and sons Manav and Gaurav. Without their understanding, encouragement, and support, I could not have completed this book.

Contents

1 Scope, Principles, and Elements of Neuroscience — 1

2 Gross Anatomy of the Central Nervous System — 21

3 Internal Anatomy of the Central Nervous System — 76

4 Embryological Development of the Central Nervous System — 111

5 Nerve Cells — 125

6 Diencephalon: Thalamus and Associated Structures — 142

7 Somatosensory System — 153

8 Visual System — 173

9   Auditory System   195

10   Vestibular System   210

11   Motor System 1: Spinal Cord   219

12   Motor System 2: Cerebellum — 241

13   Motor System 3: Brainstem and Basal Ganglia — 252

17 Vascular System — 337

18 Cerebrospinal Fluid — 354

19 Cerebral Cortex: Higher Mental Functions — 359

Scope, Principles, and Elements of Neuroscience

Learning Objectives

After studying this chapter, students should be able to do the following:
- Describe the subject matter of neuroscience and its relationship to speech–language–hearing pathology
- Appreciate the rationale behind and the benefits provided by a training in neuroscience
- List the major branches of neuroscience and describe the scope of each branch
- Explain the components of a neurological examination
- Describe common types of neurological diseases
- Explain basic principles that govern functioning of the human brain
- Define technical terms used for directional reference, planes of brain section, and movement
- Describe basic neuroanatomical terms
- List major structures of the central nervous system and describe their functions
- Describe the functional components that are used to categorize the functions of the nervous system
- Describe common hurdles in learning neuroscience
- Incorporate strategies for overcoming difficulties encountered in learning neuroscience
- List the architectural layers of the cerebral cortex
- Describe the functions of important Brodmann areas
- Appreciate the rationale underlying common neurological rules used for localizing lesions in the nervous system

RELATIONSHIP BETWEEN NEUROSCIENCE AND SPEECH–LANGUAGE–HEARING PATHOLOGY

Speech–language–hearing pathology and neuroscience are closely related disciplines. This relationship was underscored by the observations of Paul Broca and Carl Wernicke on the localization of specific expressive and receptive language functions in particular areas of the human brain. After examining a series of patients without motor problems of speech muscles, who could understand spoken language, but could not speak, Broca proposed that "We speak with the left hemisphere." An examination of patients' brains during autopsy revealed a lesion in the posterior frontal region (a region now called Broca's area). Wernicke in 1876 described a different type of aphasia caused by impaired auditory comprehension as opposed to impaired expression. He related this type of aphasia to a lesion in the posterior temporal lobe, an area different from the one described by Broca. These observations of Broca and Wernicke significantly enhanced our knowledge of the brain–behavior relationship. In doing so, they established the groundwork for neurolinguistic studies in which other language functions were assigned to different brain regions and their interconnections. Language and speech disturbances have since become sensitive indicators of structural and physiological impairment in the brain. The human brain, the most advanced in phylogenetic development, is uniquely equipped to analyze and synthesize information in the context of past, present, and future. Through its biological interaction with the environment, the brain generates substrates for **cognition, consciousness, learning, knowledge, personality, emotions, thoughts, creative ability, imagination, symbolic communication, attention,** and **sensorimotor functions.**

Domain of Neuroscience

The goal of neuroscience is to explain the mechanism the brain uses to regulate higher mental functions and to produce actions. The biological basis of such functions interfaces with both the cellular activities and the mind. The scope of neuroscience includes the study of the anatomical structures, cellular functions, and physiological processes of the nervous system. Neuroscience provides a foundation in normal anatomy and physiology of the brain, making it possible to identify sites of structural and functional abnormality. The lesion site is indicated by sensory, motor, cognitive, and behavioral changes, all of which reflect one or more areas of brain involvement. Consequently, neuroscience is indispensable for understanding the physiological correlates of speech, language, gestures, and cognition.

Domain of Speech–Language–Hearing Pathology

Speech–language–hearing pathology deals with developmental and acquired disorders of human cognition, language, and speech. Speech–language–hearing pathologists receive comprehensive training in normal development as well as abnormal aspects of communicative processes and in the assessment and management of communication disorders. With an extensive background in physiology of communication, speech–language–hearing pathologists are also trained to undertake or assist in neurolinguistic assessments, research, and management.

Need for Training in Neuroscience

An understanding of both the development and clinical nature of communicative disorders necessitates a background in neuroscience. Recent advances in medical care have prolonged the life span of many patients. This care has required comprehensive rehabilitative intervention, especially in the field of speech–language–hearing pathology. There is an ever-increasing number of patients with cognitive and communicative disorders that result from **head trauma**, **vascular accidents**, **embryological malformations**, **degenerative conditions**, **senility**, **tumors**, **epilepsy**, and other **congenital and acquired organic disorders**. Such patients require special rehabilitative intervention, and this emphasizes not only the interaction of speech–language–hearing pathology with neuroscience, but also the need for training in neuroanatomy, neurophysiology, and neurology. The application of training in neuroscience is not restricted to conditions related to adults alone; rather, it relates to communicative disorders across a spectrum of all ages. Training in neuroscience can similarly be integrated across the speech–language–hearing curriculum, or it can be taught in a separate course if possible. However, because of its comprehensiveness, it is desirable that neuroscience be taught in a separate course.

Nature of Training in Neuroscience

A well-trained professional in communicative disorders must obtain a working knowledge of neuroanatomy, neurophysiology, and neurology. Knowledge of how nerve cells communicate, how their axons serve as pathways for transferring information to other regions, and at what point they cross provides a basis for understanding the neurological correlates of higher mental functions and sensorimotor behavior. Training in fundamental neuroscience facilitates a grasp of the neurolinguistic properties of the human brain and provides clinicians in communicative disorders with a broader and better understanding of the etiology of illness, sensorimotor pathways, and structural properties and potentials of the brain. This contributes to a more effectively structured rehabilitation for communication disorders. The commonly prevailing attitude that there is a simpler version of neuroscience that is related to hearing and speech is *not accurate*. The very fundamental sensorimotor rules that apply to locomotion also apply to speaking. Similarly, the mental processes in the brain are represented by their elementary operations. Thus, some depth of discussion is unavoidable in learning neuroscience.

However, students of behavioral science need not undergo the extensive training in neuroscience generally given to neurologists and neurosurgeons. Audiologists, speech–language pathologists, psychologists, and neurolinguists need basic familiarity with the functional and anatomical organization of the nervous system, including the cerebral cortex, subcortical structures, and spinal cord.

Benefits of Training in Neuroscience

On a technical level, familiarity with the fundamentals of neuroscience does more than provide professionals in behavioral science, such as speech–language–hearing pathologists, with an understanding of the etiology of medical conditions associated with communicative disorders. Training also enables these clinicians and researchers to appreciate signs and symptoms associated with abnormalities of subcortical and cortical areas, to comprehend the principles of differential diagnosis, and to interpret neuroimaging. This training will also facilitate recognition of clinically significant symptoms—covert and overt—and the detection of life-threatening conditions associated with various cortical and subcortical pathological processes.

Students of communicative disorders trained in neuroscience are known to have achieved an improved ability to provide clinical services. The training makes them creative partners on a diagnostic team and promoters of a constructive working relationship with medical colleagues (neurologist, neurosurgeon, radiologist, pediatrician, and physiatrist). Their knowledge further enables them to follow and appreciate scientific literature, minimizes the complexity of medical terminology, enhances skills for solving neurological problems, promotes neurolinguistic research, and consequently provides a broader view of the profession.

SCOPE OF NEUROSCIENCE

Neurological assessment and management involve many branches of neuroscience. A neurological diagnosis means identifying symptoms that characterize the disease and answering key questions: What is the cause? Is it inflammatory, traumatic, genetic, psychological, or a combination? Which anatomical structures are involved? As mentioned earlier, knowledge of the anatomy of the nervous system is often essential to diagnosing a neurological problem, determining the etiology, and localizing the lesion. The key for understanding the distribution and localization of deficits is knowledge of neuroanatomical pathways in the nervous system, their cortical projections, sites of decussation, and interactions with other functional systems. Combining the signs and symptoms with the localization of the lesion facilitates arriving at a diagnosis and recommendation for treatment. Access to the family history provides information about the onset, susceptibility, and severity of the deficit. The most important branches of neuroscience are listed in Table 1-1.

Neurology

Neurology deals with diseases that disrupt the normal structural and physiological properties of the nervous system. Neurological problems include the following: **vascular disorders** (thrombosis, embolism, hemorrhage), **neoplastic conditions** (benign or malignant tumor), **degenerative conditions** (amyotrophic lateral sclerosis, multiple sclerosis, Pick's disease, and Alzheimer's disease), **motor disorders** (Parkinson's disease, chorea, and dystonia), **deficiency disorders** (Wernicke's encephalopathy and Korsakoff's syndrome), **bacterial and viral infections** (meningitis, poliomyelitis, and

encephalitis), and **epileptic disorders** (Table 1-2). The neurologist derives from the clinical history crucial information about the disease process and uses data obtained from clinical examination of sensory and motor functions and laboratory testing to diagnose and determine the site, nature, and cause of pathology to recommend proper treatment. The neurologist, with a keen interest in human behavior, also uses information from assessment of higher mental functions (Table 1-3) before making the final diagnosis. For comprehensive assessment and treatment of higher mental functions (language, speech, memory, attention, and cognition), the neurologist depends on

Table 1-1. Branches of Neuroscience

Branch	Domain
Neurology	Diagnosis and treatment of nervous system disorders.
Neurosurgery	Surgery for removal and remediation of pathologic structures that impair functional organization of the nervous system.
Neuroanatomy	Structural framework of the nervous system, consisting of nerve cells (neurons) and their tracts (fibers).
Neuroradiology	Imaging techniques for differentiating pathologic changes of the CNS; radiation therapy for nervous system tumors is a subspecialty of neuroradiology.
Neuroembryology	Embryological origins and development of the nervous system.
Neurophysiology	Chemical, electrical, and metabolic functions of the nervous system.
Neuropathology	Characteristics and origins of diseases and their effects on the nervous system.

Table 1-2. Major Brain Diseases

Disorder	Description
Cerebrovascular accident	A loss of brain (sensory, motor, speech, and language) functions caused by interruption of the blood supply
Neoplasm	Abnormal or new formation of tissue (benign or malignant tumor), which may infiltrate, invade, and destroy normal structures.
Demyelination Multiple sclerosis	Progressive autoimmune disease in which degeneration of axonal myelin in the CNS affects nerve conduction. Clinically characterized by symptoms such as weakness, incoordination, and speech disturbance, which often come and go.
Degeneration Alzheimer's disease	Progressive degenerative disease of the brain; leading cause of dementia.
Amyotrophic lateral sclerosis	Degenerative condition in which atrophy of motor neurons of the spinal cord and cortex results in muscular weakness and spasticity.
Motor disorders Huntington's chorea	Progressive brain disease of dominant inheritance appearing in person's mid-30s; leads to dementia and chorea.
Parkinson's disease	Progressive disease of the brain characterized by involuntary tremor, slowness of movement, and reduced muscular strength affecting motor speech.
Cerebral palsy	Motor disorder with or without language and cognitive deficit in children; caused by damage to the cerebrum before, during, or after birth.
Deficiency disorders	Wernicke-Korsakoff syndrome, characterized by amnesia, confabulation, and psychosis; caused by thiamine deficiency; observed among chronic alcoholics.
Bacterial and viral infection	Meningitis is an inflammatory condition of the spinal and cortical membranes.
Epilepsy	Condition of sensory, motor, cognitive, and affective disorders that is caused by seizures, abnormal electric activity in the brain.

Table 1-3. Common Areas Included in a Neurological Assessment

Motor Examination	Sensory Examination	Higher Mental Functions
Reflexes	**Reflexes**	**Language**
Superficial, tendon		Understanding
Testing of Motor Functions	**Testing of Sensory Functions**	Speaking
Gait	Pain and temperature	Naming
Muscle coordination	Touch	Repetition
Involuntary movements	Nonlocalized touch	Reading
Muscle tone (resistance to passive limb manipulation)	Two-point touch	Writing
Muscle strength	Kinesthetic sensation	**Memory**
	Proprioceptive sensation	Short term
	Sensation of vibration	Long term
	Stereognosis	**Nonverbal tasks**
Cranial Nerve Examination	Graphesthesia	Block design
Lens accommodation and pupil light reflex (CN II, III)	**Cranial Nerve Examination**	Drawing
Eye movements (CN III, IV, VI)	Smell (CN I)	Calculation
Facial movement	Vision (CN II)	Abstraction
Jaw movement (CN V)	Visual acuity	
Facial strength and articulation (CN VII)	Visual fields	
Resonance, phonation, and speech (CN IX,X, XII)	Sensation from face, mouth, nose, eye (CN V)	
Head rotation and shoulder elevation (CN XI)	Hearing, equilibrium (CN VIII)	
Tongue movement (CN XII)		

CN, cranial nerve.

the speech–language–hearing pathologist. The neurologist also employs data from disordered processes of communication and cognition to understand normal aspects of the neurolinguistic organization.

Neurosurgery

Neurosurgery is surgical intervention to treat a disease of the nervous system. Surgical access to the nervous system requires penetration of structures such as the skull, vertebral column, and meninges (brain and spinal cord coverings). Neurosurgical intervention is used for common conditions such as removal of **neoplastic** (tumor) tissue, extraction of **blood clots** (hematoma), excision of **vascular aneurysm**, removal of **carotid arterial plaque**, ablation of functionally impaired **"convulsing" tissues** (epileptogenic scars), **placement of selective lesions** in the thalamus (thalamotomy) for Parkinson's disease, placement of stereotactic therapeutic brain stimulation electrodes in the mesothalamus (midbrain and thalamus) for chronic pain, and removal of **herniated disks** in the spine. Neurosurgery also involves intensive care management of neurologically ill patients from traumatic injury and other neurologic diseases. Pediatric neurosurgery has a special place in neurosurgery because of the high frequency of surgically amenable diseases that children and infants get.

Neuroanatomy

Neuroanatomy relates to the structural organization of the nervous system. It grossly and microscopically defines the structural elements of the nervous system, specifically neurons, fiber tracts, nerves, ventricular structures, vascular networks, and supporting glial and meningeal tissues.

Neuroradiology

Neuroradiology enables the diagnosis of cranial, spinal, and peripheral nervous system abnormalities without intrusion into the cranial cavity and body tissues. It uses emission or transmission imaging to identify intact and pathological structures of the nervous system. Some modern neuroradiological techniques are **x-ray**, **angiography**, **computed tomography** (**CT**), **magnetic resonance imaging** (**MRI**), **single photon emission computed tomography** (**SPECT**), and **positron emission tomography** (**PET**). Therapeutic radiation is also used to treat various malignant body and brain tumors and is often combined with drug treatment (chemotherapy) and tumor excision.

Neuroembryology

Neuroembryology deals with growth of the nervous system during the embryonic period of development extending from conception to 7 weeks, at which time all brain structures have anatomically emerged. **Teratology** is the study of fetal malformations and monstrosities.

Neurophysiology

Neurophysiology focuses on the functional properties of the nervous system with respect to its structural, chemical, and electrical composition that are essential to living organisms.

Neuropathology

Neuropathology deals with the nature and etiology of diseased tissue that structurally and functionally disrupts the nervous system.

PRINCIPLES GOVERNING FUNCTIONAL ORGANIZATION OF THE HUMAN BRAIN

Although the human brain has a complex anatomical organization, its functions are regulated by a set of simple principles. Taken together, these simple organizational principles account not only for complex anatomical details but also for all brain functions. Eight common regulating principles of the human brain are shown in Table 1-4.

Interconnectivity in the Brain

All functionally specific primary sensory and motor regions in the cerebrum are connected through association and commissural fibers. The cortical association areas are directly connected to each other, whereas the primary cortical areas are indirectly connected through the cortical association areas. The homologous areas of the two hemispheres are connected through the interhemispheric commissural fibers. This integrated network allows constant interaction within each hemisphere and between the two hemispheres of the brain and explains how messages from multiple sources are rapidly integrated for an appropriate response to given stimuli.

Centrality of the Central Nervous System

The central nervous system (CNS) is responsible for integrating all incoming and outgoing information and for generating appropriate responses to the information received. The response can be volitional (internally generated), such as a spontaneous motor movement. Conversely, the response can be a reflex (environmentally elicited), such as withdrawal of a limb.

Because of the centrality of decision making and the all-encompassing response, no two parts in the pe-

Table 1-4. Organizational Principles of the Brain

Interconnectivity in the brain
Centrality of CNS
Hierarchy of neuraxial organization
Laterality of brain organization
Structural and functional specialization
Topographical organization in cortical pathways
Plasticity in the brain
Nonmythical brain

ripheral body can directly communicate with each other, regardless of the distance between them. Even the simplest form of communication between two adjacent body parts, such as the thumb and palm (as exemplified in the basic reflexes), is mediated through the CNS. The outgoing motor response is always different from the sensory information. A motor command in response to a sensory stimulus contains a directive that was refined and synthesized with additional informative stimuli from other sources of the neuraxis. The ability to analyze and synthesize multiple sources of information and to generate distinct responses exemplifies the centralized organization and function of the brain.

Hierarchy of Neuraxial Organization

The neuraxis of the CNS is hierarchically developed in complexity and organization of functions. Lower segment levels perform inherent specific functions that are modified to varying degrees by axial segments above. The spinal cord, the lowest segment level, serves simple sensory motor functions in the form of basic reflexes that are partly influenced by the upper axial levels. The complexity of information processing increases as the level of processing becomes more cephalic. The cerebral cortex, the highest segment level, is responsible for complex sensorimotor integration and higher mental functions (cognition, language, and speech). Functionally different neuronal structures also exist in the brainstem and diencephalon, the intermediate segment level. They consist of autonomic, chemical, and visceral systems, all of which contribute to the regulation of blood pressure, respiration, sleep, temperature, endocrine, and neurotransmitter interactions. Together these systems react to nonspecific stress and adverse bodily changes to maintain homeostatic states. The intermediate segment, which may be considered the nonthinking part of the brain, is tightly integrated with the cerebral cortex, that serves the highest segment level of decision making.

Laterality of Brain Organization

The three most important aspects of brain organization are (a) bilateral anatomical symmetry between the two hemispheres, (b) unilateral functional differences, and (c) contralateral sensorimotor control of the nervous system.

BILATERAL ANATOMICAL SYMMETRY

Anatomically the two cerebral hemispheres are essentially similar, with only minor differences. A difference related to language is that one region of the temporal lobe (planum temporale) is larger in the left hemisphere than in the right hemisphere. Both hemispheres are connected through the corpus callosum, the largest of the commissural fibers.

UNILATERAL FUNCTIONAL DIFFERENCES

Immediately after birth, the two cerebral hemispheres are functionally equipotential; each hemisphere has the functional capacity to develop all types of skills. However, after the first few years, each hemisphere acquires an advantage over the other for different specialized functions. Most people's left hemisphere becomes dominant for language, speech, and analytic processing irrespective of handedness; the right hemisphere dominates emotions, musical skills, metaphors, and humor. The right half of the brain is also involved with temporospatial attributes and regulating paralinguistic features, such as stress and intonation.

CONTRALATERAL SENSORIMOTOR CONTROL

A unique aspect of brain organization is that all sensory and motor fibers in the nervous system decussate (cross) the body's midline. The left motor cortex controls movements in the right half of the body; the sensory information from the left half of the body projects to the right sensory cortex (Fig. 1-1). Most sensory and motor fibers cross the midline in the caudal medulla of the brainstem. Fibers carrying pain and temperature cross the midline in the spinal cord. Some pathways, such as those for hearing, cross at numerous levels in the brainstem.

Structural and Functional Specialization

One striking feature of cortical organization is that the neuronal systems are functionally specialized. Sensory and motor systems possess specialized nerve cells that are functionally specific and separable. Consequently, white matter in the brain is composed of many parallel and adjacent pathways conducting various types of information. For example, sensory fibers carry sensations of pain, fine touch, and temperature; these fibers run parallel to one another and serve distinct functions that are determined by sensory receptive terminals in the peripheral body parts. The motor system also consists of several distinct pathways that transmit differentiated motor information. For example, one path mediates skilled hand movements from cortical and subcortical structures to the upper spinal cord, whereas the second transmits postural adjustment messages throughout the spinal cord and brainstem for trunk and limb movements. A third pathway controls speech muscles in the face and neck through cranial nerves in the brainstem. The functional specialization of nerve cells refers to their increased adaptivity, processing speed, and ability to make detailed analysis of selected signals.

Topographical Organization in Cortical Pathways

A remarkable aspect of the somatosensory system is that the spatial arrangement of peripheral receptors

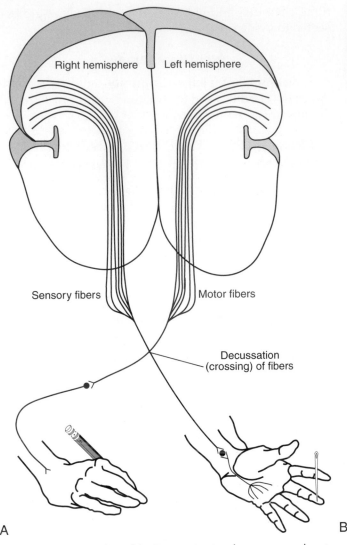

Figure 1-1. Contralateral brain organization for sensory and motor functions. **A.** The motor fibers descend from the motor cortex and decussate before synapsing upon the motor nuclei that activate muscles. **B.** The ascending fibers mediating sensation for pain and temperature decussate before projecting to the sensory cortex.

on the body is discretely maintained within the information-carrying pathway and is projected to the brain. The spatial organization of neurons, tracts, and terminals reflects the spatial relationships of the body surface and functionally related muscle groups. Therefore, the cerebral cortex is organized with a **somatosensory homunculus**. For example, an orderly visual map is discretely projected to the visual cortex by way of the thalamus. The distinctive visual map is retained throughout the brainstem, thalamus, and visual cortex. There is also continuity of representation; adjacent visual fields are represented in adjacent areas of the visual cortex. A similar relationship exists between a delineated area in the auditory cortex and the frequency specific cells in the cochlea. Similarly, there is a topographical organization in the brain for sensory and motor functions. These topographic maps of functions help to precisely locate lesions in the CNS.

Plasticity in the Brain

Functional plasticity is the ability to reorganize and modify functions and adapt to internal and external changes. The inherent plasticity of brain cells permits repair of cortical circuitry, integrates other cortical areas to serve changed functions, and responds to various pathologies. This adaptive property of the brain explains the organizational rearrangement of cellular functions and pathways after strokes, for example, and other pathologies. Regeneration of nerves (sprouting) occurs to varying degrees in the central and peripheral nervous systems. Scar tissue in the CNS prevents the establishment of axonal connections, whereas the peripheral nervous system has a greater opportunity to reestablish connection.

The brain's ability to adapt to external and internal changes has important implications for learning. Because functional plasticity and adaptivity are greatest in the early years and gradually diminish with age, learning is better accomplished if one is given early experience. Early exposure to stimuli not only facilitates learning but also results in a finer and more efficient processing of information. Fine tuning of the internal system is best illustrated by acquisition of a second language in early years.

A related observation concerns regions of the brain that are genetically committed or uncommitted to specific functions. For example, the brainstem possesses automatic control systems that are genetically acquired and cannot be modified. The cortical functions are programmed through daily experience and learning and are modifiable in the young age group.

Nonmythical Brain

Although the brain contains complex architectural organization, multiple interconnected pathways, and functionally independent specialized areas, its basic functioning is straightforward. Its operations are not governed by any personal characteristics of gender, color, or cultural variations. Its power is judged by the efficiency with which it remembers, processes information, generates responses, attends to tasks, plans, programs, makes decisions, and projects information. The brain's functioning is unaffected by normal variations in size, shape, or weight.

ORIENTATION TO BASIC TERMINOLOGY

A set of descriptive terms is used in neuroscience to indicate direction and position of structures with respect to their relative orientation within the brain. Special terminology is also used for visually delineating anatomical structures according to the various planes of brain sections.

Directional Brain Orientation

To understand the directional orientation of the human nervous system, it is important to consider first the brain of a mammal such as a dog, which because of its quadrupedal posture exemplifies a simpler axial organization. The CNS of the dog is organized in a straight (anteroposterior) line in the horizontal plane of the body. The term **rostral** refers to locations toward the nose; **caudal** refers to locations toward the tail; **dorsal** refers to locations toward the back, and **ventral** refers to locations toward the abdomen (Fig. 1-2).

This directional terminology is consistently used for referring to structures in the CNS; however, usage is slightly different in humans. During phylogenetic development, the longitudinal CNS system bends just above the brainstem. This flexure results in the spinal cord and brainstem developing vertically and the forebrain developing horizontally (Fig. 1-2). Therefore, in humans, the CNS (brain and spinal cord) is organized along two axes: horizontal (brain) and vertical (spinal cord).

Because of this axial difference in structural orientation, the terms used for describing the positions of structures in the CNS vary (Table 1-5). For the forebrain above the bend, rostral refers to locations toward the nose and caudal refers to locations toward the back of the brain, while dorsal refers to the top of the brain and ventral refers to the lower brain toward the jaw. The directions of these terms below the neuraxial bend systematically change and are similar to the ones used for lower vertebrates. For the spinal cord and brainstem, rostral refers to locations toward the brain, caudal refers to the coccygeal end of the spinal cord, dorsal refers to locations toward the back of the body, and ventral refers to locations toward the abdomen.

Planes of Brain Section

Not all cortical structures are on the brain's surface. Some can only be examined after sectioning the brain. The brain may be cut into three primary planes: **sagittal**, **coronal**, and **horizontal** (Fig. 1-3). The sagittal plane, named after the sagittal suture in the skull, is a vertical cut that passes longitudinally and divides the brain into left and right portions. A sagittal section at the center separates the brain into two equal halves and is called the **midsagittal** (median) cut. A coronal plane, a vertical section made perpendicular to the sagittal section, divides the brain into front and back parts. A horizontal plane, a cut perpendicular to both coronal and sagittal planes, divides the brain into upper and lower parts. A cross-section of the spinal cord at a right angle to its longitudinal axis divides the cord into upper and lower portions (Fig. 1-3, Table 1-6).

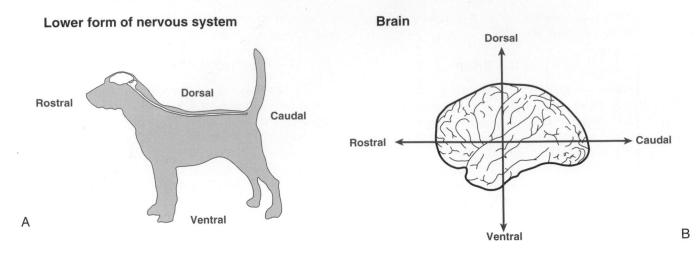

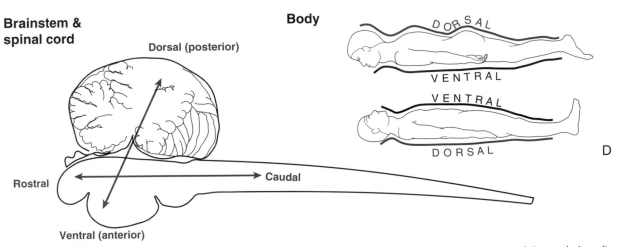

Figure 1-2. Axes of nervous system and directional terms. **A.** The nervous system in lower primates develops along a straight line. **B.** The human nervous system is organized along horizontal and vertical axes because of the cephalic flexure at the junction of the cerebral hemisphere and midbrain. For cerebral hemisphere and diencephalon, directions of these terms change systematically. **C.** Directional terms used for the spinal cord and brainstem are similar to those employed for lower vertebrates. **D.** Directional terms on the body surface.

Table 1-5.   Terms Indicating Direction

Cerebrum	
Rostral	Near front of head
Caudal	Back of brain or head
Dorsal	Top of brain
Ventral	Bottom of brain
Brainstem and Spinal Cord	
Rostral	Near or toward the brain
Caudal	Coccygeal end of spinal cord
Dorsal	Back of brainstem or spinal cord
Ventral	Belly or anterior in quadrupeds and bipeds

There are three other important orientation terms regarding brain planes: **transverse**, **lateral**, and **medial**. A transverse plane is a cross-cut at a right angle to the longitudinal axis on a bend. Because of the curvature of the brainstem, this plane is diagonal to the horizontal (cross) plane (Fig. 1-3, Table 1-6). *Lateral* and *medial* derive their meanings from their context in a midsagittal section: *lateral* refers to structures away from a mid or midsagittal plane, whereas *medial* refers to a plane approaching the midsagittal plane.

Terms Relating to Movement

Several technical terms are used to denote specific aspects of directional movement involving muscular structures (Fig. 1-4). **Flexion** refers to the bending movement of a limb. **Extension** refers to the straightening movement of a limb. **Abduction** denotes a movement in which a limb is moved away from the central axis of the body. **Adduction** denotes a movement that brings a limb toward the central axis of the body. **Pronation** is the movement that turns the palm downward, and **supination** is the action that turns the palm upward.

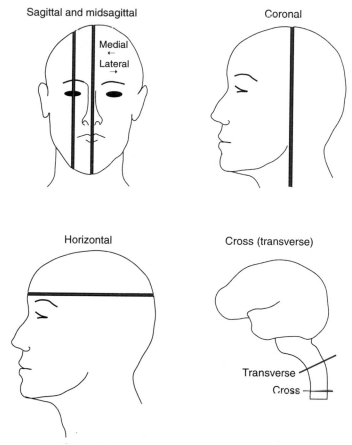

Figure 1-3. Sections of planes for brain and spinal cord.

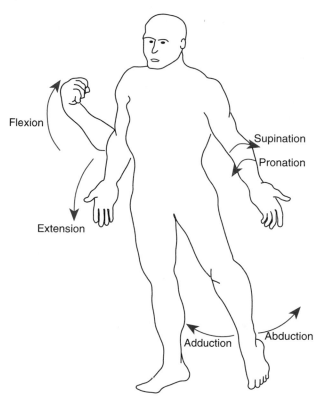

Figure 1-4. Body movements.

Table 1-6. Terms for Brain Sections

Coronal	Vertical division into front (rostral) and back (caudal)
Sagittal	Vertical division into left and right
Midsagittal	Vertical division into two equal parts
Horizontal	A cross-section division into upper and lower portions
Transverse	Diagonal to cross-plane at the curving brainstem
Lateral	Structures away from midline
Medial	Structures toward midline

Terms Relating to Muscles

The three kinds of muscle fibers in the body are differentiated on the basis of histological structure: **skeletal, cardiac,** and **smooth. Skeletal muscles** consist of striated fibers and are under voluntary control. **Cardiac muscles,** although containing striated fibers, are not under voluntary control. They are controlled by the cardiovascular reflexes of the autonomic nervous system. **Smooth muscles** consist of nonstriated fibers and are considered involuntary. Smooth muscle is found in the internal organs of the digestive system, respiratory passages, urinary and genital tracts, urinary bladder, and walls of blood vessels.

Additional Terms

The bony cavity of the skull restricts expansion of the cortical mantle; consequently, the human cortex is highly convoluted, giving the brain a folding appearance. The crest of every fold is called a **gyrus** (pl. gyri) or **convolution.** The groove or valley separating adjacent gyri is called the **sulcus** (pl. sulci) or **fissure** (in case of greater depth). **Opercular** refers to the margins of the cerebral convolutions serving as a cover. For example, the margins of the operculum of three lobes cover the **insular cortex** (Fig 2-13). A **commissure** is a band of fibers connecting part of the brain or spinal cord on one side with the same structures on the opposite side of the midline.

The brain consists of billions of nerve cells (neurons, grossly identified as **gray matter**) and their processes (axons, grossly identified as **white matter,** and dendrites). Gray matter refers to the gross appearance of the brain, which consists of nerve cells, supporting glia cells, and many unmyelinated fibers. Nerve cells are concentrated in the cerebral cortex as layers and in the subcortex as nuclei. The cells appear gray in the absence of myelin. White matter is made of nerve fibers that form tracts and carry information from one brain site to another. It is white because of the white appearance of the myelin lipid (fatlike) substance surrounding many of the axons. A **neuron** is the basic building block in the brain, and it is responsible for generating, receiving, transmitting, and synthesizing electrical impulses as well as influencing other neurons or effector tissue; **glial cells** protect and support the nerve cells. A typical neuron is bounded by a continuous plasma membrane and consists of a **cell body**, **dendrites**, and an **axon** (Fig. 1-5). The cell body, also called **soma** (pl. somata) or **perikaryon** (pl. perikarya), contains the cytoplasm with important organelles including **mitochondria, ribosomes, rough endoplasmic reticulum**, and **Golgi complex** that are needed for cellular metabolism. Also contained in the cytoplasm is a nucleus, which contains ladderlike micromolecules of DNA with a genetic blueprint and is responsible for vital cellular activities. Dendrites, highly specialized processes that look like trees, receive neural signals from other neurons through contacts (synapses). The axon, arising from the cell body at an elevation called an **axon hillock**, transmits neural messages to other neurons through its synapses (contacts). **Synaptic terminals** (terminal boutons, or knobs or buttons) are the end portions of the axon, which contain many vesicles that release neurotransmitters between the end of the axon and the surface of the next nerve cell. This narrow space is called the **synaptic cleft**. Once a neuron is adequately stimulated, a neural impulse travels along the axon, and the terminal boutons (knobs) release the neurotransmitters in the synaptic cleft to activate the receptor site of the next nerve cell. The **synapse** includes the boutons, synaptic cleft, and receptor site of the next nerve cell. A neuron that ends at the synapse is a **presynaptic nerve cell**. A neuron that receives an impulse from a presynaptic neuron is a **postsynaptic neuron**. Impulse transport in the axon is only unidirectional, such as **anterograde**, in which an impulse travels from the cell body to the axonal terminal.

However, the axonal transport within the cellular cytoplasm is bidirectional, so that it may be anterograde (with a flow from the cell body to the axon) and **retrograde**, so that the flow is from the axonal terminals to the cell body.

A well-defined collection of nerve cells in the **CNS** is called a **nucleus** or **cell column**; a similar collection of nerve cells in the **peripheral nervous system (PNS)** is called a **ganglion** (Table 1-7). A sensory ganglion contains cell bodies of the sensory nerves, and there are no synapses around cell bodies. A motor ganglion of the **autonomic nervous system** (ANS) contains cell bodies of fibers that supply the smooth muscles and glands.

Nerve fibers transmit information; a collection of nerve fibers all having a common origin is called a **tract** or **fasciculus** in the CNS. Another name for a bundle of connecting pathways is **brachium**, which specifically is used for the pathway connecting the cerebellum to the brainstem. **Stria** is used to denote a band of fibers, which may differ in color and/or texture. **Colliculus** refers to a small prominence of nervous tissues. A bundle of fibers in the PNS called a **nerve** or **nerve trunk**.

The prefix **inter-** denotes *between* and describes a structure common to both hemispheres. The interhemispheric fissure, for example, is a sulcus that divides the two hemispheres. Similarly, a fiber bundle that connects the two hemispheres is called an interhemispheric pathway. The prefix **intra-** denotes *within*; consequently, an intrahemispheric structure is one that is located within the substance of that hemisphere. Fibers connecting two areas within the same hemisphere are called an intrahemispheric pathway. The prefix **ipsi-** denotes *same*, and *ipsilateral* is used to describe lesions on one side of the brain that affect the same side of body. Conversely,

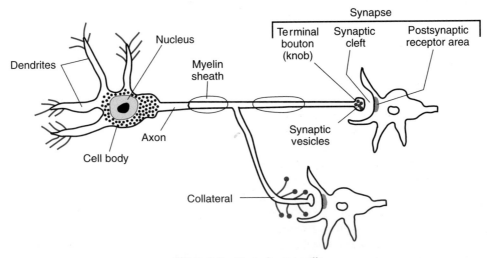

Figure 1-5.   Typical nerve cell.

Table 1-7.   Terms Used for Describing Neuronal Structures in the Nervous System

Central Nervous System	Peripheral Nervous System
Nucleus (pl. nuclei) is a mass of neurons usually deep in the brain. Examples are caudate nucleus and lateral geniculate nucleus (body). Tract is a bundle of parallel running axons with a common point of origin and termination, such as the corticospinal tract. Fasciculus (pl. fasciculi, funiculi) includes several parallel running tracts.	Ganglion (pl. ganglia) is a collection of neurons. An example is the ganglion of the trigeminal nerve or dorsal root. A nerve is a bundle of axons, as in the facial nerve. The optic nerve is the only collection of axons in the CNS that is called a nerve.

contra- denotes *opposite*, and *contralateral* is used to describe involvement of the body on the side opposite a brain lesion.

Information-carrying fibers in the nervous system are **sensory** (afferent) or **motor** (efferent). Afferent fibers carry sensory information from the body to the CNS. Efferent fibers carry motor impulses from the brain and spinal cord to the periphery of the body to contract muscles and activate gland secretion. **Decussation** refers to the crossing of incoming or outgoing fibers at the midline (Fig. 1-1). **Proximal** and **distal** are defined by their relation to the CNS. Proximal refers to structures relatively close to a specific anatomical site of reference, whereas distal identifies the position of structures farther from the same anatomical site of reference.

A **somite** is a series of mesodermal tissue blocks on each side of the neural tube during the embryonic period (see Chapter 4). Somatic structures include most axial skeletal and associated muscles that are derived from the somite. **Viscera** refers to internal organs containing nonstriated muscles, such as the digestive, respiratory, and urogenital organs; smooth glands; spleen; heart; and great vessels.

Furthermore, familiarity with terms used to describe the temporal profile of neurological symptoms is helpful. Neurological symptoms can be classified as **transient** or **persistent**. Transient symptoms resolve completely; persistent ones do not. There are three types of persistent symptoms: symptoms that reach a maximum level of severity and do not change are **static** or **stationary**; symptoms that reach maximum severity but begin to resolve are **improving**; symptoms that continue to worsen are **progressive**. Other terms referring to the rapidity of changes in the temporal profile are **acute**, **subacute**, and **chronic**. Acute symptoms evolve over minutes to hours. Subacute symptoms develop over days to weeks, whereas chronic symptoms develop over months to years.

Gross Structures of the Central Nervous System

The human nervous system is divided into the **central nervous system** and **peripheral nervous system**. The CNS consists of the **brain** and the **spinal cord**. The brain is made of three major structures: the **cerebrum**, **brainstem (midbrain, pons, and medulla)**, and **cerebellum** (Fig. 1-6, Table 1-8). Each of these structures performs specific functions. The cerebrum consists of two hemispheres separated by the longitudinal (interhemispheric) fissure; each hemisphere contains the **cerebral cortex**, **basal ganglia**, and **diencephalon (thalamus and hypothalamus)**.

The cerebral cortex refers to the 3- to 5-mm thick layer of neurons (gray matter) covering the entire surface of the cerebrum. The nerve cells in the cerebral cortex are arranged in six layers (Fig. 1-7), representing the highest level of phylogenetic development. With more than 15 to 20 billion neurons, the cerebral cortex

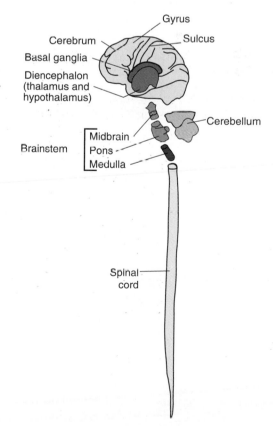

Figure 1-6.   Major structures in CNS.

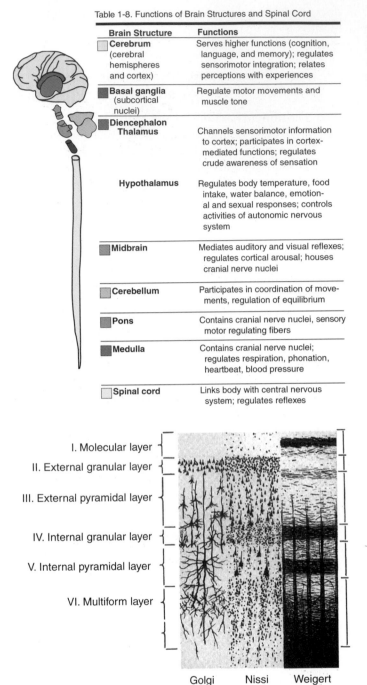

Table 1-8. Functions of Brain Structures and Spinal Cord

Brain Structure	Functions
Cerebrum (cerebral hemispheres and cortex)	Serves higher functions (cognition, language, and memory); regulates sensorimotor integration; relates perceptions with experiences
Basal ganglia (subcortical nuclei)	Regulate motor movements and muscle tone
Diencephalon Thalamus	Channels sensorimotor information to cortex; participates in cortex-mediated functions; regulates crude awareness of sensation
Hypothalamus	Regulates body temperature, food intake, water balance, emotional and sexual responses; controls activities of autonomic nervous system
Midbrain	Mediates auditory and visual reflexes; regulates cortical arousal; houses cranial nerve nuclei
Cerebellum	Participates in coordination of movements, regulation of equilibrium
Pons	Contains cranial nerve nuclei, sensory motor regulating fibers
Medulla	Contains cranial nerve nuclei; regulates respiration, phonation, heartbeat, blood pressure
Spinal cord	Links body with central nervous system; regulates reflexes

I. Molecular layer
II. External granular layer
III. External pyramidal layer
IV. Internal granular layer
V. Internal pyramidal layer
VI. Multiform layer

Golgi   Nissi   Weigert

Figure 1-7. Six cellular layers in brain stained by three methods.

serves all symbolic functions required of homo sapiens, such as language, orientation, thinking, memory, and attention.

The basal ganglia are the masses of gray matter in the depth of each cerebral hemisphere; the basal ganglia serve as an auxiliary motor system and play an important role in the regulation of motor activities by modifying the information received from the motor cortex and returning it to the motor cortex.

The thalamus is a collection of subcortical nuclei; these nuclei work closely with the cerebral hemispheres in sensorimotor functions and evaluate incoming sensory signals before directing them to the cortex. The hypothalamus is the central site of neuroendocrine production and the central structure for the control of various metabolic activities, such as water balance, sugar and fat metabolism, and body temperature. The brainstem is collectively composed of the midbrain, pons, and medulla.

Besides linking the brainstem with the brain, the midbrain controls eye movements and pupil size. The pons regulates facial movements and sensation. It also contains a center responsible for controlling the rhythm of respiration. The medulla controls respiratory activity, heart rate, and blood pressure. In addition to serving the specialized functions and controlling cranial nerves, the midbrain, pons, and medulla contain common sensorimotor fibers and the **reticular formation**, which regulates cortical arousal and attention. The cerebellum is dorsal to the brainstem, and is attached to but not part of the brainstem. The cerebellum is important in the regulation of skilled movements. The spinal cord serves as the reflex-controlling center containing fibers to and from the brain and connects the brain with peripheral structures.

The PNS is formed by nerves that connect the brain and spinal cord with peripheral structures. These include both sensory and motor nerves. Carrying pain, touch, and temperature information, the sensory fibers enter the spinal cord via the dorsal roots. The motor fibers that innervate muscles and glands exit through the ventral roots.

Functional Classification of Nervous System

The human nervous system processes information using two types of cells: **general** and **special**. General information originates from the surface of the body and is processed by general receptors. Special information is mediated by receptors to specialized cells in the nervous system. Pain and temperature are examples of general information, whereas vision and audition are examples of special information. Each type (general and special) is involved with body structures that are either **somatic** or **visceral**. As mentioned earlier, *somatic* refers to striated skeletal muscles that are embryologically derived from somites. Visceral nonstriated muscles are concerned with involuntary and vegetative tasks and relate to the internal vital body organs that are concerned with the respiratory, vascular, and digestive systems. General and special information is divided into somatic and visceral subtypes, both of which include **efferent** (mo-

Table 1-9.   Functional Components of Nervous System

General		Special	
Somatic Efferent	Visceral Afferent	Somatic Efferent	Visceral Afferent
Efferent (Motor) GSE activates muscles derived from somites, including skeletal, extraocular, and glossal (tongue) muscles. GVE projects to muscles of visceral organs, including pupillary constriction, gland secretion, and regulation of heart and tracheal muscles.		**Efferent (Motor)** SVE projects to muscles of face, palate, mouth, pharynx, larynx; does not include eye and tongue muscles. SSE does not exist.	
Afferent (sensory) GSA mediates sensory innervation from somatic muscles, skin, ligaments, and joints. GVA mediates sensory innervation from visceral organs, including larynx, pharynx, and abdomen.		**Afferent (sensory)** SSA mediates special sensations of vision from the retina, and audition and equilibrium from the inner ear. SVA mediates visceral sensations of taste from tongue, olfaction from nose.	

GSE, general somatic efferent; GVE, general visceral efferent; SVE, special visceral efferent; SSE, special somatic efferent; GSA, general somatic afferent; GVA, general visceral afferent; SSA, special somatic afferent; SVA, special visceral afferent.

tor) and **afferent** (sensory) fibers. The only exception to this classification is the lack of a **special somatic efferent system**. This functional classification consists of seven components and is important for understanding cranial nerve function (Table 1-9).

Cellular Organization (Cytoarchitecture) and Brodmann Areas

The cerebral cortex consists of six cellular layers, which are classified by their neuronal density and architecture as seen under a light microscope: **molecular layer, external granular layer, external pyramidal layer, internal granular layer, internal pyramidal layer,** and **multiform layer** (Fig. 1-7, Table 1-10). These layers of the cortex function as a physiological module, processing input and giving rise to axons. Some axons project to other cortical areas, and others form the descending tracts. Different cortical regions contain varied configurations of the cellular layers, reflecting the specialized functions served by each brain area.

Various cytoarchitectural maps of the cellular architecture of the cortex have been constructed. The most frequently used cytoarchitectural map in neurological, neuropsychological, and neurolinguistic literature is that of Brodmann (1909). Brodmann's architectural map of the cerebral cortex divides the brain into approximately 50 regions and serves as a standard for referring to specific brain areas by a number (Fig. 1-8). For example, Brodmann area 4 is the primary motor cortex, which contains very large pyramidal cells (Betz cells). Sensory cortical areas have more densely packed granular cells and only a few pyramidal cells. Primary sensory areas include the somatosensory cortex in the post-

Table 1-10.   Six-Layered Cerebral Gray Matter

Cellular Layer	Cellular Characteristics
Layer I Molecular	Terminal dendrites and axons from cortical and fusiform neurons forming interconnections.
Layer II External granular	Small granular interneurons receiving input from other cerebral regions.
Layer III External pyramidal	Small pyramidal neurons with projections to other cerebral regions.
Layer IV Internal granular	Small granular interneurons; receives input from thalamus and other subcortical nuclei.
Layer V Internal pyramidal	Large pyramidal neurons (**Betz cells** of the primary motor cortex). Their axons project to subcortical sites, such as brainstem, cerebellum, and spinal cord.
Layer VI Multiform	Fusiform neurons with projections to thalamus.

central gyrus (Brodmann areas 1–3), the primary visual cortex (Brodmann area 17), and the primary auditory cortex, or Heschl's gyri (Brodmann areas 41 and 42 in the superior temporal gyrus). Tertiary areas of the temporal, parietal, and prefrontal cortex are called association areas of the brain. The association areas are concerned mostly with processing of cross-modality input from other cortical areas, integrating and elaborating complex functions. Familiarity with commonly used Brodmann areas is necessary for working in medical speech–language hearing pathology (Table 1-11).

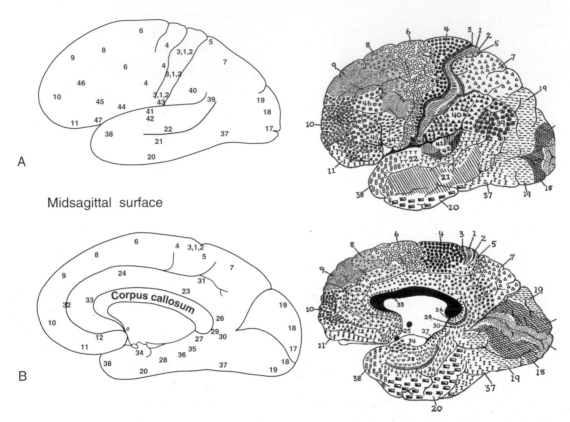

Figure 1-8. Cytoarchitectural map illustrating Brodmann areas on lateral (**A**) and medial (**B**) brain surfaces: *1-3*, primary sensory cortex; *4*, primary motor cortex; *5* and *7*, sensory association cortex; *6*, premotor cortex; *17*, primary visual cortex; *18* and *19*, visual association cortex; *22*, association language cortex (Wernicke's area); *41*, primary auditory cortex; *42*, association auditory cortex; *44*, motor speech cortex (Broca's area).

Table 1-11. Important Brodmann Areas

Functional Areas	Brodmann Areas
Primary sensory cortex (postcentral gyrus)	1, 2, 3
Primary motor cortex (precentral gyrus)	4
Primary visual cortex (medial occipital lobe)	17
Primary auditory cortex (Heschl's gyrus)	41, 42
Sensory association cortex (superior parietal lobule)	5, 7
Association language cortex of Wernicke (superior temporal gyrus)	22
Motor speech cortex of Broca (lower third frontal convolution)	44
Supramarginal gyrus	40
Angular gyrus	39

TECHNIQUES FOR SOLVING PROBLEMS WHEN LEARNING NEUROSCIENCE

Students in communicative disorders and related disciplines need not feel overwhelmed by the technical terminology, abstract nature, intricate connections, multiplicity of neuroanatomical structures, or amount of material to be learned. However, remaining confident and progressively adding knowledge in a methodical and persistent fashion is the best strategy for learning neuroscience. The following practical suggestions will simplify technical terminology and the abstractness of the material presented. These will facilitate the learning process and will also make the time spent more enjoyable (Table 1-12).

Simplification of Technical Terminology

1. Learn the definitions and functions of each new technical term. Keep a list of new words in a notebook. If possible, use one word to define each term. The definition word should preferably portray an anatomical or physiological function or description. Repeat that word mentally, write it several times, and pronounce it audibly so that it becomes familiar.
2. Relate each technical word to its synonyms. For example, frequently used words, such as *fissure* and *sulcus*, refer to the same structure. The superior cerebellar peduncle and the brachium conjunctivum refer to the same cerebellar pathway, and the cerebral aque-

Table 1-12.   Strategies for Overcoming the Complexity of Neuroscience

Relate each structure to its definition and function.
Be familiar with synonyms for each structure.
Relate each term to other functionally related terms.
Be familiar with idiosyncratic patterns for coining technical terms based on the following:
  Visual appearance
  Researcher's name
  Anatomical projections
  Roots in Greek and Latin
Undertake a visual approach to neuroanatomy:
  Visually learn the shape, size, function, and location of each structure
  Develop an orientation to each structure in relation to its adjoining structures
Find a functional context for neurological concepts and structures and rank the relationship.
Discover meaning and purpose for each new concept by solving clinical problems.
Be familiar with the rules of lesion localization.

duct and sylvian aqueduct refer to the canal connecting the third and fourth ventricles in the brain. *Iter* is also used as a synonym for the cerebral aqueduct.

3. Relate each technical term to other functionally related terms. For example, peduncle refers to the fiber bundles connecting the cerebellum to the brainstem; thus, the superior, middle, and inferior cerebellar peduncles are functionally related anatomical structures.

4. Become familiar with common principles of formulating medical terms.
   - Some neuroanatomical structures are named after their visual appearance: **lenticular** because of its lens shape; **colliculus** because of its hill-like form; **corona radiata** because the sensory and motor fibers radiate in the form of a crown; **internal capsule** because of the capsulelike formation by the sensory and motor fibers deep in the brain between the diencephalon and basal ganglia; **amygdaloid nucleus** because of its almond shape; and **hippocampus** because of its sea horse shape.
   - Some terms are eponyms, coined from the names of researchers, for example circle of Willis, Babinski reflex, Brodmann area, Huntington's chorea, foramen of Monro, sylvian fissure, fissure of Rolando, and Parkinson's disease.
   - Names of pathways may be established according to sites of origin and termination. The corticospinal tract, for instance, originates in the cortex and terminates in the spinal cord. The corticobulbar tract originates in the cortex and terminates in the bulbar area (medulla and adjacent brainstem areas). The reticulospinal system extends from the reticular formation of the brainstem to its termination in the spinal cord. Although the names of fiber tracts primarily emphasize the points of origin and ter-

mination, they sometimes include unnamed brain structures along the entire length of the tract.
   - Most neurology terms are derived from Greek or Latin. Familiarity with roots and derivational morphemes can simplify the learning task. Some examples follow.

      Ataxia: *A-* means without, and the Greek root *taxis* means order; thus, ataxia is loss of motor coordination.
      Chorea: the Greek root *choros* means dance; thus, chorea is a dancelike movement characterized by involuntary motor movements.
      Lemniscus: the Greek root *lemniskos* means a fillet or ribbon; thus, lemniscus refers to a bundle of nerve fibers in the CNS. See Appendix B for common lexical roots.

   Many medical terms derived from Greek or Latin roots have a combining form of the word that is different from its root form. For example the combining form of the Greek root *skleros* (hard) is **scler-**, as in *sclerosis*; the combining form of Greek root *soma* (body) is **somat-**, as in somatic; the combining form of Greek root *stethos* (chest) is **stetho-**, as in stethoscope. Also see Appendix B for a list of such combining forms.

Visual Approach to Neuroscience

The human nervous system is complex, but it is organized logically. Most concepts can be understood and remembered after the learner has acquired the basics in neuroscience. Some concepts and facts, however, must be memorized and repeated until they become incorporated in a readily available bank of knowledge. Neuroanatomy is best learned by persistent repetition and visual orientation. Neuroanatomical structures are not abstract entities; they are real, occupy space, and serve specific functions. All brain structures are anatomically and physiologically integrated to form a whole entity with one purpose—preservation of the species. The visual learning of anatomical structures with reference to shape, size, texture, function, and location in the nervous system and relationship to bordering structures is the most successful tool. No other effective way has been found. Consequently, developing a visual memory by correlating written descriptions of cortical and subcortical structures with their anatomical illustrations, charts, and figures has been found to be invaluable. As a student learns more, he or she should become better equipped to solve clinical problems, a highly valued activity. Thus, some practical suggestions for learning the concepts and functions of neuroscience follow:

1. Take a visual approach to learning brain structures in the context of their locations. Each gross and internal neuroanatomical structure has its own visually

distinguishing appearance. Visual familiarity with a structure as it appears in space facilitates learning neuroanatomy and reduces the fear of learning. For example, widely dispersed sensory and motor fibers are responsible in part for the bulging appearance of the pons; the four adjacent egg-shaped structures located dorsally in the midbrain are the **corpora quadrigemina** (four bodies), and the slit cleavage between two football-shaped thalami is the **third ventricle**. The fillet-shaped sensory fibers at the midbrain course through the **medial lemniscus**, and the motor fibers, through the **pes pedunculi**, or **crus cerebri**.

2. Familiarity with adjacent structures and landmarks helps form a three-dimensional image that further facilitates learning. For example, it is easier to remember the location of various cortical and subcortical structures if they are visualized in relation to the **ventricular system**. Another important anatomical landmark is the shape of the sensorimotor fibers throughout the neuraxis.

Functional Context for Learning Neuroanatomy

Every gross and microscopic structure in the nervous system has a purpose and is part of a functional system with ascending and descending projections. Determine how each newly introduced structure fits into the broader organization of the brain. To what other structures is it functionally and/or anatomically related? For instance, the medial lemniscus in the brainstem conducts sensory information from the peripheral body parts to the thalamus, whereas the lateral lemniscus refers to fibers of the brainstem that conduct auditory impulses to the thalamus. The superior colliculi are concerned with visual reflexes, whereas the adjacent inferior colliculi are the auditory relay structures in the midbrain.

Deductive Reasoning and Problem Solving

The most important aspect of training in neuroscience is to learn to localize a lesion in the nervous system using a multistep problem-solving approach. The process of localizing a lesion involves finding the point of breakdown in the neural circuitry by examining both the functions that are spared and those that are disrupted. Basic knowledge of coexisting anatomical structures and understanding of the axonal pathways with respect to their origin, termination, and decussation help in determining how a patient with a selective lesion would exhibit a combination of symptoms. For example, third (oculomotor) nerve palsy on the left side and hemiparesis on the right side of the body (alternating ophthalmohemiplegia) are most likely to result from a midbrain lesion in the left **pes pedunculi** (crus cerebri).

A lesion affecting the oculomotor nerve before it emerges from the brainstem produces paralysis of eye muscles on the same side (ipsilateral) but contralateral paralysis of the limbs because of the involvement of the corticospinal tract, which has not yet crossed in the medulla.

Further, loss of sensation (pain and temperature) and paralysis in a single limb implies a lesion either in the spinal roots or nerves or in the brain. This is because these two are the points where sensory and motor fibers are together. The bilateral presence of paralysis and sensory loss below a certain level on the trunk while there is normal function above suggests a spinal cord injury; a spinal disorder is likely to interrupt the fibers below the lesion while sparing them above. Reduced tone and reflexes are likely to result from a lesion in the PNS or one involving the lower motor neurons. On the other hand, increased muscle tone and hyperactive reflexes are always associated with lesions involving the upper motor neurons in the forebrain or brainstem. Gradually expanding on such an analytical approach can make learning neuroanatomy and neurology enjoyable and invaluable.

Rules for Lesion Localization

Lesion localization is crucial to differential diagnosis in neurology. Most of the systems in the brain are considered to be line systems, vertically organized to connect the CNS to the peripheral body region. Each abnormal sign in a patient presumably reflects a breakdown at a point in the linear (ascending or descending) pathway. If the implicated linear fibers mediating sensory and motor information intersect, a lesion involving this single point impairs both sensory and motor functions. However, the intersection of fibers at two anatomical sites signifies two potential lesion sites. Localizing a lesion becomes somewhat complex in cases with multiple clinical symptoms, implicating numerous pathways and multiple points of intersections. Lesion localization in such cases requires a systematic analysis of symptoms and profound understanding of neuroanatomy; only neurologists are able to resolve it.

Nevertheless, common neurological symptoms are accountable by a set of simple rules. These rules will become more meaningful as students become familiar with neuroanatomy and sensorimotor pathways. Common rules that assist in localizing a lesion are presented in Box 1-1.

An understanding of the lesion-localizing rules facilitates the grasp of the rationale for using selected tasks and activities when examining a patient with left or right hemiplegia. Testing of specific sensorimotor activities and behavioral functions helps to localize a lesion at different levels in the nervous system. For example, establishing a left cortical lesion in a patient with right

---

Box 1-1.
Ten Rules That Assist in Localizing a Lesion

Rule 1: Symptoms Suggesting a Cortical Lesion
Presenting symptoms: Contralateral hemiplegia, contralateral hemianesthesia of face, trunk and upper extremity, and cortical sensory loss (failure to identify an object through touch or identify a letter or word written on the surface of the skin) suggest a cortical lesion.

Dominant hemisphere: In addition to these deficits, a dominant hemisphere lesion results in aphasia, left–right disorientation, apraxia, finger agnosia, and acalculia.

Nondominant hemisphere: Besides the presenting symptoms of a lesion in either hemisphere, an injury in the nondominant (right) hemisphere can also result in left-sided neglect or inattention, constructional and/or dressing deficits (apraxia), spatial and temporal disorientation, impaired prosody of speech, and impaired ability to recognize faces.

Rule 2: Symptoms Suggesting a Subcortical Lesion
Presenting symptoms: Contralateral hemiplegia and diminution or loss of pain and temperature equally for the face, arms, and legs is associated with a subcortical (internal capsule) lesion. Emergence of involuntary movements suggests a basal ganglia lesion.

Rule 3: Symptoms Suggesting a Central Gray Spinal Lesion
Presenting symptoms: Bilateral loss of pain and temperature sensation with preserved sense of touch in the same limbs (usually the two upper limbs) implies a lesion (e.g., cavitation or syringomyelia) in the spinal central gray.

Rule 4: Symptoms Implicating a Visual Pathway Lesion
A. Presenting symptoms: Blindness in one eye suggests an optic nerve lesion anterior to the optic chiasm.
B. Presenting symptoms: Bitemporal hemianopsia (one does not see things laterally in the visual fields) results from a lesion compressing or otherwise interrupting crossing fibers from the nasal retina of each eye in the optic chiasm.
C. Presenting symptoms: Homonymous hemianopsia is associated with a lesion in the optic tract fibers; this lesion can lie between the optic chiasm and the occipital lobe.
D. Presenting symptoms: Visual agnosia, alexia (failure to comprehend written word), and homonymous hemianopsia, along with spared macular vision, are associated with a lesion of the primary visual cortex (area 17) and visual association cortex (areas 18–19).

Rule 5: Symptoms Suggesting a Complete Spinal Cord Lesion
Presenting symptoms: Paralysis and sensory loss bilaterally below the level of the lesion with spared functions above this level indicates a complete spinal cord transsectional injury.

Rule 6: Symptoms Suggesting a Spinal Hemisection Lesion
Presenting symptoms: Ipsilateral loss of position and vibratory sensation below the level of lesion, ipsilateral body paralysis, and contralateral loss of pain and temperature sensation indicate a spinal hemisection (Brown-Séquard's syndrome).

Rule 7: Symptoms Suggesting a Peripheral or Central Lesion
Presenting symptoms: Paralysis and sensory (pain, temperature) loss involving the same single limb suggests a lesion either in the peripheral nerve or in the cortex.

Rule 8: Symptoms Suggesting an Upper or Lower Motor Neuron Lesion
Presenting symptoms: Increased reflexes in a symptomatic (sensorimotor) limb indicate an upper motor neuron lesion; reduced reflexes and weakness in the same symptomatic limb imply a peripheral or lower motor neuron lesion.

Rule 9: Symptoms Suggesting a Brainstem Lesion
Presenting symptoms: An altered level of consciousness, cranial nerve impairments (facial paralysis, hearing impairment, nystagmus, dysarthria, dysphagia) on the same side (ipsilaterally), hemianesthesia and paralysis of the body on the opposite side, (alternating or crossed hemiplegia) all imply a brainstem lesion.

Rule 10: Symptoms Suggesting a Disorder in Vascular System
A. Presenting symptoms: Sudden development of contralateral paralysis of the lower face, arm, and upper extremity more than the leg—with accompanying sensory loss—results from an occlusion of the middle cerebral artery that may be caused by either thrombosis or embolism. Additional symptoms may include the symptoms discussed under rule 1. (An abrupt onset of symptoms usually indicates vascular disease, while gradual progression of symptoms indicates a mass lesion.)
B. Presenting symptoms: Toe, foot, and leg paralysis along with sensory loss and mental impairments (distractibility, indecisiveness, and lack of spontaneity) is associated with ischemia due to embolism or thrombosis in the anterior cerebral artery distribution.
C. Presenting symptoms: Homonymous hemianopsia is associated with posterior cerebral artery involvement. Low pain threshold is also seen because of the thalamic involvement.

---

hemiplegia requires that the patient be tested for aphasia (naming, verbal output, reading, and writing); the differential paralytic involvement of face, arm, and leg; right-sided cortical sensory loss; and homonymous hemianopsia. To determine a lesion in the nondominant hemisphere, testing should include the assessment of inattention to the left body space, left sensorimotor involvement, denial of disease, spatial orientation, constructional and/or dressing activities, and speech prosody. Determining a subcortical lesion requires that the patient be tested for contralateral hemiplegia and equal sensorimotor involvement of face, arm, and leg, dystonic postures, and reduced pain threshold. To con-

firm a brainstem lesion, one must test the patient for alternating hemiplegia, which is characterized by ipsilateral cranial nerve symptoms (left ear hearing loss, left tongue deviation, swallowing, and dysarthria) and crossed hemiplegia. Establishing a spinal cord lesion requires that the patient be examined for muscle tone, reflex quality, and paralysis and sensory loss on the opposite sides of the body.

SUMMARY

Neuroscience and communicative disorders are two closely related disciplines. Basic understanding of neurosciences is essential for a comprehensive training in speech–language pathology and audiology. The rationale for training in neuroscience is that it provides a broad framework for diagnosing the disorders of communication and for providing effective remediation. Such background will also help students in communicative disorders become creative partners in a team approach to managing a patient's clinical condition and will nurture good working relationships with colleagues in medical and paramedical professions.

Although neuroscience is admittedly complex, there are ways to overcome its technical terminology. Familiarity with the rules of word formation and an approach that emphasizes persistent repetition, visual orientation, and deductive reasoning can make learning neuroscience easier. Visual familiarity with the graphic details in Chapters 2 and 3 is necessary to develop the foundation for understanding the functional organization of the nervous system.

Technical Terms

abduction	ganglia
adduction	glial cell
afferent	interhemispheric
anterograde	intrahemispheric
caudal	malignant
cerebral cortex	nerve cell
cerebral hemisphere	neuraxis
cerebrum	pronation
cognition	retrograde
coronal	rostral
cytoarchitecture	sagittal
decussation	somatic
dorsal	supination
efferent	teratology
extension	ventral
flexion	visceral

Review Questions

1. Define the following terms:

abduction	general function
adduction	gray matter
afferent	interhemispheric
Brodmann area	intrahemispheric
cerebral cortex	ipsilateral
contralateral	nerve cell
convolution	plasticity
cytoarchitecture	pronation
decussation	somatic
efferent	special function
extension	tract
fissure	visceral
flexion	white matter
ganglia	

2. How can training in basic neuroscience make you a better speech–language pathologist?

3. List the major branches of neuroscience and briefly describe their scopes.

4. With a labeled diagram, illustrate directional references and planes of a brain section.

5. Match the following functional categories to the associated lettered statement:

i. GSA	a. Pain and temperature
ii. SSA	b. Autonomic nervous system controlled activity
iii. GVA	c. Limb movement
iv. SVA	d. Vision
v. GSE	e. Organ content
vi. GVE	f. Taste and smell
vii. SVE	g. Articulation and facial expression

6. Define the following **prefixes** and **suffixes** (see Appendix B):

a-	-algia
ab-	-cyst
ad-	-ectomy
ambi-	-emia
bi-	-genic
contra-	-graph
di-	-itis
dys-	-ology
hemi-	-oma
hyper-	-opia
inter-	-pathy
intra-	-rrhea
ipsi-	-tomy
neo-	
peri-	
sub-	
trans-	

7. Define the following **lexical roots** (see Appendix B):

athetos	phagein
durus	plege
enkephalos	presbys
glia	pros
gnosis	prattien, praxis
graphein	quadri
idios	somatikos
kinesis	soma
mesos	taxis
metron	tectum
opsis	teratos

8. Label the major structures of the nerve cell on Figure 1-9.

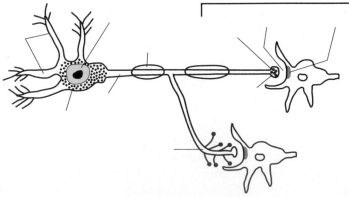

Figure 1-9. Exercise figure.

9. Locate principal brain structures (cerebrum, basal ganglia, diencephalon, cerebellum, midbrain, pons, medulla, and spinal cord) on Figure 1-10. Discuss the functions of the CNS components identified in the figure.

Lateral surface

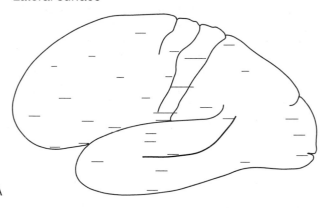

A

Midsagittal surface

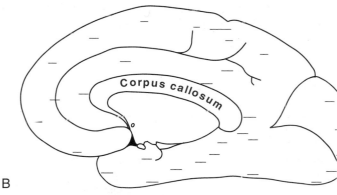

B

Figure 1-11.   Exercise figure.

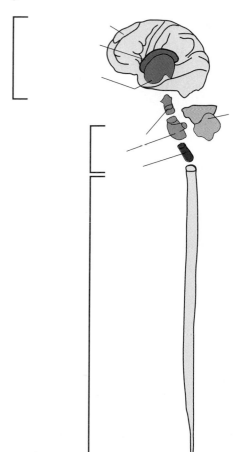

Figure 1-10.   Exercise figure.

10. Provide Brodmann area numbers for these cortical regions on Figure 1-11: **primary motor cortex, primary sensory area, primary visual cortex, and primary auditory cortex.**
11. Define four neurological diseases or conditions.
12. Describe the major components of a neurological examination.
13. The neuraxial bend at the juncture of the cerebrum and the midbrain creates two axes: horizontal axis for the forebrain and vertical axis for the brainstem and spinal cord. Provide the appropriate terms here:
    A. Above the neuraxial bend (the brain):
    _____ toward the nose
    _____ toward the top (vertex of the skull)
    _____ toward the back
    _____ toward the bottom (jaw)
    B. Below the neuraxial bend (the brainstem & spinal cord):
    _____ toward the abdomen
    _____ toward the nose (head)
    _____ toward the back
    _____ toward the spinal tail (coccyx)
14. Explain the clinical significance of the decussation of sensory and motor fibers.

15. Discuss implications of myelin degeneration on the transmission of nerve impulses.
16. Starting from the outermost, sequentially name the cellular layers of the cerebral cortex.
17. Match the following branches of neuroscience to the associated lettered statement.

   i. neurology   a. nervous system and its diseases.
  ii. neurosurgery   b. structure and anatomy of the CNS.
 iii. neuroanatomy
 iv. neuroradiology   c. imaging techniques.
  v. neuroembryology   d. embryological origin and development of the CNS.
 vi. neurophysiology
vii. neuropathology   e. chemical and physical processes of the CNS.
                           f. pathological changes in the CNS.
                           g. surgical procedures involving the structures of the nervous system.

18. Match the following numbered neurological conditions to the associated lettered statement.
    - i. Huntington's disease
    - ii. cerebral palsy
    - iii. Parkinson's disease
    - iv. Alzheimer's disease
    - v. stroke
    - vi. epilepsy
    - vii. multiple sclerosis

    a. A progressive degenerative disease of the brain associated with dementia.
    b. A motor disorder caused by damage to the cerebrum before, during, or after birth.
    c. A condition of abnormality in brain's electrical activity.
    d. A progressive hereditary disease of the brain leading to chorea and dementia.
    e. A progressive CNS disease that results from the degeneration of myelin.
    f. A progressive disease of the brain characterized by involuntary tremor and reduced muscular strength.
    g. A loss of brain (sensory, motor, speech, and language) functions caused by interruption of the blood supply.

19. Match the following numbered terms to the associated lettered statement.
    - i. tract
    - ii. nerve trunk
    - iii. nuclei
    - iv. ganglia
    - v. decussation
    - vi. motor fibers
    - vii. sensory fibers

    a. cell column on the CNS
    b. cell column in the PNS
    c. a bundle of nerve fibers in the CNS
    d. a bundle of nerve fibers in the PNS
    e. afferent fibers
    f. efferent fibers
    g. crossing of fibers

Gross Anatomy of the Central Nervous System

Learning Objectives

After studying this chapter, students should be able to do the following:

- Differentiate the central and peripheral nervous systems
- List structures in the central and peripheral nervous systems and describe their functions
- List principal embryonic divisions of the brain and gross anatomical structures related to each division
- Identify gross anatomical structures of the brain, describe their locations, and explain their functions
- Identify gross anatomical structures of the spinal cord and explain their functions
- Identify internal structures of the cerebral cortex, midbrain, pons, medulla, and spinal cord and describe their functions
- Identify parts of the ventricular cavities
- Describe the meninges, their locations, and their functions
- Differentiate the various medullary fibers and describe their functions
- List the cranial nerves, cite their anatomical locations, and describe their major sensory and motor functions
- Discuss the anatomy and functions of the autonomic nervous system

STRUCTURES OF CENTRAL AND PERIPHERAL NERVOUS SYSTEMS

The human nervous system can best be described as the generator of the electrical and chemical energy distributed throughout the body for the control of various body functions. The nervous system performs four important roles: **sensor, effector, integrator,** and **regulator**. As the sensor, it receives all environmental and bodily generated changes. As the effector, it initiates all body movements. As the integrator, it combines information received from all sources and modalities. As the regulator, it maintains the homeostatic state for the optimum control of peak body performance and repair.

Anatomically, the nervous system consists of two major parts: the **central nervous system** (**CNS**) and the **peripheral nervous system** (**PNS**). The CNS consists of the brain and spinal cord (Fig. 2-1A). The brain is responsible for initiating, controlling, and regulating all sensorimotor and cognitive (mental) functions that generate and regulate human behaviors. The spinal cord is primarily a wire cable structure in the CNS that transmits motor commands to various body parts that interact with the environment. Also the sensory information that is collected from the peripheral body parts and the environment is transmitted to the brain via the spinal cord. Some sensory input is processed locally in the spinal cord and regulates peripheral reflex motor activity.

The CNS is protected by a bony shell. The brain is encased in a tough bony skull, and the spinal cord is similarly protected by the vertebral column, which consists of a series of bones and tough cartilaginous washerlike structures; the washers buffer body movements and weight bearing. The CNS is encased in three membranous coverings, the **meninges**. They may be visualized as three "diapers," covering the CNS from the top of the brain to the tip of the spinal cord. Between the two inner diapers there is **cerebrospinal fluid** (CSF), which serves both as a protective mechanical buffer and a chemical mediator for metabolic functions. The meninges also provide the supporting framework for the CNS vessels that carry blood to and from the heart.

The PNS consists of sensory and motor nerves that are connected to the spinal cord (**spinal nerves**) and the brainstem (**cranial nerves**). These nerves extend to the organs, muscles, joints, blood vessels, and skin surface, forming an extensive network of cables and fine wires throughout the body (Fig. 2-1B). The PNS consists of two major systems: **somatic nervous system** and **autonomic**

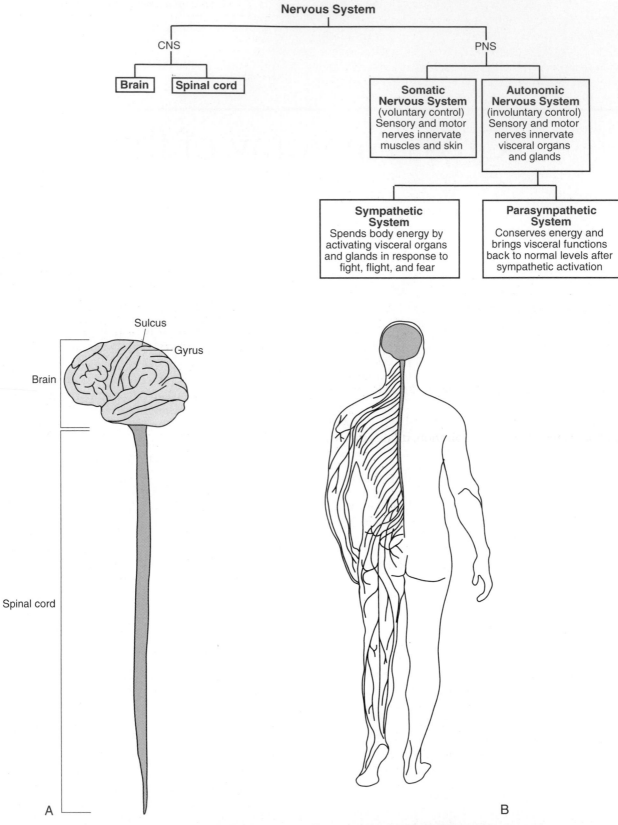

Figure 2-1. Human nervous system. CNS (**A**) consists of brain and spinal cord; PNS (**B**) consists of cranial nerves and spinal nerves through which CNS transmits commands to and receives information from end organs.

nervous system (ANS). Each of these systems of the PNS consists of two subsystems: **sensory** (afferent) and **motor** (efferent) fibers. The afferent fibers consist of nerves and cells that transmit sensory information to the CNS from receptors in the skin, muscles, and visceral organs. The efferent fibers transmit commands from the CNS to activate the muscles and glands located throughout the body.

The **somatic** afferents and efferents mediate skeletal muscle reflexes. **Visceral sensory** inputs of the ANS communicate with **visceral motor** outputs to activate visceral organ reflex and glands. The ANS regulates the activity of organs such as the salivary glands, heart, lung, blood vessels, stomach, intestines, kidneys, and bladder.

The ANS (also called visceral, involuntary, or vegetative system) is made up of two divisions: the **sympathetic nervous system** and the **parasympathetic nervous system**. Sympathetic ganglia (clusters of nerve cells) usually innervate many organs, whereas parasympathetic ganglia innervate a single organ. These systems produce opposite effects when innervating the same organ. For example, the sympathetic system tends to accelerate heart rate, and the parasympathetic tends to slow it down. The sympathetic system spends energy and prepares for fight and flight. In so doing, it constricts blood vessels of the skin, visceral organs, and bronchial passages, induces perspiration, dilates pupils, and mobilizes glucose. The parasympathetic system conserves energy; dominant during relaxing or sleeping, it constricts the pupils and slows the heart rate. Together the sympathetic and parasympathetic systems monitor, regulate, and sustain optimum visceral functions essential to survival (see Chapter 16).

PRIMARY DIVISIONS OF THE BRAIN

Familiarity with the **three major vesicles** of the embryonic brain facilitates understanding the development of the human brain and its structures. The 4- to 5-week embryonic brain is well developed in terms of structures. It has three vesicles: **prosencephalon** (forebrain), **mesencephalon** (midbrain), and **rhombencephalon** (hindbrain). These vesicles are demarcated by three brain flexures: **midbrain**, **pontine**, and **cervical** (Fig. 2-2). The **midbrain flexure** demarcates the midbrain region in the brainstem. The **cervical flexure** is at the junction of the hindbrain and the spinal cord. An unequal development of the hindbrain produces the **pontine flexure**, which results in the thinning of the roof of the hindbrain.

The prosencephalon develops into the **telencephalon** and **diencephalon**. The **cerebral hemispheres**, **limbic lobe**, and **basal ganglia** are the principal derivatives of the telencephalon, whereas the **thalamus** and **hypothalamus** are derived from the dien-

Table 2-1.   Adult Brain Structures Derived from Embryonic Vesicles

Embryonic Brain Vesicles	Major Divisions of the Brain	Gross Anatomical Structures
Prosencephalon (forebrain)	Telencephalon	Cerebral cortex, basal ganglia, limbic system, lateral ventricles
	Diencephalon	Thalamus, hypothalamus Third ventricle
Mesencephalon	Mesencephalon (midbrain)	Midbrain structures Cerebral aqueduct
Rhombencephalon (hindbrain)	Metencephalon	Pons, cerebellum, fourth ventricle
	Myelencephalon	Medulla oblongata, no ventricle

cephalon. The midbrain structures are the developmental derivatives of the **mesencephalic vesicle**. The **rhombencephalon** further divides into **metencephalon** and **myelencephalon**. The metencephalon further develops into the **cerebellum** and **pons**, whereas the **myelencephalon** evolves into the **medulla oblongata** (Table 2-1). The **brainstem**, the upward extension of the spinal cord, vertically intersects the horizontal brain and includes as a contiguous unit the **midbrain** (mesencephalon), **pons**, and **medulla** (rhombencephalon).

GROSS STRUCTURES OF THE BRAIN

Telencephalon

The human brain, which weighs approximately 1100 to 1400 g (2 lb) and represents only 2% of the total body weight, is the most elaborated recent structure in the nervous system. Its phylogenetic development is most significant in humans, as it alone accounts for higher mental functions such as *language, cognition, emotion, reasoning, attention, memory, temporospatial orientation, judgment,* and *reflective thinking*. These functions, however, are integrated by the combined activities of the cerebral hemispheres and diencephalon.

CEREBRAL HEMISPHERES

The **cerebrum** consists of two **cerebral hemispheres**, which make up the largest part of the brain (Fig. 2-3). Composed of a 3.5-mm thick layer of neurons, the cerebral cortex is the convoluted surface of the brain; it overlies internal white matter and more deeply located basal ganglia. The convolutions form ridges and valleys: the cortical ridges are called **gyri**, and the grooves are **fissures** or **sulci**. The convolutions allow for the accommodation of a large cellular volume within a limited cranial space. The cerebral hemispheres are separated along the midline by the **longitudinal fissure**, also called the **interhemispheric fissure**. The paired cerebral hemispheres are essentially mirror images, containing similar centers for processing sensory and motor

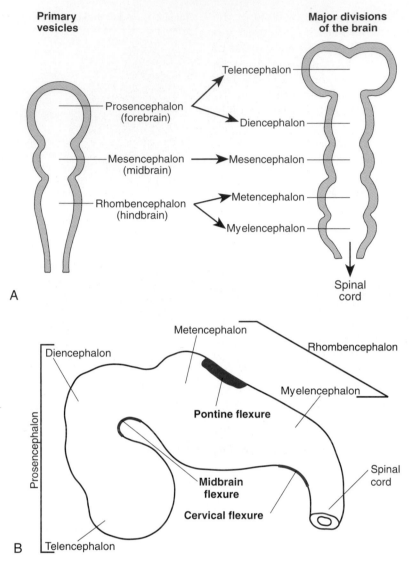

Figure 2-2. A. Three primary vesicles (*left*) in embryonic brain from which structures of CNS are derived (*right*). **B.** Lateral view of three flexures in developing brain at end of embryonic week 5; these flexures di-vide the brain into proencephalon, mesencephalon, and rhomben-cephalon.

functions. Each hemisphere controls the opposite side of the body. In addition to basic sensorimotor functions, each hemisphere possesses specialized skills. For example, the left hemisphere is superior in processing language, speech, and verbal memory, whereas the right hemisphere is better equipped to process pragmatic skills, visual and spatial concepts, music, and emotions.

Each cerebral hemisphere consists of five lobes: **frontal**, **parietal**, **occipital**, **temporal**, and **insular**. The first four, the primary lobes, are named after the overlying bones of the skull (Fig. 2-4). Considered a secondary lobe, the insular lobe is a small cortical island in the depths of the lateral sulcus, overlapped by frontal, parietal, and temporal folds of cortex. The primary lobes are divided by various sulci; the boundaries of these lobes, although well marked, are arbitrary, especially in the temporal, parietal, and occipital areas. The sulci and gyri markings of the brain are highly variable, particularly on the medial and basal surfaces of the brain. Consequently, maps of hemispheric lobe boundaries serve as only rough frames of reference.

CORTICAL SURFACES

Dorsolateral Surface

Some sulci and gyri are always present in the human brain and therefore serve as important landmarks for describing the gross external topography and for dividing the hemisphere into lobes. Three major sulci are present on the dorsolateral surface of the brain: the **central sulcus (fissure of Rolando)**, the **lateral fissure (sylvian fissure)**, and the **parieto-occipital sulcus** (Figs. 2-4

Left hemisphere

Right hemisphere

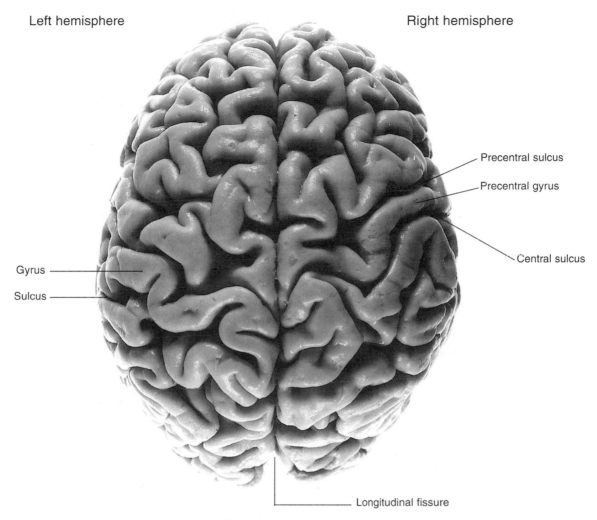

Precentral sulcus

Precentral gyrus

Central sulcus

Gyrus

Sulcus

Longitudinal fissure

Figure 2-3.   Dorsal view of human brain showing cerebral hemispheres and their major sulci and gyri.

and 2-5). The central sulcus begins at the top of the brain midway between the front and back, extends along the dorsolateral surface in a downward and rostral (anterior) direction, and ends at the lateral fissure. The central sulcus is about 2 cm deep, a depth that marks the boundary between the frontal and parietal lobes. It also separates the primary motor cortex from the primary sensory cortex. The lateral fissure, which is the most constant feature of the dorsolateral surface of the brain, begins rostrally below the frontal pole and extends posteriorly up toward the inferior parietal lobe. Anteriorly, the lateral fissure separates the frontal and temporal lobes; posteriorly, it extends partially between the parietal and temporal lobes. The parieto-occipital sulcus separates the parietal lobe from the occipital lobe.

Frontal Lobe. The frontal lobe is rostral to the central sulcus and dorsal to the lateral fissure. It is the largest lobe, occupying about one-third of the hemisphere. It contains four important gyri: the vertical **precentral**

gyrus and three horizontal gyri. The precentral gyrus lies rostral to the central sulcus with its anterior boundary marked by the **precentral sulcus,** which runs parallel to the central sulcus. The precentral gyrus is the site of the primary motor cortex (Brodmann area 4), in which the entire human body is represented (Fig. 2-6). Note the disproportionate representation of various body parts. Bioelectrical activity of nerve cells in this area is responsible for activating and controlling motor acts on the contralateral half of the body. The area immediately rostral to the precentral sulcus is the **premotor cortex** (Brodmann, area 6), which serves complex and skilled movements. There are specific areas for controlling speech, hand, and finger movements and eye–head coordination. The remaining anterior portion of the lobe is the **prefrontal cortex** (Brodmann areas 10–12) which contributes to various cognitive functions such as reasoning, abstract thinking, self-monitoring, decision making, planning, and pragmatic behaviors. Consequently, the prefrontal cortex is considered the major

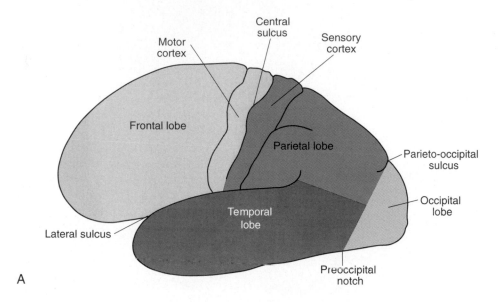

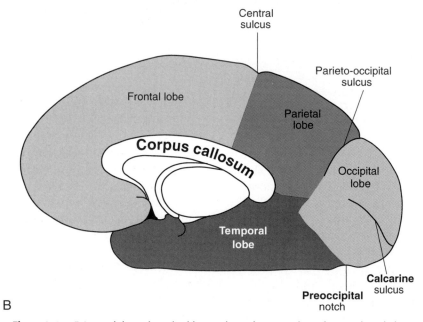

Figure 2-4.   Primary lobes of cerebral hemisphere shown on lateral (**A**) and medial (**B**) surfaces.

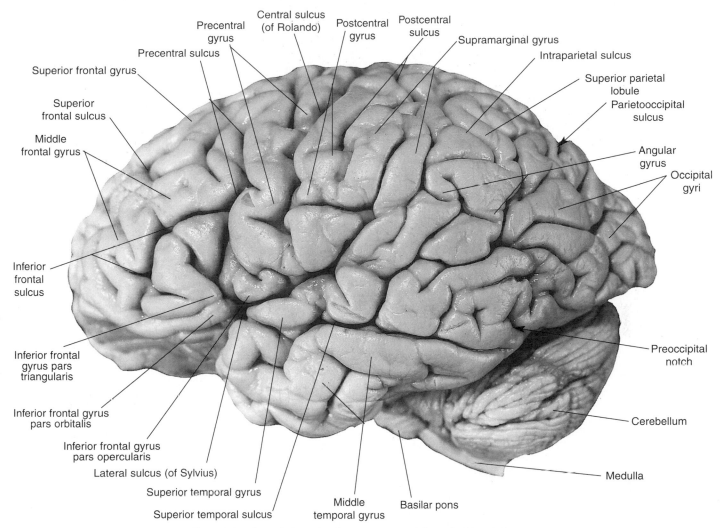

Figure 2-5.   Lateral view of major structures on left cerebral hemisphere.

biological correlate of human intelligence. Patients with prefrontal lobe lesions, commonly seen in cases of traumatic brain injury, are usually impulsive, uninhibited, apathetic, lazy, or confused. They are unaware of social expectations and consequences of their actions and cannot regulate their behavior (Table 2-2).

There are three large horizontal gyri in the frontal lobe: the **superior, middle,** and **inferior frontal gyri** (Fig. 2-5). These are also referred to as the **first, second,** and **third frontal convolutions**. The ascending rami of the lateral (sylvian) fissure intersect the inferior frontal gyrus and divide it into three sections: **pars opercularis, pars triangularis,** and **pars orbitalis**. The opercular and triangular portions of the inferior frontal gyrus in the dominant hemisphere constitute the **anterior language cortex,** or **Broca's area** (Brodmann area 44). Broca's area is important in spoken language. It is in front of the area of the primary motor cortex (Brodmann area 4) that controls jaw, lip, tongue, and vocal cord movements.

Parietal Lobe. The parietal lobe is between the frontal and occipital lobes and above the temporal lobe. The central sulcus marks the anterior boundary of the parietal lobe. An arbitrary line from the ramus of the **parieto-occipital sulcus** extending to the **preoccipital notch** marks its posterior boundary (Figs. 2-4 and 2-5). The inferior boundary of the parietal lobe is represented by a line drawn from the posterior ramus of the lateral fissure to the middle of the line connecting the **occipital notch** to the parieto-occipital sulcus.

The parietal lobe is primarily concerned with the perception of somatic sensation and with interpretation and elaboration of sensory experience. The **postcentral gyrus** (Brodmann areas 1–3), parallel to the central sulcus, is the **primary sensory cortex,** in which all modalities of somatic sensation are received; these sensations are elaborated to awareness in the parietal sensory association cortex, probably Brodmann areas 5 and 7 (Figs. 1-8 and 2-6). The sensory representation of the en-

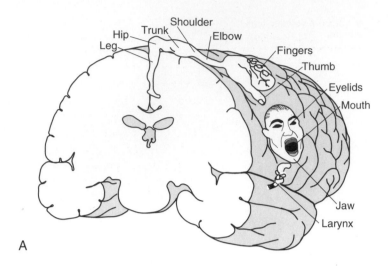

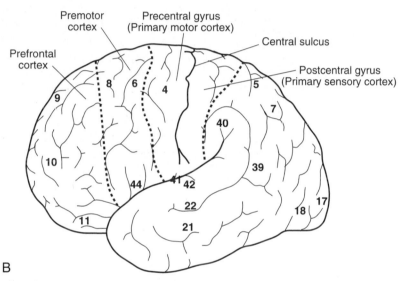

Figure 2-6. **A.** Distorted and disproportionate representation of body parts is called the motor or sensory homunculus; area allocated to each structure is based on its ability to participate in complex and/or skilled motor movements, not mere size of limbs. This representation is identi-cal in precentral gyrus (motor cortex) and postcentral gyrus (sensory cortex). **B.** Primary motor, premotor, prefrontal, and primary sensory cortices and central sulcus on lateral surface of brain.

tire body, like the motor representation in the precentral gyrus, is disproportionately represented in the postcentral gyrus, beginning with the face and head in the lower third of the postcentral gyrus and the trunk, hands, arms, and legs on the upper portion of the gyrus. The oblique **intraparietal sulcus** divides the remaining parietal lobe into the **superior** and **inferior parietal lobules** (Fig. 2-5). The entire parietal lobe is important in perceptual synthesis, spatial orientation, cross-modality integration, memory, and cognition. The analysis and integration of sensory information in the **inferior parietal lobule** contributes to complex perceptual experiences. Pathology of the parietal lobe results in contralateral sensory loss; complex perceptual disorders of constructional skills, spatial orientation, and body schema; memory deficit; and inattention to and neglect

of the contralateral half of the body (Table 2-2). Lesions affecting the **angular** (Brodmann area 39) and **supramarginal** (Brodmann area 40) **gyri** in the inferior parietal lobule of the dominant hemisphere result in disorders of reading (alexia), writing (agraphia), and calculation (acalculia).

Occipital Lobe

Only a small portion of the occipital lobe lies on the lateral surface (Figs. 2-4 and 2-5), although it is more fully developed along the medial surface of the hemisphere. Containing the primary (Brodmann area 17) and secondary (Brodmann area 18) visual cortical areas, the anterior boundary of the occipital lobe is marked by an imaginary line extending from the **ramus** of the parieto-occipital sulcus to the preoccipital notch.

Table 2-2. **Syndromes and Associated Neuroanatomic Localization of Lesions**

Anatomical Structure	Associated Symptoms
Frontal lobe	Contralateral paralysis, impaired cognition (reasoning, self-monitoring, attention, abstraction, problem solving), decreased spontaneity, impaired judgment, limited concentration, apathy, inappropriate or uninhibited social behavior, expressive (Broca's area) aphasia
Parietal lobe	Contralateral hemisensory loss, agnosia, inattention, constructional deficits, impaired tactile discrimination, contralateral hemianopsia, aphasia (involvement of left parietal lobe)
Occipital lobe	Blindness in opposite visual field, impaired recognition, visual agnosia, alexia, impaired visual memories and recognition of color
Temporal lobe	Contralateral homonymous hemianopsia, receptive aphasia (Wernicke's area in the left lobe), memory disturbance, epilepsy
Thalamus	Impaired contralateral unpleasant or painful sensation
Hypothalamus	Impaired autonomic functions; disturbance in regulation of temperature, salt, water metabolism, sleep-wake cycle; hormonal disorders; altered sexual functioning
Basal ganglia	Reduced (hypokinesia) movement, increased involuntary movement, sustained abnormal posture
Brainstem	Altered consciousness, vertigo, nystagmus, impaired ocular movement, cranial nerve involvement, crossed sensorimotor deficits
Cerebellum	Limb coordination
Spinal cord	Reduced reflex, paralysis, sensory loss

Temporal Lobe. The large temporal lobe is ventral to the frontal and parietal lobes (Figs. 2-4 and 2-5). The lateral fissure and an arbitrary line extending from its posterior ramus toward the **occipital pole** mark the dorsal limit of the temporal lobe and separate it from the frontal and parietal lobes. The ventral continuation of the imaginary line connecting the parieto-occipital fissure to the preoccipital notch separates the temporal lobe from the occipital lobe. The lateral surface of the temporal lobe contains three prominent gyri: the **superior, middle,** and **inferior** (also called the **first, second,** and **third) temporal gyri**. The superior temporal gyrus and sulcus run parallel to the lateral fissure and posteriorly turn upward in the parietal lobe, where they are surrounded by the **angular gyrus**. The dorsal surface of the superior temporal gyrus, the area hidden by the opercular portions of the frontal, parietal, and temporal lobes, dips into the **insular cortex** and houses a few short, oblique convolutions, **Heschl's gyri**. These gyri form the **primary auditory cortex** (Brodmann area 41), which is buried within the lateral sulcus in front of the insular cortex. It receives projections from both ears. Consequently, a lesion in the **primary auditory cortex** may cause only a partial attenuation in the hearing sensitivity in both ears. The **language association cortex** (Wernicke's area, or Brodmann area 22) lies in the posterior superior portion of the first temporal gyrus, the area surrounding the primary auditory cortex. This association area is concerned with the analysis and elaboration of speech sounds and verbal memory and is considered to be functional only in the dominant hemisphere. The association cortex on the nondominant side of the brain is primarily concerned with the perception of nonverbal material, such as music and environmental sounds.

Ventral Surface

The inferior surface of the brain displays structures of the frontal, temporal, and occipital lobes (Figs. 2-7 and 2-8). No parietal structure is seen on this surface. The two most important visible structures on the ventral surface are the orbital portion of the frontal lobe and the basal portion of the temporo-occipital lobes. The interhemispheric longitudinal fissure extends to the ventral surface separating the orbital portions of both frontal lobes. The **olfactory sulcus**, the site of the **olfactory bulb** and **tract**, serves the sense of smell. The **gyrus rectus** is medial to the olfactory structures at the ventromedial area of the frontal lobes. The area lateral to the olfactory region is occupied by many small orbital gyri.

The posterior structures in the temporal and occipital lobes are the inferior temporal gyrus, a large **occipitotemporal gyrus, lingual gyrus, collateral sulcus, parahippocampal gyrus,** and the **uncus**. The inferior temporal gyrus is on the lateral and ventral surfaces of the temporal lobe. The hippocampus, a structure identified with the encoding of memory, is beneath the **parahippocampal gyrus** and can be seen after removal of this gyrus. The **hippocampal gyrus** is posteriorly connected to the **cingulate gyrus** by a narrow isthmus beneath the splenium (posterior part) of the **corpus callosum** (Figs. 2-10 and 2-14). These structures (hippocampus, isthmus, and cingulate gyrus) are components of the **limbic lobe**. The collateral sulcus marks the lateral limit of the parahippocampal and lingual gyri (Figs. 2-7 and 2-8).

Midsagittal Surface

Cortical structures on the medial surface of both hemispheres are easily examined after the cerebral hemispheres are separated by section of the fibers of the **corpus callosum** (Figs. 2-9 to 2-11). Although portions of all four lobes are on the midsagittal surface, their sulci and gyri, except for the **cingulate** and **parahippocampal gyri,** do not present consistent boundaries of the lobes.

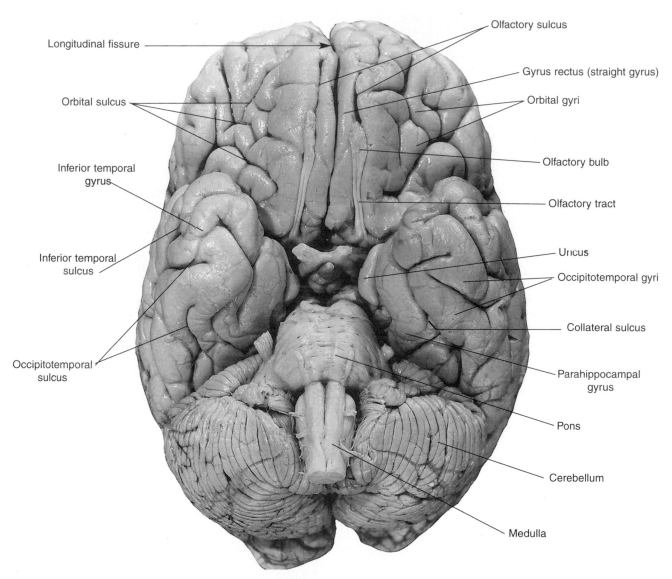

Longitudinal fissure

Orbital sulcus

Inferior temporal gyrus

Inferior temporal sulcus

Occipitotemporal sulcus

Olfactory sulcus

Gyrus rectus (straight gyrus)

Orbital gyri

Olfactory bulb

Olfactory tract

Uncus

Occipitotemporal gyri

Collateral sulcus

Parahippocampal gyrus

Pons

Cerebellum

Medulla

Figure 2-7.   Ventral surface of cerebral hemispheres with pons, medulla, and cerebellum in place.

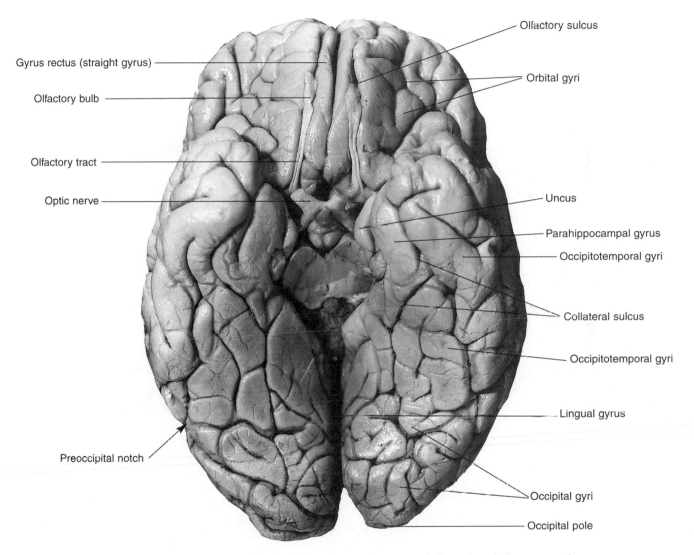

Figure 2-8.   Ventral surface of cerebral hemispheres with pons, medulla, and cerebellum removed.

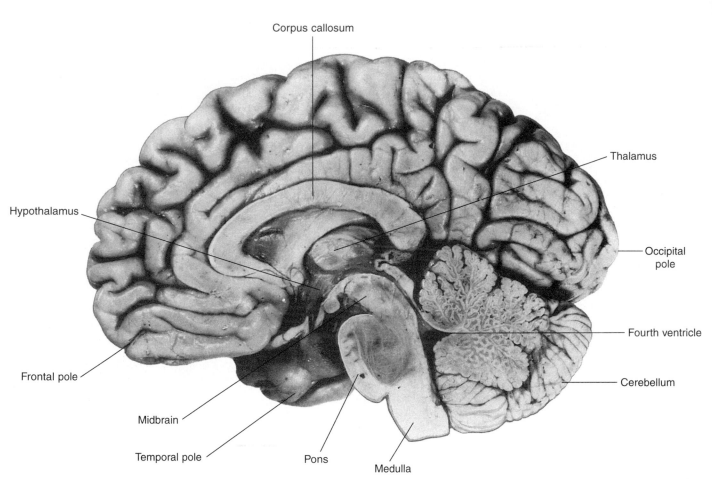

Corpus callosum

Thalamus

Hypothalamus

Occipital pole

Frontal pole

Fourth ventricle

Cerebellum

Midbrain

Temporal pole

Pons

Medulla

Figure 2-9. Midsagittal section of brain with intact brainstem structures; important midsagittal parts of brainstem are identified in Figure 2-11.

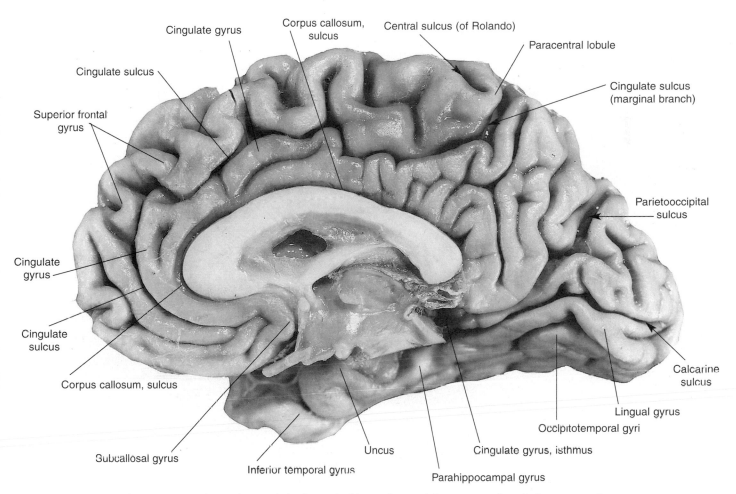

Figure 2-10.   Midsagittal section of right cerebral hemisphere with brainstem and cerebellum removed.

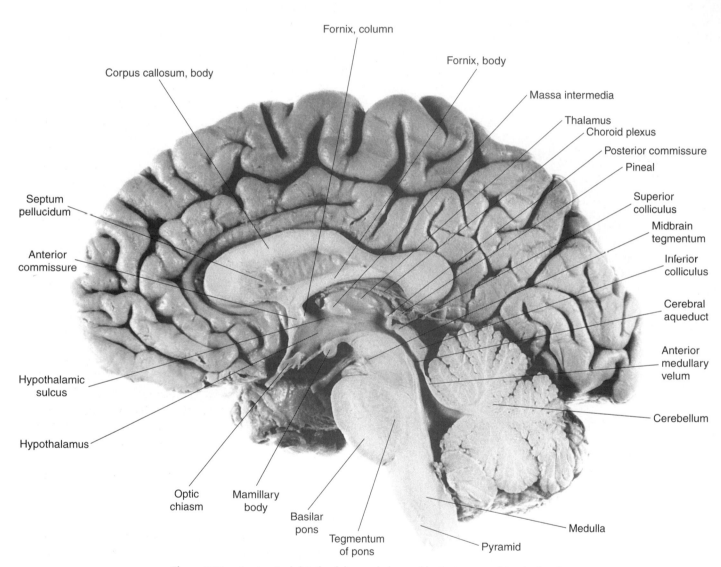

Figure 2-11.   Anatomical details of diencephalon and brainstem on midsagittal surface.

Frontal Lobe.   A line drawn from the notch of the central sulcus to the cingulate sulcus marks the caudal boundary of the frontal lobe (Fig. 2-4). A portion of the frontal lobe, on the medial surface, is part of the superior frontal gyrus extending from the dorsolateral surface.

Parietal Lobe.   Portions of the parietal lobe on the midsagittal surface extend from the superior parietal lobule of the lateral surface (Fig. 2-4). The line drawn from the notch of the central sulcus to the cingulate sulcus also demarcates the rostral boundary of the medial parietal lobe. The posterior boundary of the medial parietal lobe is marked by the **parieto-occipital sulcus** on the medial as well as the lateral surface. The precentral and postcentral gyri from the lateral surface continue midsagittally and constitute the **paracentral lobule**, an area notched by the central sulcus (Fig. 2-10).

Occipital Lobe.   A larger portion of the occipital lobe is visible on the medial surface than on the lateral surface. The parieto-occipital sulcus and a line extending from it to the preoccipital notch separate the occipital lobe from the parietal lobe and the temporal lobe (Fig. 2-4). The occipital lobe has two important structures on the medial surface: the **calcarine sulcus** and **lingual gyrus** (Fig. 2-10). The calcarine sulcus divides the primary visual cortex (Brodmann area 17) into the **upper** and **lower operculum**, which in turn are surrounded by the **visual association cortex** (Brodmann areas 18 and 19). There are spatial patterns of representation in the primary visual cortex; the **upper calcarine operculum** receives information from the lower quadrants of the visual field, whereas the **lower calcarine operculum** receives visual impulses from the upper quadrants of the visual field. A destructive lesion in the primary visual cortex in one hemisphere causes blindness in the opposite visual field. A lesion in the visual association area, which participates in the recognition and appreciation of visual stimuli, results in visual agnosia, alexia (inability to read), and impaired visual memories and recognition of color (Table 2-2). The structure below the calcarine sulcus is **lingual gyrus**.

Temporal Lobe

The medial temporal structures are contiguous with the ones that are visible on the ventral (basal) surface. They include the uncus, parahippocampal gyrus, collateral sulcus, isthmus of cingulate gyrus, and occipitotemporal gyrus (Fig. 2-10).

ADDITIONAL STRUCTURES

Among other important structures on the midsagittal surface is the corpus callosum (Figs. 2-9 to 2-12), the largest horizontal interhemispheric commissural fiber bundle. This massive, half-moon-shaped myelinated fiber bundle interconnects most cortical areas of both hemispheres. The myelinated fibers of the corpus callosum form the floor of the longitudinal (interhemispheric) fissure and the roof of the underlying ventricular cavities.

The corpus callosum consists of four parts. From its rostral to caudal extent, they are the **rostrum**, the most anterior portion; the **genu**, the anterior bend; the **body**, the large portion caudal to the genu; and the **splenium**, the posterior region (Fig. 2-12). Memories, experiences, and actions of both hemispheres are shared and integrated by way of the corpus callosum. A complete sectioning of the corpus callosum (**commissurotomy**) makes both hemispheres independent and unable to communicate or share experiences. Using patients with commissurotomy, researchers examined the discretely localized neurolinguistic functions in each hemisphere independent of interference from the other half of the brain. Their findings revealed that the left hemisphere is dominant for analytic skills and receptive and expressive language. The nondominant right hemisphere was found to have merely adequate receptive language capacity but superior skills for facial recognition, music, temporal and spatial information, and paralinguistic functions, such as stress and intonation.

Major structures dorsal to the callosal fibers are the **callosal sulcus**, the **cingulate gyrus**, and the sulcus of the cingulate gyrus. The callosal sulcus separates the corpus callosum from the overlying cingulate gyrus and surrounds the corpus callosum, curving ventrolaterally to become the **sulcus of the hippocampus**. The cingulate sulcus marks the inferior boundary of the frontal lobe. Running rostrocaudally, the cingulate sulcus turns dorsally to become its marginal branch (Fig. 2-10), which ascends and continues as the postcentral sulcus on the lateral surface. The cingulate gyrus, a part of the **limbic** or **visceral–emotional brain**, circles the corpus callosum and posteriorly curves ventrally to continue as the parahippocampal gyrus in the medial temporal lobe (Fig. 2-10).

Important structures ventral to the corpus callosum are the **septum, fornix, thalamus, hypothalamic sulcus, hypothalamus, massa intermedia (thalamic adhesion), anterior commissure, posterior commissure, mamillary body, hypophysis (pituitary gland), subcallosal gyrus, pineal body**, and **optic chiasm**. The septum, consisting of a midline membrane and nuclear structure, separates the lateral ventricles anteriorly. Bidirectionally connecting the mamillary body of the hypothalamus, septum, and hippocampus, the fornix is important in regulating limbic brain functions. The thalamus is important in sensorimotor integration and speech–language functions. The hypothalamus, ventral

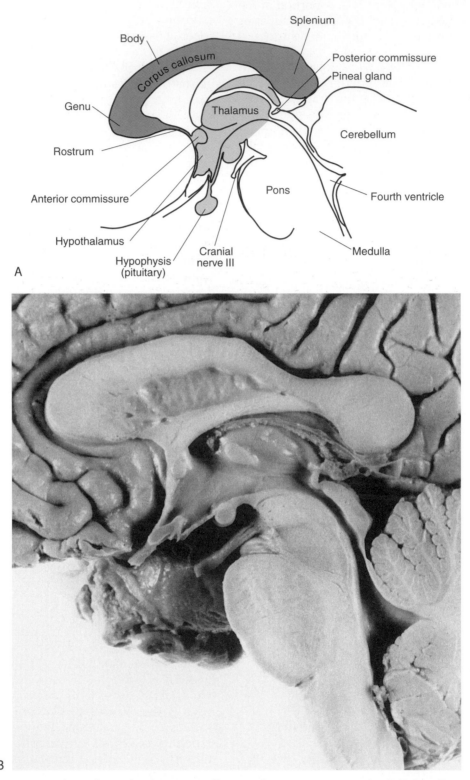

Figure 2-12. **A.** Midsagittal view showing corpus callosum and its major parts. **B.** Midsagittal view of brainstem, diencephalon, and corpus callosum.

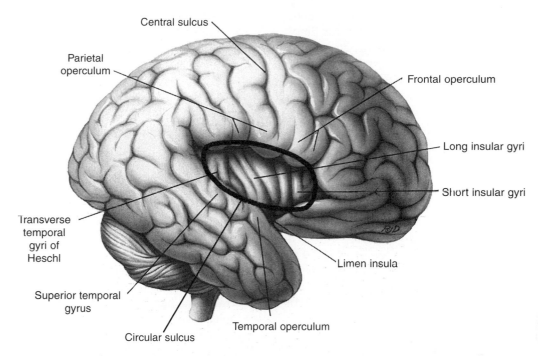

Figure 2-13.   Lateral view of right cerebral hemisphere with both banks of lateral fissure separated to illustrate insular cortex and transverse Heschl's gyrus.

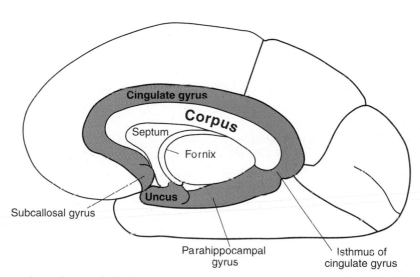

Figure 2-14.   Midsagittal view. *Shaded area,* limbic structures, including cingulate gyrus, parahippocampal gyrus, and uncus.

to the thalamus, controls various endocrine and autonomic functions. Specifically, it controls food and water intake, sexual behavior, and body temperature. The boundary between the thalamus and the hypothalamus is identified by the hypothalamic sulcus, an indentation along the medial wall. The anterior commissure connects the two olfactory bulbs and the basal and temporal cortices. The posterior commissure contains crossing fibers from the **pretectal nuclei**, the midbrain's visual

reflex center. The massa intermedia consists of interthalamic adhesions between the medial walls of the two thalami, which are found in only 70 to 80% of humans. The mamillary body, a hypothalamic nucleus, connects the anterior thalamus, septum, and hippocampus. The hypophysis (pituitary gland), another hypothalamic structure commonly called the master gland of the body, secretes hormones that regulate metabolic, sexual, pain, emotional drive, temperature, and electrolyte control systems. The subcallosal gyrus, also known as the paraolfactory area, may be considered part of the limbic lobe. The pineal body is a cone-shaped structure at the level of the posterior commissure. It secretes important neurotransmitters (**serotonin**, **melatonin**, and **norepinephrine**) that regulate the circadian rhythm and control sexual reproduction cycles. The **optic chiasm** is the site at which optic fibers from the medial retina of each eye cross the midline, join uncrossed fibers of the lateral retina, and continue to the opposite hemisphere.

Insular Lobe

The **insular cortex (isle of Reil)** is concealed within the depth of the lateral fissure by the opercula of the frontal, parietal, and temporal lobes (Fig. 2-13). The removal or spreading apart of these opercular tissues exposes structures of the insular cortex. Outlined by the **circular sulcus**, the insular cortex consists of short and long gyri that run parallel to each other. The **limen insula** is the opening of the insula toward the lateral fissure. Its anatomical location suggests that it is related to limbic and sensorimotor functions.

LIMBIC LOBE

The limbic lobe, phylogenetically one of the older parts of the brain, includes the mammalian brain structures that form a ring around the most medial margins of the frontal, parietal, and temporal lobes (Fig. 2-14). The limbic lobe consists of the cingulate gyrus, hippocampal formation, parahippocampal gyrus, uncus, and subcallosal gyrus. All of these structures, through their connections with diencephalic and brainstem nuclei, provide emotional drive to many visceral, behavioral, and vegetative functions. These behaviors, fundamental to survival, include **instinctual reflexes**, **feeding**, **defensive behaviors**, **mating**, **aggression**, **anxiety**, and **fear**. The parahippocampal gyrus is the direct continuation of the cingulate gyrus through the isthmus of the cingulate gyrus, a narrow strip of the cortex below the splenium of the corpus callosum. The fornix is the principal hippocampal output to the septum and the cingulate output to the mamillary body of the hypothalamus. The proximity of the hippocampal gyrus to the **amygdala**, uncus, and **olfactory system** emphasizes the importance of smell in visceral and emotional behaviors. The **Papez circuit**, which includes the thalamus, cingulate cortex, hippocampus, and their projections to the hypothalamus, has been implicated in emotional expression because its lesion may produce profound deficits in emotional behaviors.

BASAL GANGLIA

Basal ganglia structures, such as the cerebral hemispheres, are the derivatives of the telencephalon and are important in regulating motor functions and muscle tone. The nuclear masses of the basal ganglia are subcortical and can best be seen on either horizontal or coronal sections of the brain (Figs. 2-15 to 2-17). The basal ganglia consist of five nuclear masses: **caudate nucleus**, **putamen**, **globus pallidus**, **claustrum**, and **amygdaloid nucleus**. Various anatomical terms are used for grouping basal ganglia nuclei (Table 2-3). The caudate nucleus and putamen, as a group, constitute the **neostriatum** or **striatum**. The **lenticular nucleus** includes the putamen and globus pallidus. The globus pallidus is also called the **pallidum**. Pathology in the basal ganglia does not cause paralysis or paresis. Rather, it produces involuntary movements, such as the tremors of Parkinson's disease and chorea of Huntington's disease (Table 1-2).

Caudate Nucleus

The caudate nucleus is a large **C**-shaped nucleus. It has a massive pear-shaped head and a long, curved tail. Rostrally, the head of the caudate forms the lateral wall of the anterior horn of the lateral ventricle into which it bulges. The tail of the caudate extends caudally (posteriorly) from the head, curves around the ventricular trigone to enter the inferior horn, and ends at the level of the amygdala in the temporal lobe (Fig. 2-17).

Putamen

The putamen, a half-moon shaped basal ganglia nucleus with a role in motor functions, lies within the subcortical white core of the brain. The putamen is located caudal and lateral to the caudate nucleus, to which it is attached, and lateral to the globus pallidus. Lateral to the putamen is the **external capsule**, a long, slender white fiber bundle. Other structures lateral to the putamen are the claustrum and **extreme capsule** underlying the insular cortex (Figs. 2-15 and 2-16).

Globus Pallidus

The wedge-shaped globus pallidus is medial to the putamen. It consists of medial and lateral components. The globus pallidus is bordered by the optic tract fibers and amygdala ventrally and by the internal capsule medially (Figs. 2-15 and 2-16).

Claustrum

The claustrum is a slender mass of gray matter buried in the white matter of the brain between the insular cortex and the lateral margin of the lenticular nucleus. It is connected with sensory cortical areas and contributes to visceral functions and sensory integration (Figs. 2-15 and 2-16).

Table 2-3. Correlating Terms for Basal Ganglia Structures

Neostriatum or striatum	Caudate nucleus and putamen
Lenticular nucleus	Putamen and globus pallidus
Pallidum	Globus pallidus

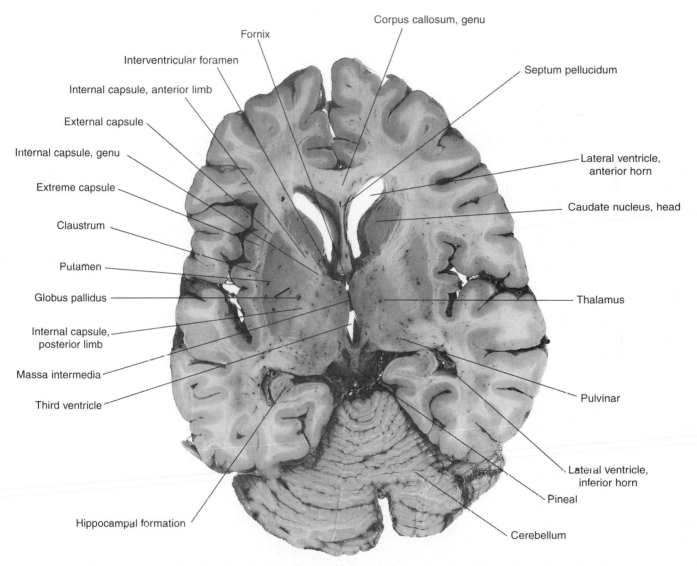

Fornix

Corpus callosum, genu

Interventricular foramen

Internal capsule, anterior limb

External capsule

Internal capsule, genu

Extreme capsule

Claustrum

Putamen

Globus pallidus

Internal capsule, posterior limb

Massa intermedia

Third ventricle

Hippocampal formation

Septum pellucidum

Lateral ventricle, anterior horn

Caudate nucleus, head

Thalamus

Pulvinar

Lateral ventricle, inferior horn

Pineal

Cerebellum

Figure 2-15.   Horizontal section showing subcortical basal ganglia structures in relation to internal capsule and its parts.

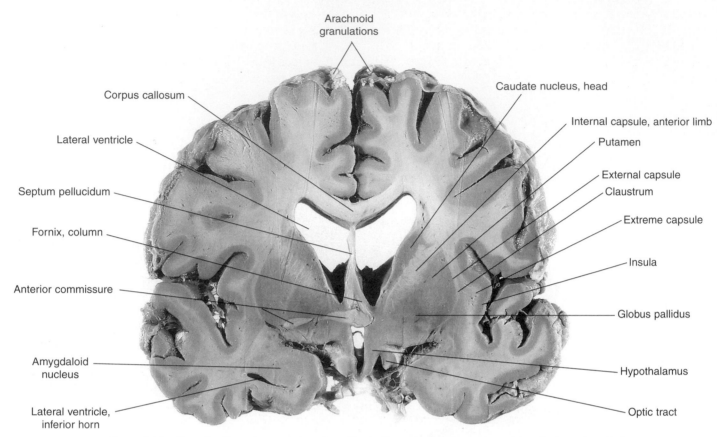

Figure 2-16. Rostral surface of a coronal section of brain illustrating basal ganglia nuclei and other subcortical structures in relation to internal capsule.

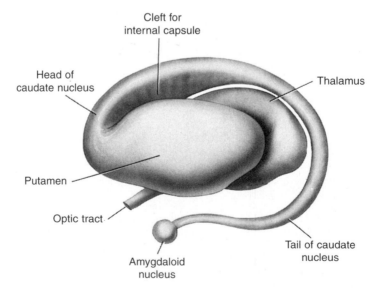

Figure 2-17. General anatomy of isolated striatum. Rostrally, caudate nucleus merges with putamen. Because of the C shape of the caudate nucleus, it contains a head and a tail. Tail of caudate nucleus travels in floor of lateral ventricle and ends in the amygdaloid nucleus. Fibers of internal capsule pass through cleft between putamen and thalamus.

Amygdaloid Nucleus. The amygdaloid nucleus is a small round nucleus that lies in the rostromedial temporal lobe at the end of the temporal horn and is contiguous to the tail end of the caudate nucleus (Fig 2-17). Although anatomically included in the basal ganglia nuclei, the amygdaloid nucleus is usually discussed in conjunction with the functionally related limbic system structures.

The **substantia nigra**, **red nucleus**, and **subthalamic nucleus** are important subcortical nuclei that participate in motor activity (Figs 2-18 and 2-24). These are not basal ganglia structures, although they are functionally

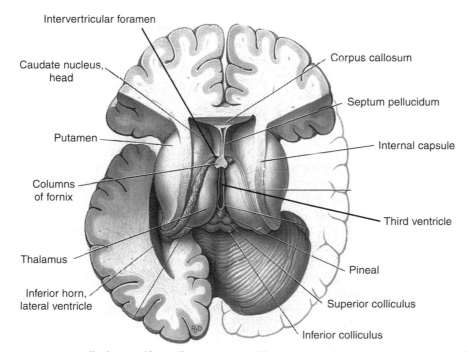

Figure 2-18.   Horizontally dissected brain illustrating general locations of thalamus, striatum (caudate and putamen), internal capsule, and cavity of lateral ventricle.

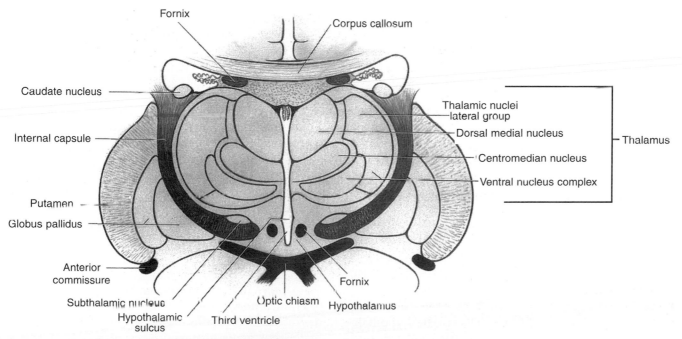

Figure 2-19.   Coronal section through diencephalon showing thalamus and hypothalamus in relation to third ventricle. Additional structures are internal capsule, striatum, corpus callosum, and fornix.

related to the basal ganglia. The structural and functional details of these structures are discussed in Chapter 13.

Diencephalon

The diencephalon includes the subcortical nuclear masses that form the central core of the brain. The thalamus and hypothalamus are two major substructures of the diencephalon, and they both can be seen in sagittal and coronal sections of the brain (Figs. 2-11, 2-18, and 2-19). The diencephalon is divided in half by a vertical slit of the third ventricle that demarcates the medial limit of the diencephalon. The **interventricular foramen**, bilaterally located at the rostral end of the third ventricle, marks the rostral limit of the diencephalon. The caudal boundary of the diencephalon is contiguous with the rostral end of the midbrain, and its dorsal boundary is delineated by the lateral ventricles. Laterally, the diencephalon extends to the internal capsule.

THALAMUS

The thalamus, an oval nuclear mass, is above the hypothalamus in the floor of the lateral ventricle. The interventricular foramen and the posterior commissure, respectively, mark the anterior and posterior limits of the thalamus (Fig. 2-11). The third ventricle delineates the medial border, and the internal capsule delineates the lateral border (Figs. 2-15, 2-18, and 2-19). Both thalami are bridged by a loose fibrous tissue, massa intermedia (thalamic adhesion), that crosses the midline through the third ventricle (Fig. 2-11).

The thalamus is made up of numerous small specific and nonspecific nuclei, each serving definite functions and projecting to different parts of the brain. A major function of the thalamus is to relay sensorimotor information to the cortex. Research evidence from patients with thalamic infarcts and thalamotomy (surgically induced lesion of the thalamus for treatment of intractable pain and motor disorders) suggests that the thalamus also contributes to cortically mediated speech and language functions. Vascular or neoplastic thalamic lesions produce impaired contralateral somatic sensation, a burning sensation of pain, and a low threshold of pain (Table 2-2). The anatomy and function of the thalamus are discussed in Chapter 6.

HYPOTHALAMUS

The hypothalamic sulcus is the border between the hypothalamus and the dorsal thalamus (Fig. 2-19). The optic chiasm and anterior commissure mark the anterior limit, and the mamillary body marks the caudal limit of the hypothalamus (Fig. 2-11). The hypothalamus consists of many nuclei that regulate various autonomic and endocrine functions, such as body heat production, water intake, hormone production, emotional expression, food consumption, and reproduction. Its structures and functions are discussed in Chapter 16. Hypothalamic pathology results in impaired control of body temperature regulation, food intake, salt metabolism, sleep–wake cycles, and endocrine functions (Table 2-2).

Brainstem

The brainstem is a short extension of the brain that connects the diencephalon to the spinal cord (Figs. 2-20 to 2-22). It consists of three structures: the midbrain, pons, and medulla oblongata. The brainstem does not include the cerebellum. Integrating and coordinating both centrally and peripherally acquired information, the brainstem monitors all brain outputs. It possesses automatic control systems that are genetically acquired, whereas the cortex contains largely voluntary control systems that are programmed through daily experience and learning and are especially modifiable at an early age. Brainstem syndromes include impaired ocular control, altered consciousness, and sensorimotor deficit of the opposite half of the body (Table 2-2).

The entire ventral surface of the brainstem is shown in Figure 2-20. Dorsal and lateral surfaces are exposed only after the overlying cerebellar tissues are removed (Figs. 2-21 and 2-22). The ventral surface of the midbrain consists of a midline **peduncular groove** and a **pes pedunculi** (crus cerebri) on each side. Caudal to the peduncular groove and pes pedunculi is the large protruding body of the pons. Caudally attached to the pons is the medulla, the cone-shaped and most caudal portion of the brainstem, which becomes contiguous with the spinal cord at the level of the **foramen magnum**.

The superior surface of the brainstem is seen after the removal of the cerebellum (Fig. 2-21). The brainstem structures on its dorsal surface are the **corpora quadrigemina** (**superior** and **inferior colliculi**), the floor of the **fourth ventricle**, and three **cerebellar peduncles**. The floor of the fourth ventricle contains many cranial nerve nuclei. Caudal to the ventricular floor is the dorsal view of the medulla. The **cuneate tubercle** and the **fasciculus gracilis** and **fasciculus cuneatus** are the most evident structures of the medulla. These structures contain the tactile sensory relay nuclei, **nucleus gracilis** and **nucleus cuneatus**, which mediate fine discriminative touch from the body (see Chapter 7). Figure 2-22 provides a lateral view of the entire brainstem and its gross anatomical structures.

Internally, the brainstem predominantly consists of **cranial nerve nuclei**, **longitudinal fiber tracts**, and the **reticular formation**. The reticular formation collectively represents groups of specialized nerve cells that are interconnected with parallel and serial running neu-

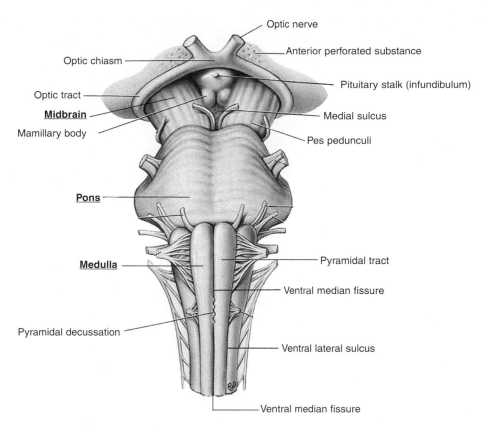

Figure 2-20.   Ventral brainstem marking locations of midbrain, pons, and medulla and showing various cranial nerve rootlets.

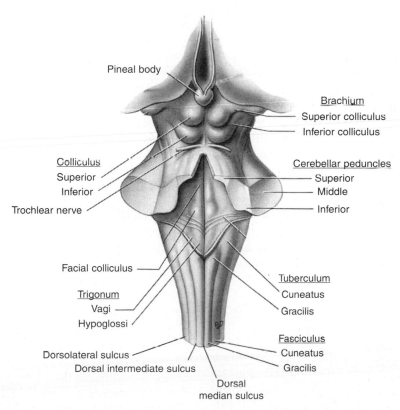

Figure 2-21.   Dorsal view of brainstem and exposed cavity of fourth ventricle after removal of overlying cerebellum.

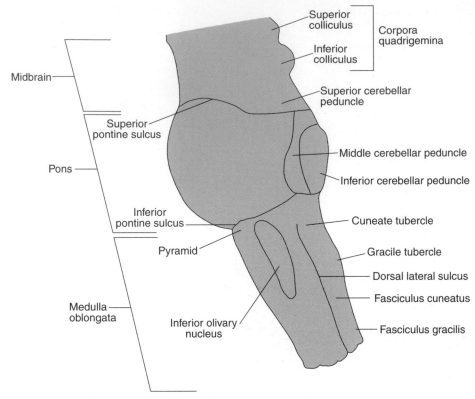

Figure 2-22. Lateral brainstem illustrating midbrain, pons, and medulla in relation to cerebellar peduncles.

ronal circuits. Composing most of the brainstem, it is functionally wired to nuclei in the thalamus and spinal cord (Fig. 2-23). By virtue of their central locations, these neuronal circuits inhibit, facilitate, modify, and regulate all cortical functions. The reticular formation integrates all sensorimotor stimuli with internally generated thoughts, emotions, and cognition. It is also responsible for maintaining the homeostatic state of the brain, which is essential for regulating visceral, sensorimotor, and neuroendocrine activities, including arousal, consciousness, sleep, blood pressure, and movement. It energizes the reticular activating system (RAS) that controls arousal and consciousness. A lesion of the RAS can produce altered states of arousal or prolonged unconsciousness (coma). While the hemispheres are sleeping, the specialized nuclei of the brainstem turn on the body's metabolic repair systems; after the body repair is completed and energy replenished, the reticular formation clock turns and reawakens the brain. Two of the functions of the reticular formation that are closely related to communicative disorders are the regulation of **respiration** and **swallowing**. The **pontine pneumotaxic center** regulates the depth and rhythm of the **medullary respiratory center**, which in turn is regulated by the carbon dioxide level in the blood. Damage to the respiratory centers in the medulla and pons can be life threat-

ening. The reticular formation regulates swallowing by integrating the sensorimotor functions of the **trigeminal**, **facial**, **glossopharyngeal**, **vagus**, and **hypoglossal nerves**. See Chapter 16 for a detailed discussion of the anatomy and physiology of the reticular formation and its functions.

MIDBRAIN

Located between the diencephalon and pons, the midbrain is a link between the cerebral hemispheres and peripheral and cranial sensory input systems. It contains all incoming sensory and outgoing motor fibers and important reticular and cranial nerve nuclei. It is also responsible for generating neurotransmitters vital to telencephalic, diencephalic, brainstem, and spinal cord functions.

Ventrally, the midbrain has an **interpeduncular fossa** that is divided by a longitudinal indentation (peduncular groove). The elevation on each side is formed by the pes pedunculi tracts of pyramidal motor fibers (Fig. 2-20). Dorsally, the midbrain has four rounded elevations (corpora quadrigemina). These round structures, just beneath the overlapping pineal gland of the thalamus, form the roof (tectum) of the midbrain (Fig. 2-21). The upper two rounded elevations are the superior colliculi (sing. colliculus), which participate in reflex

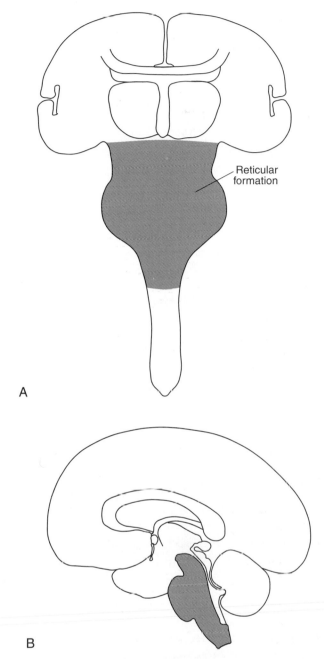

A

B

Figure 2-23. Brainstem reticular formation. A. frontal view. **B.** lateral view.

Reticular formation

the visual relay nucleus of the thalamus, whereas fibers of the **brachium of the inferior colliculus** connect the inferior colliculi with the auditory relay nucleus of the thalamus.

Internally, the midbrain contains many important nuclei and bundles of sensory and motor fibers; these can be seen on a cross-section of the midbrain (Fig. 2-24). There are three subdivisions in the midbrain: **tectum** (roof), **tegmentum**, and **basis pedunculi**. The tectum is the most dorsal portion of the midbrain; it is dorsal to the **cerebral aqueduct**, a small tubular connection between the **third** and **fourth ventricles**. The tectum is important for mediating visual reflexes. The tegmentum, the central part of the midbrain, contains numerous scattered nuclei, such as the red nucleus, cranial nerve nuclei, reticular formation, and central gray region. The basis pedunculi is ventral to the tegmentum; it consists of the substantia nigra, a nuclear group of cells, and **pes pedunculi** (crus cerebri), a group of cortical pyramidal fiber tracts that terminate in the brainstem and spinal cord.

PONS

The pons, a metencephalic structure, is identified by its bulging appearance on the ventral surface. The pons is separated from the midbrain by the **superior pontine sulcus** and from the medulla by the **inferior pontine sulcus** (Fig. 2-22). The ventral pontine surface is convex both longitudinally and horizontally, whereas dorsally the pontine structures are hidden by the overlying cerebellum. The pons contains all descending motor fibers and ascending sensory fibers, numerous cranial nuclei, reticular formation, and transverse fibers that form the middle cerebellar peduncle that attaches the cerebellum to the brainstem. The rhomboid fourth ventricle is dorsal to the pons and is visible after removal of the overlying cerebellum. The ventricular floor is broad in the middle and narrows toward its caudal end. The floor is divided in half by the dorsal median sulcus, and it contains important cranial nerve nuclei (Fig. 2-21). Along the medial eminence of the ventricular floor is a small round protrusion, the **facial colliculus**, formed by the facial nerve fibers.

Internally, the pons consists of two parts: the **pontine tegmentum** and the **basis pontis** (base of the pons) (Fig 2-25). The tegmentum of the pons contains ascending and descending fibers and numerous diffusely scattered pontine reticular nuclei. The fibers of the **medial lemniscus** are responsible for mediating fine discriminative touch. The basis pontis contains the cortical descending fiber tracts, pontine nuclei, and pontocerebellar fibers. The base of the pons also contains descending corticospinal fibers, which form the medullary pyramids in the medulla and continue in the spinal cord.

control of eye movements, visual reflexes, and coordination of vestibular-generated head and eye movements. The lower two rounded elevations are the inferior colliculi, which form the relay center for the transmission of auditory impulses from the ear to the thalamus and auditory cortex. The inferior colliculi also mediate reflexes triggered by auditory stimuli. Lateral to the corpora quadrigemina are swellings of the two **brachia** (sing. brachium). Fibers of the **brachium of the superior colliculus** connect the superior colliculi with

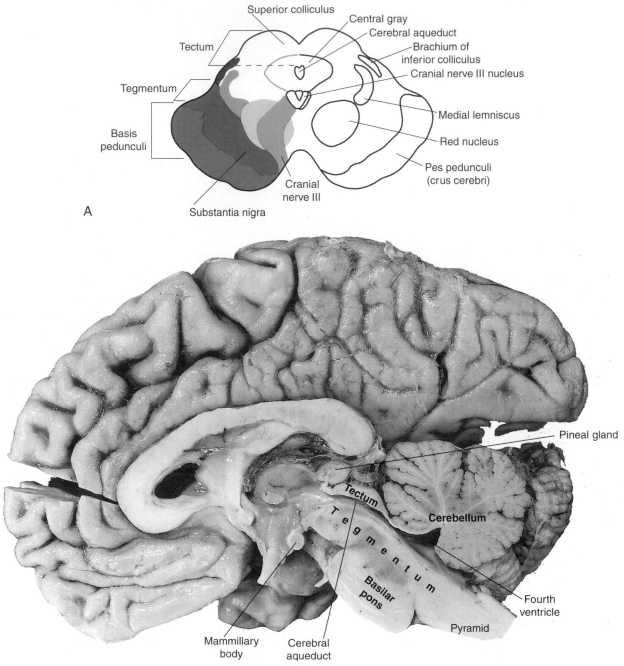

Figure 2-24.   A. Transverse section of rostral midbrain at level of superior colliculus illustrating internal anatomy of midbrain. Tectum, containing superior and inferior colliculi, is dorsal to cerebral aqueduct. Tegmentum contains sensorimotor nuclei, many passing tracts, and reticular formation. Pedunculi region contains motor fibers of corticospinal and corticobulbar systems. **B.** Sagittal view of the brainstem.

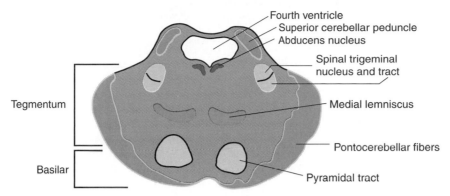

Figure 2-25. Transverse section of mid pons illustrating internal anatomy of pons, which consists of tegmentum and basilar pons. Tegmentum of pons contains diffusely scattered sensorimotor nuclei of cranial nerves, core of reticular formation, and multiple ascending and descending fibers. Basilar pons largely contains pyramidal fibers of corticobulbar and corticospinal systems.

MEDULLA OBLONGATA

The medulla oblongata, the most caudal part of the brainstem, is between the pons and the spinal cord (Fig. 2-20 and 2-22). The rostral limit of the medulla is at the level of the pontine protrusion. The caudal limit is at the level of the first cervical nerve rootlets and the crossing of the corticospinal fibers (**pyramidal decussation**). The medulla is shaped like a cone with its apex extended to the spinal cord. It contains all motor fibers that descend to the spinal cord and all sensory fibers that carry sensory information from the body to the more rostral brain areas. Surface features of the medulla that serve as important landmarks are the **ventral median sulcus**, **pyramidal tract**, **inferior olivary nucleus**, and **dorsal tuberculum** (fasciculus gracilis and fasciculus cuneatus).

The ventral median fissure divides the medulla in half. Parallel to the ventral median fissure is the **ventrolateral sulcus**. Between both of these sulci is the pyramidal tract, which carries motor information from the motor cortex to the spinal cord for activation of skeletal muscles. The descending fibers of the pyramidal pathway decussate at the level of the caudal medulla. After the motor fibers cross the midline, they form the **lateral corticospinal tract**, a motor pathway of the spinal cord.

The **dorsal median sulcus** divides the dorsal surface of the medulla in half; the caudal floor of the fourth ventricle forms a **trigonum**, which contains the **hypoglossal** and **vagus nuclear complexes** (Fig. 2-21). The **dorsolateral sulcus** runs parallel to the dorsal median sulcus. Between these two sulci are two sensory pathways, fasciculus gracilis and fasciculus cuneatus, which carry fine discriminatory sensory information from the body to the gracilis and cuneatus nuclei of the medulla and then to the thalamus. On the lateral medullary surface is an oval protrusion produced by the underlying enlarged inferior olivary nucleus. Fibers from the inferior olivary nucleus project to the cerebellum by way of the inferior cerebellar peduncle.

Internally, the medulla consists of two parts: the dorsal **tegmentum** and ventral **pyramid** (Fig. 2-26). The **tegmental** area contains several nuclei, reticular formation, fibers of the medial lemniscus, and fibers projecting to the cerebellum. Numerous cranial nerve nuclei are anchored and interconnected through the reticular bed that extends up and down the brainstem tegmentum. Some nuclei of the medullary reticular formation form three vital reflex centers. The **cardiac center** regulates the rate and strength of heartbeat. The **vasomotor center** monitors and alters the diameters of blood vessels. The **respiratory center**, in conjunction with the pontine pneumotaxic center, controls the rhythm and rate of breathing. Consequently, injuries to the medulla that implicate those centers may be fatal. The pyramid contains the descending motor fibers that are ventral in the medulla and cross the midline in the caudal medulla.

Cerebellum

The cerebellum is dorsal to the pons and medulla (Figs. 2-9, 2-11, and 2-12). It is separated from the cerebral hemispheres above by a meningeal layer of dura mater and from the brainstem by the fourth ventricle.

Although the cerebellum does not initiate motor activity, it contributes to the maintenance of equilibrium and coordination of motor activity by modifying cortical motor functions. Through direct and indirect links to the motor cortex, basal ganglia, and spinal cord, the cerebellum coordinates and modifies the tone, speed, and range of muscular excursions in the execution of motor functions. For example, it adjusts the strength needed to lift 10 versus 200 pounds and ensures smooth movement. The cerebellar projections to the vestibular system make crucial contributions to equilibrium-maintaining mechanisms. A lesion in the cerebellum leads to mild weak-

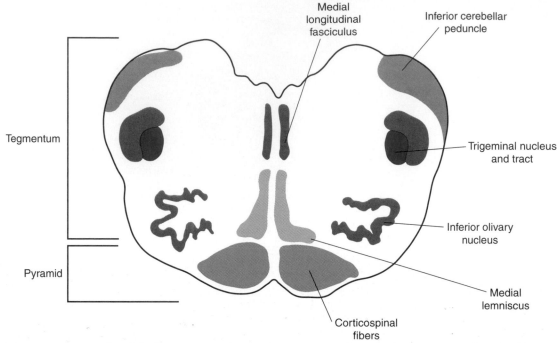

Figure 2-26. Transverse section of medulla showing internal anatomical regions of tegmentum and pyramid. Tegmentum contains sensorimotor nuclei, reticular formation, and passing fibers; pyramidal region contains pyramidal motor fibers.

ness, tremors, paucity of movement, ataxia (muscular incoordination), and impaired equilibrium.

The cerebellum has a highly distinctive appearance; its surface consists of a large number of transverse thin sulci formed by narrow rows of tightly packed gyri called **folia** (sing. folium). The wedge-shaped cerebellum is divided into two **cerebellar hemispheres** (Fig. 2-27). The structures in the midline portion of the cerebellum are grouped into the **vermis** (Fig. 2-28). Each cerebellar hemisphere is divided into three lobes: the **anterior**, **posterior**, and **flocculonodular** (Figs. 2-27 and 2-28). The portion of the cerebellum rostral to the primary fissure is the anterior lobe. The posterior lobe lies between the primary fissure and the posterolateral fissure. The flocculonodular lobe, the oldest part of the cerebellum, is on the inferior surface; it consists of two vermal structures: the **nodulus** and the paired **flocculi** (Fig. 2-29). A midsagittal section of the vermis reveals its central structures and provides a better view of the overall internal anatomy of the cerebellum. The nodulus portion of the flocculonodular lobe is medial; the remaining part of this older lobe, the paired flocculi, is ventrolateral on the inferior surface of the cerebellum (Fig. 2-29).

Structurally, the cerebellar lobes consist of a surface area of gray matter and a medullary core of white matter. Within the core of the white matter are important intrinsic cerebellar nuclei that participate in the analysis and synthesis of sensorimotor information and project motor modulating impulses to all motor control centers.

CEREBELLAR PEDUNCLES

The cerebellum is connected to the brainstem through three fiber bundles called the **superior** (brachium conjunctivum), **middle** (brachium pontis), and **inferior** (restiform body) **cerebellar peduncles**. The lateral inferior surface of the cerebellum reveals the connections of these peduncles to the brainstem (Figs. 2-29 and 2-30). The superior peduncle is stem shaped. Ventrally, the middle and inferior peduncles appear as a bulging thick semicircular collar attached to the pontine ventrolateral brainstem.

INPUT TO CEREBELLUM

The cerebellum receives its afferent information from two sources. Afferents from the motor cortex enter through fibers of the middle cerebellar peduncle. Fibers of the inferior cerebellar peduncle transmit proprioceptive afferent information from the trunk and limbs to the cerebellum (Fig. 2-30).

OUTPUT FROM CEREBELLUM

After analysis and synthesis of the received sensorimotor information, the cerebellum projects its corrective feedback predominantly to the opposite motor cortex through the superior cerebellar peduncle (Fig. 2-30).

Spinal Cord

The spinal cord is the transmission link between the brain and the body. As a bidirectional pathway, it

Rostral (upper) View

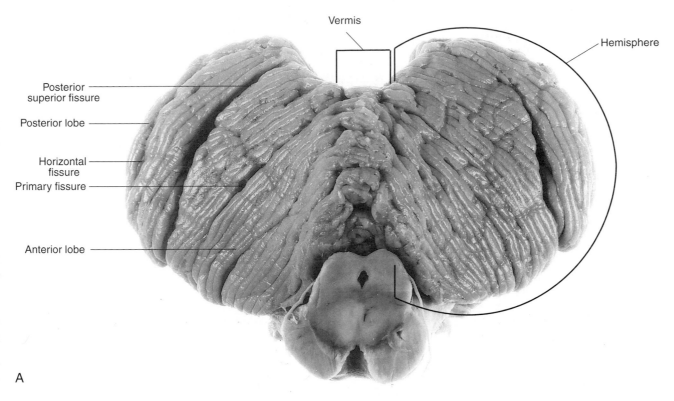

A

Caudal View

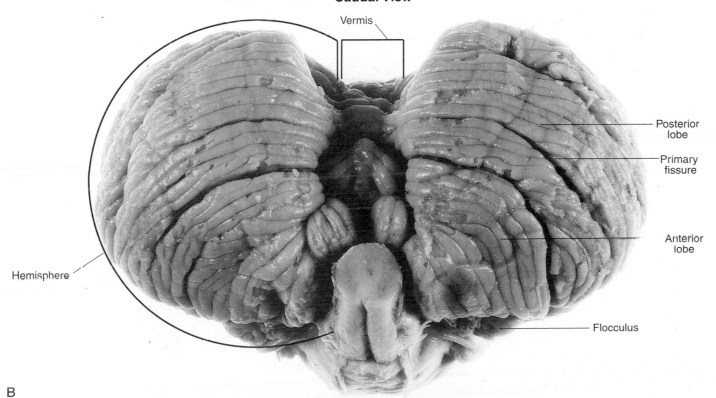

B

Figure 2-27.   Rostral (**A**) and caudal (**B**) views of cerebellum illustrating cerebellar hemispheres, primary lobes, vermis, and fissures.

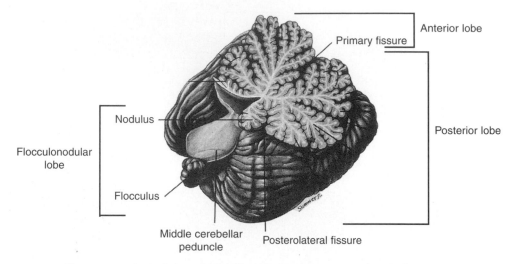

Figure 2-28.   Sagittal view of cerebellum illustrating structures of cerebellar vermis.

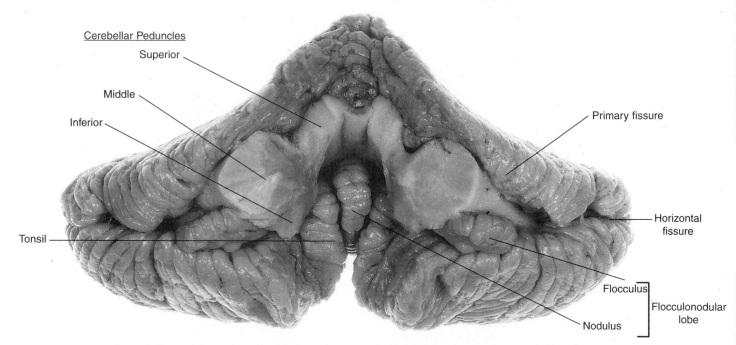

Figure 2-29.   Inferior surface of cerebellum after removal of brainstem to expose three cerebellar peduncles and vermal structures.

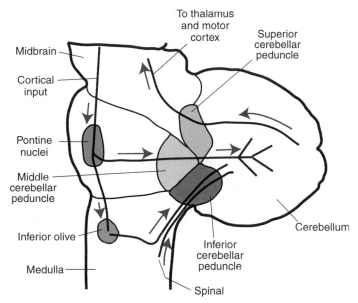

Figure 2-30. Lateral view of brainstem and a midsagittal section of cerebellum with three connecting cerebellar peduncles.

The **ventral median fissure** divides the cord into anterior halves. The **dorsal median sulcus** divides the cord into dorsal halves. The spinal cord has a series of nerve roots attached to it. A continuous series of dorsal rootlets enters the cord on its posterolateral surface. Similarly, a series of rootlets exits the cord from its anterolateral surface. There is one spinal nerve on each segment of a spinal cord. The dorsal and ventral nerve roots from the same side join to form the peripheral

transmits motor impulses from the brain to various visceral organs, muscles, and glands, and it transmits sensory information such as pain, touch, temperature, and proprioception from various body parts to the brain. Sensory input that requires an immediate response may not reach the level of awareness. Instead, the spinal cord locally integrates sensory information via collaterals and thereby generates its own sensorimotor reflex, an immediate response to environmental changes.

The spinal cord begins as the caudal continuation of the medulla oblongata. The spinal cord is cylindrical and approximately 42 to 45 cm (16 to 18 inches) long; it has a diameter of about 1 cm (Fig. 2-31). Wrapped in the three meningeal layers of **pia**, **arachnoid**, and **dura-maters** (Fig. 2-32), it is housed in the bony vertebral column. On cross-section, the internal anatomy of the spinal cord is composed of gray matter and white matter (Figs. 2-32 and 2-33). The gray matter has a butterfly-shaped appearance and contains all spinal nerve cells. It is surrounded by the white matter, which is made up of the ascending and descending fibers arbitrarily divided into three **myelinated funiculi** (fasciculi): dorsal, lateral, and ventral. The gray matter consists of two **dorsal horns** and two **ventral horns**. The dorsal horns contain the nerve cells that receive sensory information from the body through the **dorsal root fibers**. The ventral horn contains motor nerve cells whose axons leave the cord through the anterior roots to activate visceral and skeletal muscles and glands. After exiting through the intervertebral foramina, the fibers of the dorsal and ventral roots join to form the spinal nerves. In the center of the spinal cord there is a small opening of the **central canal**.

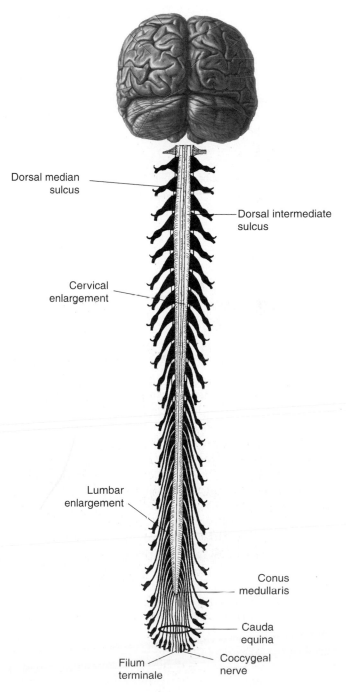

Figure 2-31. Posterior view of spinal cord as it extends from brainstem, showing a series of dorsal root ganglia and spinal nerves.

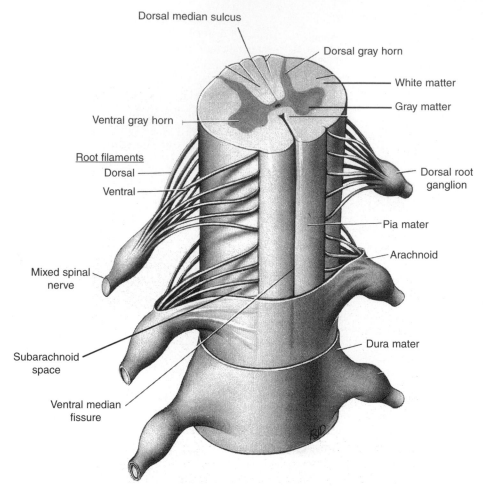

Figure 2-32.   Structures of spinal cord showing fibers of dorsal and ventral roots; dorsal root ganglion, spinal nerves, meninges, and subarachnoid space; and internal anatomy of spinal gray and white matter.

nerve, which innervates that side of the body (Figs. 2-32 and 2-33). The cell bodies of the dorsal root fibers form the **dorsal root ganglion**; this ganglion is proximal to the site at which the dorsal root fibers join the **ventral root fibers** to form a spinal nerve. The region of spinal cord that gives rise to the fibers making up a spinal nerve is a spinal cord segment. Without the rootlet fibers, the spinal cord would show no signs of its segmental nature; rather it would appear as continuous columns of gray and white matter.

There are 31 segments in the spinal cord (Fig. 2-34) and 31 spinal nerves on each side. These segments are grouped in five divisions of the spinal cord: **cervical** (n = 8), **thoracic** (n = 12), **lumbar** (n = 5), **sacral** (n = 5), and **coccygeal** (n = 1). The segmental sensorimotor organization of the spinal cord is reflected by peripheral overlapping of sensory and motor innervations for body parts and areas. The area of body innervated by the neurons in a single dorsal root ganglion (DRG) or a single dorsal root is a **dermatome**. The entire body is divided into numerous dermatomes. However, the muscles or parts of muscles innervated by all the axons exiting the cord via single ventral root is called a **myotome**. Knowing the chart of dermatomes and their corresponding spinal segments plays an important role in clinical diagnosis (Fig. 2-35; Table 2-4).

The 31 pairs of spinal nerves, named after the regions from which they arise, are formed by the merging of the dorsal (sensory) and ventral (motor) roots of the spinal cord. After traveling hardly a centimeter, each nerve divides into two rami: **dorsal** and **ventral**. Each ramus, like a spinal nerve, contains both sensory and motor fibers. Thus, a lesion of a ramus or spinal nerve results in both paralysis and loss of sensation for a specific limb. The dorsal rami serve sensorimotor functions of the posterior trunk. However, the ventral rami have a different pattern of distribution. Other than those originating from T-1 through T-12, ventral rami do not go directly to body structures. They form a plexus near the cervical and lumbar enlargements of the spinal cord by merging with the adjacent ventral rami (Fig. 2-33, B). There are four major plexuses: **cervical**, **brachial**,

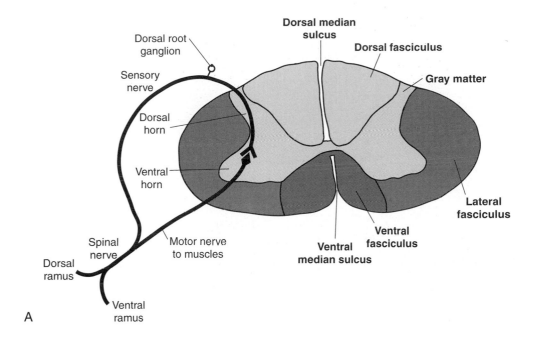

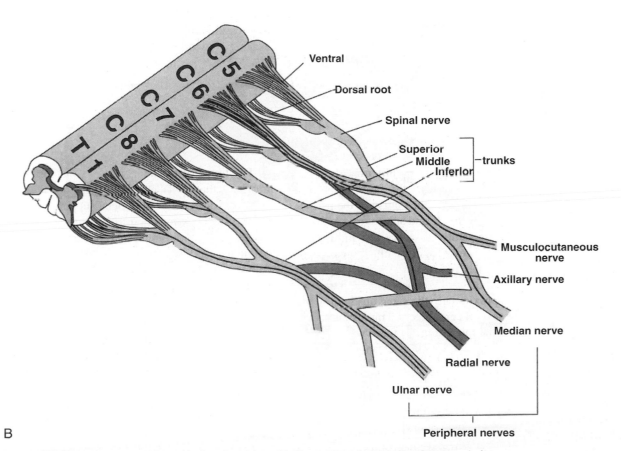

Figure 2-33.   A. Internal topography of spinal cord and entering and exiting fibers. **B**. Spinal plexuses.

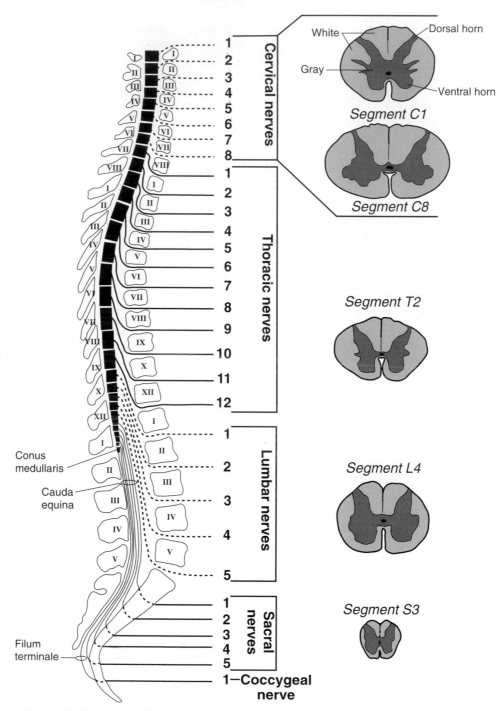

Figure 2-34. **A**. Positions of spinal nerves in relation to vertebrae. **B**. Cross-section of spinal cord illustrating varying size of the cord and differing shape of gray matter at different levels.

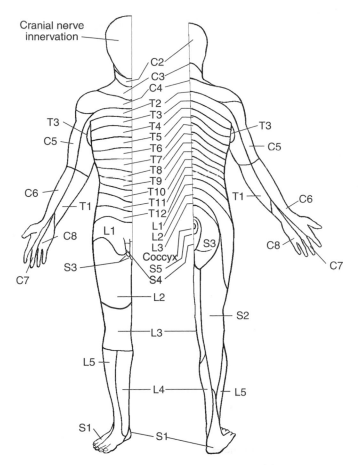

Figure 2-35.   Pattern of dermatomal distributions and their innervation by spinal nerves.

Table 2-4.   Spinal Roots and Primary Muscles Functions

Roots	Actions
C-5	Shoulder abduction
C-5	Body rotation
C-5, C-6	Flexion of forearm
C-6	Wrist extension
C-7	Finger extensions; forearm extension at elbow
C-8, T-1	Digital abduction and adduction (Check: have patient move fingers apart and together against resistance)
L-2–L-4	Knee extension, thigh and hip extension, thigh adduction
L5	Ankle and large toe dorsiflexion (have patient walk on heels)
S1	Ankle plantar flexion (have patient walk on tiptoes)

lumbar, and **sacral** (Table 2-5). Therefore, peripheral nerves contain mixed sensory and motor fibers from several adjacent spinal roots.

Understanding the spinal control of the muscles of respiration (Table 2-6) is an important aspect of training for students in communicative disorders. In addition to being vital for our survival, respiration entails a patterned cycle of inhalation and exhalation,

which regulates our speaking. The contraction of the **diaphragm** and **external intercostal muscles** increases the intrathoracic volume, triggering the process of inspiration. An increase in intra-abdominal pressure by **abdominal muscles** and rib depression by **internal intercostals** initiates exhalation. The motor nuclei from the anterior horns of the C-3 to C-5 segments (predominantly from C-4) innervate the diaphragm, the primary muscle of inspiration. The efferents to the intercostals (internal and external) exit from thoracic segments 1 to 12. The motor nuclei from thoracic segments 6 to 12 innervate the abdominal muscles (rectus abdominus, internal oblique, external oblique, and transversus abdominus). Spinal lesions involving these motor nuclei have different implications for respiration. For example, a patient with a spinal lesion above C-4 has complete paralysis of the respiratory muscles and may lose the ability to breathe, requiring artificial respiration for life support. A patient with a spinal injury below C-4 has paralysis of the lower intercostal muscles but not the diaphragm. With basic control of the diaphragm, this patient may quietly inhale and exhale because of muscle elasticity. Similarly, a patient with a thoracic lesion may be able to breathe quietly; however, he or she may have to learn to compensate to cough and exhale forcefully.

In earthworms and fish, the body area (dermatome) related to each spinal segment is not only equal in width to the spinal cord but is also parallel to the spinal segment. The segmental organization of spinal innervation has not changed during phylogenetic development. What has changed is the level of the innervated area that used to be parallel to the cord. In humans, prior to approximately the fourth fetal month, the location of cord segments matches corresponding segments of the vertebral column. In later months, however, the bony column grows faster than the cord. Consequently, the lumbar and sacral nerve roots descend below the level of the **conus medullaris** and form the **cauda equina**. The nerves from the caudal segments of the spinal cord continue to exit from the same intervertebral foramina as they did in early development; however, they progressively stretch and appear as a bundle of nerve roots descending in a fluid-filled spinal canal before exiting the spinal column. The **filum terminale** is a fibrous extension from the cord that is attached to the **coccyx** (Fig. 2-34).

VENTRICLES

The primary function cerebral spinal fluid (CSF) of the ventricular cavities in the brain is to circulate the **CSF,** which is produced by the **choroid plexus.** Circulating around the CNS, the CSF forms a spongy cushion to protect the CNS from excessive accelerating and decelerating head movements.

Table 2-5. Nerve Plexus and Motor Functions

Plexus and Origin	Nerves	Served Body Areas	Clinical Characteristics
Cervical (C-1–C-5)	Phrenic	Diaphragm; muscles of shoulder, neck	Respiratory paralysis
Brachial (C-5–C-8, T-1)	Radial	Triceps, other arm extensors	Wrist drop, inability to extend hand at wrist
	Median	Flexors of forearm; muscles of hand	Inability to pick up objects because of inability to abduct thumb and index finger
	Ulnar	Wrist; many hand muscles	Inability to spread fingers
Lumbar (T-12, L-1–L-4)	Femoral	Lower abdomen, buttocks, anterior thigh	Inability to extend leg and flex hip
Sacral (L-4–L-5, S-1–S-4)	Sciatic	Lower trunk, posterior surface of thigh and leg	Inability to extend hip and flex knee
	Peroneal	Foot and lateral leg	Footdrop, inability to dorsiflex foot

Table 2-6. Spinal Control of the Muscles of Respiration

Spinal Roots	Muscles	Functions
C3–5	Diaphragm	Contracts to increase the thoracic diameter for inspiration
T1–12	External intercostals	Contract to raise the ribs for inspiration
T1–12	Internal intercostals	Assist in rib depression for forced expiration
T6–12	Abdominal muscles Rectus abdominus Internal oblique External oblique Transversus abdominus	Increase intrathoracic pressure for forced expiration

There are four interconnected ventricles within the brain (Figs. 2-36 and 2-37): two **lateral ventricles**, one **third ventricle**, and one **fourth ventricle**. Both lateral ventricles are connected by way of the interventricular foramen to a midline third ventricle. The third ventricle, by way of a small opening of the **cerebral aqueduct**, is connected to the fourth ventricle in the brainstem. The inner wall of these interconnected **ventricular cavities** is lined with a layer of **ependymal cells**. These glial cells in part prevent diffusion of substances from the CSF into the brain. A common pathological condition associated with CSF circulation is **hydrocephalus**. Hydrocephalus in childhood is characterized by an enlarged skull caused by dilation of the ventricles. In adults, when the sutures of the skull have fused and the skull can not enlarge, the ventricles may enlarge at the expense of the surrounding cerebral hemispheres. In both children and adults, this pathological condition is usually caused by an obstruction in the flow of the CSF from its sites of origin (choroid plexus) to its site of reabsorption into the bloodstream, the superior sagittal sinus, a structure of the dura meninges at the top of the skull between the cerebral hemispheres. The dural sinuses are described

later in this chapter. Hydrocephalus is a treatable condition.

Lateral Ventricles

The lateral ventricles, one in each hemisphere, are C-shaped structures that form an arch. Each lateral ventricle consists of the central part, or **body**, and three extensions: the **anterior**, **posterior** (occipital), and **inferior** (temporal) **horns**. The roof of the body of the lateral ventricle is formed by the fibers of the corpus callosum. The superior surface of the thalamus constitutes the floor of the lateral ventricle. The body of the lateral ventricle extends from the interventricular foramen (of Monro) to an imprecisely defined point near the splenium of the corpus callosum. The arch-shaped body of the lateral ventricle enlarges near the **collateral trigone area**, the broader portion in the posterior floor of the lateral ventricle. Here, the ventricular body diverges into the posterior and inferior horns. The anterior horn refers to the extension of the lateral ventricle in the frontal lobe rostral to the interventricular foramen. The membranous thin part of the septum forms the medial wall of the anterior ventricular horns (Figs. 2-11 and 2-16). The posterior horn, shaped like an elongated slender finger, is the caudal extension of the ventricle from the trigone area into the occipital lobe. The inferior horn is the curved inferior extension of the lateral ventricle from the trigone area into the temporal lobe. Some important anatomical structures in the floor of the inferior horn are the hippocampus, amygdala, tail of the caudate nucleus, and crus (leg) of the fornix.

Third Ventricle

The third ventricle is a narrow vertical space between the two thalami and is rostrally connected to the lateral ventricles through the foramen of Monro. The hypothalamic nuclei form the floor of the third ventricle. Caudally in the midbrain, the cavity of the third ventri-

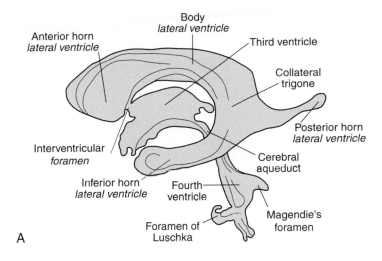

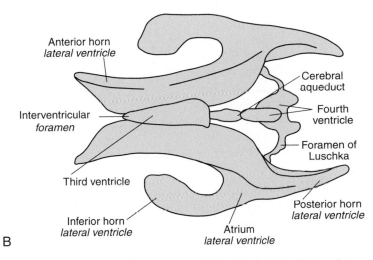

Figure 2-36.   Entire ventricular system in brain. **A.** Lateral view of ventricles. **B.** Dorsal view of ventricles.

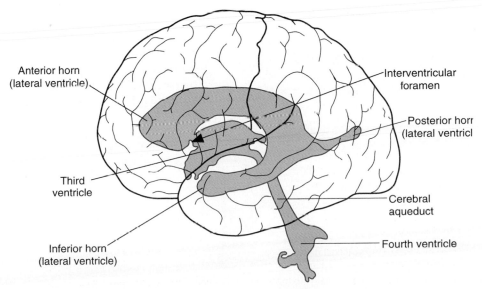

Figure 2-37.   Ventricular system in relation to brain in lateral view.

cle narrows to become the cerebral aqueduct, which connects the third ventricle with the fourth ventricle of the brainstem.

The cerebral aqueduct is ventral to the corpora quadrigemina in the midbrain and is surrounded by the central gray matter (Fig. 2-24). The cerebral aqueduct is an important reference point for the transition between dorsal and ventral midbrain areas. The area dorsal to the cerebral aqueduct, the tectum, includes the corpora quadrigemina in addition to the tectal nuclei (Fig. 2-24). The midbrain region ventral to the cerebral aqueduct is the tegmentum, which contains important structures, such as the red nucleus and reticular formation nuclei.

Fourth Ventricle

The triangular floor of the fourth ventricle is in the brainstem. The tegmentum of the pons and medulla constitute the floor of the fourth ventricle; the cerebellum forms its roof. The rhomboid floor of the fourth ventricle can be completely seen after removal of the cerebellum (Fig. 2-21). Beneath the floor of the ventricle are the nuclei of the fifth to twelfth cranial nerves. At the widest portion of the fourth ventricle, there are three openings: two lateral apertures (**foramina of Luschka**) and one medial aperture (**foramen of Magendie**) (Fig. 2-36). Through these three openings, the CSF gains access to the subarachnoid space surrounding the CNS.

MEDULLARY CENTERS IN THE BRAIN

Besides containing the cellular gray matter and ventricular cavities, each cerebral hemisphere includes a large volume of white fibers. The myelinated fibers form the medullary center of the brain and account for all **interhemispheric** (between) and **intrahemispheric** (within) connections. The comprehensive and efficient connectivity through the medullary centers within and between both cerebral hemispheres accounts for the efficiency with which external information is quickly analyzed, synthesized, and transferred from one modality to another and adequate responses are formulated and executed promptly with left, right, or both limbs. These interconnecting fibers keep all brain areas informed of activities undertaken, actions performed, information processed, and decisions made. The medullary center in the brain consists of three types of fibers: **projection**, **association**, and **commissural**.

Projection Fibers

While carrying sensory and motor information, the projection fibers travel vertically to connect the cortex with the brainstem and spinal cord structures. These fibers are concentrated in the internal capsule and project through the **corona radiata** to the brain. The internal capsule, a subcortical band of fibers, contains all ascending and descending fibers as they pass between the basal ganglia and thalamus. The internal capsule, which can be seen on a coronal or horizontal section, consists of an **anterior limb**, **genu**, and **posterior limb** (Figs. 2-15 and 2-16).

The **motor fibers** of the corticospinal (pyramidal) tract primarily originate from the precentral gyrus and descend through the corona radiata, internal capsule between the basal ganglia and thalamus, and pes pedun-

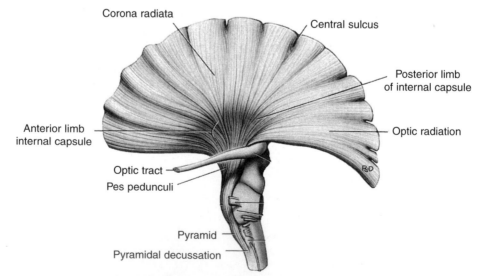

Figure 2-38.   Continuity of longitudinally arranged projection fibers from cortex through corona radiata, internal capsule, and midbrain pedunculi to pyramids in medulla.

culi in the midbrain (Fig. 2-38). They form the pyramid in the medulla before crossing the midline and entering the spinal cord. The **sensory projection fibers** collect cutaneous and proprioceptive sensation from the skin and joints and project to the CNS. These sensory fibers enter the spinal cord, ascend through the brainstem and internal capsule, then fan out through the corona radiata and project to the primary sensory cortex in the parietal lobe.

Motor projection fibers include **corticospinal** and **corticobulbar fibers**. Corticospinal fibers originate from the motor cortex and terminate in the spinal cord. Corticobulbar fibers originate from the motor cortex and terminate in the brainstem, the bulbar area. Interruption of the projection fibers results in sensorimotor syndromes.

Association Fibers

Association fibers, the most numerous of the three types of fibers, are confined within the hemisphere. Some of the association fibers are short and connect adjacent gyri, whereas some are long and connect distant cortical areas. Functionally, they share the same goal, which is to provide efficient bidirectional channels for communication among cortical areas within each hemisphere. They are also important in refined and integrated behavioral responses. Lesions involving these pathways result in disconnections between two areas within a hemisphere. Selective involvement of one or more of these pathways may result in a peculiar symptom complex, such as the cortical disconnection syndrome.

Short association fibers are **U-shaped arcuate** fibers that bend sharply around a sulcus and connect two adjacent gyri. The important **long association fiber bundles** are the following: the **superior longitudinal fasciculus, cingulum, superior occipitofrontal fasciculus, inferior longitudinal fasciculus,** and **uncinate fasciculus**. The general location of these pathways can be best seen on a coronal section of the brain (Fig. 2-39).

The superior longitudinal fasciculus, also known as the **arcuate fasciculus**, lies anteroposterior above the insular cortex. This associational fasciculus connects the frontal lobe with the occipital lobe. Many of its fibers diverge from the parietal lobe, curve around as the arcuate fasciculus, and project to the temporal lobe (Fig. 2-40). This fasciculus is an important communication link among the frontal, parietal, occipital, and temporal lobes. The curved arcuate fibers of the fasciculus are known to connect the classical Wernicke's area (posterior language cortex) in the temporal lobe with Broca's area (anterior language cortex) in the frontal lobe. This pathway is significant in the normal acquisition of language functions, auditory–verbal (repetition) memory, and propositional communication.

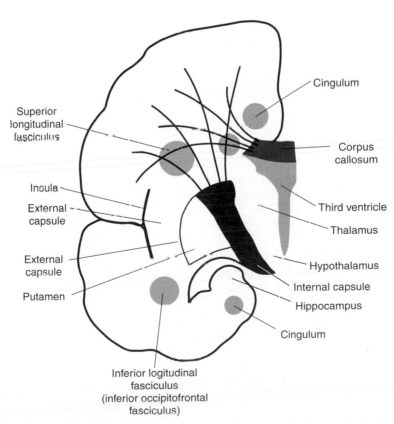

Figure 2-39.   Intrahemispheric location of major associational pathways on a coronal section.

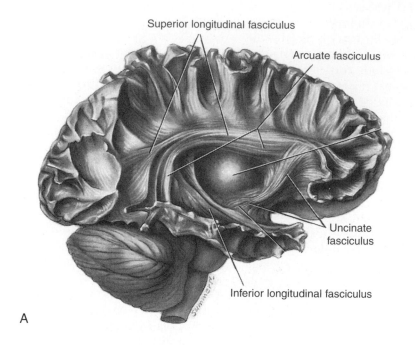

Superior longitudinal fasciculus

Arcuate fasciculus

Uncinate fasciculus

Inferior longitudinal fasciculus

A

Cingulum

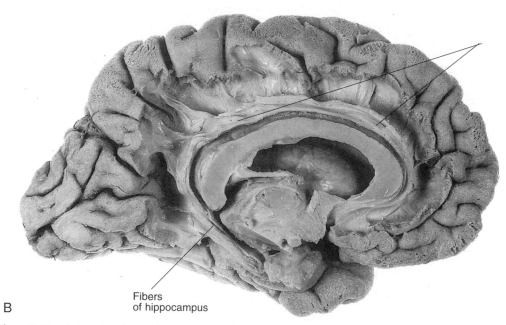

Fibers
of hippocampus

B

Figure 2-40. **A.** Long intrahemispheric association fibers on lateral surface. **B.** Dissected view of medial aspect of left
hemisphere illustrating cingulum and fibers of hippocampus.

The superior occipitofrontal fasciculus, a subcallosal fiber bundle, is deep within the white substance of the hemisphere beneath the fibers of the corpus callosum. Its fibers provide a communication link between the occipital and frontal lobes.

The inferior longitudinal fasciculus is a well-defined compressed bundle of fibers beneath the sylvian fissure and the insular cortex. It connects the temporal and occipital lobes. Its fibers travel anteroposteriorly from the occipital to the temporal lobe. Traveling parallel to the inferior longitudinal fasciculus are the short fibers of the uncinate fasciculus (Fig. 2-40, *A*); some consider it to be an extension of the inferior occipitofrontal fasciculus. These fibers connect the orbital frontal gyri with the rostral region in the temporal lobe.

The cingulum, a C-shaped association fiber bundle, is beneath the cingulate gyrus, which lies above the corpus callosum. The cingulum is an association fiber bundle of the limbic lobe connecting the medial, frontal, and parietal cortices with the temporal cortex. Its fibers originate in the subcallosal area beneath the genu of the corpus callosum, circle around the corpus callosum within the cingulate gyrus, and terminate in the parahippocampal gyrus of the medial temporal lobe (Fig. 2-40, *B*).

Commissural Fibers

Commissural fibers in the brain run horizontally and connect the corresponding cortical areas in both cerebral hemispheres. Most neocortical commissural fibers are included in the corpus callosum, and the remainder of the fibers constitute the anterior commissure. The corpus callosum, the largest commissural bundle of fibers, is a thick plate of more than 300 million to 400 million fibers (Figs. 2-15, 2-16 and 2-41). The fibers of the corpus callosum are known to connect the corresponding cortical areas in both hemispheres except for the primary centers for motor, sensory, auditory, and visual functions. The primary centers in both hemispheres are connected to each other only through the association cortical areas, which in turn are interconnected through the callosal fibers.

The corpus callosum contains four parts: **rostrum**, **genu**, **body**, and **splenium** (Fig. 2-12). The fibers in the genu and rostrum of the corpus callosum interconnect the anterior and orbital regions of the frontal lobes. The fibers from the posterior frontal lobes and the parietal lobes pass through the body of the corpus callosum. The fibers forming the splenium originate from the occipital and temporal lobes. Because the corpus callosum is shorter than the hemispheres from front to back, its fiber radiations extend anteriorly and posteriorly to the frontal and occipital poles.

The fibers of the corpus callosum allow each hemisphere to access the memory traces, experiences, and unique learning abilities of the contralateral hemisphere. This close interaction underlying normal behavior was best illustrated by the neurosurgical procedure commissurotomy, producing a so-called split brain. Surgical sectioning of the callosal fibers, undertaken as a medical treatment, renders the cerebral hemispheres functionally independent. This hemispheric separation has provided researchers with a unique opportunity to map independently the neurolinguistic functions of each hemisphere with no interference from the other. That each hemisphere has exclusive skills and functions remains the outstanding neurolinguistic observation from that study. The left hemisphere is dominant for verbal expression. The right hemisphere is known to process some receptive language; however, it is uniquely equipped to serve nonverbal, visuospatial,

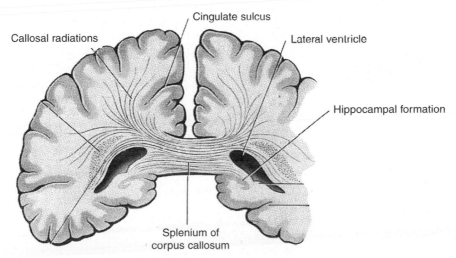

Figure 2-41.   Coronal view illustrating course of corpus callosal fibers at level of its splenium; callosal fibers lateral to ventricles are called tapetum.

and musical skills. Dr. Roger W. Sperry has extensively studied functions of the commissural fibers in humans. In 1981 he received a Nobel prize in physiology and medicine for examining the neurolinguistic organization of the human brain in patients with commissurotomy.

The smaller anterior commissure, a second commissural bundle, contains crossing fibers other than the neocortical ones (Fig. 2-11 and 2-16). It is rostral to the thalamus. The bulk of the fibers that form the anterior commissure originate from the middle and inferior temporal gyri and terminate in the same gyri in the contralateral hemisphere. Some fibers of the anterior commissure originate in the olfactory bulb and terminate in the opposite olfactory tract.

MENINGES OF THE BRAIN

The soft and gelatinous nature of the CNS makes the brain and spinal cord susceptible to trauma. The structures that provide the basic protections to the CNS include the three meningeal layers, the cushioning CSF, the bony wall of the skull, and the vertebral column. The meninges consist of three concentric fibrous tissue membranes that encase the CNS: **dura mater**, **arachnoid membrane**, and **pia mater** (Fig. 2-42; Table 2-7).

Dura Mater

The dura mater, the gray outermost membrane, consists of dense, fibrous connective tissue and provides the maximum meningeal protection to the CNS. It is thick and tough in comparison with the pia and arachnoid. The dura is attached to the inner surface of the skull and overlies the underlying arachnoid. There are

Table 2-7. Cerebral versus Spinal Meninges

Cerebral Meninges	Spinal Meninges
Dura adheres to inner skull composed of two fused layers (periosteal and meningeal), which split to form sinuses	Dura separates from vertebrae by potential epidural space composed of only meningeal layer (vertebrae have their own periosteum)
Arachnoid attaches to dura in living condition (no subdural space); subarachnoid space with several cisterns	Arachnoid attaches to dura in living condition (no subdural space); subarachnoid space with sacral cistern
Pia adheres to surface of brain with extension within depth of sulci; follows vessels as they pierce cerebral cortex	Pia adheres to surface of cord specializations in the form of denticulate ligaments; filum terminale follows vessels as they pierce the cord

two spaces around the cranial dura, the **epidural** and **subdural spaces**. The epidural refers to the potential space between the dura and the bone. The subdural is the potential space between the dura mater and the arachnoid. Dura mater consists of two fibrous layers, the external **periosteal** and internal **meningeal**. The two layers are attached to each other except where they separate to form sinuses that carry the blood from veins and absorb the circulated CSF (Fig. 2-43). The outer periosteal layer of the dura mater is attached to the inner surface of the cranium, and its meningeal layer forms various **septa** (**dural extensions**) that form two lateral compartments for the cerebral hemispheres and one posterior compartment for the cerebellum (Fig. 2-44).

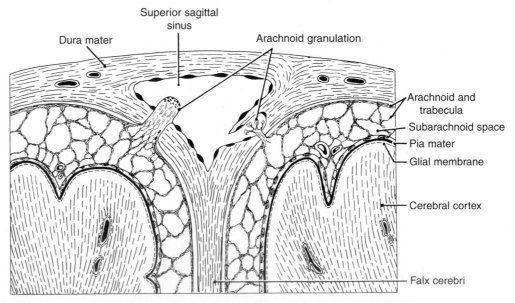

Figure 2-42.   Three meninges in relation to surfaces of brain, subarachnoid space, and sagittal sinus. Also shown are arachnoid villi (granulations) that drain CSF in sagittal sinus.

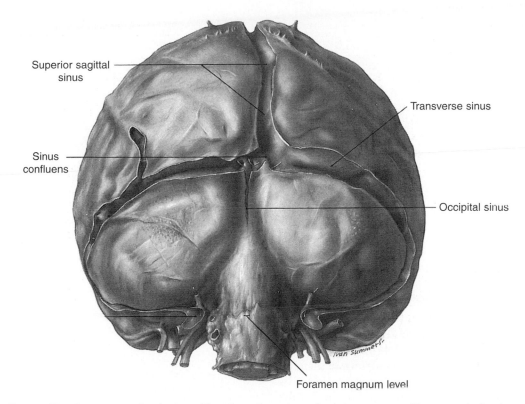

Superior sagittal sinus

Transverse sinus

Sinus confluens

Occipital sinus

Foramen magnum level

Figure 2-43.   Dura surrounding brain and locations of prominent dural sinuses exposed by removal of periosteal layer of dura mater.

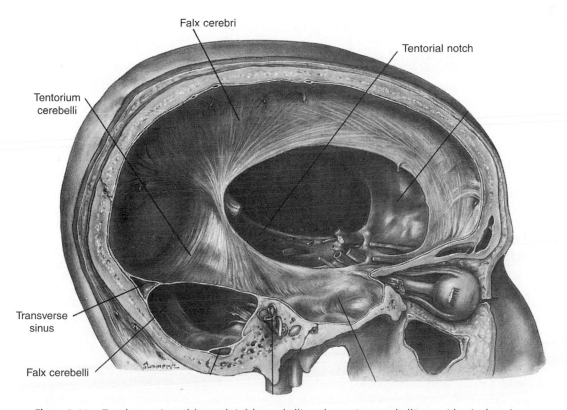

Falx cerebri

Tentorial notch

Tentorium cerebelli

Transverse sinus

Falx cerebelli

Figure 2-44.   Dural extensions (falx cerebri, falx cerebelli, and tentorium cerebelli) on midsagittal section.

FALX CEREBRI

This dural extension, named for its sickle shape, is the largest dural reflection. It extends longitudinally in the interhemispheric fissure between the two hemispheres, and it forms a vertical partition in the cranial cavity between two cerebral hemispheres (Fig. 2-44). Anteriorly, this dural reflection is attached to the **crista galli** of the **ethmoid bone** in the inner cranium; posteriorly, it extends to the internal occipital protuberance and the **tentorium cerebelli,** another dural reflection. At the dorsal edge of the interhemispheric fissure, the falx cerebri forms the cavity for the **superior sagittal sinus**. Inferior within this fissure above the corpus callosum is the **inferior sagittal sinus** along the free inferior margin of the falx cerebri.

TENTORIUM CEREBELLI

The tentorium cerebelli, a dural extension, arises from the petrous portion of the temporal bone. Its attachments to the falx cerebri along the midline pull it up, giving it the shape of a tent over the posterior fossa, which houses the cerebellum (Fig. 2-44). Its margins are between the cerebellum and the basal surface of the temporal and occipital lobes, so that the occipital lobes lie over it and the cerebellum is below it. Anteriorly, the free borders of the tentorium cerebelli constitute the opening named the **tentorial incisure,** or **tentorial notch**. The brainstem descends through the tentorial notch toward the foramen magnum. The space above the tentorium, the **supratentorial space,** it contains the cerebral cortex. The space below the tentorium, the **infratentorial space,** contains the cerebellum and brainstem (Fig. 2-45).

FALX CEREBELLI

The falx cerebelli is a small triangular vertical extension from the tentorium cerebelli that separates two cerebellar hemispheres (Figs. 2-44 and 2-45).

Arachnoid Membrane

The arachnoid membrane is a thin, nonvascular membrane between the internal pia mater and the external dura mater. It does not adhere to the cortical surface like the pia mater (Figs. 2-42 and 2-46) but bridges the cortical surface and the pia mater. The space between the pia and the arachnoid is traversed by the **arachnoid trabeculae,** which consist of fibrous and elastic connective tissue (Figs. 2-42 and 2-46). The **subarachnoid space** between the arachnoid and pia mater is filled with CSF. The CSF is produced in the ventricular system and enters the subarachnoid space through openings in the fourth ventricle. The subarachnoid space envelops the entire nervous system.

The arachnoid membrane is separated from the dura mater by the potential subdural space. However, the arachnoid pushes through the dura to form flower-

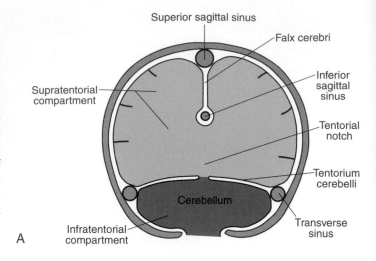

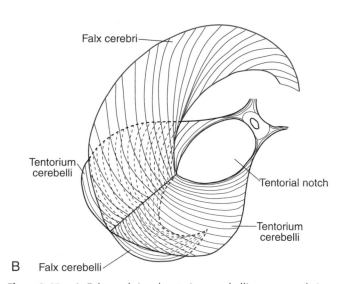

Figure 2-45. **A.** Falx cerebri and tentorium cerebelli on a coronal view. Also depicted are supratentorial and infratentorial compartments. **B.** Locations of three dural extensions.

shaped **arachnoid granulations** (villi) near the vertex of the brain (Figs. 2-16 and 2-46). The arachnoid granulations, through which CSF drains into the vascular system, are predominantly located around the superior sagittal sinus on the dorsal surface of the brain.

Pia Mater

The pia mater, a thin, transparent, collagenous (connective tissue) membrane, is closely attached to the surface of the brain (Fig. 2-42). It adheres to the entire surface of the brain and thus follows the contours of the gyri and the sulci (Fig. 2-46). It has a network of blood vessels that penetrate the pia before entering the cortical substance. The pia mater also surrounds the blood vessels and forms a perivascular space. Both the pia and arachnoid membranes are relatively delicate, and together they are called the **leptomeninges**.

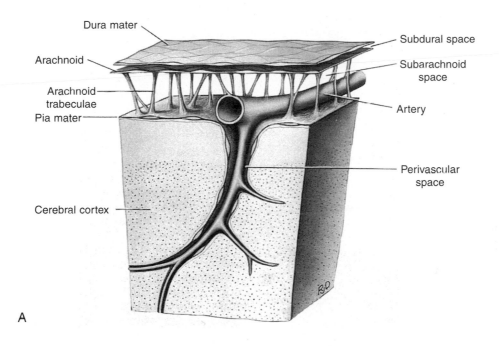

A

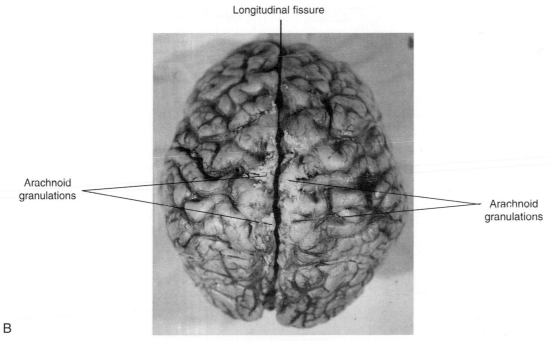

B

Figure 2-46.   A. Meningeal structures of brain illustrating order and locations of meninges in relation to subarachnoid and perivascular space. **B.** Arachnoid granulations.

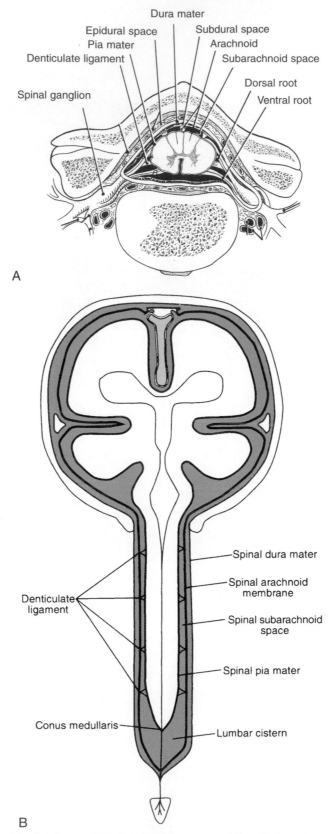

Figure 2-47. **A**. Spinal cord and its meningeal coverings on a cross-section. **B.** Complete view of the meningeal relationship to the brain and spinal cord.

MENINGES OF THE SPINAL CORD

Spinal Dura Mater

As a part of the CNS, the spinal cord is equally protected by the three meningeal membranes, the CSF, and the bony vertebral column (Figs. 2-32 and 2-47B). However, the spinal dura mater is a single-layer meningeal membrane; it lacks the cranial periosteal layer (Table 2-7). The periosteum of the vertebrae is the outer layer of the cranial dura. The spinal dura looks like a loose tube pierced by the spinal nerve roots. It is rostrally attached to the foramen magnum, an opening in the occipital bone through which the spinal cord passes. The spinal dura is separated from the wall of spinal canal by an extradural space and extends in a sack formation to the S-2 vertebral level, at which point it merges with the filum terminale to form the coccygeal ligament, a thin fibrous cord. The spinal dura is surrounded by an actual epidural space, which is normally obliterated (Figure 2-47). Anesthetic agents are injected to the epidural space for anesthetizing the lower body by blocking nerve transmission of pain.

Spinal Arachnoid Membrane

The arachnoid covering for the spinal cord begins at the **foramen magnum** and extends to the cauda equina. The subarachnoid space around the cord is filled with CSF. The arachnoid also invests the tubular projections of the spinal nerve roots from the cord to their foramina of exit. At the lumbar level of the spinal column, with the diminished cord size, the subarachnoid space extends into the **lumbar cistern**. With no cord structure present, the lumbar level forms the best site for the **lumbar puncture** (spinal tap). Anesthesiologists use this sac to administer anesthetics to produce spinal anesthesia. Removal of CSF (spinal tap) for chemical examination is done at the level below the first or second levels by puncturing the dura and arachnoid to enter the subarachnoid space (Fig. 2-48).

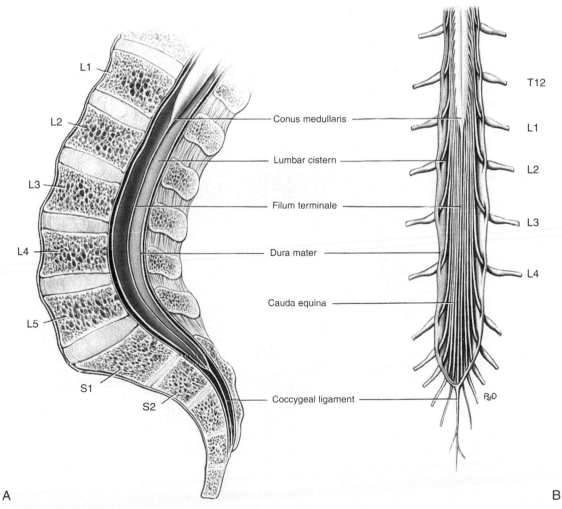

L1
L2
L3
L4
L5
S1
S2

Conus medullaris

Lumbar cistern

Filum terminale

Dura mater

Cauda equina

Coccygeal ligament

T12
L1
L2
L3
L4

RjD

A

B

Figure 2-48.   A. Sagittal view of caudal spinal cord, conus medullaris, lumbar cistern, and lumbosacral vertebral column. **B.** Posterior view of lumbosacral cord, conus medullaris, and lumbar cistern.

Spinal Pia Mater

The pia, the innermost protective layer, surrounds and tightly adheres to the spinal cord. The fibers of the dorsal and ventral spinal roots pierce the pia membrane. The cord suspended within the dural tube is not free; it is attached to the surrounding dura mater by a series of **denticulate ligaments** on both sides. These fibrous ligaments originate from the lateral surface of the spinal cord between the dorsal and ventral roots and are connected to the inner dura. Below the termination of the cord at the conus medullaris, the pia mater continues with the filum terminale and eventually merges with the dura at the sacral level.

CRANIAL NERVES

The PNS consists of **spinal** and **cranial nerves**. The efferent fibers of the spinal nerves innervate skeletal muscles and the visceral organs, whereas the afferent fibers transmit sensory information from the skin and visceral organs to the CNS. The cranial nerves originate from the brainstem and innervate muscles of the head, neck, face, larynx, tongue, pharynx, and glands. The cranial nerves are essential for speech, resonance, and phonation. In addition, they also serve the special senses vision, audition, smell, and taste. Of the 12 pairs of cranial nerves, some mediate either sensory or motor functions, whereas others serve both (Table 2-8).

Nomenclature

Two sets of names are used for cranial nerves. Roman numerals from I to XII indicate the sequence in which the cranial nerves exit and/or enter the brain. The other nomenclature is specific names that contain information describing some or all the functional characteristics of the nerve in question (Table 2-8). An acronym clustering of three initial letters has been used to facilitate learning the specific names:

OOO	olfactory, optic, oculomotor
TTA	trochlear, trigeminal, abducens
FAG	facial, acoustic, glossopharyngeal
VAH	vagus, accessory, hypoglossal

One common acrostic used to facilitate learning of the names and the order of nerves:

On	olfactory
old	optic
Olympus's	oculomotor
topmost	trochlear
top	trigeminal
a	abducens
Finn	facial
and	auditory (acoustic)
German	glossopharyngeal
viewed	vagus
a	accessory
hop.	hypoglossal

Functions

Cranial nerves exit and/or enter the CNS at various points. Consequently, the cranial nerves have also been categorized in relation to their anatomical locations in the CNS (Table 2-9). The first 2 cranial nerves (olfactory and optic) are related to the cerebral cortex; the remaining 10 nerves originate from the brainstem. Cranial nerves are best seen on the ventral or lateral surface of the brainstem (Figs. 2-49 and 2-50).

The **olfactory (I) nerve** is a sensory nerve responsible for the perception of smell. It originates from the receptor cells in the mucosa of the nasal cavity and synapses in the olfactory bulbs on the orbital surface of the frontal lobe. The axons from the bulb travel in the olfactory tract and terminate in the olfactory area (pyriform cortex) of the basal medial temporal lobe (Figs. 2-7 and 2-8). An interruption of olfactory fibers produces anosmia, a condition of impaired sense of smell.

Table 2-8. Cranial Nerves and Their Functions

	Cranial Nerves	Major Motor Function	Major Sensory Function
I	Olfactory		Smell: transmits information from nasal mucosa to olfactory bulb
II	Optic		Vision: conveys messages from retina to visual cortex
III	Oculomotor	Eye movement; regulation of pupil; accommodation of lens for near vision	
IV	Trochlear	Eye movement	
V	Trigeminal	Mastication	Facial, orbital, oral sensation
VI	Abducens	Eye movement	
VII	Facial	Facial expression, secretions of saliva	Taste, anterior two-thirds of tongue
VIII	Vestibuloacoustic		Equilibrium and audition
IX	Glossopharyngeal	Swallowing	Taste, posterior one-third of tongue
X	Vagus	Phonation and swallowing	Sensation from thoracic, abdominal organs
XI	Accessory	Head movement	
XII	Hypoglossal	Tongue movement	

Table 2-9.   Anatomical Classification of Cranial Nerves

Anatomical Locations		Cranial Nerves
Prosencephalon (forebrain)		
Telencephalon	I	Olfactory
Diencephalon	II	Optic
Mesencephalon (midbrain)	III	Oculomotor
	IV	Trochlear
Rhombencephalon (hindbrain)		
Metencephalon (pons)	V	Trigeminal
	VI	Abducens
	VII	Facial
	VIII	Vestibulo-acoustic
Myelencephalon (medulla oblongata)	IX	Glossopharyngeal
	X	Vagus
	XI	Spinal Accessory
	XII	Hypoglossal

The **optic (II) nerve** is a sensory nerve concerned with visual sensation. Optic nerves originate from the retina in both eyes and unite at the optic chiasm at the base of the brain. The crossed and uncrossed optic fibers continue in the optic tract and via the thalamus project visual information from each eye to the visual cortex in the occipital lobes. With direct projections to the thalamus, it is considered a diencephalic nerve (Figs. 2-7 and 2-8). Injury to any part of the visual pathway results in a selective visual field loss (scotoma).

The **oculomotor (III) nerve** is a motor nerve that controls four of the six muscles responsible for moving the eyeball. It emerges from the ventral surface of the midbrain medial to the pes pedunculi and enters the interpeduncular fossa. Complete interruption of the oculomotor nerve results in ptosis of the eyelid, dilation of the pupil, and an abducted (laterally deviated) position of the eye. This eye deviation is produced by unopposed action of the lateral rectus muscle, which is supplied by abducens, the sixth cranial nerve.

The **trochlear (IV) nerve** is a motor nerve. It controls one of the muscles responsible for eye movement. The trochlear nerve exits from the brainstem below the inferior colliculus. It is the only motor nerve to exit the brainstem from the dorsal surface. A trochlear lesion or injury is associated with impaired downward gaze.

The **trigeminal (V) nerve** and the next three nerves (VI to VIII) originate from the tegmentum of the pons. The trigeminal is a functionally mixed nerve with both sensory and motor functions. Primarily, it is a sensory nerve for the face, head, and oral structures and a motor nerve for jaw movements. It is a large nerve in the pons, and its sensory and motor roots leave the brainstem from the ventrolateral surface of the pons. Loss of trigeminal function is associated with facial sensory loss and paralysis of the jaw.

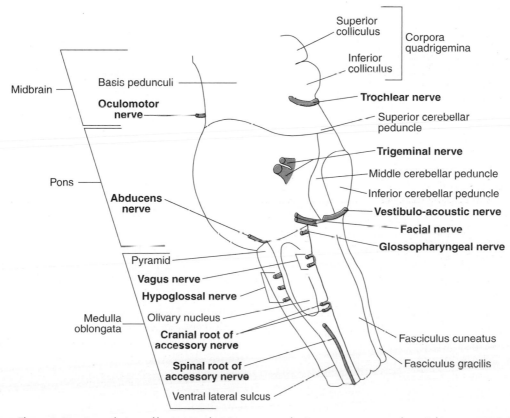

Figure 2-49.   Lateral view of brainstem showing common brainstem structures and cranial nerve roots.

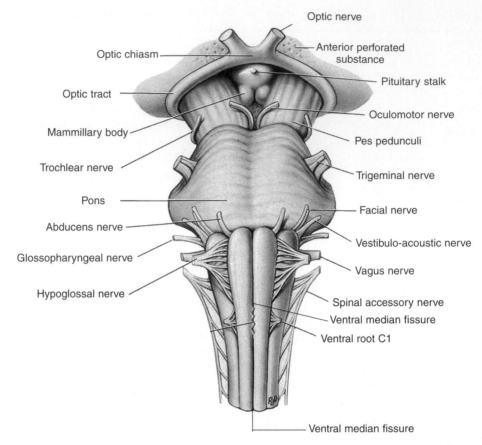

Figure 2-50.   Ventral view showing cranial nerves exiting from midbrain, pons, and medulla.

The **abducens (VI) nerve** is a motor nerve that controls one of the muscles responsible for eye movement, the lateral rectus muscle, which turns the eyeball away from the nose. Fibers of the abducens nerve originate from the tegmentum of the pons and emerge ventrally from the junction of the pons and the medulla oblongata. Interruption of this nerve results in partial ocular paralysis with a medially fixed eye.

The **facial (VII) nerve** is primarily a motor nerve, but it also has some sensory functions. As the name implies, this nerve controls all muscles of facial expression. It also serves the sense of taste from the anterior two-thirds of the tongue. Fibers of this nerve exit from the ventrolateral surface of the pons at its border with the medulla. A facial nerve lesion results in facial paralysis and loss of taste sensation. It may also interfere with production of tears and saliva.

The **vestibulo-acoustic (VIII) nerve** is a sensory nerve. It has two divisions: **vestibular** and **acoustic**. The vestibular division is concerned with the position of the head in space; the acoustic portion is concerned with hearing. This is a large nerve, and its fibers enter the brainstem at the ventrolateral surface of the pons at its junction with the medulla. Its rootlets are lateral to the roots of the facial nerve, and its location is the landmark of the pontomedullary junction. Interruption of the vestibulocochlear nerve is associated with impaired hearing and equilibrium.

The **glossopharyngeal (IX) nerve** originates from the medulla oblongata. It serves both sensory and motor functions. Its motor function is to contribute to swallowing, and its sensory function is to process the sensation of touch and taste from the posterior third of the tongue. Its nuclei are in the rostral medulla, and its fibers leave the medulla just below the acoustic nerve from the lateral surface. A glossopharyngeal lesion results in the loss of taste sensation from the posterior third of the tongue and mild dysphagia (swallowing disorder). It may also cause loss of the gag reflex.

The **vagus (X) nerve**, the largest cranial nerve, has a wide distribution of its fibers serving both sensory and motor functions. Its fibers leave the brainstem from the lateral medulla just below the point of exit for the glossopharyngeal nerve. The vagus is primarily a sensory nerve, but it has a motor component. Its motor fibers activate the muscles of the pharynx, larynx, and soft palate. Vagus nerve pathology results in decreased sensation from and activation of visceral organs and paralysis of the larynx and pharynx.

The **spinal accessory (XI) nerve** consists of spinal and cranial fibers. It innervates muscles for controlling head movement. The spinal roots exit from the four cervical segments; the cranial root exits the lateral medulla and contribute to the innervation of neck and shoulder muscles. A spinal accessory nerve injury causes restricted neck movement and weakness of the shoulder.

The **hypoglossal (XII) nerve** is a motor nerve. Its nucleus is in the medulla, and its fibers exit the medulla just lateral to the pyramid (axons of corticospinal tract). The branches of this nerve innervate all intrinsic and some extrinsic muscles of the tongue. A pathological condition of the hypoglossal nerve results in paralysis of half of the tongue.

AUTONOMIC NERVOUS SYSTEM

The ANS controls the activity of smooth muscles and regulates the secretion of glands in the viscera (internal organs), which include the salivary glands, lungs, heart, kidneys, gastrointestinal tract, and bladder. It also innervates smooth muscles in the walls of blood vessels, sweat glands, and the eye.

The ANS consists of **sympathetic** and **parasympathetic systems** (Table 2-10). Sympathetic ganglia (clusters of nerve cells) usually innervate many organs, whereas parasympathetic ganglia innervate a single organ. Together the sympathetic and parasympathetic systems monitor, regulate, and sustain optimum visceral functions essential to survival. These systems serve the same visceral organs but produce opposite effects (Table 2-11). The sympathetic system spends energy and prepares for fight and flight. In so doing, it constricts blood vessels in skin, visceral organs, and bronchial passages, induces perspiration, dilates pupils, accelerates heart rate, and mobilizes glucose. The parasympathetic system conserves energy; it dominates while relaxing or sleeping and acts by constricting the pupils, lowering body metabolism, and lowering heart rate (see Chapter 16).

Besides this functional difference, the sympathetic and parasympathetic systems are anatomically different from the somatic system (Fig. 2-51), which we use for activating the limbs and trunk. In the somatic motor system, the motor nuclei are in the spinal cord, and their axons (spinal nerves) extend to skeletal (striated) muscles. The ANS uses an additional ganglion in the PNS. The fibers from the CNS projecting to this ganglion are **preganglionic** axons and the **postganglionic** fibers from this ganglion extend to the target organs. The sympathetic and parasympathetic systems also differ in terms of the location of this peripheral ganglion, which is next to the spinal cord (in the spinal chain) in the case of the sympathetic system but closer to the target organ in the parasympathetic system.

An additional difference between the sympathetic and parasympathetic systems is the anatomical locations from which they arise (Table 2-10; Figs. 16-2 and 16-4). The sympathetic system is also called the **thoracolumbar division** of the ANS because the sympathetic preganglionic neurons are present in the lateral cell column of spinal segments T-1 through L-2. The parasympathetic system, also called **craniosacral system**, consists of preganglionic neurons that either reside in the brainstem and contribute axons to cranial nerves III, VII, IX, and X or reside in the intermediolateral cell column of spinal segments S-2 to S-4.

LESION LOCALIZATION

Rule 1: Cortical Lesion

PRESENTING SYMPTOMS

Contralateral hemiplegia; contralateral hemianesthesia of face, trunk, and upper extremity; and cortical sensory loss (failure to identify an object through touch or identify a letter or word written on the surface of the skin) suggest a cortical lesion.

Dominant hemisphere: In addition to these deficits, a dominant hemispheric lesion results in aphasia, left–right disorientation, apraxia, finger agnosia, and acalculia.

Nondominant hemisphere: In addition to the symptoms of a lesion in either hemisphere, a pathological process in the nondominant hemisphere also results in left-sided neglect or inattention, constructional and/or dressing deficits, spatial and temporal disorientation, impaired prosody in speech, and impaired ability to recognize faces.

Table 2-10.   Subdivisions of the Autonomic Nervous System

Divisions of ANS	Nuclei Locations	Functions
Sympathetic system	Thoracolumbar	Expanding energy in flight, fright, or fight
Parasympathetic system	Craniosacral	Restoration of energy

Table 2-11.   Differential Effects of Sympathetic and Parasympathetic Systems

Structure	Sympathetic System	Parasympathetic System
Glands		
Sweat	Decreased secretion	Increased secretion
Smooth muscles		
Iris	Pupil dilation	Pupil constriction
Bronchi	Dilation	Constriction
Lungs	Vasodilation	Vasoconstriction
Cardiac muscles	Increased activity	Decreased activity
Blood vessels	Vasoconstriction in viscera, skin; vasodilation in skeletal muscle, heart	None

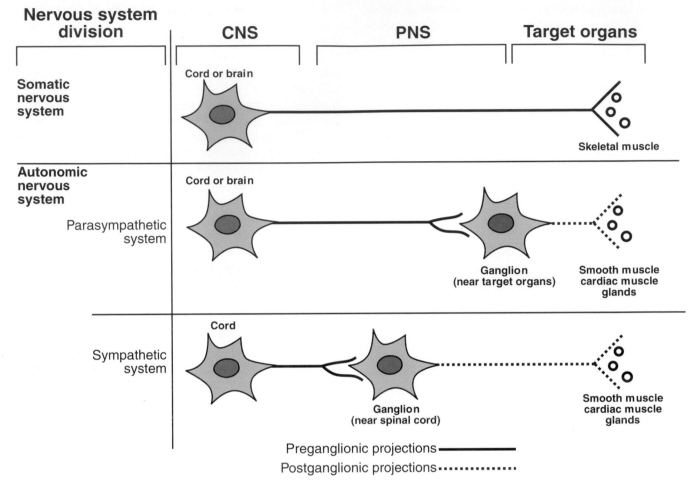

Figure 2-51. Comparison between somatic and autonomic nervous systems.

RATIONALE

- The cerebral cortex contains the language cortex (aphasia), sensory cortex (anesthesia and cortical sensory loss), and motor cortex (paralysis).
- Lateral corticospinal fibers mediating motor commands from the cortex cross the midline (decussate) in the medulla. Thus, a left cortical lesion involving the motor fibers above the level of their crossing results in right-sided paralysis.
- Fibers mediating fine discriminative touch from the body decussate at the mid medulla. Thus, a lesion in the left brain affects the sensory fibers originating from the right half of the body and results in sensory loss (anesthesia) in the right side of the body.
- The right (nondominant) hemisphere regulates visuospatial orientation, speech and prosody, attention, and sensorimotor control for the left half of the body.

See Chapter 7 for somatic sensation, Chapters 11 to 14 for the physiology of motor systems, Chapter 17 for vascular system, and Chapter 19 for neurolinguistic properties of the brain and higher mental functions.

Rule 2: Subcortical Lesion

PRESENTING SYMPTOMS

Contralateral hemiplegia and diminution or loss of pain and temperature equally for the face, arms, and legs are associated with a subcortical (internal capsule) lesion. Emergence of involuntary movements suggests a basal ganglia lesion.

RATIONALE

- All of the descending motor fibers and ascending sensory fibers pass through the internal capsule. Thus, any involvement of the internal capsule is likely to produce equal sensorimotor deficits for the contralateral face, arm, and leg.

- Involuntary movements such as tremor, athetosis, and chorea imply basal ganglia involvement.

See Chapters 7 and 11 to 14 for a discussion of the physiology of sensory and motor systems.

CLINICAL CONSIDERATIONS

Case Studies

Patient One

A 52-year-old man was taken to an emergency room because he had been progressively exhibiting confusion about time over 2 months. He had also been having difficulty organizing his thoughts and making decisions. Lately, he had begun speaking incoherently from time to time. The attending physician noticed the following signs:

- Time-related confusion
- Mild right-sided hemiparesis (face, arm, leg)
- Right hemianopsia
- Increased deep tendon reflexes and Babinski sign
- Altered personality (the patient appeared reclusive and unconcerned)
- Expressive aphasia (dysfluent verbal output consisting of a few words and limited phrases)
- Good auditory comprehension

The physician suspected a tumor (neoplastic growth) in the brain because of the progressive nature of the deficit. MRI revealed a left cortical neoplastic mass bordering the frontoparietotemporal region. The patient was referred for biopsy and surgical removal of the tumor if possible, followed by radiation treatment, if needed.

Question: Can you account for these symptoms on the basis of your understanding of the functional organization in the brain?

Discussion: The involvement of the frontoparietotemporal tissue accounts for all of the reported symptoms:

- Time-related confusion was related to parietal involvement.
- Expressive aphasia reflected premotor and language area disturbance, while the altered personality resulted from the involvement of the prefrontal projections.
- Right-sided paralysis and positive Babinski sign indicated involvement of the motor and surrounding cortex.

Patient Two

A 75-year-old man had poor control of his bladder but would not seek medical attention because of embarrassment. Finally, his family took him to the family physician, who noted that his failure to control the sphincters had resulted in impaired urinary retention and fecal incontinence. The physician suspected an interruption of the sacral spinal nerves. MRI revealed a tumor involving the cauda equina region of the spinal cord.

Question: Can you account for these symptoms from your knowledge of the myotomal and dermatomal patterns of spinal innervation of the lower half of the body?

Discussion: The spinal nerves from the sacral region (S-3 through S-5) innervate the bladder and anal sphincters (Fig. 2-35). Interruption of these nerves affects bowel and bladder functions, which are common after lower spinal cord injuries.

SUMMARY

The human nervous system is the generator of the electrical and chemical energy that controls body parts and their functions. The nervous system consists of the CNS (brain and spinal cord) and PNS (spinal and cranial nerves). The brain is responsible for initiating, controlling, and regulating all sensorimotor and cognitive (mental) functions, whereas the spinal cord mediates sensory and motor commands, both somatic and visceral, to and from body parts that interact with the environment. The bony shell of the skull and vertebral column and the dural, arachnoid, and pial layers of the meninges protect the CNS. CSF in the subarachnoid space also helps protect the brain and spinal cord by serving as a mechanical buffer. Embryologically, the brain is derived from three vesicles: prosencephalon, mesencephalon, and rhombencephalon. The cerebral hemispheres, basal ganglia, limbic lobe, thalamus, hypothalamus, and lateral and third ventricles are derived from the prosencephalon. The mesencephalon develops into the midbrain and cerebral aqueduct, whereas the rhombencephalon gives rise to the pons, cerebellum, medulla oblongata, and fourth ventricle. Each of these structures serves a specific sensorimotor or regulating function. The PNS, which includes spinal and cranial nerves, extends to organs, muscles, joints, blood vessels, and skin surfaces, forming an extensive network of cables and fine wires throughout the body. The PNS consists of the somatic and autonomic nervous systems. The somatic motor and sensory nerves innervate skeletal muscles, whereas the autonomic sensory and motor nerves innervate the visceral organs and glands. Cranial nerves regulate the sensory and motor functions of the face and head.

Technical Terms

afferent	insula
arachnoid trabecula	ligaments
basal ganglia	limbic lobe
brainstem	meninges
cauda equina	parasympathetic
choroid plexus	peduncle
conus medullaris	septum
corpora quadrigemina	septum pellucidum
denticulate ligaments	subarachnoid space
dermatome	subdural space
efferent	sympathetic
filum terminale	tectum
foramen magnum	tegmentum
fornix	thalamus
hippocampus	
homeostatic	
hypothalamus	

Review Questions

1. Define the following terms:

arachnoid trabecula
basal ganglia
brainstem
cauda equina
choroid plexus
conus medullaris
corpora quadrigemina
denticulate ligaments
dermatome
filum terminale
foramen magnum
fornix
hippocampus

homeostasis
hypothalamus
insula
limbic lobe
meninges
parasympathetic
septum
subarachnoid space
subdural space
sympathetic
tectum
tegmentum
thalamus

2. What are the three vesicles in the embryological brain that serve as the forerunner for all brain parts?

3. Match the following numbered structures to the associated lettered vesicles:

i. pes pedunculi
ii. limbic system
iii. fourth ventricle
iv. basal ganglia
v. cingulate gyrus
vi. substantia nigra
vii. medulla
viii. pons

a. forebrain (prosencephalon)
b. mesencephalon
c. rhombencephalon

4. Name the major sulci and gyri in each lobe.

5. Mark the locations of the central sulcus, lateral sulcus, frontal lobe (prefrontal lobe, premotor region, motor cortex, third frontal convolution), parietal lobe (primary sensory cortex, angular gyrus, supramarginal gyrus), occipital lobe, and temporal lobe (superior, middle, inferior temporal gyri) on Figure 2-52.

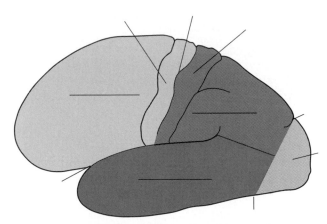

Figure 2-52. Exercise figure of lateral brain surface.

6. Identify the midsagittal locations of the calcarine sulcus, cingulate gyrus, corpus callosum, fornix, hypothalamus, thalamus, and septum on Figure 2-53.

7. Match the following numbered structures to the associated lettered lobes and surfaces:

Structures	**Lobes**	**Surfaces**
i. central sulcus	A. frontal	a. dorsal
ii. lateral sulcus	B. parietal	b. ventral
iii. precentral sulcus	C. temporal	c. lateral
iv. postcentral sulcus	D. occipital	d. sagittal
v. supramarginal gyrus		
vi. angular gyrus		
vii. calcarine sulcus		
viii. olfactory sulcus		

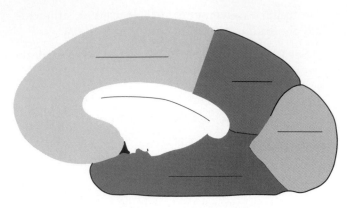

Figure 2-53. Exercise figure of midsagittal brain surface.

ix. uncus
x. parahippocampal gyrus
xi. collateral sulcus
xii. third frontal convolution
xiii. superior temporal gyrus

8. Draw the sensory and motor homunculus outlining major body parts. Also comment on the extent of area occupied by the representation for face, hand, and trunk.

9. Which primary cortex is located at the postcentral gyrus?

10. What is meant by dominant hemisphere and nondominant hemisphere?

11. What is the function of the prefrontal lobe?

12. What is the function of the parietal lobe?

13. What is the function of the occipital lobe?

14. What is the function of the temporal lobe?

15. Discuss major functions of the thalamus and hypothalamus.

16. Describe the location of basal ganglia structures and describe their functions.

17. Describe the location of the midbrain and discuss functions of its internal (red nucleus, substantia nigra, pes pedunculus) and external (superior and inferior colliculi and pes pedunculi) structures.

18. Discuss the location and functions of the reticular formation.

19. Name the three parts of the brainstem.

20. Name the midbrain regions that respectively lay dorsal and ventral to the cerebral aqueduct.

21. Name the portion of the pons located beneath the floor of the fourth ventricle.

22. Discuss the major external and internal structures of the pons.

23. What are the major internal and external medullary structures? Discuss their functions.

24. Discuss the location and functions of the limbic lobe.

25. What is the function of the cerebellum?

26. What structure connects the cerebellum to the brainstem?

27. Discuss the structures (length, shape, and divisions) of the spinal cord.

28. Discuss the functions of the spinal cord.

29. Explain the clinical implications of segmental spinal organization (dermatome and myotome).

30. Match the following numbered structures to the associated lettered dermatomes that they innervate.

i. Thumb	a. Cervical—7
ii. Middle finger	b. Cervical—6
iii. Knee	c. Lumbar—3
iv. Big toe	d. Lumbar—4
v. Little toe	e. Sacral—1
vi. Breast nipple	f. Thoracic—4

31. What forms a spinal nerve and plexus?

32. Label white and gray matter, dorsal and ventral horns, and dorsal and ventral fiber roots on a cross-section of the spinal cord.

33. What is the filum terminale?

34. What is the cauda equina?

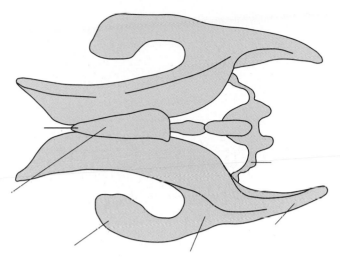

Figure 2-54.   Exercise figure of ventricles.

35. At what vertebral level does the spinal cord end?
36. Which ventricular space is found in the forebrain?
37. Which ventricular space is found in the diencephalon?
38. With a labeled diagram (Fig. 2-54), identify the major parts of the ventricular system.
39. Describe the circulation of CSF.
40. List the major association pathways and discuss their functions.

41. Discuss the function of the corpus callosum and identify its parts.
42. How many spinal nerves exit from the cervical, thoracic, lumbar, sacral, and coccygeal regions of the cord, respectively?
43. Discuss the functions of meningeal membranes and describe the location of epidural, subdural, and subarachnoid spaces.
44. Name the dural extensions in the brain and describe their relationship to the brain.
45. Label (name) the cranial nerves marked by lead lines on Figure 2-55. Describe the sensorimotor function for each of the illustrated 10 pairs of cranial nerves (2 cranial nerves related to the forebrain are not included).
46. Match the following numbered pathologies to the possible associated lettered clinical effects.

   i. small lesion in area of 17 on the left side
   ii. destruction of area 41 on the left side
   iii. destruction of area 22 on the left side
   iv. damage to the white matter of the prefrontal lobe
   v. cutting the corpus callosum

   a. Wernicke's aphasia
   b. blindness
   c. loss of executive function
   d. auditory imperceptibility
   e. disconnection of hemispheres

47. Discuss the functions of the autonomic nervous system.
48. Describe the functions of the sympathetic and parasympathetic systems.
49. Define the preganglionic and postganglionic neurons.

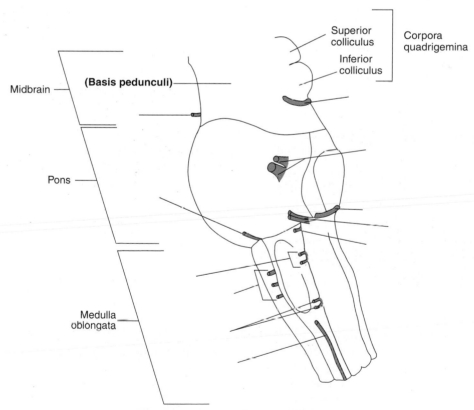

Figure 2-55   Exercise figure of brainstem.

Internal Anatomy of the Central Nervous System

Learning Objectives

After studying this chapter, students should be able to do the following:

- Identify shapes of corticospinal fibers and the ventricular cavity at various neuraxial levels
- Recognize major internal anatomical structures of the spinal cord and describe their functions
- Recognize important internal anatomical structures of the medulla and describe their functions
- Recognize important internal anatomical structures of the pons and describe their functions
- Identify important internal anatomical structures of the midbrain and describe their functions
- Recognize important internal anatomical structures of the forebrain (diencephalon, basal ganglia, and limbic structures) and describe their functions
- Follow the continuation of major anatomical structures and relate them in each sequential section of the brain

The gross anatomical (cortical and subcortical) structures relating to the meninges, ventricles, and medullary centers have been discussed in relation to their functions (see Chapter 2). The next step is to use specific and easily identified anatomical structures as signposts for developing an orientation to the **internal anatomy** of the brain in relation to surrounding structures. **Learning internal brain anatomy is the most important part of training in neuroscience**; it is often neglected in teaching neuroscience to students of communicative disorders and related disciplines. Internal anatomy is best learned by repeated exposures to the serial sections of the **spinal cord, brainstem**, and **forebrain**. In this chapter, the spinal cord, brainstem, and diencephalon are examined on stained sections, whereas the forebrain is studied in unstained sections.

Nuclear structures and fiber tracts related to various functional systems exist side by side at each level of the nervous system. Disease processes rarely strike only one anatomical structure. Consequently, there is a tendency for a series of related and unrelated clinical symptoms to occur. A thorough knowledge of the **internal brain structures**, their **shape**, **size**, **location**, and **proximity**, makes it easier to understand their functions independently. In addition, the proximity of nuclear structures and fiber tracts explains multiple symptoms that may develop from a single lesion site.

ANATOMICAL ORIENTATION LANDMARKS

The two most distinct anatomical landmarks used for visual orientation to the brain are the shapes of the **corticospinal fibers** and the **ventricular cavity** (Fig. 3-1). Both are present throughout the brain, although their shape and size vary as one progresses caudally from the rostral forebrain (telencephalon) to the caudal brainstem. Consequently, familiarity with the progressively changing shapes and sizes of structures is essential for identifying the various brain levels they represent.

Shapes of Corticospinal Fibers

Immediately after their origin in the sensorimotor cortex, the corticospinal fibers fan down through the **corona radiata** (Fig. 2-38) to enter the wedge-shaped **internal capsule** at the diencephalic level (Figs. 2-15, 2-16, and 3-1A). Along the ventral surface of the midbrain they form the **pes pedunculi** (crus cerebri), a bilaterally compact fillet-shaped mass of fibers on a cross-sectional view (Figs. 2-24 and 3-1B). The fibers of the corticospinal tract later disperse among the scattered pontine nuclei and appear as many irregular round masses scattered throughout the basal pons (Figs. 2-25 and 3-1C). The corticospinal tract fibers recombine when entering the medulla and form a **pyramid**, which is best viewed in

Motor Fibers   Ventricles

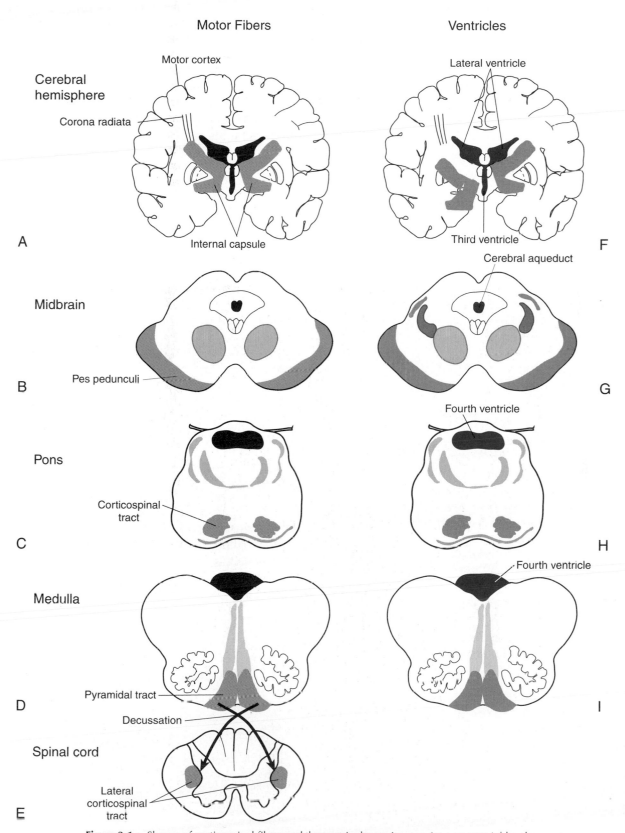

Figure 3-1.   Shapes of corticospinal fibers and the ventricular cavity at various neuroaxial levels.

gross and microscopic cross-section of the caudal brainstem (Figs. 2-26 and 3-1*D*). The term *pyramid* gave origin to the term pyramidal tract, which is synonymous with corticospinal tract. Pyramidal fibers cross the midline at the caudal medulla, and after crossing, they enter the **lateral funiculus** of the spinal cord and are known as the **lateral corticospinal tract** (Fig. 3-1*E*).

Shape of Ventricular Cavity

The **lateral** and **third ventricles** together are butterfly-shaped in a cross-section of the rostral brain (Figs. 2-16 and 3-1*F*). The wings represent the two lateral ventricles and the body; the narrow slit in the middle marks the third ventricle. The **cerebral aqueduct** of Sylvius is the small tube-shaped midbrain canal (Figs. 2-24 and 3-1*G*) that connects the **third** and **fourth ventricles**. The **fourth ventricle** overlies the pons (Figs. 2-9 and 3-1*H*); it tapers to end in the rostral medulla (Fig. 3-1*I*).

For identifying important internal anatomical landmarks, the central nervous system has been serially examined. The **spinal cord** is examined in cross-sections. **Midbrain**, **pons**, and **medulla** are reviewed in transverse sections. The **forebrain structures** (the cerebral cortex, diencephalon, and basal ganglia), are studied in both coronal and horizontal sections.

SPINAL CORD IN CROSS-SECTIONS

The internal anatomy of the spinal cord is studied in four sections with a representative section from each of the following anatomical divisions: **sacral**, **lumbar**, **thoracic,** and **cervical**. The basic internal anatomical pattern of the spinal cord remains the same throughout its extent. The **central gray matter** of the cord, made up of cell bodies, is shaped like a butterfly and appears gray in freshly cut sections. The outer part of the cord, which looks like the rim of a wheel, consists of ascending and descending fiber tracts surrounding the central gray "butterfly." The fiber tracts form functionally related longitudinal funiculi, which are demarcated by longitudinal grooves and spinal nerve attachments along the surface of the spinal cord. The only change in the internal anatomy of the spinal cord is the ratio of white to gray matter at each of the four spinal levels. That ratio gradually increases from sacral to cervical as new fibers add to the afferent tracts. Additional changes relate to the shape of the gray matter; the spinal cord enlarges in the cervical and lumbar regions because of the relatively great amount of nerve supply necessitated for sensory and motor functions by the upper and lower extremities (Fig. 2-34). The important internal structures of the spinal cord include the sensory and motor nuclei and various ascending and descending tracts (Table 3-1).

Sacral Section

This cross-section illustrates the anatomical characteristics at the **sacral level** of the spinal cord (Fig. 3-2). This level of the cord, which is small in diameter, contains a thin mantle of white matter and a larger gray region with bulky **ventral** and **dorsal horns**. The **dorsal lemniscal column** consists of the ascending fibers of the **fasciculus gracilis**, which carry information of **discriminative touch**, **pressure**, and **limb position** from the lower half of the body. The fasciculus gracilis contains sensory fibers that enter the cord from the sacral to **midthoracic** level. The lateral column of the white matter at this level contains the lateral corticospinal tract and fibers of the **anterolateral system**. The lateral corticospinal tract transmits motor commands from the motor cortex via the lower motor neurons to muscles. The anterolateral system consists of the **anterior** and **lateral spinothalamic tracts**, which mediate sensations of **diffuse touch**, **pain**, and **temperature**.

The large ventral horns are the sites of motor nuclei. The dorsal horns contain the sensory nuclei, which include the **substantia gelatinosa** and **nucleus proprius**

Table 3-1. **Anatomical Structures of Spinal Cord**

Characterizing Structures
Dorsal median sulcus
Ventral median sulcus
Dorsal intermediate sulcus
Gray matter
Dorsal horns
Ventral horns
White matter
Dorsal fasciculus
Lateral fasciculus
Anterior fasciculus
Dorsal root
Ventral root
Sensory nuclei in gray column
Motor nuclei in gray column
Fasciculus gracilis and cuneatus
Spinothalamic (lateral and anterior) tracts
Spinocerebellar (dorsal and ventral) tracts

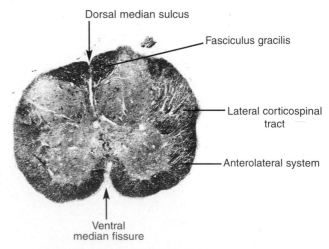

Figure 3-2. Cross-section of spinal cord at sacral level.

(see Chapter 7 for a discussion of their functions); these nuclei are present throughout the spinal cord and receive input predominantly from spinal sensory nerves. Other sensory spinal cells include the **nucleus dorsalis of Clark**. Many dorsal horn cells give rise to fibers of the spinocerebellar and anterolateral system.

Lumbar Section

Figure 3-3 shows the anatomical appearance of the **lumbar level** (L-4) of the spinal cord. The gray matter at this level contains larger dorsal and ventral horns in relation to the white matter. The dorsal lemniscal column continues to exclusively represent fibers of the fasciculus gracilis, which is lateral to the dorsal median sulcus. This level also contains the lateral corticospinal tract and the anterolateral system consisting of the spinothalamic and spinocerebellar tracts (spinocerebellar tract not identified on Fig. 3-3). The dorsal horns contain the sensory nuclei, and the ventral horns contain the motor nuclei. This cross-section presents the **dorsal root fibers** and **ventral root fibers**.

Thoracic Section

Figure 3-4 reveals the anatomical characteristics in the **thoracic** (T-4) level of the spinal cord. This level of the cord is characterized by the reduced size of the gray matter and the enlarged share of white matter. In comparison to the previous sections, the dorsal and ventral horns are smaller and tapered. The dorsal lemniscal column at this level is larger because of additional sensory fibers from higher body levels. The additional sensory fibers form the **fasciculus cuneatus**, which ascend lateral to the **fasciculus gracilis** in the dorsal columns of the spinal cord. The fasciculus cuneatus fibers carry the sensations of **fine discriminative touch**, **pressure**, and **limb position** from the upper body; its fibers enter the spinal cord at the midthoracic through cervical levels. With emergence of the fasciculus cuneatus, the **dorsal intermediate sulcus** appears; it separates the medial fasciculus gracilis from the lateral fasciculus cuneatus fibers. The lateral corticospinal tract is larger than at lower levels, although it retains the same relative lateral location. The fibers of the spinothalamic tracts (anterolateral system), which mediate sensations of diffuse touch, pain, and temperature, continue to occupy the same general space throughout the cord.

Appearing along the lateral surface are the **dorsal** and **ventral spinocerebellar tracts**. Fibers of the spinocerebellar tracts mediate **unconscious proprioception** from the limbs to the cerebellum. This proprioception, which is unconscious because it does not reach the sensory cortex, plays an important role in the acquisition and maintenance of skilled motor activities.

Cervical Section

Figure 3-5 reveals the anatomical characteristics of the **cervical** (C-7) region of the spinal cord. The volume

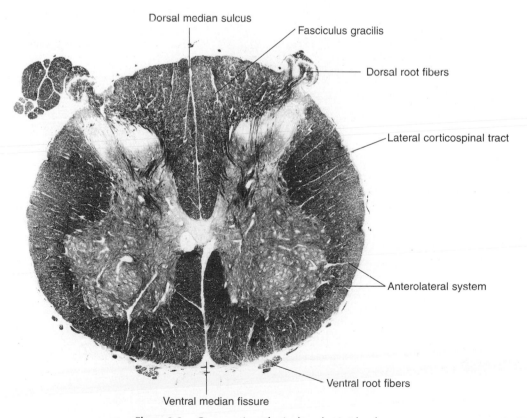

Dorsal median sulcus

Fasciculus gracilis

Dorsal root fibers

Lateral corticospinal tract

Anterolateral system

Ventral root fibers

Ventral median fissure

Figure 3-3.   Cross-section of spinal cord at L-4 level.

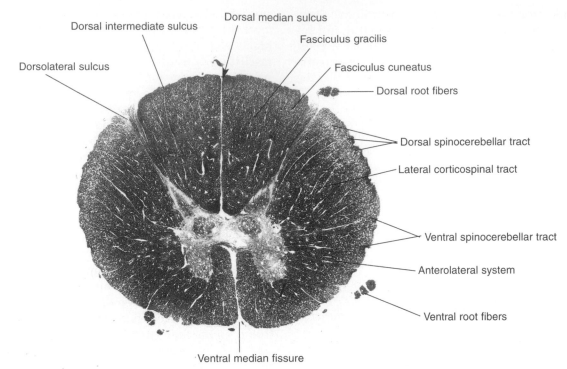

Figure 3-4. Cross-section of spinal cord at T-4 level.

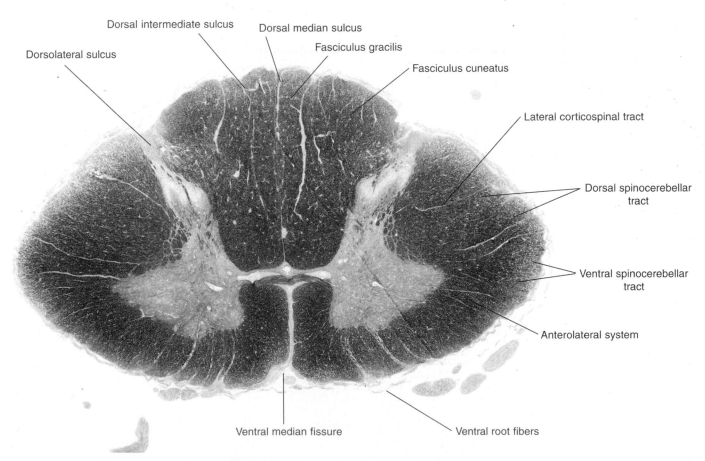

Figure 3-5. Cross-section of spinal cord at C-7 level.

of white matter at this level is much greater than at the lower spinal levels. In addition, the dorsal horns are slender, whereas the ventral horns are large and wing-shaped. In the dorsal column, the fasciculi of gracilis and cuneatus have become large and are demarcated by the dorsal intermediate sulcus. The corticospinal tract is relatively larger than at lower levels. This configuration of the lateral corticospinal tract occurs below the level of the **pyramidal decussation** (soon to take place rostral to this level at the junction of the spinal cord and the medulla). The lateral column of fibers continues to contain the **spinothalamic** and **spinocerebellar pathways**.

BRAINSTEM IN TRANSVERSE SECTIONS

The brainstem, as the axial part of the brain, protrudes from the base of the brain and consists of the following structures: **medulla oblongata**, **pons**, and **midbrain.** Besides containing all ascending and descending fiber tracts, the brainstem includes a large group of nuclei that relate to the sensorimotor functions of cranial nerves, serve various vital visceral functions, and mediate many special senses and reflexive functions. The levels of transverse sections of the brainstem are illustrated in Figure 3-6.

Medulla Oblongata

The medulla oblongata is the most caudal portion of the brainstem. It begins above the rootlets of the first cervical spinal nerve and gradually increases in size until it merges with the pons rostrally. Important structures in the medulla include the **corticospinal fibers** (pyramidal tract), **pyramidal decussation, dorsal lemniscal column** (fasciculus gracilis and fasciculus cuneatus), **sensory decussation, inferior cerebellar peduncle, principal** (inferior) **olivary nucleus, reticular formation**, and many cranial nerve nuclei (Table 3-2).

Table 3-2.   Anatomical Structures of Medulla

Characterizing Structures
Caudal (low) medulla
Pyramid
Decussation of pyramidal fibers
Lateral corticospinal tract
Fasciculus gracilis and cuneatus
Nucleus gracilis and cuneatus
Spinal trigeminal nucleus and tract
Midmedulla
Nucleus gracilis and cuneatus
Fasciculus gracilis and cuneatus
Inferior cerebellar peduncle (restiform body)
Sensory decussation
Internal arcuate fibers
Medial lemniscus
Principal inferior olivary nucleus
Pyramid
Spinal trigeminal nucleus and tract
Rostral (high) medulla
Principal inferior olivary nucleus
Inferior cerebellar peduncle
Cochlear nucleus
Vestibular nucleus
Medial lemniscus
Pyramid
Spinal trigeminal nucleus and tract

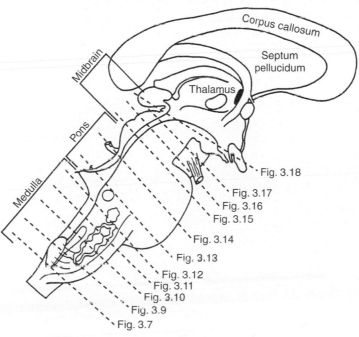

Figure 3-6.   Representative levels of brainstem transverse sections.

CAUDAL MEDULLA

The transverse section shown in Figure 3-7 is the most caudal level of the brainstem, where the medulla merges with the spinal cord. Four important structures in the dorsal medulla are the **nucleus gracilis**, **fasciculus gracilis**, **nucleus cuneatus**, and **fasciculus cuneatus**. The ascending fibers of the fasciculus gracilis synapse on the cells of the nucleus gracilis, and those of the fasciculus cuneatus synapse on the cells of the nucleus cuneatus.

In the center of this low medullary section is the crossing of the **pyramidal fibers** (pyramidal decussation). After the crossing, the descending pyramidal fibers move to a lateral position in the spinal column and become the lateral corticospinal tract. This crossing of the corticospinal fibers accounts for the motor cortex of one side of the brain controlling the opposite side of the body. Lateral to the fasciculus cuneatus is the massive formation of the **spinal trigeminal nucleus** and the **spinal trigeminal tract**.

The spinal trigeminal tract consists of fibers of the trigeminal (cranial) nerve that are responsible for pain and temperature from the face. Fibers of this tract enter the brainstem, descend ipsilaterally in the medulla, and terminate in the spinal trigeminal nucleus. Secondary fibers from the spinal trigeminal nucleus cross the midline and ascend to the thalamus from which impulses are relayed to the sensory cortex (see Chapter 7). Medial to the trigeminal tract and nucleus are diffusely located cellular and fiber components of the **reticular formation** that extend throughout the brainstem. The reticular formation (Fig. 2-23) is the integrator of complex behaviors such as sleep, awake states, respiration, aggression, and cardiovascular functions.

A discussion of the events related to the crossing of sensory fibers is important for an orientation to the course of the dorsal column fibers and their level of crossing (Fig. 3-8). The fasciculi of gracilis and cuneatus are the first-order sensory fibers with their sensory neurons in the spinal **dorsal root ganglion**. Fibers of these

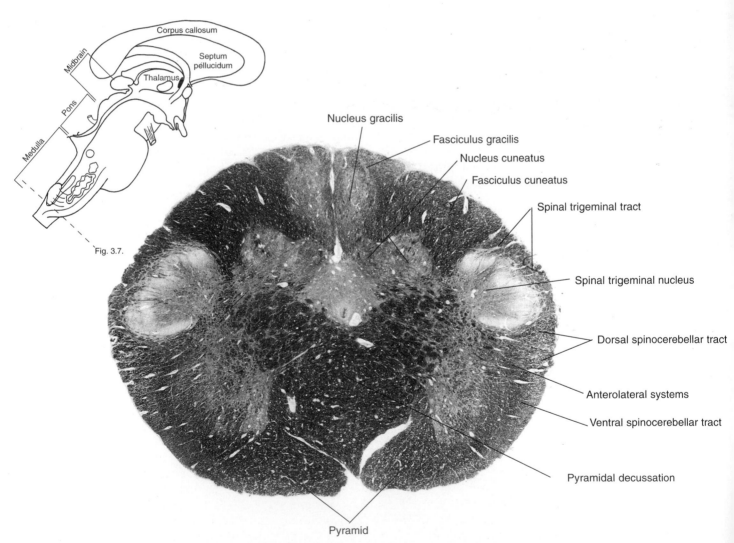

Figure 3-7.   Transverse section of medulla through pyramidal decussation.

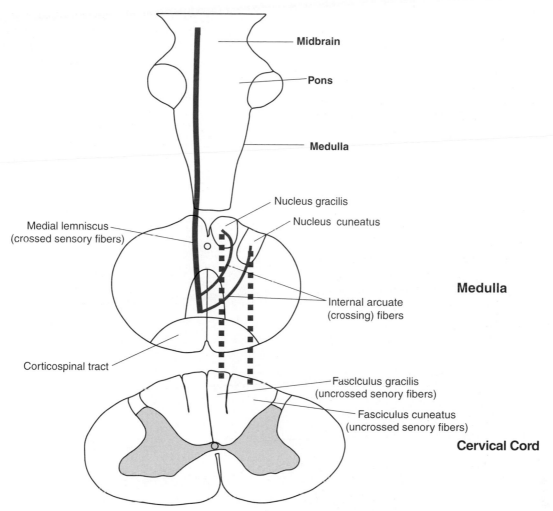

Figure 3-8.   Crossing of dorsal lemniscus fibers in caudal medulla.

two fasciculi enter the spinal cord and ascend on the same side in the **dorsal lemniscal column**. In the medulla, the fibers of these two sensory fasciculi terminate on their respective nuclei. These nuclei project secondary fibers across the midline as the **internal arcuate fibers**; after crossing the midline, they form the **medial lemniscus** and travel upward to relay to the thalamus information related to discriminative touch. The **thalamocortical** projections transmit the sensory information to the **primary sensory cortex**. This explains how different terms (e.g., dorsal lemniscal column, internal arcuate fibers, and medial lemniscus) refer to fibers that mediate the same sensory information received from the fasciculi of gracilis and cuneatus, which transmit sensation from the lower and upper body, respectively.

LOWER (CAUDAL) THIRD OF MEDULLA

The transverse section shown in Figure 3-9 is above the level described in the previous section. It provides a better view of the internal arcuate fibers that

arise from the gracilis and cuneatus nuclei and cross the midline.

At this level, the gracile and cuneate nuclei attain their largest size. The internal arcuate fibers from those nuclei cross the midline to form the medial lemniscus and travel rostrally to the thalamus. The decussation at this medullary level thus transmits tactile and discriminative sensation from one side of the body to the opposite half of the brain. The **pyramids** in the ventromedial medulla appear as a compact pyramidal bundle of fibers just above the level at which they decussate. The decussations of the **sensory arcuate fibers** and **motor pyramidal fibers** are important landmarks of the caudal medulla.

The core of the reticular formation in the central third of the medulla is continuous with lower levels. It is a netlike arrangement of cell bodies and interwoven projections (Fig. 2-23) that interact with virtually all sensorimotor systems and regulate brain functioning. The **central gray** is the **midbrain reticular-limbic area** that

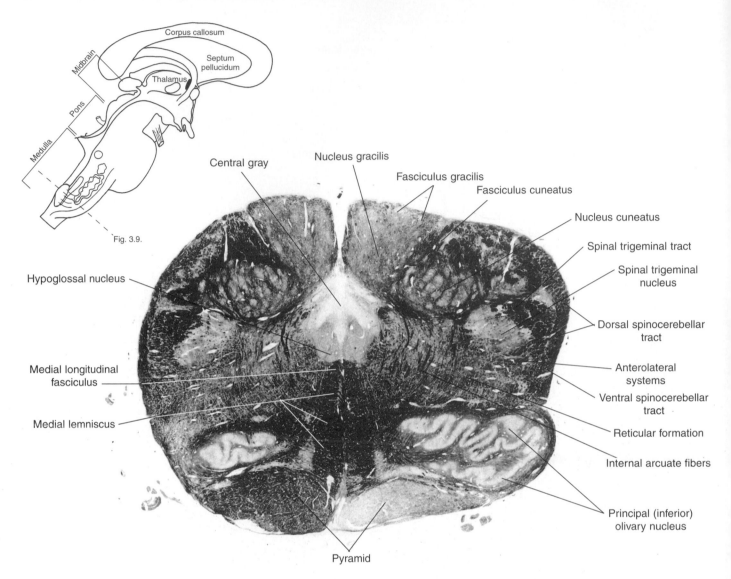

Figure 3-9. Transverse section of medulla through dorsal column (gracilis and cuneatus) nuclei, caudal portions of hypoglossal nucleus, caudal end of inferior olivary nucleus, and middle portions of sensory decussation.

regulates somatic and visceral functions. Beneath the central gray is the nucleus of the **hypoglossal nerve** (cranial nerve XII). It controls all intrinsic and most extrinsic tongue muscles and therefore is an important nerve for speech production and swallowing. The structure below the hypoglossal nucleus is the **medial longitudinal fasciculus**, a fiber bundle running longitudinally from the cervical cord to the brainstem, which receives visual and vestibular projections. It interconnects the motor nuclei of four cranial nerves (oculomotor, trochlear, abducens, and spinal accessory), which regulate head–eye coordination.

Another structure that appears in this section is the caudal tip of the **principal** (inferior) **olivary nucleus**, an important nucleus in the relay of information to the cere-

bellum. Other previously described structures are in the locations identified in the previous section.

MIDDLE THIRD OF MEDULLA

The transverse section shown in Figure 3-10 presents structures of the middle third of the medulla. The rostral portion of the hypoglossal nucleus is larger at this level than the lower third of the medulla. The fully developed principal (inferior) olivary nucleus is above the pyramidal tract and occupies a major portion of the lower half of the medulla. The principal (inferior) olivary nucleus, which is wrinkled and saggy, is an important relay center for motor and proprioceptive information that it transmits to the cerebellum. This nucleus receives input from the spinal cord (**spino-olivary**) and

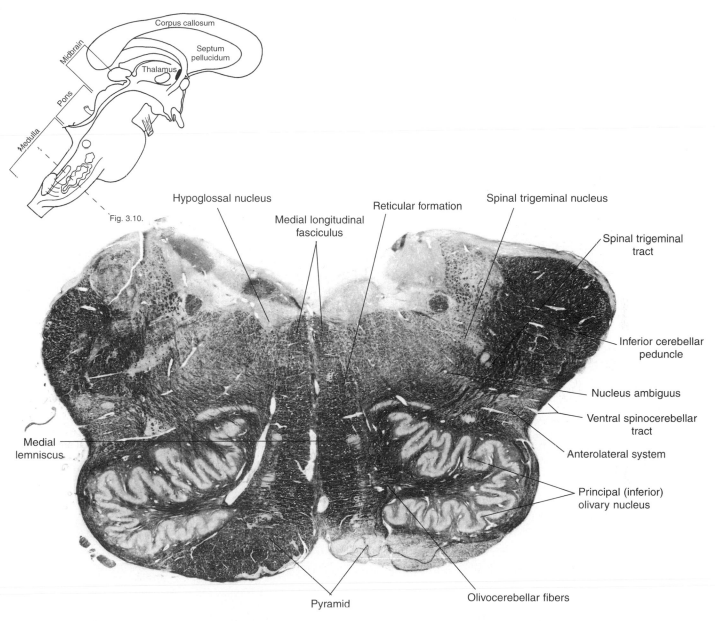

Figure 3-10.   Transverse section of medulla through rostral portions of hypoglossal nucleus and middle portions of principal (inferior) olivary nucleus.

reticular formation (**reticulo-olivary**) that is related to pain, touch, and position sense of limbs. The **olivocerebellar fibers** cross the midline and project to the opposite cerebellar hemisphere through the inferior cerebellar peduncle (**restiform body**). The inferior cerebellar peduncle appears along the lateral dorsal surface of the upper half of the medulla. It is relatively small at this level in contrast to the levels above and is the most caudal of the three peduncles that connect the brainstem to the cerebellum (Figs. 2-29 and 2-30).

In the region between the inferior cerebellar peduncle and the reticular formation are **cranial nerve nuclei**, that are related to the **glossopharyngeal** and **vagus nerves**. One of the important nuclei at this level is the **nucleus ambiguus**, the motor nucleus of the spinal accessory, glossopharyngeal, and vagus nerves; it supplies muscles of the soft palate, pharynx, larynx, and upper esophagus and controls swallowing and phonation. The nuclei of the reticular formation are scattered and occupy a larger core area in the center of the medulla.

ROSTRAL THIRD OF MEDULLA

This transverse section through the rostral third of the medulla shown in Figure 3-11 reveals an enlarged inferior cerebellar peduncle and the principal (inferior) olivary nucleus. Note the large inferior cerebellar peduncle at this level in contrast to its appearance in Figure 3-10.

Among the newly appearing structures are the **cochlear complex** and glossopharyngeal nerve. The cochlear nucleus is above the restiform body in the dorsolateral medulla, and it receives projections from the inner ear. The glossopharyngeal nerve mediates taste and contributes to swallowing.

The compact pyramidal motor fibers are in the ventral medulla. The principal (inferior) olivary nucleus is present in its fully developed form. The medial lemniscus and the medial longitudinal fasciculus lie along

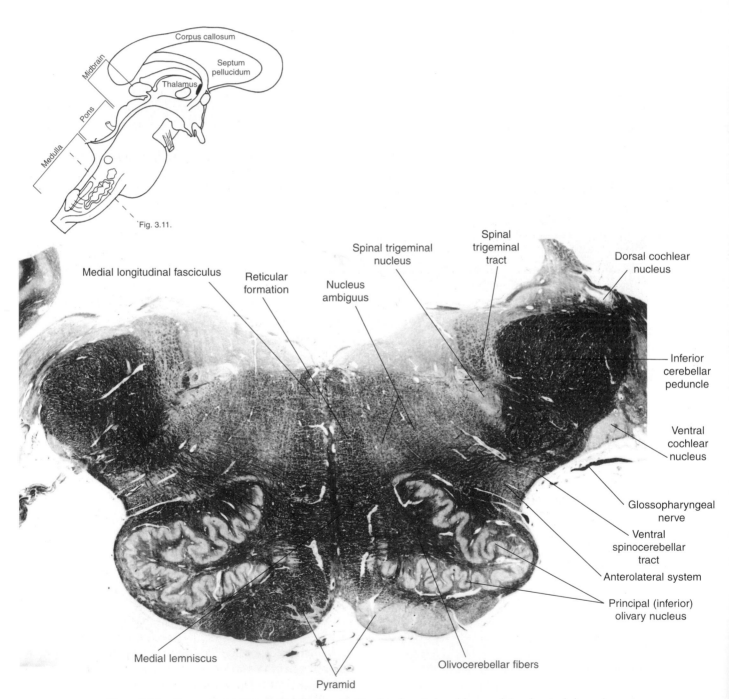

Figure 3-11. Transverse section of medulla through dorsal and ventral cochlear nuclei and root of glossopharyngeal nerve.

the midline of the medulla dorsal to the pyramids. The spinal trigeminal nucleus and its tract are also emerging. The reticular formation occupies a large core in the middle third of the medulla, spanning the area dorsal to the principal (inferior) olivary nucleus.

Pons

Major pontine structures include the following: the **corticospinal fibers** interspersed with diffused **pontine nuclei**, the crown-shaped cavity of the **fourth ventricle**, the massive **middle cerebellar peduncle (brachium pontis)**, the **medial lemniscus** that separates the **tegmental pons** from the **basal pons**, the **crossing pontocerebellar fibers**, the **trigeminal nuclear complex**, the **spinal trigeminal nucleus** and **tract**, the **superior cerebellar peduncle (brachium conjunctivum)**, and the remnants **inferior cerebellar peduncle**. Important pontine structures are listed in Table 3-3.

LOWER PONS

Illustrated in Figure 3-12 are the transitional anatomical characteristics between the medulla and pons. The enlarged fourth ventricle and diffuse pontine nuclei represent the pons, whereas the pyramid characterizes the medulla. The superior cerebellar peduncle forms part of the lateral roof of the fourth ventricle. Dorsal in the section is the convex **anterior medullary velum** that forms the roof of the fourth ventricle (Fig. 2-12). The ventral teardrop-shaped pyramid does not hug the ventromedial area as it does in the lower medullary levels.

The **vestibular nucleus** appears beneath the floor of the fourth ventricle. The cochlear nucleus, seen at the

Table 3-3. Anatomical Structures of Pons

Characterizing Structures
Lower pons
Full-size crown-shaped fourth ventricle
Diffuse pyramidal fibers piercing basal pons
Remnants of inferior cerebellar peduncle
Facial nucleus and nerve
Middle cerebellar peduncle (brachium pontis)
Medial lemniscus (marking upper limit of basal pons)
Anterior medullary velum
Spinal trigeminal nucleus and tract
Superior cerebellar peduncle (brachium conjunctivum)
Middle pons
Middle cerebellar peduncle
Trigeminal nuclear complex
Pontine nuclei
Superior cerebellar peduncle
Fourth ventricle cavity
Anterior medullary velum
Medial lemniscus
Diffuse corticospinal fibers

previous section, is no longer present. The vestibular complex receives projections from the semicircular canals in the inner ear and is important in equilibrium and head–eye coordination (see Chapter 10).

Exiting laterally from the pontomedullary junction are the fibers of the **vestibular branch** of the **vestibuloacoustic nerve** along the ventral surface of the middle and inferior cerebellar peduncles. The structures beneath the vestibular complex are the spinal trigeminal tract and spinal trigeminal nucleus.

The **spinal tract fibers of the trigeminal nerve** descend ipsilaterally to synapse with the trigeminal nucleus, which relays facial sensation through crossing fiber tracts; these fibers join the medial lemniscus to terminate in the thalamus. The nucleus of the facial nerve is in the tegmentum of the pons. The **facial cranial nerve** innervates the muscles of facial expression and controls smiling, frowning, and laughing and assists in speaking. Fibers of the facial nerve exit laterally from the pontomedullary junction.

The middle cerebellar peduncle's massive body, which is by far the largest of the cerebellar peduncles, is lateral in this section. Fibers of the middle cerebral peduncle connect the pons with the cerebellum and mediate information from the motor cortex to the cerebellum. The fibers medial to the middle cerebellar peduncle belong to the inferior cerebellar peduncle, which mediates vestibular and spinal information to the cerebellum. The crescent-shaped fibers of the superior cerebellar peduncle emerge dorsally and form the dorsolateral roof of the fourth ventricle.

MIDDLE PONS

The transverse section shown in Figure 3-13 in the middle of the pons is at the level of the trigeminal nerve, the principal sensory nerve for the face, as it exits laterally through the middle cerebellar peduncle. The most characteristic features of the pons are the interspersed **corticospinal–corticopontine fibers** and the crown-shaped lumen of the fourth ventricle. Fibers of all three cerebellar peduncles are present laterally in this section, although the inferior cerebellar and superior cerebellar peduncles are relatively small. Scattered pontine nuclei receive massive inputs from the ipsilateral primary motor and sensory cortices and project the **pontocerebellar fibers**, which cross the midline to enter the middle cerebellar peduncle. These fibers mediate information from the opposite primary motor, sensory, and visual cortices and are concerned with limb movement during skilled acts. Laterally, the crescent-shaped superior cerebellar peduncle provides cerebellar feedback to the primary motor cortex via the **red nucleus**. Located ventrolaterally are fibers of the **lateral lemniscus**, which carry information from both ears to the cortex.

This pontine section also demonstrates spatial relationships among the facial nucleus, facial nerve,

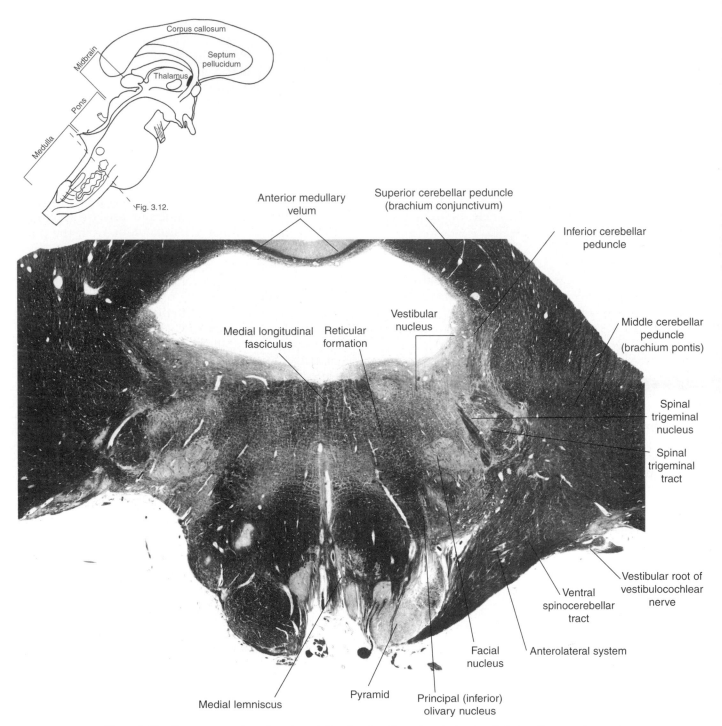

Figure 3-12.   Transverse section of pontomedullary junction through rostral pole of inferior olivary nucleus and facial nucleus.

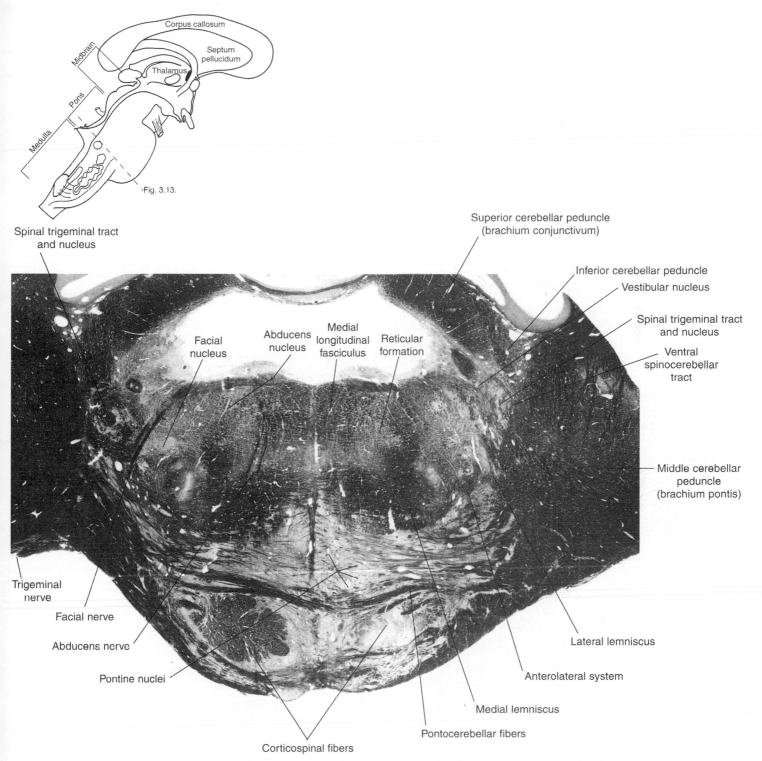

Figure 3-13. Transverse section of pons through rostral pole of facial nucleus and internal genu of facial nerve.

abducens nucleus, and abducens nerve. The internal genu refers to fibers of the facial nerve as they curve over the nucleus of the abducens nerve just below the floor of the fourth ventricle (Fig. 15-3*B*).

PONTOMIDBRAIN JUNCTION

The section shown in Figure 3-14 reveals the transition between the rostral pons and the midbrain. The transition is evident in a reduction in the size of the

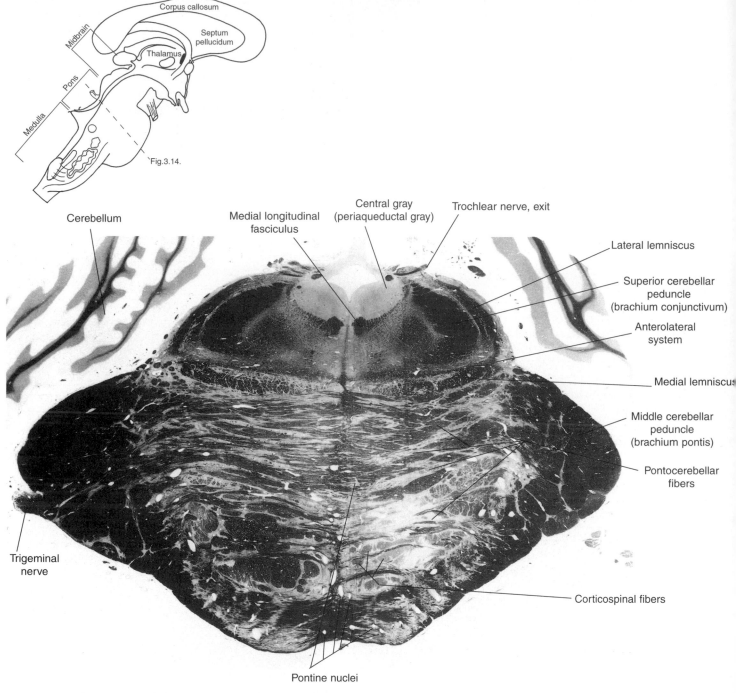

Figure 3-14.   Transverse section of rostral pons through exits of trochlear and trigeminal nerves.

fourth ventricle. The ventricular floor is formed by the enlarged central gray of the reticular formation, which contains important somatic and visceral nuclei. Located dorsally in this section is the root of the **trochlear nerve**. It is one of three cranial nerves (the other two are **oculomotor** and **abducens**) responsible for innervating the eye and is the only motor nerve that exits dorsally. The medial longitudinal fasciculus is buried within the cen-

tral gray substance of the reticular formation. The massive cerebellum is dorsal to the ventricular cavity. Ventral to the central gray of the reticular formation are fibers of the superior cerebellar peduncle, which occupy the outer third of the tegmentum and decussate at a higher level in the midbrain. These superior cerebellar peduncle fibers originate in the deep cerebellar nuclei and provide feedback to the opposite thalamic and cortical centers. Lateral to the fibers of the superior cerebellar peduncle are the lateral lemniscus fibers, which relay information from both ears to the primary auditory cortex in the temporal lobe. The ventral region in this section contains diffuse pontine nuclei, a massive amount of crossing pontocerebellar fibers that make up the large middle cerebellar peduncles, and the scattered corticospinal tract fiber bundles on each side of the midline. Located laterally is the root of the trigeminal nerve.

Midbrain

The midbrain consists of the **tectum**, **tegmentum**, and **basis pedunculi** (Fig. 2-24). The tectum consists of the **corpora quadrigemina**, which refers to four egg-shaped structures (Figs. 2-21 and 2-22). The upper two bodies of the corpora quadrigemina are the **superior colliculi**, and the lower two bodies are the **inferior colliculi**. Below the **midbrain tectal structure** is the **cerebral aqueduct**, a narrow canal that connects the third and fourth ventricles. The tegmentum is an elongated mass of nuclei and white matter in the center of the brainstem that includes decussation of the superior cerebellar peduncle, reticular formation, and red nucleus. Tectum and tegmentum are distinguishable by their locations with respect to the cerebral aqueduct. The tectum is dorsal to the cerebral aqueduct, whereas the tegmentum is beneath the aqueduct. The basis pedunculi is ventral, and it includes the **substantia nigra** and the wing-shaped fibers of the **pes pedunculi** (crus cerebri). Important midbrain structures are listed in Table 3-4.

CAUDAL MIDBRAIN

The transverse section shown in Figure 3-15 reveals the anatomical view of both the low midbrain and pons. The two round structures located dorsally are the

Table 3-4.   Anatomical Structures of Midbrain

Characterizing Structures
Low caudal midbrain
Cerebral aqueduct
Inferior colliculus
Superior cerebellar peduncle, decussation
Medial lemniscus
High rostral midbrain
Pes pedunculi (crus cerebri)
Substantia nigra
Red nucleus
Superior colliculus
Central gray
Cerebral aqueduct
Oculomotor nucleus and nerve
Medial lemniscus

inferior colliculi. The inferior colliculus is a relay center in the transmission of information from the ears to the auditory cortex; it also regulates auditory reflexes. In this section, fibers of the lateral lemniscus that carry auditory information are merging with the inferior colliculus. The fourth ventricle rostrally communicates with the cerebral aqueduct, which is a frequent site of obstruction in congenital hydrocephalus because of its small lumen. The central gray region and reticular formation lie around the cerebral aqueduct and mediate affective behavior.

Originating from the deep dentate cerebellar nucleus are the fibers of the superior cerebellar peduncle; these fibers course ventromedially below the aqueduct, where they cross the midline before they go to the thalamus and cortex. This decussation of the superior cerebellar peduncle fibers accounts for the cerebellar projections to the contralateral motor cortex. Also note the emergence of pes pedunculi. The remaining structures in Figure 3-15 have been previously identified; they include the medial lemniscus, the medial longitudinal fasciculus, the lateral lemniscus, the pontine nuclei, the pontocerebellar fibers, and the corticospinal fibers.

ROSTRAL MIDBRAIN

The slightly oblique section shown in Figure 3-16 reveals the anatomical characteristics of the high midbrain. The two dorsally located round structures at this level are the superior colliculi, the visual reflex center. The superior colliculus and the adjacent **pretectal area** mediate reflexes involving intrinsic eye muscles; they also regulate pupil constriction (light reflex) and lens accommodation (see Chapter 8).

The superior colliculi look similar to the inferior colliculi. The way to differentiate these colliculi is by relating them to the co-occurring structures. When seen on a cross or transverse section, the decussation of the superior cerebellar peduncle fibers is the important landmark of the inferior colliculus. The presence of the red nucleus and the substantia nigra identifies the level of the superior colliculus.

Lateral to the superior colliculus is the **brachium of the inferior colliculus**, which carries auditory information from the inferior colliculus to the **medial geniculate body**, the thalamic relay center for audition. The round nucleus in the midbrain tegmentum is the red nucleus, which has two important functions. First, it receives the cerebellar projections through the crossed superior cerebellar peduncle fibers and transmits the cerebellar feedback to the thalamus. Second, it transmits descending motor information to the spinal and cranial motor nuclei and regulates muscle tone.

Below the red nucleus is the substantia nigra, which is important in the extrapyramidal circuitry. Cells of the substantia nigra have been identified as producers

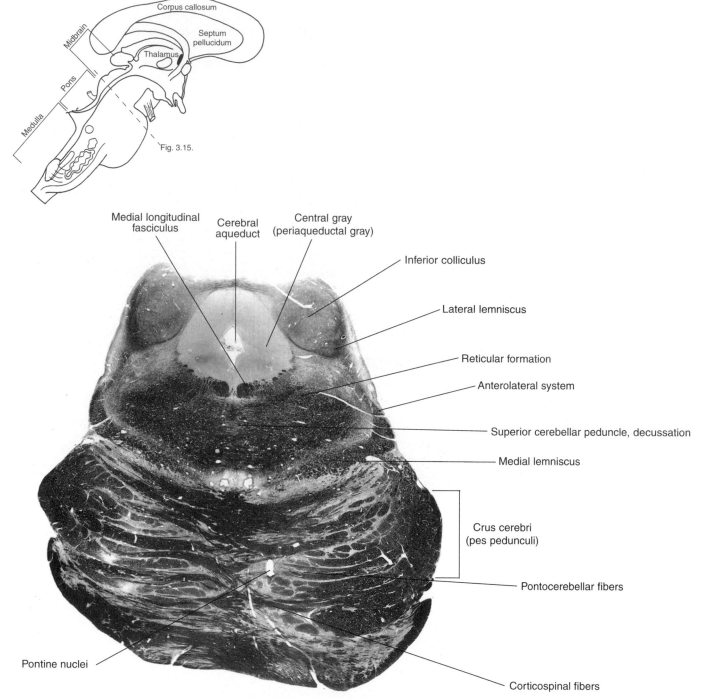

Figure 3-15.   Transverse section of pons–midbrain junction through inferior colliculus, caudal portions of decussation of superior cerebellar peduncle, and rostral parts of basilar pons.

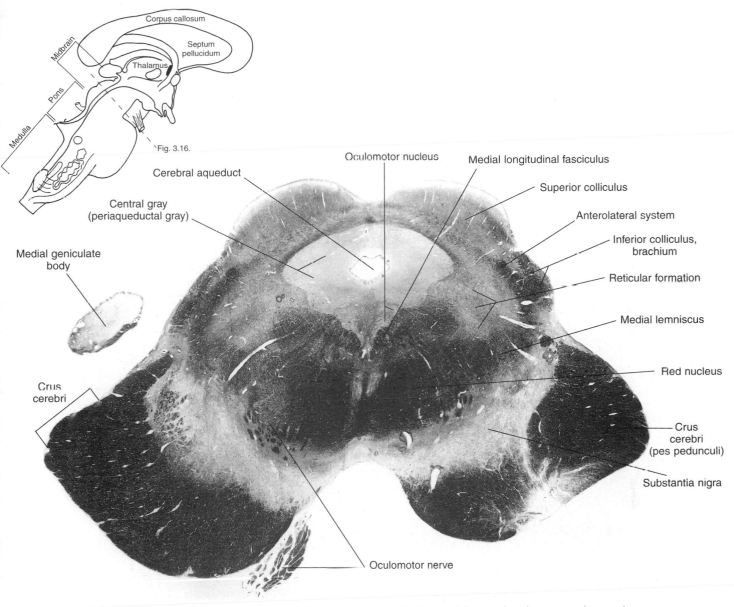

Figure 3-16. Transverse section of midbrain through superior colliculus, caudal parts of oculomotor nucleus, and red nucleus.

of **dopamine**, an inhibitory basal ganglia neurotransmitter; the nigrostriatal fibers project dopamine to the **caudate nucleus** of the **neostriatum**. The degeneration of the substantia nigra's dopamine-producing cells is associated with **Parkinson's disease**, a slowly progressive degenerative condition characterized by **resting tremor, expressionless face, muscular rigidity, flexed posture**, and moderate to severe **motor speech difficulty** (see Chapters 1 and 13). Ventrally located in this section are the wing-shaped fibers of the pes penduculi (crus cerebri), which indicate the midbrain location of the **corticobulbar** and **corticospinal fibers**.

In the floor of the central gray is the oculomotor nerve nucleus, the third cranial nerve responsible for eye movements. Fibers of the oculomotor nerve exit in the interpeduncular fossa (Fig. 15-10). The medial longitudinal fasciculus is below the oculomotor nucleus and is an important fiber bundle that interconnects three cranial nerves (oculomotor, trochlear, abducens) with the vestibular system. It is also important in coordinated eye movements.

HIGH ROSTRAL MIDBRAIN

The transverse section of the rostral midbrain contains structures that were not present at lower levels, including the **posterior thalamus**, the **optic tract**, and the **Edinger-Westphal nucleus** (Figs. 2-24, 3-17, and 15-10). The Edinger-Westphal nucleus is the visceral nucleus of the **oculomotor nerve**, which mediates pupillary constriction and lens accommodation reflexes. The

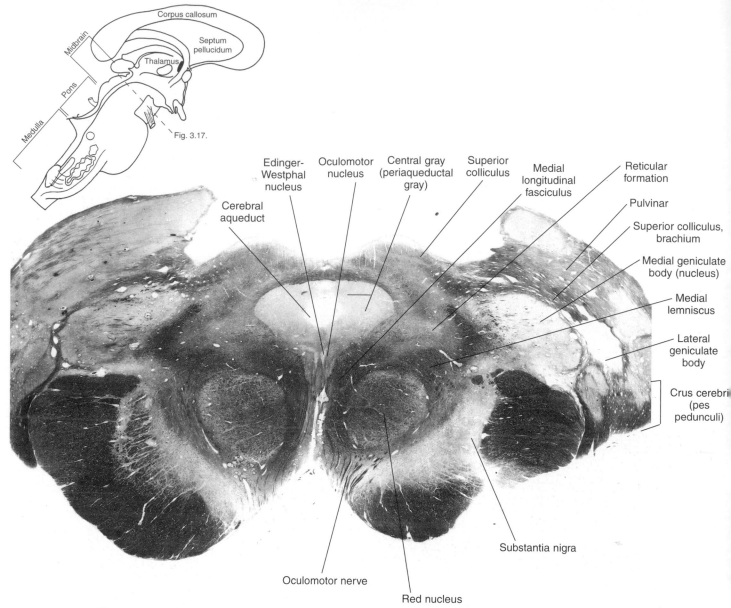

Figure 3-17. Transverse section of midbrain through superior colliculus and rostral portions of oculomotor nucleus.

posterior thalamus includes **pulvinar**, **lateral geniculate**, and **medial geniculate bodies** (see Chapter 6). The lateral geniculate body is the thalamic relay center for vision. The medial geniculate body is the thalamic relay for audition. The oculomotor nerve runs along the medial border of the midbrain next to the medial border of the large red nucleus (Fig. 2-24). The substantia nigra sits in the hammock of the pes pedunculi just beneath the red nucleus. The large red nucleus between the central gray above and the large pes pedunculi below identifies this level of the midbrain.

Midbrain–Diencephalon Junction

The oblique section shown in Figure 3-18 presents a transitional view with structures from both the **midbrain** and **diencephalon**. The important structures at this level are the **posterior commissure** with the overlying **pineal gland** in the dorsal midline, the posterior part of the **pulvinar nucleus**, the rostral end of the red nucleus flanked laterally by the medial lemniscus, and the large diagonal **internal capsule–pes pedunculi**. Fibers of the internal capsule, which were identified as the pes pedunculi below this level, are hugged by the optic tract, which runs along its ventrolateral border. The **subthalamic nucleus** is sandwiched between the internal capsule and the red nucleus, the site that was occupied by the substantia nigra at lower levels of the midbrain. Both the subthalamic nucleus and substantia nigra are major contributors to motor control, and their dysfunction is associated with movement disorders. The pineal gland, an endocrine organ, is located

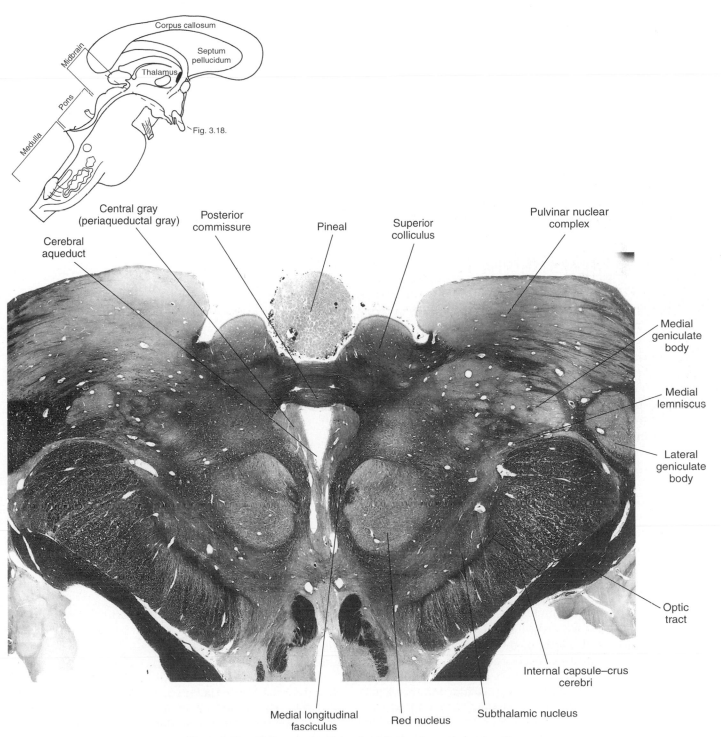

Figure 3-18. Oblique section through midbrain–diencephalon junction.

dorsally and is important in diurnal rhythm. Inhibition of its secretion has also been associated with the onset of puberty. The posterior commissure is considered to connect the two superior colliculi. The posterior thalamus includes pulvinar, lateral, and medial geniculate bodies. The lateral geniculate body is the thalamic relay center for vision. The medial geniculate body is the thalamic relay center for audition. The pulvinar—the most caudal part of the thalamus—is reciprocally connected with the association cortex in the temporal and parietal cortex. It also has speech and language functions (see Chapter 6). The subthalamic nucleus, which is mediodorsal to the crus cerebri, is an important extrapyramidal structure. Pathology in it results in **hemiballism**, characterized by violent and flinging movements. Ventrally situated in the section is the optic tract.

FOREBRAIN IN CORONAL SECTIONS

Learning the forebrain anatomy entails orientation to the subcortical structures that include the **basal ganglia** (caudate nucleus, putamen, globus pallidus, and functionally related subthalamic nucleus), **diencephalon** (thalamus and hypothalamus), **ventricular cavity** (lateral and third), and **limbic structures** (amygdala, fornix, hippocampal formation, and cingulate gyrus). Other important structures are the **corpus callosum**, **optic chiasm**, **insular cortex** (isle of Reil), **septum pellucidum**, **anterior commissure**, **cingulate gyrus**, **internal, external,** and **extreme capsules**, and **claustrum** (Table 3-5).

These structures are in fixed positions with respect to each other; a review of their relative locations on a horizontal section (Fig. 3-19) facilitates the orientation to them on subsequent coronal serial sections of the brain (Fig. 3-20).

Located rostrally in the horizontal section of the brain (Fig. 3-19) are the **frontal lobes** on each side of the midline corpus callosum (genu). The fibers of the corpus callosum connect the homologous cortical areas in both hemispheres by corticocortical fibers. The **septum pellucidum** is in the midline extending from the ventral surface of the corpus callosum and ending along the anterior limits of the thalamus. On each side of the septum pellucidum are the **anterior horns** of the **lateral ventricle**. The third ventricle is in the midline between two thalami. Each lateral ventricle communicates with the midline third ventricle through the **interventricular foramina of Monro**. The interventricular foramen is at the junction of the septum and thalamus on each side of the midline.

Two large nuclear masses projecting into the lateral ventricles are the heads of the **caudate nuclei**, which are important contributors to motor functions. Caudal to the caudate nuclei are the two thalami on each side of the third ventricle. The junctional area between the caudate and thalamus is indented by the **genu** of the inter-

Table 3-5. Anatomical Structures of Basal Ganglia and Diencephalon at Different Levels

Characterizing Structures
Posterior thalamus
Pineal gland
Corpus callosum, splenium
Pulvinar of thalamus
Cerebral aqueduct
Lateral geniculate body
Medial geniculate body
Internal capsule merging in crus cerebri/pes pedunculi
Midthalamus
Corpus callosum, body
Fornix
Midthalamus
Subthalamic nucleus
Lateral ventricle
Third ventricle
Hypothalamus
Diminishing globus pallidus and putamen
Anterior thalamus
Anterior thalamus
Anterior commissure
Caudate
Putamen
Globus pallidus
Third ventricle
Hypothalamus
Internal capsule, genu
Corpus callosum, body
External capsule
Extreme capsule
Septum pellucidum
Claustrum
Anterior limb of internal capsule
Corpus callosum, body
Head of caudate nucleus
Putamen
Attachment of caudate and putamen
Lateral ventricle, anterior horn
Septum pellucidum
Internal capsule, anterior limb
External capsule
Claustrum
Extreme capsule

nal capsule, which connects the **anterior limb** with the **posterior limb**. The anterior limb is associated predominantly with cortical motor projections and the posterior limb, with sensory cortical projections.

The bend of the internal capsule is in part produced by the **lenticular nucleus** (putamen and globus pallidus). These nuclei contribute to motor control and in conjunction with the caudate nucleus constitute the basal ganglia. Just lateral to the putamen is the claustrum, a thin, wavy line of cells that possesses two-way projections predominantly with the sensory cortical areas of the brain. The insular cortex, concerned with visceral functions, overlies the claustrum and lenticular nucleus.

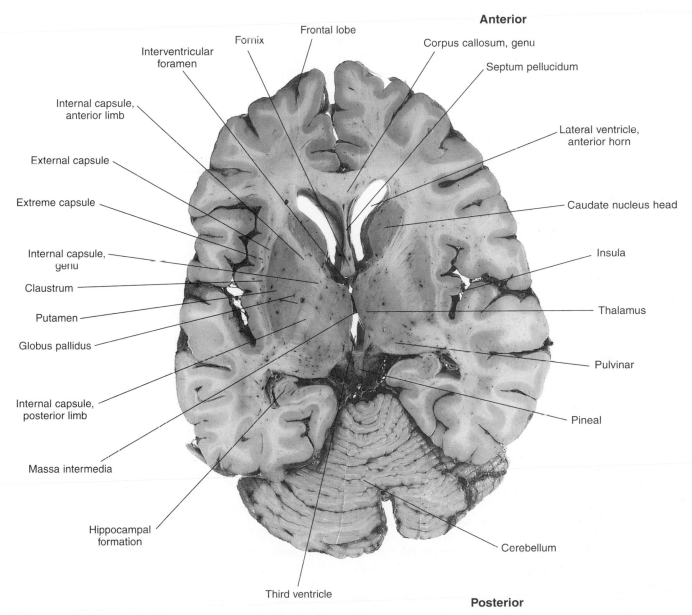

Anterior

Frontal lobe

Fornix

Interventricular foramen

Corpus callosum, genu

Septum pellucidum

Internal capsule, anterior limb

External capsule

Extreme capsule

Lateral ventricle, anterior horn

Caudate nucleus head

Internal capsule, genu

Insula

Claustrum

Putamen

Thalamus

Globus pallidus

Pulvinar

Internal capsule, posterior limb

Pineal

Massa intermedia

Hippocampal formation

Cerebellum

Third ventricle

Posterior

Figure 3-19.   Dorsal view of a horizontal section through interventricular foramina, third ventricle, and pulvinar.

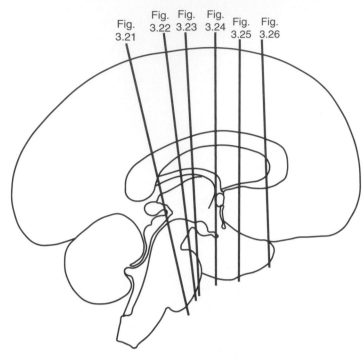

Figure 3-20. Midsagittal view displaying levels of coronal brain sections shown in Figures 3-21 to 3-26.

The caudal end of the third ventricle is identified by the **posterior commissure** and the **pineal gland** in the midline. This level is the transitional area between the posterior thalamus and midbrain. More caudally, the cerebellum is in the midline between the occipital lobes. The cerebellum overlies the fourth ventricle and is attached to the brainstem by the cerebellar peduncles.

Coronal Section Through Posterior Thalamus

The coronal brain section shown in Figure 3-21 clearly shows the distinction between white and gray matter with sulci and gyri markings. The large fissure in the middle separating both hemispheres is the inter-hemispheric **longitudinal fissure**. The body of the corpus callosum forms the roof of the lateral ventricles. The **splenium** of the corpus callosum connects both **occipital lobes**. The large cavities in this section are the bodies of the lateral ventricles; the small cavities in the temporal lobe are the **inferior horns** of the lateral ventricles. In the floor of the lateral ventricle is the **fornix**, a bundle of fibers that mediates two-way connections between the hypothalamic structures and the hippocampus. Forming the medial wall of the inferior horn of the lateral ventricles is the **hippocampal formation**, which is thought to serve memory functions. The thalamic nucleus in this section is the **pulvinar**, the most posterior nucleus of the thalamus, which is reciprocally connected with the **parietal association cortex** and participates in language functions. Ventral to the pulvinar are the **geniculate** (medial and lateral) **bodies**, which serve as thalamic re-

lay centers. The medial geniculate body mediates auditory information from the ears to the auditory cortices in **Heschl's gyrus**. The lateral geniculate body transmits visual information from homonymous halves of the retinas to the primary visual cortex in the occipital lobe. Dorsal to the inferior horn and lateral to the thalamus is the posterior limb of the internal capsule, which contains the ascending (sensory) and descending (motor) fibers. In the middle of Figure 3-21 is the brainstem section, which contains the cerebral aqueduct, the decussation of the superior cerebellar peduncle, the basal pons, and the pretectal structure. The pretectal area regulates visual reflexes (see Chapters 8 and 15).

Coronal Section Through Midthalamus

The section of the brain shown in Figure 3-22 retains most of the previously identified structures at the posterior thalamic level in addition to a few newly visible structures. A new structure emerging bilaterally from the walls of the lateral ventricle is the larger body of the caudate nucleus. The caudate nucleus, with its long tail, is a C-shaped structure in the sagittal view of the brain (Fig. 2-17) that can be seen in many sequential coronal sections of the brain. The caudate is an important nucleus that contributes to motor activity. Forming the floor of the lateral ventricles in this section are the large gray masses of the thalamus. Both thalami are connected through the **massa intermedia**, a thalamic loose fibrous tissue. In the midline, between the two lateral ventricles, is the **septum**. Through the base of the

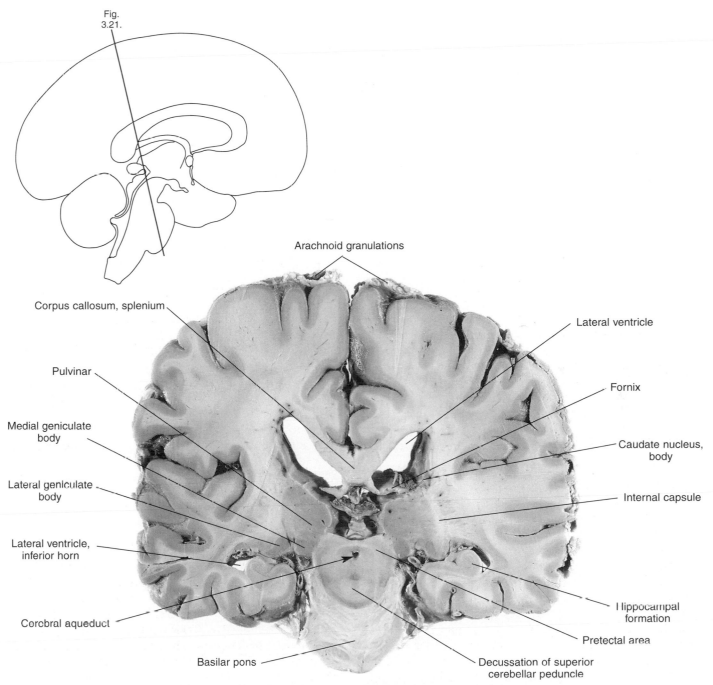

Fig.
3.21.

Arachnoid granulations

Corpus callosum, splenium

Lateral ventricle

Pulvinar

Fornix

Medial geniculate
body

Caudate nucleus,
body

Lateral geniculate
body

Internal capsule

Lateral ventricle,
inferior horn

Hippocampal
formation

Cerebral aqueduct

Pretectal area

Basilar pons

Decussation of superior
cerebellar peduncle

Figure 3-21.   Caudal surface of a coronal section through posterior thalamus.

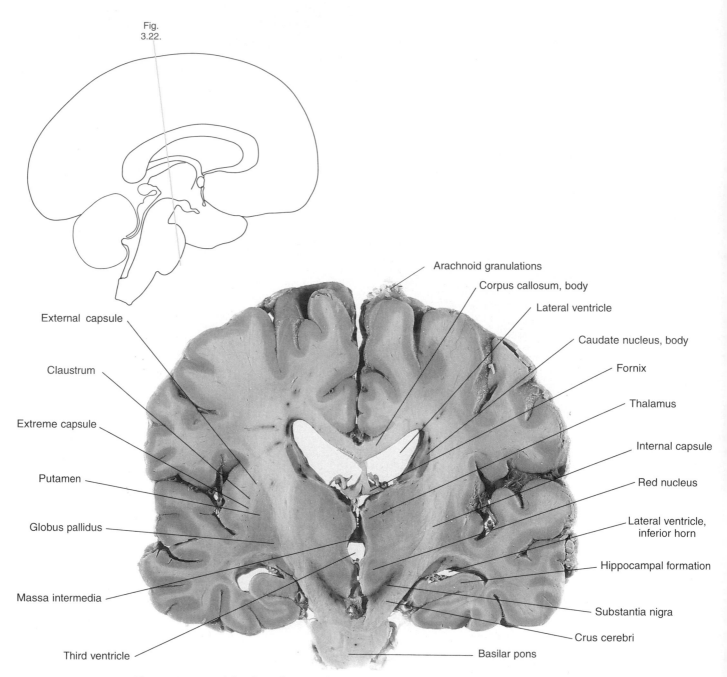

Figure 3-22.   Caudal surface of a coronal section through medial thalamus and massa intermedia.

septum courses the fornix, an important C-shaped limbic structure that connects the mamillary bodies of the hypothalamus with the hippocampus and septum and is involved in autonomic functions. The lenticular nucleus, lateral to the internal capsule, consists of the globus pallidus and putamen. The globus pallidus and putamen are parts of the basal ganglia and are important in regulating motor functions and muscle tone. The external capsule is a thin band of fibers lateral to the lenticular nucleus. Lateral to the external capsule is the claustrum, a thin layer of gray matter. The thin bundle of fibers lateral to the claustrum is the extreme capsule. The most lateral structure in this section is the insular cortex. The vertical slit in the center is the third ventricle, formed by the medial walls of each thalamus. The remaining brainstem structures in the center of the section include the crus cerebri (pes pedunculi), basilar pons, red nucleus, and substantia nigra.

Coronal Section Through Anterior Thalamus

The general orientation of the forebrain anatomy in this section is similar to that of the previous section, although it is more rostral at the anterior thalamic nucleus level (Fig. 3-23). The rough, saggy, and worm-shaped structure in the lateral ventricles is the **choroid plexus**, which produces **cerebrospinal fluid**. Forming the floor of the lateral ventricle is the **anterior nucleus**, the most rostral nucleus of the thalamus, which receives direct projections from the **mamillary bodies** of the hypothalamus. Along the lateral wall of the lateral ventricles is the caudate nucleus, a C-shaped structure. This section of the forebrain is unique because it simultaneously reveals the dorsal component (body of the caudate nucleus in the lateral ventricle) and ventral component (tail of the caudate nucleus in the lateral wall of the temporal horn). Medial to the internal capsule is the subthalamic nucleus, an important structure in the extrapyramidal network; pathology in it causes hemiballism, which is characterized by violently jerking movements on one side of the body.

Coronal Section Through Anterior Commissure

The coronal section of the forebrain through the **anterior commissure** and the internal capsule genu, shown in Figure 3-24, marks the anterior limit of the thalamus. The head of the caudate nucleus emerges in the ventricular cavity as a larger structure than at the more caudal levels. There is a clear view of the anterior commissure and its crossing. The anterior commissure is a small forebrain fiber bundle that contains bidirectional olfactory fibers and connects temporal cortices. At this level, the internal capsule fibers, which are somewhat diminished, suggest the beginning of its **anterior limb**. Centrally located is the septum, which anteriorly separates the lateral ventricles. All hippocampal projections terminate in the septum verum nuclei, which are part of the limbic system. Forming the lateral walls of the third ventricle below the level of the anterior commissure is the **hypothalamus**. Two important structures of the hypothalamus, not seen in this section, are the mamillary body and pituitary gland. **Hypothalamic nuclei** produce neurosecretions that are important in controlling water balance, sugar, fat metabolism, body temperature, and hormone production. The **amygdaloid nucleus** in this section is at the level at which the tail of the caudate nucleus terminates (Fig. 2-17). The amygdala, a massive round structure in the medial temporal lobe, is generally responsible for activating emotional behavior. Pathology in it has been known to lead to aggression and other abnormal behaviors; surgical removal in animals has caused aggressive animals to become docile and hyposexual.

The previously identified structures that are also present in this section and unchanged in basic configuration are as follows: corpus callosum, septum pellucidum, fornix, caudate nucleus, putamen, globus pallidus, internal capsule, external capsule, claustrum, extreme capsule, and insular cortex.

Coronal Section Through Anterior Limb of Internal Capsule and Caudate Head

The coronal section of the forebrain at the rostral region of the basal ganglia, shown in Figure 3-25, reveals the large head of the caudate nucleus, the anterior horn of the lateral ventricles, and the anterior limb of the internal capsule. At this level of the brain, the thalamus and globus pallidus are no longer present (Fig. 3-19). The massive caudate nucleus head forms the ventrolateral wall of the lateral ventricle at the level of the anterior horn. Laterally, the ventral component of the caudate nucleus merges with the putamen to form the **corpus striatum**. The portion of the internal capsule at this level is the anterior limb that courses between bodies of the caudate and putamen. In the middle, forming the medial ventricular wall, is the septum pellucidum, which is attached to the medial basal forebrain area. The cingulate gyrus, a limbic structure, is dorsal to the body of the corpus callosum. The **cingulum**, a bundle of mediofrontal parietal cingulate association fibers is beneath the cingulate gyrus. Also here is the septum pellucidum with its underlying nucleus, a limbic structure related to visceral functions, reward, and gratification.

The cortical regions rostral to this level undergo only a few changes. The ventricular cavity rostrally ends at the genu of the corpus callosum (Fig. 2-12). Anterior to the corpus callosum is the massive accumulation of white matter that consists of **callosal radiations** and **corona radiata**. These changes can be seen in Figure 3-26.

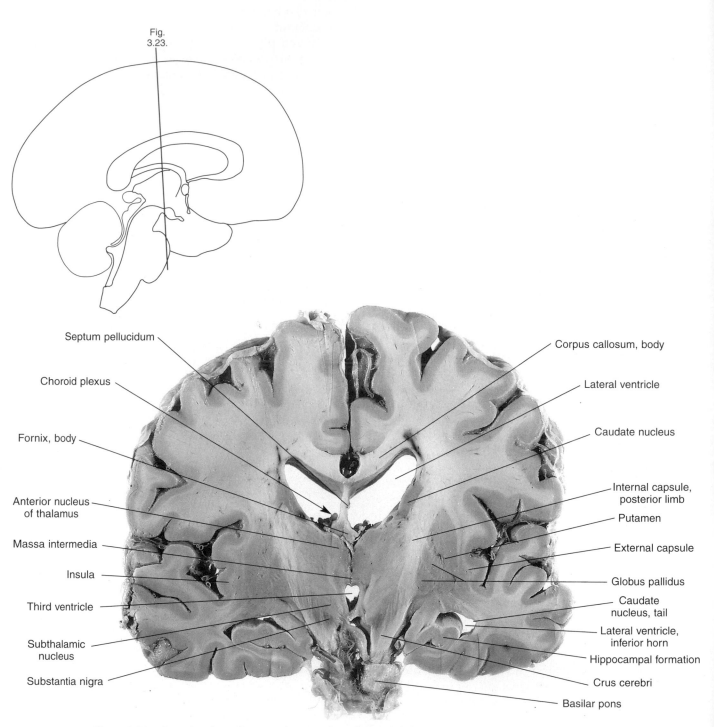

Fig.
3.23.

Septum pellucidum

Choroid plexus

Fornix, body

Anterior nucleus
of thalamus

Massa intermedia

Insula

Third ventricle

Subthalamic
nucleus

Substantia nigra

Corpus callosum, body

Lateral ventricle

Caudate nucleus

Internal capsule,
posterior limb

Putamen

External capsule

Globus pallidus

Caudate
nucleus, tail

Lateral ventricle,
inferior horn

Hippocampal formation

Crus cerebri

Basilar pons

Figure 3-23.   Rostral surface of a coronal section through rostral thalamus, massa intermedia, and subthalamic
nucleus.

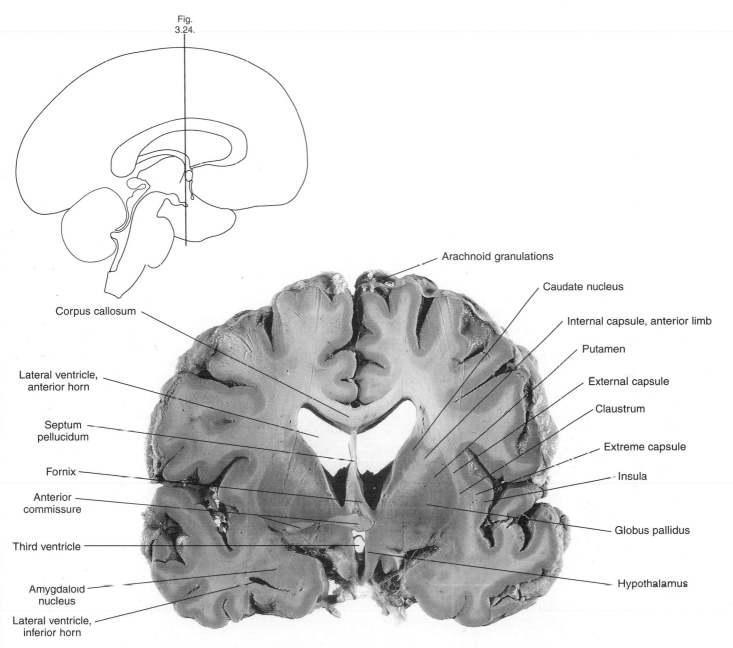

Fig.
3.24.

Arachnoid granulations

Caudate nucleus

Corpus callosum

Internal capsule, anterior limb

Putamen

Lateral ventricle,
anterior horn

External capsule

Septum
pellucidum

Claustrum

Extreme capsule

Fornix

Insula

Anterior
commissure

Globus pallidus

Third ventricle

Amygdaloid
nucleus

Hypothalamus

Lateral ventricle,
inferior horn

Figure 3-24.   Rostral surface of a coronal section through level of anterior commissure rostral to genu of internal
capsule.

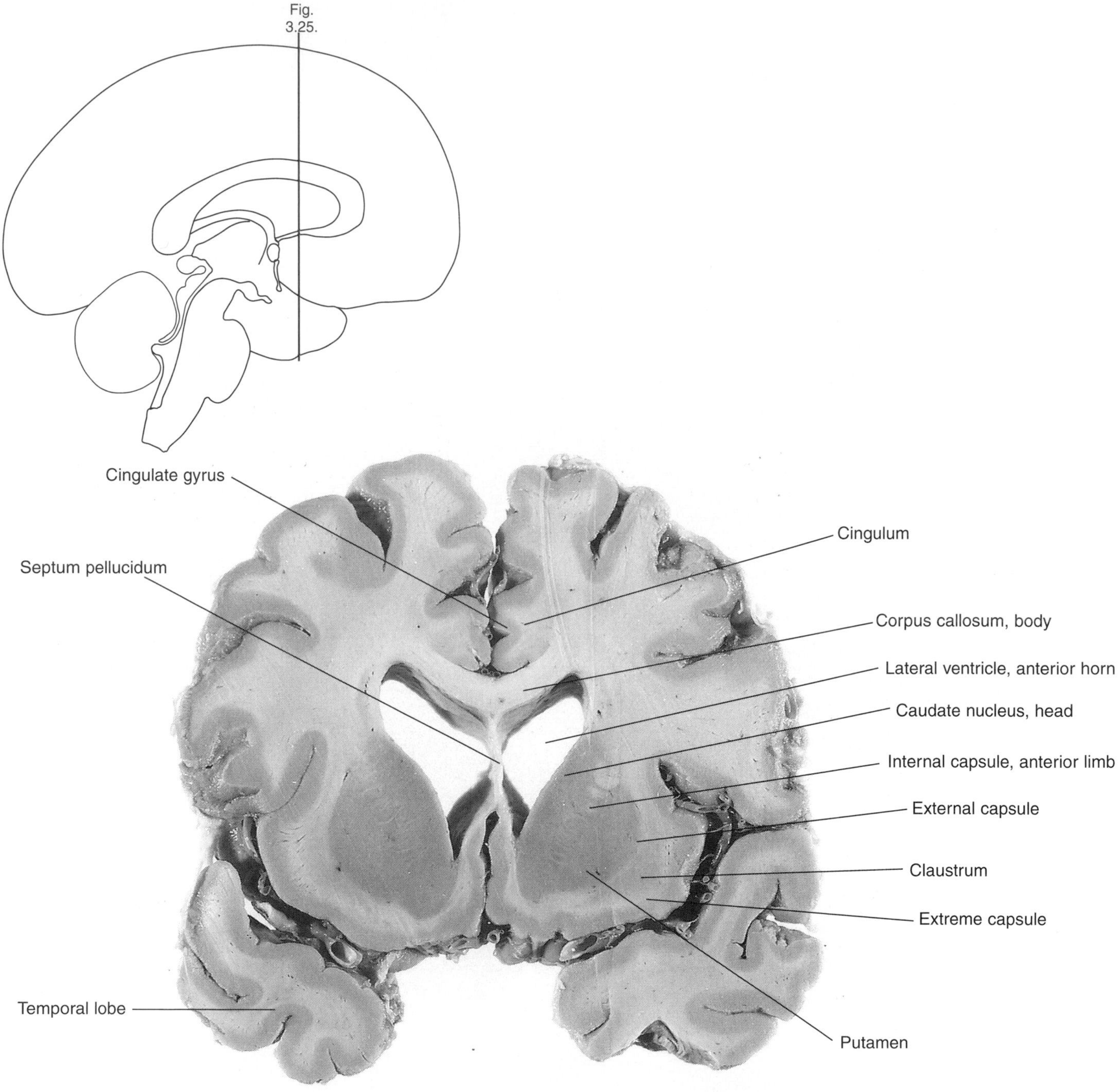

Fig. 3.25.

Cingulate gyrus

Septum pellucidum

Temporal lobe

Cingulum

Corpus callosum, body

Lateral ventricle, anterior horn

Caudate nucleus, head

Internal capsule, anterior limb

External capsule

Claustrum

Extreme capsule

Putamen

Figure 3-25. Caudal surface of a coronal section through head of caudate nucleus.

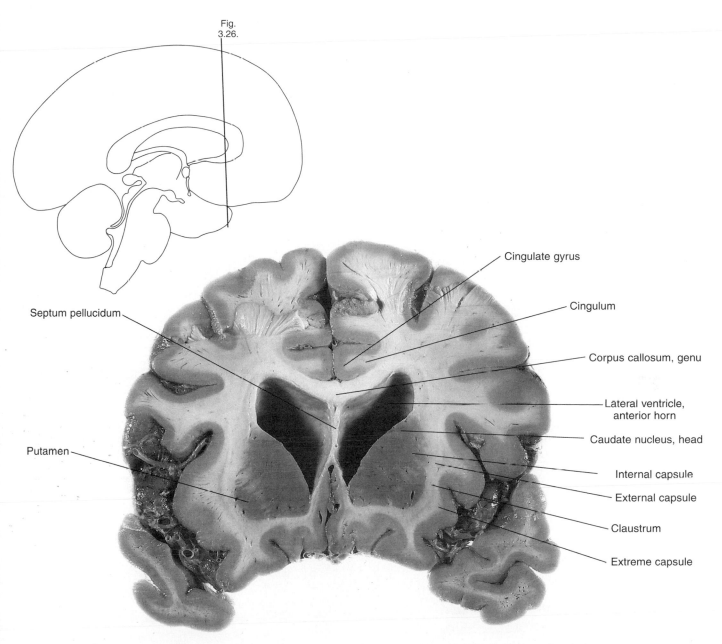

Fig.
3.26.

Cingulate gyrus

Cingulum

Septum pellucidum

Corpus callosum, genu

Lateral ventricle,
anterior horn

Caudate nucleus, head

Internal capsule

External capsule

Putamen

Claustrum

Extreme capsule

Figure 3-26.   Caudal surface of a coronal section just caudal to genu of corpus callosum and rostral end of anterior
horns.

Coronal Section Through Anterior Horn

The coronal section of the forebrain at the genu of the corpus callosum (Fig. 3-26) exhibits the end of the lateral ventricle (anterior horn) and the rostral striatum (caudate head and putamen). Other previously identified rostral structures include the septum, internal and external capsules, claustrum, cingulate gyrus, and cingulum.

FOREBRAIN IN HORIZONTAL SECTIONS

A review of the forebrain anatomy on horizontal sections further contributes to the visual orientation of the internal anatomy and helps consolidate the previous learning. In Figures 3-27 to 3-30, the human brain has been horizontally dissected to illustrate a three-dimensional view of the corpus callosum, ventricular cavity, thalamus, and basal ganglia structures.

In this first horizontal view of the brain (Fig. 3-27), a layer of the cerebral cortex approximately 1 cm thick has been removed to expose the underlying brain. The residual indentation of the **interhemispheric longitudinal fissure** is evident in the middle, with sulci and gyri, including the central sulcus, in the periphery of this section. In each hemisphere is the **semiovale center**, a massive accumulation of white matter, which contains the blended **association**, **commissural**, and **projection fibers** above the internal capsule level; it is oval in this

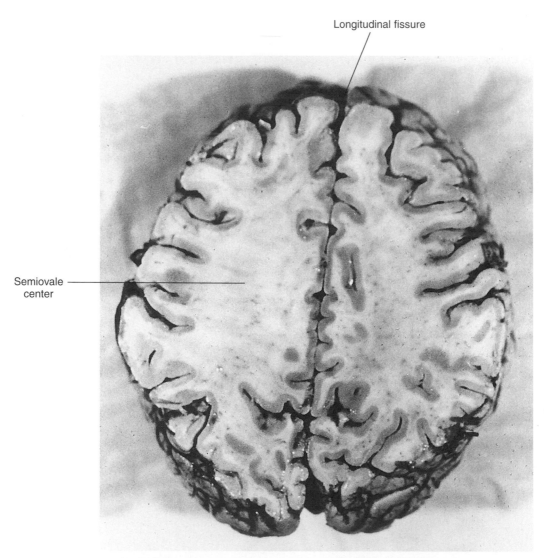

Longitudinal fissure

Semiovale center

Figure 3-27. Horizontal section of brain above corpus callosum.

horizontal section of the brain. The sensorimotor fibers form the **corona radiata**, in which descending motor fibers fan down toward the internal capsule and the ascending sensory fibers fan out to reach the cerebral cortex.

The additional removal of a 1- to 2-cm-thick cortical substance, which includes the cingulate gyrus parts and cingulum, exposes the dorsal surface of the corpus callosum (Fig. 3-28). Starting rostrally in this section are the genu, body, and splenium of the corpus callosum. The densely packed radiating fibers of the corpus callosum connect the hemispheres. The body of the corpus callosum and its lateral radiations form the roof of the lateral ventricles.

Further removal of the corpus callosum and its radiating cortical fibers reveals the large underlying sub-cortical structures and lateral ventricles (Fig. 3-29). Laterally located are the fibers constituting the **corona radiata**, the condensed projection fibers before they enter the internal capsule. The spaces on both sides of the corpus callosum mark the cavities of the lateral ventricles. The two prominent structures in the floor of the ventricles are the caudate nucleus and the thalamus. The massive balloon-shaped structure located rostrally and laterally in the ventricular cavity is the head of the caudate nucleus; its C-shaped tail is buried within the adjoining white matter. The head of the caudate nucleus forms the lateral anterior wall of the lateral ventricles. The thalamus, the largest diencephalic structure, is located posteriorly in the floor of the ventricular cavity. Removal of parietal and occipital tissues has also exposed the caudal portion of the lateral ventricles, particularly the

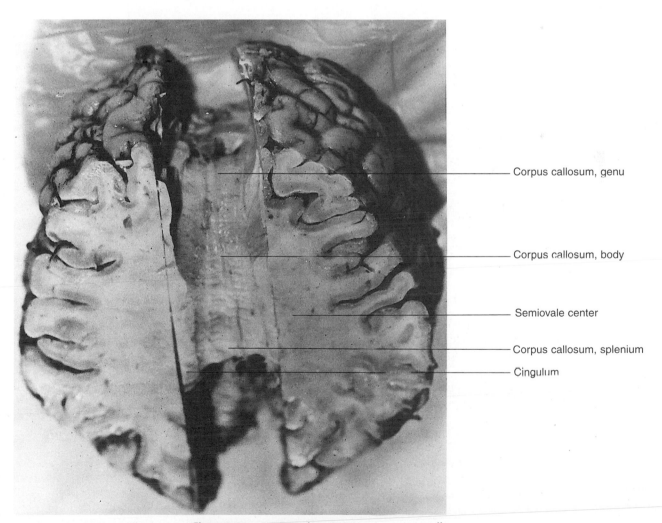

Corpus callosum, genu

Corpus callosum, body

Semiovale center

Corpus callosum, splenium

Cingulum

Figure 3-28.   Horizontal section exposing corpus callosum.

posterior horns in the occipital lobes. The remaining genu, body, and splenium portions of the corpus callosum are easily identified above the lateral ventricles. Also present is the point at which the tail of the caudate nucleus enters the temporal lobe.

Further removal of the overlying white medullary substance, caudate nucleus, and thalamus by sectioning rostral to the genu of the corpus callosum exposes the cavity of the lateral ventricles and the surrounding subcortical structures (Fig. 3-30). The exposed inner temporal lobe contains the slender temporal horns of the lateral ventricles. The **hippocampus**, **amygdala**, and **uncus** are located medially in the infe-

rior horn. The hippocampus forms the medial wall of the temporal horns. It receives direct projections from the fornix and indirect projections from the cingulum via the **parahippocampal gyrus**. Anterior to tip of the hippocampus is the amygdaloid nucleus, an important limbic structure with a protruding cortical component called the uncus. With the callosal fibers absent, the floor of the lateral ventricles becomes visible. The septum is seen rostrally, separating the anterior horns of the lateral ventricles. The structure at the base of the septum is the **fornix column**. Also present are the head of the caudate nucleus, the medial dorsal thalamus, and the third ventricle.

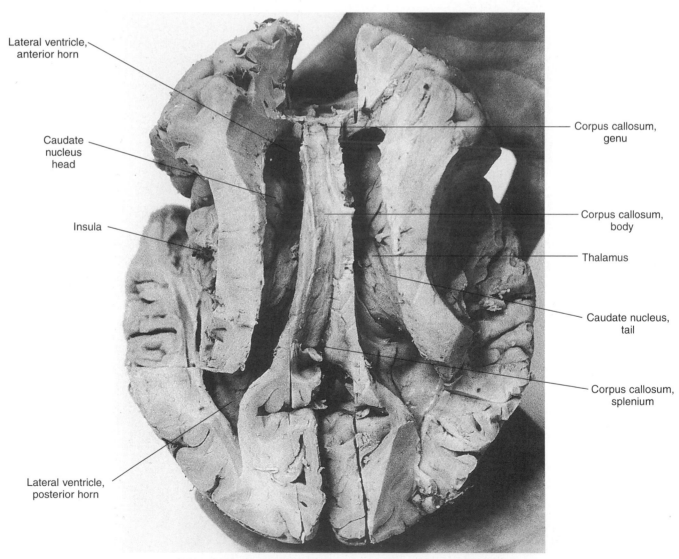

Figure 3-29.   Horizontal section exposing ventricles and basal ganglia.

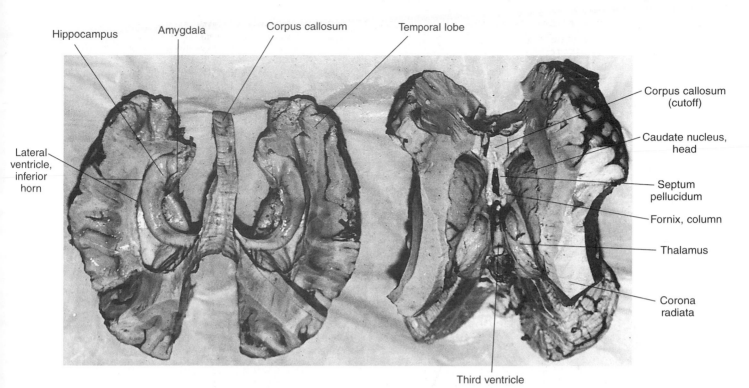

Figure 3-30. Horizontal section where sectioning of corpus callosum from adjacent cortical structure separately exposes hippocampus, ventricular cavity, and basal ganglia structure.

SUMMARY

Knowledge of the internal brain anatomy is the most important part of training in neuroscience and is best learned by repeated studying of internal structures on the serial sections of the spinal cord, brainstem, and forebrain and by relating structures to their functions. Visual orientation to structures and functional knowledge of the internal anatomy are essential, the basis for overall understanding of brain structures and their relation to clinical symptoms.

Technical Terms

amygdaloid nucleus
anterior medullary velum
caudate nucleus
central gray
cerebral aqueduct
choroid plexus
cingulate gyrus
collateral trigone
corona radiata
fornix
hippocampus (hippocampal formation)
hypothalamus
inferior cerebellar peduncle (restiform body)
inferior colliculus
insula (isle of Reil)
internal arcuate fibers
lateral geniculate body
lateral lemniscus
medial geniculate body
medial lemniscus
medial longitudinal fasciculus
middle cerebellar peduncle (brachium pontis)
pineal
principal (inferior) olivary nucleus
pyramidal decussation
red nucleus
reticular formation
semiovale center
spinocerebellar tract
substantia nigra
subthalamic nucleus
superior cerebellar peduncle (brachium conjunctivum)
superior colliculus
thalamus

Review Questions

1. Define the following terms:
   amygdaloid nucleus
   anterior medullary velum
   cerebral aqueduct
   corona radiata
   inferior cerebellar peduncle (restiform body)
   inferior colliculus
   insula (isle of Reil)
   internal arcuate fibers
   lateral geniculate body
   lateral lemniscus
   medial geniculate body
   medial lemniscus
   medial longitudinal fasciculus
   middle cerebellar peduncle (brachium pontis)
   pineal
   principal (inferior) olivary nucleus
   pyramidal decussation
   red nucleus
   reticular formation
   semiovale center
   spinocerebellar tract
   substantia nigra
   subthalamic nucleus
   superior cerebellar peduncle (brachium conjunctivum)
   superior colliculus
2. Describe changes related to the shape of descending fibers and the ventricular cavity at different neuraxial levels.
3. Discuss the clinical implications of the decussation of sensory and motor fibers in the medulla.
4. Identify three or four landmark structures of the internal medulla and describe their functions.
5. What ventricular cavity is located in the rostral medulla?
6. Identify three or four landmarks of the internal pons and discuss their functions.
7. Discuss the function of the corticopontine fibers that decussate in the pons.

8. Discuss the clinical implications of decussation of the corticocerebellar and cerebellar–cortical fibers.
9. Name structures surrounding the similar-looking inferior and superior colliculi on a cross-section of the midbrain.
10. What ventricular cavity separates the tectal and tegmental areas in the midbrain?
11. Describe the difference between tectal and tegmental regions in the midbrain.
12. Name three structures ventral to the cerebral aqueduct and dorsal to the crus cerebri (pes pedunculi).
13. Name four major internal structures of the midbrain and describe their functions.
14. What cavity forms the medial boundary of the thalamus?
15. What limb of the internal capsule separates the thalamus from the lateral basal ganglia?
16. What forms the roof of the lateral ventricles?
17. Why are the thalamus and caudate head not present on a single coronal section of the forebrain?
18. What structure forms the medial wall of the lateral ventricle at the level of the inferior ventricular horn?
19. Discuss the function of the substantia nigra and describe symptoms associated with its degeneration.
20. Describe the role of the red nucleus in cerebellar projections to the cortex and spinal cord.
21. Explain why a hemorrhage in the right caudal pons involving corticospinal fibers and facial nerves would cause right-sided facial weakness and left hemiplegia.
22. Explain the function of the medial lemniscus.
23. Name the structure medial to the lenticular nucleus but lateral to the thalamus.
24. List the structures on a cross-section of the high cervical spinal cord.
25. Cranial nerve III exits the midbrain close to the corticospinal (pes pedunculi) fibers. Vascular pathology of the nerve and motor fibers on the left result in motor symptoms on which side or sides of the body?
26. Name the most posterior thalamic nucleus.
27. What forms the medial wall of the lateral ventricles at the frontal horn level?
28. Describe the function of the fasciculus gracilis.
29. A hemorrhage in the dorsal lateral region of the caudal medulla involving the fibers of the fasciculus gracilis and cuneatus is likely to result in what symptoms?

Embryological Development of the Central Nervous System[a]

Learning Objectives

After studying this chapter, students should be able to do the following:

- Define important embryological terms
- Describe the developmental processes of sperm and ova from a single cell leading to adult form
- Explain human development during the first 3 weeks
- Discuss the ways in which central and peripheral nervous systems form
- Construct a flow diagram of human development from the zygote to derivatives of the three germ layers
- Discuss the critical periods of susceptibility to teratogenesis for central nervous system and for other related organ systems
- Describe common cerebrospinal malformations

HUMAN CHROMOSOMES, GENES, AND CELL DIVISION

The normal number of human somatic chromosomes is 46. Of these, 22 pairs are alike in both sexes and are called autosomes (Fig. 4-1). The remaining pair constitutes the sex chromosomes and is designated XY in males and XX in females. Thus, there are 24 types of human chromosomes (22 autosomes, X, and Y).

The diploid human **genome** comprises about 6 billion to 7 billion base pairs of DNA arranged linearly on the autosomes and sex chromosomes. Molecularly defined, a **gene** is the sequence of chromosomal DNA required for a functional product—a polypeptide or an RNA molecule—to be produced. The human genome

consists of 31,778 known genes and gene predictions that encode equal number of proteins. This number is still uncertain and is constantly changing (see Lander et al., 2001, Nature 409, p.902, Table 23). Except for the small mitochondrial chromosome, each chromosome is made up of a single continuous DNA double helix or DNA molecule. These DNA molecules have been estimated to range in size from about 50 million base pairs for the smallest (chromosome 21) to 250 million base pairs for the largest (chromosome 1). The DNA molecule appears along with **histones** (chromosomal proteins) and other proteins. The DNA and protein complex combined is called the **chromatin**.

Cell division is indispensable for living organisms. Whereas the embryonic cells and some adult cells divide by **mitosis** (equal division), sex cells, or gametes, form by a special type of cell division called **meiosis**. Meiosis is the reduction division that occurs during gametogenesis. In meiosis, the chromosome number is reduced to half the usual number, ensuring the constancy of chromosome numbers from generation to generation. Maternal and paternal chromosomes are independently assorted and crossed over, which shuffles the genes. This recombines genetic material.

Mitosis has four phases: prophase, metaphase, anaphase, and telophase. During prophase, the chromosomes make their appearance within the nucleus and double longitudinally (fold in half), forming two chromatids united at a centromere. The nuclear envelope breaks down, and kinetochore fibers form. This stage is also called the prometaphase. The chromosomes then arrange themselves on the equatorial plate, or metaphase plate. The chromosomes move apart during anaphase and reach spindle poles during telophase. The division of the cytoplasm takes place and leads to the formation of two sibling cells. The increase in cell

---

[a] This chapter was written by Kunwar P. Bhatnagar, PhD, Department of Anatomical Sciences and Neurobiology, University of Louisville School of Medicine, Louisville, Kentucky.

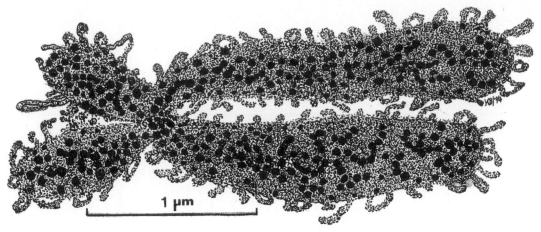

1 μm

Figure 4-1. Electron micrographic representation of an unsectioned human chromosome 12 from a dividing cell. Chromosome is divided in half along its length (into two chromatids) except at centromere. This chromosome contains about 4 cm of DNA double helix per chromatid. Some looping and coiling that allows packing of all this DNA into a chromosome 3 μm long is visible (×40,200).

numbers and hence in the growth of the tissue leads to development. Details of mitosis should be sought in other textbooks.

EARLY HUMAN DEVELOPMENT

Even though human development is a continuous process, it is best to consider it beginning with **gametogenesis**, or the formation of male and female gametes, the spermatozoa and the ova, respectively. With the union of spermatozoon and ovum (secondary oocyte), fertilization is complete. The large cell that results is called a **zygote**. The zygote undergoes repeated divisions, giving rise to the multicellular human form.

Gametogenesis

The formation of germ cells called gametes (spermatozoa and ova) involves the halving of chromosomes (i.e., they become haploid from diploid) and an alteration in cell shape. The reduction of chromosome number, from 46,XY for males and 46,XX for females to 23,Y for males or 23,X for females, occurs during a unique process of cell division called meiosis (Figs. 4-2 and 4-3). The other process of cell division is mitosis, in which the chromosome numbers remain the same.

During gametogenesis, two meiotic divisions occur one after the other. During the first meiotic division, the homologous chromosomes (one from each parent) in the primary spermatocyte or oocyte pair in **prophase** (Fig. 4-2*A*). They separate during **anaphase**, with each chromosome going to the two poles of the cell (Fig. 4-2*E*). Therefore, at the end of this process, each of the two resulting cells (the secondary spermatocyte or oocyte) contains half of the original number of chromosomes

(Fig. 4-2*G*). This **disjunction** of homologous chromosomes enables the separation of the **allelic genes** during meiosis. Without an interphase (break in the process of cell division), the second meiotic division follows. Each chromosome, consisting of two **chromatids**, divides, with each chromatid drawn to opposite poles of the cell during division (Fig. 4-2, *F* and *G*). The haploid number of chromosomes in the resulting daughter cells is maintained. Meiosis ensures that the number of chromosomes between generations remains the same and that chromosomes are recombined to create a balance of genetic material from both parents. **Nondisjunction** causes abnormal gametes that actually become congenitally malformed babies. During gametogenesis, each primary spermatocyte gives rise to four spermatozoa. However, each primary oocyte develops into only one mature ovum and three nonfunctional **polar bodies** that soon degenerate. This entire process is diagrammed in Figure 4-3, but detailed accounts of the process should be sought in an embryology textbook.

In the human male, spermatogonia lie dormant in the testes from the fetal period through puberty. Spermatogenesis begins at puberty and continues through life. Associated genes BMP8B, DAZ, and paternal effect genes influence gametogenesis. In the human female, however, oogenesis begins before birth. All oogonia develop into primary oocytes before birth and are retained as primordial follicles, possibly as many as 2 million. These begin the first meiotic division before birth. However, prophase is not complete until after puberty, at which time no more than 40,000 primary oocytes can be seen. Of these, it is estimated that only about 400 become secondary oocytes and are expelled one at a time on a monthly cycle (see Moore and Persaud in the suggested

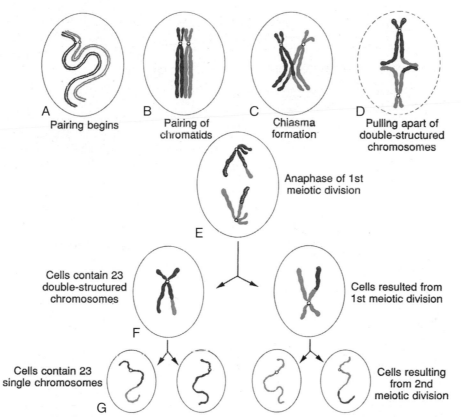

Figure 4-2. First and second meiotic divisions. **A.** Homologous chromosomes approach each other. **B.** Homologous chromosomes pair, and each member of pair consists of two chromatids. **C.** Intimately paired homologous chromosomes interchange chromatid fragments (crossover); note chiasma. **D.** Double-structured chromosomes pull apart. **E.** Anaphase of first meiotic division. **F** and **G.** During second meiotic division double-structured chromosomes split at centromere. At completion of division, chromosomes in each of the four daughter cells are different from each other.

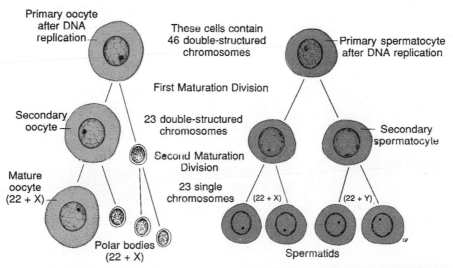

Figure 4-3. Reduction in number of chromosomes during maturation divisions. **A.** Female germ cell. **B.** Male germ cell.

reading list). Thus the entire reproductive period of a human female can be considered to last only about 400 months, or 33 years, from puberty to age 45 years. A small number of the expelled ova never reach the status of secondary oocytes.

Fertilization and First Week of Development

Once spermatozoa and the secondary oocyte are united, human development begins. Only one spermatozoon can gain entry through the thick zona pellucida surrounding the secondary oocyte. Binding of spermatozoon to zona pellucida is brought about by the molecules ZP3, SP56, ZRK, and galactosyl transferase. At the time of contact between the two gametes, the secondary oocyte completes the second meiotic division and becomes a mature ovum. Its nucleus becomes the female pronucleus. The head of the spermatozoon forms the male pronucleus. With the fusion of these pronuclei, a **zygote** is formed. Within 24 hours of ovulation fertilization is complete, the diploid number of chromosomes is restored, and sex and species variation are determined. The zygote then begins to divide slowly by mitotic division. The molecules MPF, cyclins, and cdc 25 phosphatase participate in cleavage. The new cells, called **blastomeres**, gradually become smaller because

they remain confined within the zona pellucida. After the two-, three-, and four-cell stages, the ball of 12 to 16 blastomeres is called a **morula** (Fig. 4-4).

This stage, about 3 days after fertilization, occurs when the morula enters the uterus. The morula develops a central cavity—the blastocyst cavity—that gets larger as more uterine fluid gains access to it. Cells are now clustered into an outer ringlike cell mass, or trophoblast, and a group of cell clusters, the inner cell mass, or embryoblast (Fig. 4-5). The blastocyst formation plays a role in the adhesion molecules, including cadherins. The blastocyst remains free in the uterine cavity for about 2 days, during which time the zona pellucida gradually degenerates, allowing the blastocyst to grow in all directions. About 6 days after fertilization, the blastocyst attaches to the uterine endometrium at the embryonic pole, most frequently on the upper part of the posterior fundic wall near the midsagittal plane. Week 1 of human development begins with fertilization and ends with the blastocyst superficially implanted in the uterine lining or endometrium.

Second Week of Development

In week 2, the blastocyst becomes completely implanted, and the **bilaminar embryo** develops. Other

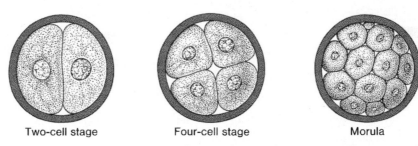

Two-cell stage   Four-cell stage   Morula

Figure 4-4.   Development of zygote from two-cell stage to late morula stage. Two-cell stage is reached approximately 30 hours after fertilization; four-cell stage, at approximately 40 hours; 12- and 16-cell stage, at approximately 3 days; late morula stage, at approximately 4 days.

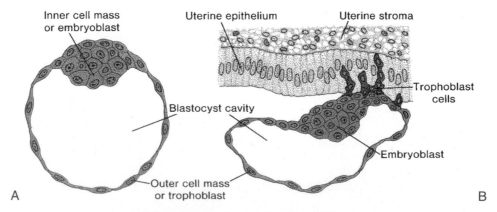

Figure 4-5.   **A.** Section through a human blastocyst recovered from uterine cavity at approximately 4.5 days. **B.** A section of a blastocyst at day 9 of development. Human blastocyst begins to penetrate uterine mucosa probably by day 5 or 6.

structures that develop during this period are the **cytotrophoblast** and **syncytiotrophoblast** (both differentiated from the trophoblast), **amniotic cavity**, **amnion**, **chorion**, **primary** and **secondary yolk sacs**, **connecting stalk**, **chorionic cavity** or **extraembryonic coelom**, ex-

traembryonic mesoderm, and the two components of the bilaminar embryo, the **epiblast** and the **hypoblast**. Another important structure develops: the prechordal plate, a thickened cranial region of the hypoblast and epiblast combined; it is the site of the future mouth (Fig. 4-6).

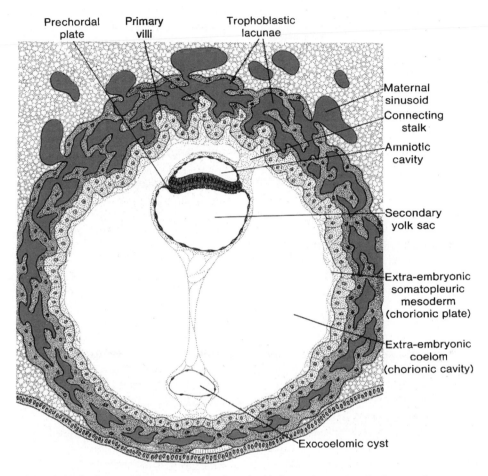

Figure 4-6. A 13-day human blastocyst completely embedded in endometrium. Dark region between amniotic cavity and secondary yolk sac is bilaminar germ disk.

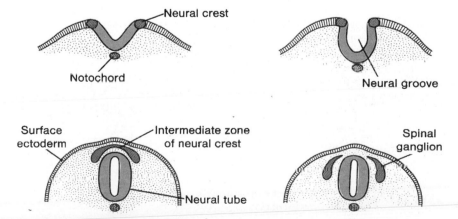

Figure 4-7. Transverse sections through successively older embryos, showing formation of neural crest (**A**), neural groove (**B**), and neural tube (**C**). Cells of neural crest, initially forming an intermediate zone between neural tube and surface ectoderm (**C**), develop into spinal and cranial sensory ganglia (**D**) and other structures.

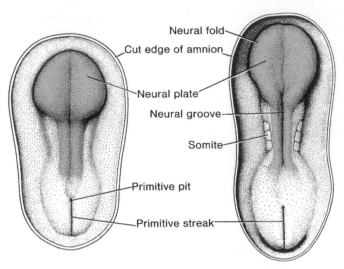

Figure 4-8. **A.** Dorsal view of a late presomite embryo (approximately 18 days); amnion has been removed, and neural plate is clearly visible. **B.** Dorsal view at approximately 20 days; note somites, neural groove, and neural folds.

Third Week of Development

Week 3 coincides with the week following the first missed menstrual period, that is, the fifth week after the onset of the last normal menstrual period. The embryo becomes **trilaminar**, having developed the three germ layers: **ectoderm**, **mesoderm**, and **endoderm**. A caudal midline thickening on the dorsal embryonic disk forms. Through this **primitive streak**, epiblastic cells move between the epiblast and the hypoblast, ultimately giving rise to the mesoderm, the shaded area lateral to the neural tube, and the **notochord** (Fig. 4-7). The notochord is the first skeletal structure that develops, and it is retained in the adult intervertebral disks as the **nucleus pulposus**. Mesodermal masses arrange themselves segmentally into paired **somites** (Fig. 4-8), which give rise to muscles and other tissues. The **allantois** appears, and the **neural plate**, the forerunner of the nervous system, develops. The **neural crest** separates as the **neural tube** closes and gives rise to numerous components of the peripheral nervous system. Any disturbance in the development of the neural plate results in severe abnormalities of the nervous system. The intraembryonic coelom, the primitive placenta, and the cardiovascular system, including the plasma and blood cells, also develop in week 3. Among the 8 weeks of embryonic development, week 3 can be considered the most significant because of the definitive beginnings of numerous structures.

DEVELOPMENT OF THE CENTRAL NERVOUS SYSTEM

Development of the brain and spinal cord begins early in week 3 of gestation under the inductive influence of the notochord and the paraxial mesoderm adja-

cent to it. Neurulation is one of several important processes that begin during the trilaminar stage of human development and is complete by the end of week 4. The entire trilaminar stage is completed in week 3.

The 2-week embryo (Fig. 4-6) is essentially in the form of a bilaminar embryonic disk having two layers: the epiblast and hypoblast. The primitive streak forms under the influence of the following molecules: **nodal**, **goosecoid**, **lim-1**, and **hnf-1**. The notochord forms under the expression of the **sonic hedgehog gene**. As the embryo enters week 3, epiblastic cells give rise to endoderm and mesoderm through the region of the primitive streak. The remaining epiblastic cells are now called ectodermal cells. The hypoblast moves to form the secondary yolk sac. Thus in week 3 three primary germ layers (ectoderm, mesoderm, and endoderm) are established. Anterior to the primitive streak, the ectodermal cells in the dorsal midline of the embryonic disk thicken to become the neuroectodermal layer, the forerunner of the entire central and peripheral nervous system.

Neural Plate, Neural Tube, and Neural Crest

The neuroectoderm overlying the midline notochord thickens to form the neural plate, cranial to the primitive knot. The neural plate later extends caudally with the receding primitive streak. On day 18, the neural plate invaginates along the midline to form a neural groove flanked by neural folds on either side (Fig. 4-7). At this time, some neuroectodermal cells on the crest of each neural fold are identifiable. These cells first fuse and later split to lie on the right and left sides of the **neural tube** when it closes on approximately day 22. The neural tube develops into the brain and the spinal cord, and the segmentally arranged **neural crest** tissue develops into the **cranial** and **spinal ganglia**, **nerve sheaths**, **postganglionic autonomic nerves**, and other structures (Figs. 4-7, 4-8, and 4-12). The neural tube soon separates from the adjacent ectoderm and differentiates into a **posterior** (**dorsal**) alar lamina or **alar plate** and an **anterior** (**ventral**) basal lamina or **basal plate**. These two regions are separated by a groove, the sulcus limitans, midway on the inner surface of the lateral walls of the neural tube. The gap over the neural tube is bridged dorsally by ectoderm that will become skin. Mesoderm will later develop into the bony cranial vault and the vertebral column around the central nervous system.

Brain

Early in week 4 (days 22–23), the cranial two-thirds of the neural tube represents the future brain, whereas the caudal third represents the future spinal cord. The fusion of the neural folds occurs irregularly. The resulting neural tube is open first at both cranial and caudal ends (Fig. 4-9). The cranial opening (rostral or anterior neuropore) closes on day 25. The caudal, or posterior,

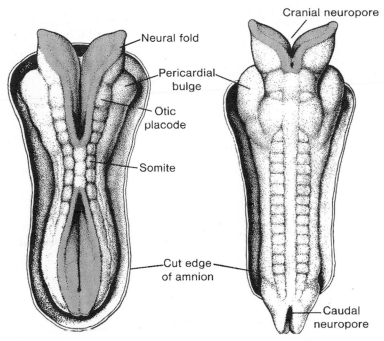

Figure 4-9.   A. Dorsal view of a human embryo at approximately day 22. Seven distinct somites are visible in each side of neural tube. **B.** Dorsal view of human embryo at approximately day 23. The central canal is in communication with the amniotic cavity through the open cranial and caudal neuropores.

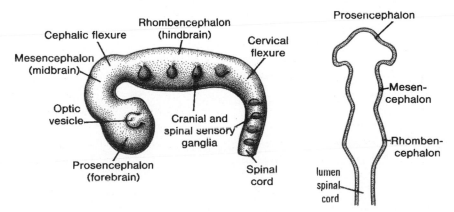

Figure 4-10.   A. Lateral view of brain vesicles and part of spinal cord in a 4-week embryo. Note sensory ganglia formed by neural crest on each side of rhombencephalon and spinal cord. **B.** Lumina of three brain vesicles and spinal cord.

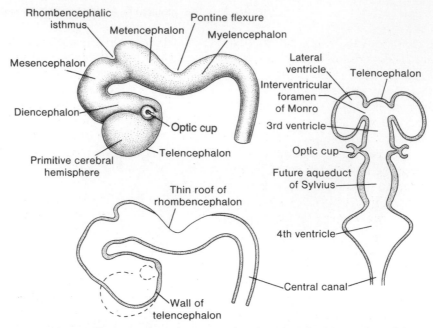

Figure 4-11. **A.** Lateral view of brain vesicles in beginning of week 6. **B.** Midline section through brain vesicles and spinal cord in beginning of week 6; note thin roof of rhombencephalon. **C.** Lumina of spinal cord and brain vesicles in beginning of week 6.

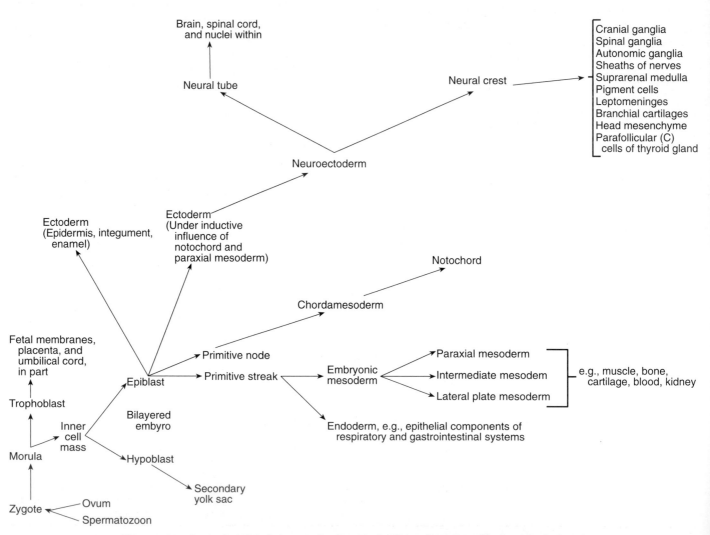

Figure 4-12. Stages during early human development leading to formation of brain and spinal cord.

neuropore closes 2 days later. In the brain, the final closure of the anterior neuropore is represented by the **lamina terminalis**; the representation of the closure of the posterior neuropore would have to be sought within the filum terminale. As the neural folds fuse dorsocranially and the rostral neuropore closes, three primary brain vesicles form. The brain proper develops from the following vesicles that are formed during week 4: prosencephalon, or forebrain; mesencephalon, or midbrain; and rhombencephalon, or hindbrain (Figs. 4-10 and 4-11). A week later, the prosencephalon develops into two secondary vesicles, the telencephalon and the diencephalon. Likewise, the rhombencephalon develops into the metencephalon and myelencephalon. The mesencephalon does not divide. The brain is now represented by five secondary brain vesicles, each with its own wall of neuroectoderm that gives rise to motor, sensory, association, and preganglionic autonomic neurons, glia, and ependyma. Cavities in each vesicle differentiate into brain ventricles (Table 4-1).

Three brain flexures, or bends, develop with the rapid growth and folding of the brain. The midbrain and cervical flexures develop ventrally in the midbrain region and at the junction of the hindbrain and spinal cord. The pontine flexure develops dorsally between these two flexures, thinning the roof of the hindbrain.

PROSENCEPHALON, OR FOREBRAIN

The forebrain develops into two subdivisions, the telencephalon and the diencephalon.

Telencephalon

Early in week 4, a pair of lateral outgrowths from the forebrain appears. These optic vesicles are the primordia for retinas and optic nerves (Fig. 4-10). Soon another pair of diverticula, the telencephalic vesicles, appears dorsal and rostral to the optic vesicles. These grow into cerebral hemispheres, each with a lateral ventricle. The median connection between the cerebral vesicles develops into the lamina terminalis, the site of closure of the rostral neuropore. The cerebral vesicles give rise to three main structures: olfactory lobe, corpus striatum (caudate nucleus and lentiform nucleus), and cerebral cortex.

The olfactory lobe consists of the olfactory bulb, olfactory tract, anterior perforated substance, and certain other olfactory structures collectively known as the pyriform lobe. The olfactory parts of the brain constitute the rhinencephalon (see Chapter 15).

The entire forebrain is considered to be an alar lamina derivative. The cerebral cortex in early development consists of three concentric zones: a germinal zone surrounding the lateral ventricles, an intermediate zone that becomes the white matter, and an outer cortical zone that develops into the six-layered isocortex. The olfactory cortex, together with the hippocampal formation and dentate gyrus, constitutes the allocortex, because these do not have six layers.

The cerebral hemispheres are smooth (lissencephalic) up to about 20 weeks. By week 24, various sulci and gyri gradually appear. At birth, all topographical features of the adult brain are present. The various lobes (frontal, parietal, occipital, temporal, and insula) become clearly identifiable during the third trimester. Commissures connecting the right and left hemispheres develop. The principal ones are the anterior commissure, commissure of the fornix, corpus callosum, habenular commissure, and posterior commissure. The last two develop in relation to the pineal body.

Table 4-1. Development of Human Brain (See Figs. 4-10 and 4-11)

Week 3	Week 4	Week 5	Weeks 6–12[a]		
			Cavity	Alar Lamina	Basal Lamina
Neural tube	Prosencephalon	Telencephalon	Lateral ventricles, choroid plexus; rostral third ventricle	Cerebral hemispheres, cortex, corpus striatum	None
		Diencephalon	Caudal part of third ventricle, choroid plexus	Thalamus, hypothalamus, epithalamus, including pineal body	None
	Mesencephalon	Mesencephalon	Cerebral aqueduct	Tectum: superior and inferior colliculus	Cerebral peduncles, tegmentum
	Rhombencephalon	Isthmus rhombencephali	Rostral part of fourth ventricle	Superior cerebellar peduncles	
		Metencephalon	Middle part of fourth ventricle	Cerebellum, middle cerebellar peduncles, sensory nuclei of cranial nerves V, VIII (in part)	Pons
		Myelencephalon	Posterior fourth ventricle, choroid plexus	Inferior cerebellar peduncles, sensory relay nuclei of cranial nerves VII, IX, X (in part)	Medulla oblongata

[a] "Many embryologists consider that the prosencephalon is formed of alar laminae alone" (Hamilton et al., 1972:470 in suggested reading list).

Diencephalon

The caudal forebrain develops into the diencephalon. Its cavity is the third ventricle, to which small contributions are added from the telencephalic cavities. The epithalamus, thalamus, metathalamus, hypothalamus, and subthalamus develop in the lateral walls of the third ventricle that constitute the diencephalon. The epithalamus differentiates into the pineal body, habenular trigone, stria medullaris, tenia thalami, and posterior commissure. The posterior commissure separates the diencephalon from the mesencephalon. The thalamus is a huge structure. Its rapid development reduces the third ventricle to a narrow cavity. In about 70% of humans the two thalami fuse, forming the massa intermedia. The medial and lateral geniculate bodies constitute the metathalamus. The hypothalamus develops into the inferior lateral wall and floor of the third ventricle. The optic chiasm, infundibulum, tuber cinereum, mamillary bodies, and neurohypophysis are grossly identifiable hypothalamic structures. The subthalamus is small, and it lies between the thalamus and the tegmentum.

The pituitary gland, or hypophysis, develops during weeks 4 and 5. An ectodermal diverticulum grows dorsally from the roof of the mouth cavity and comes into close contact with the ventral diencephalic diverticulum, the infundibulum. These two diverticula develop into the adenohypophysis, which consists of the pars distalis, pars tuberalis, and pars intermedia, and the neurohypophysis, which consists of the pars nervosa, infundibular stem, and median eminence, respectively. The commonly known anterior lobe consists of the pars distalis and pars tuberalis. The posterior lobe comprises the pars intermedia and pars nervosa.

MESENCEPHALON, OR MIDBRAIN

The midbrain is the least modified subdivision. The superior and inferior colliculi form in its roof, or tectum. The superior colliculi relay visual impulses. The inferior colliculi relay auditory impulses. The basal laminae become the tegmentum, which includes red nuclei, substantia nigra, reticular nuclei, and nuclei of cranial nerves III and IV. The substantia nigra and cerebral peduncles develop anteriorly.

RHOMBENCEPHALON, OR HINDBRAIN

The hindbrain develops into the metencephalon (pons and cerebellum) and the myelencephalon (medulla oblongata), whereas its cavity develops into the fourth ventricle and central canal, respectively, both of which continue into the spinal cord.

Metencephalon

The region of the brainstem (pons, medulla oblongata, mesencephalon, and diencephalon) through which nerve fibers connect the cerebellar and cerebral cortices with the spinal cord develops in the anterior region of the metencephalon as the pons. The tegmental part of the pons is derived from the basal laminae. The pons receives contributions from the alar laminae of the myelencephalon.

The cerebellum is derived from the dorsal alar laminae of the metencephalon that comes together as the rhombic lips. The cranial region of each rhombic lip thickens, forming the cerebellar rudiment that later fuses with its opposite. The extraventricular portion, which does not project into the fourth ventricle, becomes larger. By the end of the fourth month, it develops a small midline vermis, the lateral lobes, and surface fissures. Development of secondary fissures gives rise to the characteristic folia of the cerebellum.

Myelencephalon

The future medulla oblongata develops from the most caudal brain region, the myelencephalon. It is continuous with the brainstem superiorly and the spinal cord inferiorly. Here, the sulcus limitans divides the alar lamina and the basal lamina in such a manner that the alar region lies lateral to the basal lamina. The bilaminar roof plate in the region of the fourth ventricle consists of an outer thin layer of pia mater and an inner layer of ependymal cells. Together these two layers constitute the tela choroidea, which projects into the fourth ventricle (and into other ventricles in a similar manner) as the choroid plexus. Two lateral apertures (foramina of Luschka) and a median aperture (foramen of Magendie) connect the fourth ventricle as well as the entire ventricular system, including the spinal central canal, with the cerebellomedullary cistern.

Spinal Cord

As the neural tube begins to close, its walls thicken and stratify. Three layers, an inner ependymal, a middle mantle, and an external marginal, differentiate. As the layers develop by proliferation of neuroblasts, they give rise to alar and basal laminae, roof and floor plates, and a sulcus limitans that separates the alar from the basal regions. With the formation of the anterior median fissure, the central canal is greatly reduced in size. The large neuroblasts near the central canal rapidly divide and form neurons and neuroglia. The mantle layer develops into gray matter, and the marginal layer becomes the white matter of the spinal cord.

CLINICAL CONSIDERATIONS

Abnormal Development of the Central Nervous System

The brain and spinal cord, with the exception of the cerebellum, reach the full complement of neurons by week 25 of gestation. After this point and well into the postnatal years, glial cells develop and multiply, various neuronal processes develop, and synaptogenesis occurs. Glial cells proliferate from midgestation to the end of the second postnatal year and beyond. Myelinogenesis begins at the end of the first trimester (month 3 of gestation) and extends to age 4. In embryogenesis, the timing is more detrimental than the nature of the insult in causing cerebrospinal malformation; hence **teratogenesis** is a timing specific (Table 4-2) and insult nonspecific phenomenon. Of the patients with cerebrospinal disorders admitted to hospitals, some 90% relate to neural tube

closure, notably spina bifida cystica and anencephaly. Table 4-3 summarizes the critical periods and relative vulnerability of neural regions to insults leading to specific defects.

ANENCEPHALY

Defective fusion of the neural tube results in anencephaly, in which the cranial vault is congenitally absent. Cerebral hemispheres are either missing or highly reduced and attached to the base of the skull. This

Table 4-2. Teratogenic Sensitivity of Some Developing Human Organ Systems

Preembryonic (Weeks 1–2)	Embryonic (Weeks 3–8)	Fetal (Weeks 9–38)	Postnatal[a]
Either not susceptible to teratogens when only few cells are damaged and embryo recovers or most cells are affected, resulting in death	3–16	CNS	Cerebellum[a]
	4–8	Eyes	
	4–9	Ear 16	
	6–8	Teeth	
	6–8	Palate	
	3–6 Heart		
	5–6 Lip		

Dark red, major congenital defects; light red, minor defects or functional malformations. CNS, central nervous system.
[a] DNA synthesis has been reported in cerebellar granular layer during first few years after birth; antiviral therapy in infants may cause extensive damage to developing cerebellar neurons (Langman et al., 1972). Other brain regions are also known to continue mitotic division of neurons postnatally.

Table 4-3. Critical Periods of Development of Human Central Nervous System

Age (days)	Developmental Stage	Malformation
14	Bilaminar germ disk	Not vulnerable; either all cells are damaged resulting in death or only few cells affected and may recover fully
18	Neural plate and neural groove	Anterior midline defects
22	Optic vesicles	Hydrocephalus
25	Rostral neuropore (anterior neuropore) closes	Anencephaly (after 23 days to ?), exencephaly, meroanencephaly
27	Caudal neuropore (posterior neuropore) closes	Cranium bifidum, spina bifida cystica, spina bifida occulta (after 26 days to ?)
32	Cerebellar primordium	Microcephaly (30–130 days)
33–35	Five cerebral vesicles, choroid plexuses, dorsal root ganglia	
56	Differentiation of cerebral cortex, meninges, ventricular foramina, cerebrospinal fluid circulation	
70–100	Corpus callosum	
140–175	Neuronal proliferation in central nervous system (except cerebellum) fully completed	Defects of cellular circuitry, myelin defects
175 days–4 years postnatally	Neuronal migration, glia, and myelin formation, synaptic connections	

abnormality has an incidence of 1:1,000 deliveries, occurring most commonly in female infants. Affected infants do not survive beyond a few hours or days after birth. Indications of the defects include absence of the optic nerves, although the eyes appear normal (Fig. 4-13), and exposure or herniation of cerebral tissue. Folic acid with a multivitamin preparation taken by the mother even before conception has been used to prevent such a defect. Anencephaly is incompatible with extrauterine existence; survival in many cases lasts between 3 to 48 hours after birth.

CRANIUM BIFIDUM

Cranium bifidum is a condition in which bone fusion is prevented in the posterior midline of the skull. As a result, the brain or spinal cord protrudes through this opening.

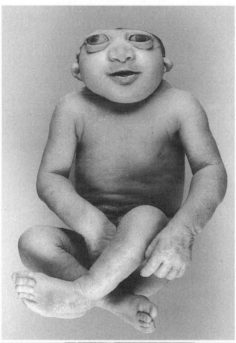
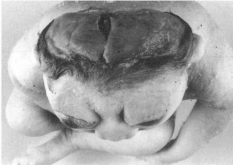

Figure 4-13. Female anencephalic newborn. **A.** Front view; note large eyes and absence of cranial vault. **B.** Dorsal view of head showing exposed, poorly formed brain.

SPINA BIFIDA

When a defect similar to cranium bifidum occurs in the vertebral column, it is called spina bifida. The latter condition has several subtypes depending on severity and tissue involvement. In **spina bifida cystica**, posterior vertebral arches fail to fuse, and meninges herniate but neural tissues do not; lumbar or lumbosacral defects are very common. In **spina bifida occulta**, the skin of the back is epithelialized and always shows a surface marking in the form of a dimple, a dermal sinus, or a hairy region. Several skin, spinal cord, and bone deformities of this kind can be revealed through radiograms. These defects are extremely common.

HYDROCEPHALUS

Hydrocephalus is characterized by an enlarged head, a prominent forehead, brain atrophy, mental deficiency, and convulsions. Cerebral ventricles enlarge because of excessive production of cerebrospinal fluid and/or obstruction of the cerebrospinal fluid drainage pathways. Hydrocephalus is caused by the obstruction of cerebrospinal fluid circulation. The ventricles are enlarged and the cerebral mantle is thin. Neurologic findings are abnormal.

MICROCEPHALY

Microcephaly is an uncommon condition in which the brain and calvaria (skull cap) are small but the face is normal. Because the brain is underdeveloped, infants with this condition are mentally retarded. Environmental disturbances, genetic abnormalities, and ionizing radiation during the critical period of central nervous system development have been implicated as primary causes of the defect.

Other less common abnormalities of the nervous system include craniorachischisis, encephalocele, meningocele, cyclopia, and agenesis of the cortex, corpus callosum, and cerebellum.

Peripheral Nervous System

NORMAL DEVELOPMENT

The peripheral nervous system is composed of cranial and spinal ganglia and nerves and the ganglia and nerves of the autonomic nervous system. The suprarenal gland medulla, which is derived from the postganglionic sympathetic neurons, also falls in this category. Of the 12 pairs of cranial nerves, 4 (III, VII, IX, and X) belong to the cranial parasympathetic system. Likewise, the S-2, S-3, and S-4 spinal nerves form the components of the sacral parasympathetic system.

The peripheral nervous system as a whole is derived from the neural tube. This is the case because the motor nuclei for all cranial and spinal nerves, along with all preganglionic neurons for the autonomic nervous system, are derived from the neural tube. Both are within the brain and the spinal cord. Therefore, axons of all such neurons, even though they collectively form peripheral nerves, are derived from the central nervous system. The spinal or dorsal root ganglia, sensory ganglia of the cranial nerves, all autonomic ganglia, and postganglionic autonomic neurons are derived from the neural crest in a similar manner from tissue that separated from the closing neural tube. The suprarenal medulla, the mucosal and submucosal enteric ganglia, the capsular cells that enclose the sensory nerve bodies, and myelin-producing Schwann cells also develop from the neural crest. Some cranial ganglia (cranial nerves IX and X) and the first order olfactory and accessory olfactory (vomeronasal) neurons arise not from the neural tube but from the surface ectoderm, that is, a placode origin.

Variations in muscles are fairly common. In these cases, the nerves to such muscles develop abnormally. Sternocleidomastoid muscle fibrosis, absence of the head of the pectoralis major muscle, and appearance of the sternalis muscle are all examples of muscle abnormalities that cause abnormal development of nerves.

ABNORMAL DEVELOPMENT

Abnormal development of the peripheral nervous system cannot ordinarily be distinguished from the developing central nervous structures. Anencephalic fetuses lack optic nerves, but externally the eyes, although large, appear normal. Another example of such a disorder is congenital aganglionic megacolon (Hirschsprung's disease). In this condition, the colon is greatly dilated because of lack of muscular tone and contractile activity of the bowel segment, which causes fecal retention. This is because the postganglionic parasympathetic neurons are congenitally decreased in the myenteric plexus, which is located in the distal segment of the large intestine. The innervation of the muscle layers is defective even when ganglionic neurons are present. Only the rectum and sigmoid colon are generally involved, but occasionally more proximal parts of the colon are affected.

SUMMARY

There are 46 human somatic chromosomes. Estimates of gene numbers encoding proteins are given as 31,778. Human sex cells divide by meiosis. Growth occurs through mitosis. Human development begins with the union of spermatozoon and the secondary oocyte. During week 1 of development, a zygote forms and divides into blastomeres that pass through the 2-, 3-, and 4-cell stages. In the 12- to 16-cell stages, on about day 6, the morula becomes the blastocyst and attaches to the endometrium.

During week 2, trophoblast differentiation and formation of the amnion and chorion, the 2 yolk sacs, and the 2 germ layers (epiblast and hypoblast layers) occur. In week 3, the mesoderm and endoderm form through the primitive streak, and the ectoderm differentiates. Somites and the neural tube develop at this time. The 5 brain vesicles appear early in week 4 and gradually differentiate into corresponding brain structures and ventricles. Sulci and gyri appear in approximately week 24. Abnormal development of the central nervous system causes deficits such as anencephaly, cranium bifidum, spina bifida, hydrocephaly, and microcephaly. The peripheral nervous system is derived from a specialized portion of the neural tube, the neural crest. The nervous system continues to develop for many years after birth.

Technical Terms

abembryonic (or vegetal) pole	lamina terminalis (lamina
allantois	terminalis hypothalami)
allelic gene	meiosis
amnion	mesoderm
anaphase	metaphase
anlagen	mitosis
basal lamina	morula
bilaminar embryo	neural crest
blast	neural plate
blastocyst	neural tube
blastomere	nondisjunction
chorion	notochord
chromosomes	nucleus pulposus
cleavage	oogonia
coelom	polar bodies
conceptus	prechordal plate
connecting stalk	primitive streak
cytotrophoblast	primordium
disjunction	prophase
ectoderm	somite
embryoblast	spermatogonia
embryonic (or animal) pole	syncytiotrophoblast
endoderm	telophase
epiblast	trilaminar embryo
extraembryonic	trophoblast
gametes	vesicle (brain)
gametogenesis	yolk sac (primary and
genes	secondary)
genome	zygote
hypoblast	

Review Questions

1. Define the following terms:

abembryonic (or vegetal) pole	basal lamina
allantois	bilaminar embryo
allelic gene	blast
amnion	blastocyst
anaphase	blastomere
anlagen	chorion

chromosomes
cleavage
coelom
conceptus
connecting stalk
cytotrophoblast
disjunction
ectoderm
embryoblast
embryonic (or animal) pole
endoderm
epiblast
extraembryonic
gametes
gametogenesis
genes
genome
hypoblast
lamina terminalis (lamina terminalis hypothalami)
meiosis
mesoderm
metaphase

mitosis
morula
neural crest
neural plate
neural tube
nondisjunction
notochord
nucleus pulposus
oogonia
polar bodies
prechordal plate
primitive streak
primordium
prophase
somite
spermatogonia
syncytiotrophoblast
telophase
trilaminar embryo
trophoblast
vesicle (brain)
yolk sac (primary and secondary)
zygote

2. What is the normal number of human somatic chromosomes?
3. What are the two major parts of the central nervous system?
4. Name the primary germ layer from which central nervous system is derived.
5. Name the rostral end of neural tube, which gives rise to anterior wall of third cerebral ventricle.
6. Name the derivatives of the neural crest.
7. What days, respectively, does the neural tube close rostrally and caudally?
8. How many secondary brain vesicles are there?
9. Name the primary brain vesicle from which cerebral cortex is derived?
10. Discuss the following conditions: anencephaly, cranium bifidum, hydrocephaly, microcephaly, spina bifida.
11. Describe the sensitive period for the developing CNS when it is susceptible to teratogenesis.

True–False Questions

12. Normally developing humans have *46* somatic chromosomes.
13. There are *24* types of human chromosomes; *22* autosomes, and one *X* and one Y chromosome.

14. The reduction of chromosomes by half occurs during the cell division process called meiosis. During the *first* meiotic division one homologous chromosome from each parent pairs during *prophase* and subsequently separates during *anaphase*.
15. The neural *plate* is the forerunner of the nervous system.
16. The neural *tube* develops into the brain and the spinal cord.
17. Two ends of the neural tube that are separated by the sulcus limitans are the *alar* lamina and the *basal* lamina.
18. The anterior (dorsal) end of the neural tube, the *alar* lamina, gives rise to the anterior wall of the *third* ventricle.
19. The anterior end of the neural tube is closed on day *25* and the caudal end is closed on day *27*.
20. There are five brain vesicles; three primary vesicles are the *prosencephalon*, *mesencephalon*, and *rhombencephalon*.
21. Teratogenesis consists of *timing* specific and *insult* nonspecific disorders.
22. The CNS is most susceptible to major congenital defects during weeks *3* to *16* of development.
23. The palate is most susceptible to major congenital defects during weeks *6* to *8* of embryonic development.
24. In spina bifida, the failure of bone fusion results in many conditions, such as **spina bifida cystica** (meninges and or neural tissues do not protrude) and **spina bifida occulta** (where the skin over the area has hair).
25. In cranium bifidum, bone fusion is prevented in the posterior midline of the skull resulting in the protrusion of the brain.
26. Trisomy of the autosomes is associated primarily with three syndromes: trisomies of 21, 18, and 13, all of which are associated with mental retardation.
27. Teratogenesis is an insult specific, timing nonspecific phenomenon.
28. All neurons of the brain and spinal cord are present by the twenty-fifth week of gestation.
29. Glial cells proliferate from midgestation through the fourth postnatal year.
30. Myelinization is primarily a postnatal event.
31. Match the following numbered disorders to the associated lettered definition:

i. anencephaly	a. failure of brain to form two hemispheres
ii. holoprosencephaly	
iii. lissencephaly	b. developmental failure of gyri and/or sulci formation
iv. microencephaly	
	c. miniature brain and small skull cap with normal face size
	d. defective fusion of the neural tube resulting in the congenital absence of the cranial vault with missing or reduced forebrain

Learning Objectives

After studying this chapter, students should be able to do the following:

- Explain parts of a typical nerve cell and describe their functions
- Discuss common types of nerve and glial cells
- Describe functions of nerve and glial cells
- Explain electrical and chemical properties of nerve cells
- Describe the mechanism of impulse generation and its conduction
- Explain nerve cell responses to injuries in the nervous system
- Explain differential regenerative processes between the central and peripheral nervous systems
- Discuss common neurotransmitters and their functions

A **nerve cell** is the basic functional unit in the central nervous system (CNS). Each nerve cell participates in activities vital to the life of the cell and organ. Each cell uses identical mechanisms to synthesize protein, thereby using and transforming energy. More than 15 billion nerve cells in the human brain generate nerve impulses and are the main means of communication in the nervous system and between the nervous system and body parts. The CNS consists of two primary types of cells: **nerve cells** (neurons) and **neuroglial cells** (associational cells). These cells form the structure of the nervous system responsible for functional behavior. Through excitatory and inhibitory nerve impulses, nerve cells also serve all sensorimotor activities and higher mental functions, including attention, problem solving, memory, thinking, reasoning, calculation, and language. Neuroglial cells support and protect nerve cells by proliferating and participating in tissue repair in response to brain injury and disease.

NEURON

A nerve cell primarily consists of three elements: **cell body** (perikaryon, or soma), **dendrites**, and **axon** (Fig. 5-1A). Cells receive impulses primarily via the dendrites and secondarily through the soma and the initial segment of the axons. Cells conduct excitatory or inhibitory nerve impulses through their axonal fibers. The axons travel various distances and synapse on the receptive ends of other nerve cells, muscles, and glands. Nerve cells are highly specialized in responding to excitatory and inhibitory impulses. Factors that add to the operational complexity of nerve cells are the various ways they are interconnected and respond to electrochemical signals.

Nerve Cell Structure

CELL BODY

The cell body of a neuron consists of two major components: a **nucleus** and **cytoplasm**. The term **protoplasm** refers to both these components. The nucleus and cytoplasm work closely together to maintain the viability of the organ. Cytoplasm consists of protein molecules and an aqueous substance and is enclosed within the cell membrane. The cytoplasmic material of the cell contains many **microscopic organelles** (Fig. 5-1B), which include structures such as **neurofibrils, mitochondria, ribosomes, lysosomes,** and **Golgi complexes**. The primary function of these organelles and associated structures is to metabolize protein essential for the maintenance and growth of a cell body and its processes and add to the viability of the cell and the organ. Nerve cells have a high metabolic activity that depends on the availability of glucose. Cells also manufacture their own proteins, which are either incorporated into the cell membrane or exported. Cell bodies transport proteins through cylindrical **microtubules** that run the length of the axons and provide them with metabolic and structural support. Retrograde (axon to cell body) transport also occurs.

The nucleus is the controlling center of the cell and

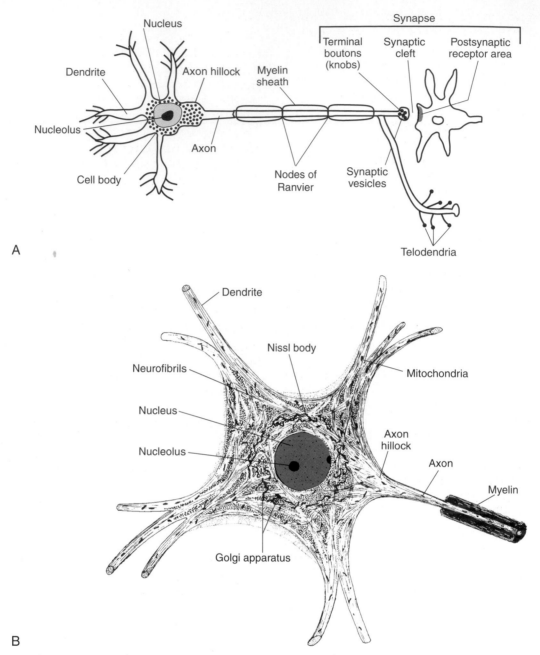

Figure 5-1.   A. Nerve cell and its major parts: body, dendrites, and axon. **B.** Soma organelles, the most important of which are neurofibrils, mitochondria, Nissl bodies, and Golgi apparatus.

is responsible for all vital cellular activities. The nucleus contains **DNA**, the micromolecules with genetic information. The transformation and replication of DNA through cell division provide the mechanism for genetic inheritance (see Chapter 4). Visible within the nucleus is the **nucleolus**, which is the site of assembly of ribosomes and contain ribosomal RNA. The ribosomes play a key role in protein synthesis.

Much chemical activity happens in the cellular cytoplasm, and relates to the changes in the organelles in the cytoplasm. **Neurofibrils** (neurofilaments) or **microfilaments** are small and delicate fibers within the

cytoplasm that serve as the channels for intracellular communication among the cytoplasmic organelles. **Mitochondria**, scattered throughout the cell body, contain enzymes involved with cellular metabolic energy. **Lysosomes** contain the enzymes that participate in intracellular digestion. The **Golgi complex** is primarily responsible for protein secretion and its transportation.

DENDRITIC AND AXONAL PROCESSES

Dendrites and axons are cytoplasmic extensions that extend from the cell body and mediate impulses.

Dendrites are afferent (receptive), transmitting information to the cell body from other cells via synaptic sites. They tend to be short and have many branches. The branching dendrites sometimes have small spikes that add to their arborization (subbranching); this increases the surface available for synapses with other nerve cells.

The term **nerve fiber** means an axon and its covering sheath. Axons are efferent (motor) structures that transmit information away from the cell body to other neurons. Because axons do not produce their own protein, they depend on the cytoplasmic substance of the cell body for survival. Axons originate from a cone-shaped region of the cell, the **axon hillock** (initial segment), and extend longer distances than dendrites. On their way to a terminal destination, axons give off collaterals that communicate with many intervening nerve cells along the way. Axons terminate by branching into smaller multiple filaments, **telodendria**, that include synaptic knobs at their ends. The synaptic knobs contain various neurotransmitters, which are released with impulse transmission.

MYELIN SHEATH

The speed of nerve conduction is determined by the diameter of the nerve and its myelin sheath. **Myelin** is a multilayered lipid material that insulates and protects the nerve fiber. Important functions of this insulation are to prevent the escape of electrical energy during impulse transmission and to regulate the speed of nerve impulses. **Oligodendroglial cells** produce the myelin sheath in the CNS. The myelin sheath is formed in small segments that are interrupted by intervals called the **nodes of Ranvier**. The segment of myelin between two nodes is the **internode**. In a longitudinal section, the nerve fiber looks like a string of sausages. Electrical impulses jump from one node of Ranvier to the next (saltatory conduction), which facilitates rapid nerve fiber conduction, up to 120 m/sec. The myelin formation process begins during the fetal period and continues to maturity. The growth rate and time span for myelin formation (myelogenesis) are directly related to that of our sensorimotor and cognitive development (Lecours, 1975; Lenneberg, 1967; Yakovlev and Lecours, 1967). The incomplete or impaired maturation process of myelination has definite implications for the development of sensorimotor functions and speech–language–cognitive skills. Damaged myelin in the CNS impairs nerve impulse conduction, a deficit found in **multiple sclerosis**.

In the peripheral nervous system (PNS), the myelin sheath is produced by the **Schwann cells** that lie along the axons. One characteristic of myelin formation in the PNS is that each Schwann cell is associated with only one axon, whereas an oligodendroglial cell contributes to the myelination of a group of adjacent axons of the CNS.

SYNAPSE

The synapse is the connection point between neurons. It includes three parts: the **knob**, or **bouton**, containing synaptic vesicles; **synaptic cleft**; and **receptive sites** of the connecting nerve cells. The synaptic knobs contain vesicles filled with neurotransmitters that are released for impulse transmission. The receptive ends of the receiving (postsynaptic) cell are chemically activated and generate the electric impulses that stimulate the nerve cell body. The synaptic cleft is the space between the axon of the presynaptic nerve cell and the receptive ends of the postsynaptic cell. The nerve impulses do not actually cross the synapse. Communication at the synapse occurs through a neurotransmitter released from the bouton terminals. The presynaptic cell transmits a nerve impulse, whereas the postsynaptic cell generates an impulse from synaptic chemical transmission. Electrical impulse transmission through the axon causes the vesicles at the axon terminals to release stored neurotransmitters into the cleft area. These neurotransmitters influence the receptive surface of the postsynaptic nerve cell and initiate an action potential.

The terminal ends of the axons have enlargements called boutons that serve as presynaptic endings. Thickened axonal shafts also establish contacts with other neurons, thus forming additional synapses. Axons usually synapse with dendrites (**axodendritic synapse**) but may also synapse with axons (**axoaxonic synapse**) or directly on cell bodies (**axosomatic synapse**).

Nerve Cell Types

The ability of a cell to process specialized information depends not only on how it is connected with other cells but also on its shape, size, and structural configuration. Accordingly, this structural diversity serves as the basis for nerve cell classification. Nerve cells are classified according to the number of receptive processes coming out of their bodies and by the length of their axons. Both dendritic and axonal processes add to cells' abilities to respond differentially to various types of sensorimotor information. Based on the number of processes arising from the cell body, the cells can be classified into three types: **multipolar**, **bipolar**, and **unipolar** (Fig. 5-2). Multipolar cells have many dendrites and one axon. Differing in size and shape, they make numerous synaptic contacts with other cells. Most multipolar cells are in the CNS. Spinal interneurons and cerebellar Purkinje cells are the best examples of the multipolar type. Bipolar cells have two processes, one extending from each pole of the body: a peripheral process (dendrite) and a central process (axon). Unipolar cells are T-shaped, with one process that extends from the body. It divides into central and peripheral portions. The central portion serves the axonal process, whereas the peripheral portion serves as the dendritic process. Cells in the spinal dorsal roots, for example, are unipolar.

The two types of cells, **Golgi type I** and **Golgi type II**, are distinguished by axonal length. Golgi type I cells have a long axon ranging from inches to feet; many form the sensory or motor tracts connecting cells across long distances. Golgi type II cells, such as the interneurons that connect with other adjacent cells, have a short axonal process.

Neuronal Circuits

The CNS contains billions of cells that are organized into specific patterns of neuronal pools. Each pool or circuit processes information differently and is concerned with the facilitation, excitation, and inhibition of information. The common neuronal circuits include networks used for divergent and convergent processing, lateral inhibition, and reverberating information feedback (Fig. 5-3). A **divergent circuit** amplifies an impulse when an impulse from a single presynaptic cell activates several postsynaptic cells. A **convergent circuit** has two patterns of connections. In the first neuronal circuit of convergence, the postsynaptic neuron receives impulses from several diverged fibers of the same presynaptic nerve cell. In the second pattern, impulses from different nerve cells converge on one postsynaptic nerve cell. In **lateral inhibition**, the signal or cellular message is sharpened by inhibiting the adjacent nerve cells. The **reverberating circuit** is a self-propagating system between cells that if activated, can discharge the signal continuously until its operation is blocked by an external source. In the reverberating circuitry, neurons are arranged in a chain formation. The incoming impulse activates the first nerve cell, which activates the second cell, which stimulates the third, and so on. Branches from the second, third, and fourth cells send impulses back to activate the previous nerve cell, forming a closed neuronal loop.

Neuroglial Cells

The function of neuroglia (glia means glue) cells is to support and protect the nerve cells (Table 5-1). Glial cells are in the gray and white matter of the brain, and there are approximately 40 to 50 times as many glial cells as nerve cells. However, the glial cells are small and do not participate in the generation and transmission of nerve impulses. There are four types of glial cells in the CNS: **astrocytes, oligodendroglia, ependymal cells**, and **microglia** (Fig. 5-4). Glial cells of the PNS include **Schwann cells** and **satellite cells**. Schwann cells may be capable of acting as fibroblasts (connective tissue).

Predominant in the white matter, the **astrocytes** function like connective tissue and provide skeletal support for the brain cells and their processes. In the gray matter, they protect the brain by forming **external** and **internal limiting membranes**. By contacting capillary surfaces with their end feet and by using tight junctions, astrocytes contribute to the **blood–brain barrier**. This refers to the selective permeability of capillaries and arteries that restricts the movement of certain substances from the blood to the brain (see Chapter 17). Astrocytes also regulate the extracellular concentration of ions and in some instances can degrade released neurotransmitters. After an injury to the brain, astroglial cells are important in recovery. In cerebrovascular accidents, the astrocytes and microglial cells proliferate and migrate to the lesion site. Microglia phagocytose (engulf) cellular debris, leaving a cavity. In the case of a large lesion, astrocytes seal the cavity, which is called a **cyst**. In the case of a limited-size lesion, astrocytes fill the space with a glial scar that is called **replacement gliosis**.

Oligodendroglia cells form and maintain the myelin sheath in the CNS. Each of the processes that

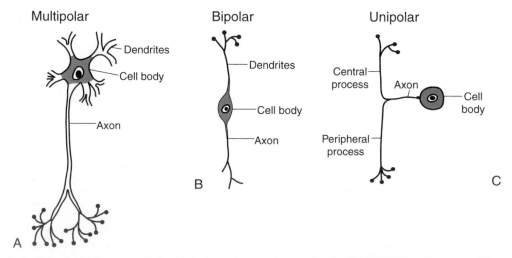

Figure 5-2. Types of nerve cells based on their processes. **A.** Multipolar cell. **B.** Bipolar cell. **C.** Unipolar cell.

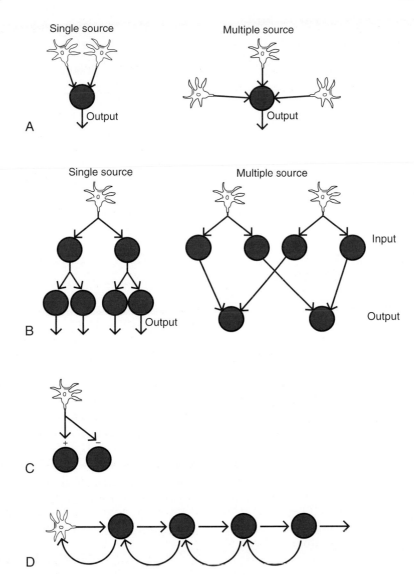

Figure 5-3.   Common types of neuronal circuits. **A.** Convergent circuit. **B.** Divergent circuit. **C.** Lateral inhibition. **D.** Reverberating circuit.

Table 5-1.   Neuroglia and Their Functions

Glia Cells	Locations	Functions
Astrocytes	CNS (gray and white matter)	Provide supporting network in brain by forming complete lining around external surface of brain and blood vessels in CNS. With attached endings to blood vessels, contribute to blood–brain barrier by regulating transmission of substances. Form scars around dead brain tissue.
Oligodendrocytes	CNS	Form myelin sheaths around axons in CNS.
Microglia	CNS	Travel to site of lesion and engulf cellular debris before removing it.
Ependymal cells	Ventricular cavity	Form a lining around ventricular surface.
Schwann cells	PNS	Form myelin sheath around axons in PNS. Constitute fibrous connective tissue around fibers in PNS.

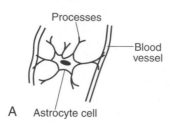

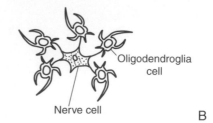

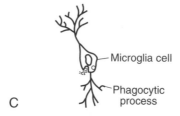

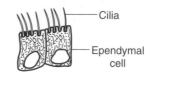

Figure 5-4. Glia cells. **A.** Astrocyte. **B.** Oligodendroglia. **C.** Microglia. **D.** Ependyma.

radiate from the oligodendrocyte contributes to forming myelin. Thus, each oligodendrocyte may supply myelin for as many as 25 or more axons. The sheath of myelin insulates the axons and speeds up impulse conduction. The myelin that covers PNS fibers is formed by Schwann cells, which are derived from the neural crest.

Ependymal cells primarily form the inner surface of the ventricles. In conjunction with the astrocytes, the ependymal cells form the internal limiting membrane. The **choroid plexus**, which secretes cerebrospinal fluid and is in the ventricular cavity, consists of vascular pia surrounded by an epithelial layer of ependymal cells.

Microglial cells are multipotential because they sometimes act as phagocytes and other times act like astrocytes or oligodendrocytes. These cells are the scavengers of the CNS. Their primary function is to phagocytose (digest) dead tissue debris and remove it from a lesion site.

CENTRAL AND PERIPHERAL NERVOUS SYSTEMS

The two important cytological differences between the CNS and the PNS are (*a*) different myelin-forming cells and (*b*) the presence in the PNS of endoneurium, a fibrous connective tissue covering for axons. Schwann cells myelinate the fibers in a jelly roll manner; that is, the myelin consists of layers of Schwann cell membranes. One Schwann cell forms myelin exclusively for one internode of a peripheral nerve fiber, whereas one oligodendrocyte myelinates many axons in the CNS. Myelin formation by these two types of cells is otherwise similar. Also, the composition of nerve fibers varies between the CNS and PNS. Peripheral nerve fiber bundles

are held together by connective tissues. These include the collagen fibers of the fibroblasts and other cells that form an **endoneurial membrane** (Fig. 5-5). This is a fragile covering that surrounds each peripheral nerve individually. This fibrous connective tissue is not known to exist in the CNS. This endoneurial wrapping around a peripheral axon merges with **neurilemma**, the most external layer of the multilayered myelin, which contains the nucleus of the Schwann cell. The neurilemma, which is found only in the PNS, is important in the regeneration of injured axonal fibers in the PNS.

NERVE IMPULSE

Nerve cells communicate with one another through nerve impulses that represent all neuronal activity. The nerve impulses have a chemical component that underlies the electric potential of the cells (Fig. 5-6). The excitability of nerve cells depends on their ionic channels in the neuronal membrane. An action potential results from charged particles (ions) moving through the cell membranes. Nerve impulses activate the release of a neurotransmitter in a presynaptic neuron. The transmitter causes the adjacent postsynaptic receptors to open an ion channel. By selectively opening or closing an ion channel, the released neurotransmitter controls the excitability of the interconnecting neuron.

A cell is in a **resting state** when it is not excited or excitable and not conducting an impulse. In this resting state, there is a specific level of **membrane potential** in which the distribution of positive and negative ions on each side of the membrane is unequal (polarized). Consequently, there is a difference between electrical charges on the inner and outer sides of the cell membrane (Fig. 5-6*A*). The resting membrane potential is

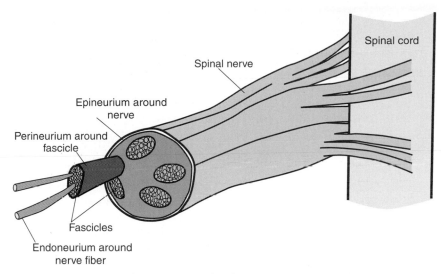

Figure 5-5. Peripheral nerve components

arbitrarily defined as −70 mV inside the cell membrane. This membrane potential is maintained by an unequal distribution of positively charged sodium and potassium ions and negatively charged chloride ions and proteins across the membrane. The ionic channels consist of several polypeptide units arranged around a central pore. The negative ions are in higher concentration inside the cell, whereas the positive ions are in higher concentration outside the cell.

Even during a resting state, when the nerve cell is not conducting an impulse, some ions constantly pass through the membrane. The membrane channels are gated (opened or closed) by electric potential or neurotransmitters. The flow of ions through the membrane depends on the **density** of the channels, the **size** of the opening, and the **ion concentration gradient** across the membrane. The steeper the gradient across the membrane, the greater the flow of ions from high to low concentration. The membrane potential and the concentration gradient together determine the flow of ions through the membrane. The distribution of **sodium** and **potassium** across the cellular membrane is constantly adjusted by the **sodium–potassium pump**, which pumps sodium out of the cell and transports potassium into the cell. Because of the membrane pore size, the cell membrane maintains selective permeability to these ions. Potassium ions can easily leave the cell interior, whereas sodium has restricted access to the cell interior. Similarly, the membrane is not permeable to negative ions inside the cell. Because of the selectivity of ionic transportation, the positively charged potassium easily diffuses through the membrane, and only a few sodium components get inside the cell. Not many large, negatively charged ions can diffuse out through the cell membrane. Furthermore, with the attraction of opposite ions and the repulsion of identical ions, the sodium concentration outside the cell repulses the potassium, driv-

ing it back into the cells. Similarly, the negative protein molecules and chloride attract the positively charged sodium and potassium ions. This tug of war forms an electrochemical gradient along the cell membrane in which the external surface is positive and the internal surface is negative. This gradient is the cell's resting potential (Fig. 5-6A).

Nerve Excitability

Excitability is a cell's response to various stimuli and conversion of this response into a nerve impulse or **action potential** (Fig. 5-6). Stimuli can include a chemical or temperature change, electrical pulse, or nerve tapping. During its resting state, the neuron undergoes several short changes in intracellular potential. When the neuron becomes **hyperpolarized** (with the cell interior becoming more negative), it returns to the resting level. When this change is in the other direction (**depolarization**), it triggers a large spike. A change of at least 10 mV, bringing the cell interior to −60 mV, is required to trigger an action potential and depolarize a nerve cell. The depolarization of a cell membrane alters its permeability to external positively charged sodium, which begins flowing into the cell. It changes the membrane potentials from −70 to −60 mV, and the changed membrane potential triggers an action potential resulting in a nerve impulse or message (Fig. 5-6B). In membrane depolarization there is a constant flow of sodium to the inside. This flow continues until the cell's interior potential becomes positive and shoots up to 30 or 40 mV before reversing the cellular interior environment (Fig. 5-6D). Membrane potential from this peak first returns to the **absolute refractory period**, in which the cell interior drifts to −80 to −90 mV, and it cannot fire another action potential until the membrane potential returns to the resting potential.

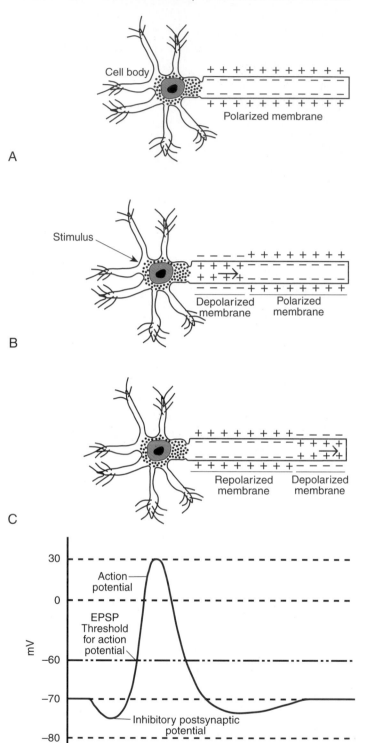

A

B

C

D

Figure 5-6. Action potential. **A.** Resting potential with polarized membrane. **B.** Generation of action potential with depolarized membrane. **C.** Conduction of action potential along membrane. **D.** Recorded changes in membrane potentials, threshold excitatory postsynaptic potential (*EPSP*), and inhibitory postsynaptic potential (*IPSP*).

Not all stimuli are strong enough to change the membrane potentials by 10 mV. Accordingly, many stimuli with subthreshold strength, if temporally and spatially summated, can initiate a nerve impulse. In summation, weak stimuli arrive in sequence, and their cumulative effect is strong enough to initiate an impulse.

Impulse Conduction

A nerve impulse is passively conducted a short distance in the axon by sodium entering the cell membrane. The interior of the axon becomes more positive than the adjacent neighboring area (Fig. 5-6*B*). This gradually changes the membrane potential in the neighboring area, and the impulse continues to allow positively charged ions to enter the cell membrane as it moves distally along the axon (Fig. 5-6*C*). Impulse conduction in a myelinated axon is the same as in an unmyelinated axon except that the impulse conduction in the myelinated axon is faster as the impulse jumps from one node of Ranvier to the other (saltatory conduction).

An action potential or nerve impulse is either excitatory or inhibitory to the postsynaptic neuron. An excitatory impulse lowers the postsynaptic neuron's membrane potential and creates the environment for a new impulse. This change in the next cell is called the **excitatory postsynaptic potential (EPSP)**. An inhibitory nerve impulse works in the opposite manner on the postsynaptic potential. An inhibitory nerve impulse makes the postsynaptic neuron membrane potentially hyperpolarized. The more negative the inside membrane potential, the more difficult it is for the postsynaptic neuron to generate an action potential. This is called the **inhibitory postsynaptic potential (IPSP)**.

Most cells have their own frequency and pattern of action potentials that serve as codes for transmitted messages. This keeps messages for cells separate, because many cells fire spontaneously and simultaneously.

Conduction velocities of myelinated neurons can be determined by multiplying the axonal diameter by 6 m/sec. Thus, a myelinated axon with a diameter of 3 μm conducts an impulse at 18 m/sec. Another axon with a diameter of 20 μm conducts an impulse at 120 m/sec. In contrast, an unmyelinated axon with a diameter of 1 μm conducts an impulse at less than 1 m/second.

NEURONAL RESPONSES TO BRAIN INJURIES

Nerve cells in the human brain are incapable of further cell division and regeneration. This lack of cellular regeneration restricts the recovery of sensorimotor functions and mental processes after lesions in the CNS. The nerve cell synapses serve as good points of reference for discovering the effects of cellular injuries, because in addition to conducting an impulse, the cells transmit nutritive (trophic) substances between neurons. Trophic factors are crucial for normal cell maintenance on both sides of the synapse. A neuron may degenerate if either the presynaptic or postsynaptic terminal degenerates.

Understanding the physiological events that cells undergo subsequent to injuries is important because the effects explain the processes of spontaneous recovery after traumatic injuries, vascular accidents, tumors, and metabolic insufficiency. The two types of degenerative changes that follow axonal sectioning are the **axonal** or **retrograde reaction** and **wallerian (anterograde)** degeneration (Fig. 5-7A; Table 5-2). During axonal reactions, retrograde degenerative changes occur in the cell body in response to sectioning the axon (axotomy). This is due to the interruption of trophic factors that flow from the axon to the cell body and to reprogramming of the cell body in the face of metabolic changes. Axonal injury extends from the site of injury to the cell body. In wallerian degeneration, the degenerative changes occur in the axon region detached from the cell body. The axonal segment still attached to the cell body is the **proximal segment**, whereas the detached axonal segment is the **distal segment** (Fig. 5-7C).

Axonal Reaction

Degenerative responses of nerve cells to injuries pass through a series of internal changes (Fig. 5-7B, Table 5-3). After an injury, the microscopic structures (organelles) of the soma undergo structural changes that are evident within 24 to 48 hours after the injury. The first cytological signs of changes in the cell body are swelling of the organelles and dissolution of coarse clumps of Nissl substance into fine granules. Cellular edema, brought about by an altered blood–brain barrier, obliterates structural details of the gray and white matter and triggers nuclear shrinking (pyknosis). It is maximal within 90 to 100 hours. This reactive or degenerative process in individual cells, called **chromatolysis**, begins between the axon hillock and the cell nucleus. It is followed by the degeneration of Nissl bodies and the displacement of the cell nucleus from the center to the periphery of the soma. Depending on the severity of injury, the chromatolytic process may continue for 10 to 18 days. While the cell is injured and undergoing reactive or degenerative changes, cellular RNA production and protein synthesis increase, as does the formation of the plasma membrane, to regenerate the severed axon and to prevent the cell body from dying. Specifically, free ribosomes in the postchromatolysis phase synthesize increased structural proteins, which are needed for restoring cellular structure and rebuilding Nissl bodies and cellular fibers. If the connection of the severed axon is properly restored, the chromatolysis ends, and the cell may return to its normal appearance. Some cells, if not seriously damaged, may respond to the natural recovery process and survive the injury. In such cases, all cell

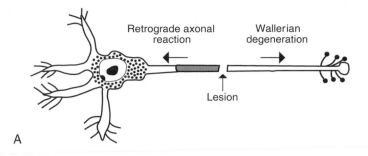
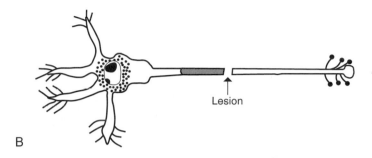
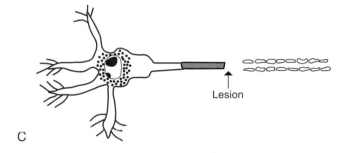
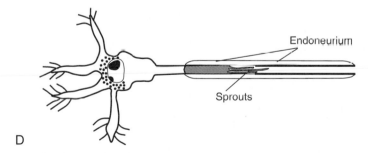

Figure 5-7. Neuronal response to injury as illustrated by severed axon. Recovery process in PNS is also depicted. **A.** Types of neuronal response to injury. **B.** Axonal retrograde reaction. **C.** Wallerian degeneration. **D.** Peripheral nerve regeneration.

body organelles resume their normal appearance, and the nucleus again assumes a central location. However, this restitution may take months. Cells that are severely injured do not survive. They shrink and assume irregular shapes because of the degenerated organelles. They gradually atrophy and leave only debris.

Cellular swelling, if not medically treated, can lead to death by elevating intracranial pressure. By the end of

Table 5-2. Neuronal Response to Injury

Sites of Degeneration	Types of Degenerative Changes
Axonal (retrograde) reaction	Chromatolysis in cell body
	Dissolution of cellular organelles
	Displacement of cell body to periphery
	Possible cellular death
	Recovery process
	Increased protein synthesis to regenerate severed axon, prevent cell body from dying
Wallerian (anterograde) degeneration	Axonal degeneration
	Myelin degeneration for sectioned axon
	Degeneration of axon beginning with its distal end
	Macrophagic process
	Recovery
	Increased protein synthesis to promote recovery
	Formation of endoneurium tube by Schwann cells
	Closing of cleft by sprouting of cut ends of axons
	Establishing sprout connections between both axonal ends

Table 5-3. Sequence of Pathological Features in Necrotic Process

Time	Pathological Changes
1 day	No visible sign of tissue death
2–4 days	Cellular edema and shrinking of cells eliminating the structural details between gray and white matter
4 days and afterwards	Maximum swelling in necrotic tissues due to impaired blood–brain barrier
	Infiltration of infection-fighting blood monocytes
1 week	Attenuation of swelling, astrocytic and capillary proliferation (hyperplasia and hypertrophy)
1 week–3 mo	Liquefaction of necrotic tissues and their phagocytosis by macrophagic microglial cells
3–6 mo and onward	Formation of a cystic cavity; scar formation in case of a small infarct

a week, swelling may begin to go down, but necrotic tissues are invaded by a considerable number of new capillaries (hyperplasia) and a proliferation of macrophages (astrocytes and microglia). The period following the first week is marked by liquefaction of necrotic tissue and **phagocytosis**, in which lipid-laden macrophagic microglia cells engulf and remove the dead tissue. Macrophagy may take 3 months or more depending on the size of the lesion. In the case of a large lesion, tissue removal is likely to leave a cavity filled with fluid and some macrophagic cells and outlined by a sheet of astro-

cytes. The presence of this cystic cavity in the brain of stroke patients has made many feel pessimistic about the benefit of speech–language treatment and other rehabilitative efforts. However, the recovery process is highly dynamic and presumably involves multiple steps.

Wallerian Degeneration

Survival of the axon depends on cytoplasmic flow from the cell body. Deprived of the metabolic activity from the cell body, an axon cannot survive. The wallerian reaction (Fig. 5-7C) refers to the degeneration of the axonal part that is separate from its cell body. The distal portion of the sectioned axon swells and begins to degenerate within 12 to 20 hours. Axons degenerate before the myelin sheath, and within 2 to 3 days the connected muscles become denervated. Within 7 days, the axon and its myelin are broken into small pieces that gradually disintegrate, setting the stage for the macrophagic action of microglia cells. Macrophagy begins in 7 days and is complete in 3 to 6 months (Table 5-3).

Neuroglial Responses

Neuroglial cells react to cellular injuries and brain tissue necrosis by multiplying in number (**hyperplasia**) and by increasing their size (**hypertrophy**). The infection-fighting **neutrophils** (scavenger white blood cells) arrive at the lesion site within a few days of the injury. This is followed by the migration of microglia and the proliferation of the astrocytes and other histiocytes in the region of the dying cells. The blood–brain barrier breakdown also allows monocytes to invade brain tissues. In the case of a small lesion, the astrocytes form a glial scar called replacement **gliosis**. In large lesions, they outline the fluid-filled space, forming a **cystic cavity**.

Microglia are the scavengers of the nervous system. In case of inflammation or injury, they rapidly proliferate and migrate toward dead tissue within 24 hours. Their function is to phagocytose the cellular debris. Normally microglia cells are small, but they become large after phagocytizing dead cells; their cytoplasm becomes less dense and their nucleus, more prominent. Within 1 week, they look like typical macrophages, with pale cytoplasm and no visible processes. As the macrophages ingest debris of myelin, cells, and lipid droplets, the nucleus is pushed to the side. The phagocytic cells dominate the injury site from the first week, and it may take several months to years to remove the debris of dead brain tissue (Table 5-3).

In addition, the proliferation and migration of glial cells displace presynaptic and postsynaptic terminals and cell bodies of axotomized neurons, thus impairing transmission between neurons. After normal input to the cell body is removed, new synaptic trigger zones develop on its dendritic tree and begin to excite the cell.

Axonal Regeneration in Peripheral Nervous System

The regeneration of fibers in the PNS has been clinically confirmed (Fig. 5-7D). The sectioned nerve endings proximal to the cell body begin regenerating within 3 to 4 days. This regeneration is facilitated if proximal and distal ends of the severed nerve are cleaned and attached. The Schwann cells and fibroblasts contribute significantly to axonal regeneration in the PNS. In the first few days, the proliferating Schwann cells fill the interval between opposing ends of the nerve fiber. The sheath of Schwann, or neurilemma, in conjunction with the endoneurial connective tissue, forms a tube from the proximal fiber end leading to the distal end. This neurilemmal tube guides growth of the peripheral axon. As the proximal end of the axon regenerates, many sprouts (regenerated processes of axons) form. One or more axonal sprouts may grow along the tube and pass through the cleft. Some axonal sprouts that cross the scar may grow to connect to the distal portion of the axon at a rate of 4 mm a day. However, the axonal regeneration may encounter problems, one being that the probability of the regenerated axon reaching its previously attached fiber is small. The attachment of the regenerated axon to a different sensory or motor fiber poses additional problems. For example, the connection of a pain-mediating fiber to a touch receptor results in the sensation of pain from touch. The nerve fibers that are incorrectly connected usually atrophy.

Axonal Regeneration in Central Nervous System

Nerve growth in the CNS would have tremendous implications for the natural and assisted recovery of brain-damaged patients. The physiological concept that most intrigues and frustrates health professionals is the minimal restoration of function after a lesion in the CNS. As a result, the prognosis for recovery of axotomized neurons in the brain is poor. Axons severed in the CNS also undergo regrowth and sprouting similar to those in the PNS; however, unknown factors prevent damaged neurons from reconnecting to the distal axonal segments and reinnervating their target structures. One factor may be the lack of growth protein in the CNS that is present in the PNS. The proximal ends of axons in the CNS exhibit some growth (sprouting). However, this growth is not significant because the regenerated axons cannot cross the astrocytic scars. Furthermore, there are no Schwann cells and no endoneural tissue tubes (Fig. 5-5) to guide axonal growth. With no guiding structure, the regenerated axons form an axonal ball.

In spite of the limited regeneration in the CNS, recovery is highly dynamic and may involve multiple steps, such as restitution of partially injured adjacent neuronal structure and functional reorganization within the hemispheres and across the hemispheres involving the homotopic cortex.

NEUROTRANSMITTERS

Understanding neurotransmitters is important for students of communicative disorders. Neurotransmitters help to regulate brain mechanisms that control cognition, language, speech, hearing, moods, attention, memory, personality, motivation, and physiological tuning of the brain (Fig. 5-8).

A neurotransmitter is a chemical substance released at a synapse to transmit signals across neurons (Table 5-4). There are two types of transmitters in the nervous system: **small molecules** and **large molecules** (peptides). Small-molecule neurotransmitters include **acetylcholine, dopamine, norepinephrine, serotonin, glutamate,** and **γ-aminobutyric acid** (GABA). The last five listed are called **monoamines** because they are derived from **amino acids**. They are known to have short-lasting effects. Large-molecule peptides produce long-lasting effects on postsynaptic nerve cells. Most neurotransmitters have more than one receptor type and may have different effects on different synapses. Also, more than one neurotransmitter may be secreted by a single terminal bouton. It is therefore difficult to identify the specific behavioral effect of a given neurotransmitter definitely at all times.

Acetylcholine

Acetylcholine was the first identified and is still one of the most studied neurotransmitters. It is synthesized from choline by **acetylcoenzyme** in a reaction catalyzed by the enzyme. When released in synapses, it is broken down and destroyed by the enzyme **acetylcholinesterase**. Dissolution of acetylcholine is necessary to permit repetitive nerve impulses to be effective and to allow for muscle repolarization. It is the primary neurotransmitter of the PNS. Acetylcholine is also an important neurotransmitter of the CNS; cholinergic neurons are concentrated in the **reticular formation**, the **basal forebrain**, and the **striatum** (Fig. 5-8A).

The actions of acetylcholine are slow and diffuse in the CNS, whereas they are brief and precise in the PNS. The cholinergic neurons in the forebrain (**nucleus basalis of Meynert**), together with related nuclei in the nearby septal area, supply the neocortex, hippocampus, and amygdala. These cholinergic projections are thought to participate in regulating levels of forebrain activity. In addition, together with the projections from the reticular formation to the thalamus, they are critical in the cycle of sleep and wakefulness. The reticular cholinergic neurons of the forebrain with their connections with the basal ganglia, also influence stereotyped movements.

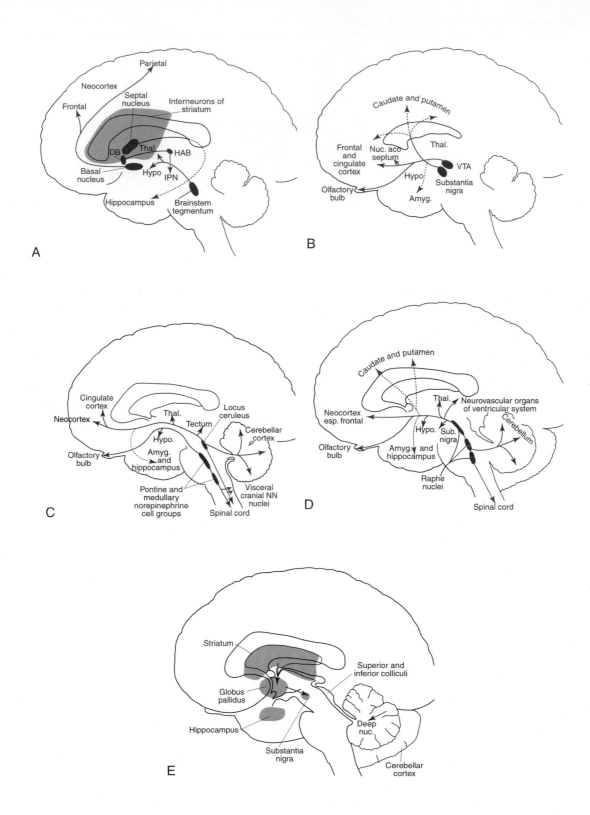

Figure 5-8. Sites of cell bodies and their projections in brain for acetylcholine, dopamine, norepinephrine, serotonin, GABA. **A.** Acetylcholine. **B.** Dopamine. **C.** Norepinephrine. **D.** Serotonin. **E.** GABA. *Amyg*, amygdala; *DB*, diagonal band of Broca; HAB, habenula; Hypo, hypothalamus; IPN, interpeduncular nucleus; NN, nerves; nuc, nucleus; Nuc acc, nucleus accumbens; Sub, substantia; Thal, thalamus; VTA, ventral tegmental area.

Table 5-4.   Neurotransmitters and Their Functions

Neurotransmitters	Functions	Site of Secretion
Acetylcholine	Regulates forebrain activity; inhibits basal ganglia activity	Basal forebrain, brainstem, myoneural junctions
Dopamine	Modulates limbic and prefrontal functions; regulates basal ganglia motor functions	Brainstem and forebrain
Norepinephrine	Along with reticular projections, regulates sleep, attention, moods	Reticular formation and autonomic nervous system
Serotonin	Regulates arousal, emotions, pain perception	Brainstem and limbic system
GABA	Regulates pain perception; inhibits basal ganglia movements	Diffusely in CNS
Peptides (endorphins, enkephalins, substance P)	Regulates pain perception	CNS

In the PNS, acetylcholine is released by α- and γ-motor neurons and by autonomic (preganglionic and parasympathetic postganglionic) neurons. Acetylcholine binds to receptor sites on the muscle fiber membrane and increases its permeability to sodium and potassium ions. This depolarizes the muscle membrane, causing the muscle to contract. Because acetylcholine is the major chemical messenger in the PNS, release of it controls voluntary movements of motor fibers of the spinal and cranial nerves. Antibodies that interfere with the action of acetylcholine on muscle cells at the myoneural junction are found in **myasthenia gravis**. Deficient cholinergic projections in the hippocampus and orbitofrontal cortex have also been implicated in **Alzheimer's disease**, a degenerative condition characterized by atrophy of the neocortex and hippocampus that causes memory loss, personality change, and dementia. In Alzheimer's disease, however, acetylcholine replacement therapy has not been successful, since multiple transmitter systems, such as somatostatin-containing neurons, are also implicated in the degenerative process.

Monoamines

Monoamines are a subgroup of small molecular transmitters derived from amino acids. They consist of **norepinephrine, epinephrine, dopamine**, and **serotonin**. All monoamine-producing cell clusters lie in the brainstem (Fig. 5-8). Despite the restricted area of origin, these neurons have wide areas of brain projections, which suggests that they participate in regulating or tuning the activity of large portions of the CNS.

DOPAMINE

Dopaminergic cells are found mainly in the upper midbrain and project ipsilaterally. Clinically, the two most important dopaminergic projections are the **mesostriatal** (midbrain and striatum) and **mesocortical** (midbrain to cortex) systems (Fig. 5-8B). Mesostriatal projections include the dopaminergic projections from the substantia nigra to the putamen and caudate nucleus of the basal ganglia. Degeneration of the substantia nigra reduces production and transmission of dopamine and is associated with **Parkinson's disease**, a degenerative condition characterized by **resting tremor, reduced movement, dysarthria**, and **stooped posture**.

Dopamine mesocortical projections originate in the substantia nigra, and their terminals are in the cortex, nucleus accumbens, and amygdala. The cortical projections innervate the medial, frontal, anterior cingulate, and olfactory cortices. Dopamine projections to the cortex and limbic structures support their involvement in cognition and motivation. Impairments of these projections are involved in some mental illnesses. Drugs of abuse directly or indirectly cause dopamine release in the nucleus accumbens, suggesting that mesolimbic (midbrain to limbic lobe) projections are involved in pleasurable feelings. Excessive dopamine activity in the forebrain contributes to schizophrenia. Thorazine and related drugs that block dopamine receptors are used in the treatment of schizophrenia, which suggests that the midbrain–limbic and midbrain–cortical dopaminergic projections contribute to this psychiatric disorder.

NOREPINEPHRINE

Norepinephrine-containing neurons are in the pons and medulla (Fig. 5-8C). Most norepinephrine cells are in the **reticular formation** in the brainstem, **locus ceruleus**, and **lateral medullary reticular formation**. **Noradrenergic neurons** project to the thalamus, hypothalamus, limbic forebrain structures, and the cerebral cortex. Descending noradrenergic fibers project to other parts of the brainstem, cerebellar cortex, and spinal cord.

Clinically, noradrenergic neurons are thought to be involved in generating paradoxical sleep and maintaining attention and vigilance. Drugs used for the treatment of depression act by enhancing norepinephrine transmission. When examined in postmortem brains, norepinephrine has been found to be richly distributed in the left pulvinar and right ventrobasal nuclear complex of the thalamus. This norepinephrine asymmetry at the thalamic level is intriguing, since it may be related to handedness and the prevalence of one-sided vascular lesions.

SEROTONIN

Although serotonin is an important neurotransmitter of the CNS, 95% of it is found peripherally in blood platelets and the gastrointestinal tract. Serotonin neurons are found at most levels of the brainstem (Fig. 5-8D). The serotonergic terminals are in the reticular formation, hypothalamus, thalamus, septum, hippocampus, olfactory tubercle, cerebral cortex, basal ganglia, and amygdala. The rostral reticular serotonergic projections are active in sleep, and the caudal reticular serotonin terminals with afferents from the periaqueductal gray matter interact with spinal enkephalin interneurons and exert some control over pain input.

Clinically, the firing rate of serotonin and noradrenergic neurons fluctuates with sleep and wakefulness and thus may be involved in the general activity level of the CNS. Serotonin is thought to be concerned with the overall level of arousal and slow-wave sleep. It also contributes to the descending pain control system. Severe depression is thought to be associated with low serotonin. It was found to be low in persons who committed suicide as compared with accident victims. Antidepressant drugs appear to enhance the concentration of serotonin at the synapse by reducing its uptake.

γ-AMINOBUTYRIC ACID (GABA)

GABA, a derivative of glutamate, is a major neurotransmitter for the CNS, just as acetylcholine is in the periphery. GABA is the major transmitter of brief inhibitory synaptic events in the CNS. Neurons containing glutamate or GABA are widespread in the nervous system. Cortical pyramidal cells and other cortical outputs are rich in glutamate. Examples of GABA local-circuit neurons are cells found in the hippocampus, cerebral cortex, and cerebellar cortex (Fig. 5-8E). GABA serves as the inhibitory neurotransmitter from the striatum to the globus pallidus and substantia nigra, from the globus pallidus and substantia nigra to the thalamus, and from the Purkinje cells to the deep cerebellar nuclei. GABA projections suppress the firing of projection neurons and sharpen contrast by inhibiting nearby elements.

Clinically, GABA is implicated in **Huntington's chorea**, a degenerative disease characterized by involuntary movements. It is due to the loss of GABA-producing neurons in the striatum (caudate and putamen). Decreased GABA-containing **striatonigral** (striatum to substantia nigra) projections result in a reduced presence of GABA in the substantia nigra. The GABA reduction causes an abnormal elevation of the ratio of dopamine to acetylcholine, which produces abnormal movements. In contrast, a lowered ratio of dopamine to acetylcholine ratio resulting from loss of nigral dopaminergic cells is associated with the reduced movement (bradykinesia) or lack of movements of parkinsonism.

Peptides

Peptides are large-molecule chemicals that can function as neurotransmitters or neuromodulators. Most neurons that contain a neuropeptide also contain one of the classical small-molecule transmitters. For example, GABA-ergic striatal neurons that project to the globus pallidus also contain peptides such as **enkephalin**, **endorphins**, and **substance P**. This suggests that a single synapse can mediate multiple effects. These peptides consist of opioidlike compounds, and their projections are important in pain management.

Drug Treatment Principles

Drug treatment modifies the action of neurotransmitters at synapses either by blocking their effects or by simulating their actions. Two important principles that explain the nature of drug treatment follow.

- **Blocking enzymatic breakdown of a neurotransmitter.** Neostigmine, an anticholinesterase drug, for example, is used to impede acetylcholine breakdown by the enzyme acetylcholinesterase; this allows the level of available acetylcholine to rise. Anticholinesterase drugs are standard treatment for **myasthenia gravis**, which is characterized by reduced synthesis and or effectiveness of acetylcholine in myoneural junctions.
- **Regulating the activity of the postsynaptic membrane.** This is exemplified by the administration of atropine, a drug commonly used for dilating the pupil; it blocks the effects of the normally released acetylcholine on the constrictor fibers of the iris, thus causing pupil dilation.

Curare is another drug with postsynaptic effects. It prevents the excitatory effects of acetylcholine on muscle fibers. Commonly used by Indians in South America on their arrows for hunting, curare causes paralysis by inhibiting the normal contraction of muscles in response to efferent impulses. Paralysis of the respiratory muscles ensures death by suffocation.

CLINICAL CONSIDERATIONS

Multiple Sclerosis

Multiple sclerosis is a chronic degenerative disease of the CNS of unknown cause (Fig. 5-9). However, it has been linked to abnormalities in the immune system. It usually begins in young adults. It accounts for 5 to 10% of organic neurological disease. The myelin sheath degenerates, but the axon remains intact. The sparing of axons probably accounts for the remissions (recovery) of varying periods that occur in many cases. Haphazard demyelination and glial proliferation occur simultaneously. The broken-up myelin is transported by microglial cells to the regional perivascular spaces. Intense proliferation of fibrous glia exceeds the ordinary reparative process. As a result, the glia form dense plaques or patches, predominantly at sites in the white matter of the brain and/or spinal cord. Plaques are a few millimeters to several centimeters in diameter and may become coalescent. In advanced cases, the plaques cause secondary degeneration of the axons, which in the spinal cord usually results in spasticity. In the brain, there is predilection for the plaques to occur in the region of the ventricles, brainstem, and cerebellar peduncles. The optic nerves and optic chiasm are also often sites of plaque formation. Brain plaques cause axon degeneration that may result in mental symptoms in addition to various sensory and motor deficits.

Among the symptoms of multiple sclerosis, the most common initial symptoms are weakness and fatigue, followed by paresthesias (abnormal sensations) and then oculovisual disturbances. Although less frequent, other early complaints are tremor, ataxia, speech impairment, dizziness, and disorders of urination. The diagnostic triad described by Charcot in 1862 (nystag-mus, scanning speech, and intention tremor) is sometimes seen in the later stages of illness. Life expectancy after onset of the disease is probably 20 to 25 years. Treatment has been largely supportive and psychotherapeutic, but steroids are used to shorten attacks. Also, **β-interferon injections** are used to reduce the frequency and severity of new attacks and slow the progression of the disability.

Myasthenia Gravis

Myasthenia gravis is a chronic disease characterized by muscle weakness that becomes worse with exercise and temporarily improves with rest. An impairment of impulse transmission is caused by an inadequate amount of acetylcholine at the myoneural junction. The cause of the disease is unknown, although it is thought to be autoimmune. In this condition, antibodies bind to cells or proteins that are normal components of one's own body. The antibodies bind with the acetylcholine receptors at motor end plates and prevent the normal effects of acetylcholine. The antibody-producing cells are derived from the thymus. Half of patients with myasthenia gravis have enlarged thymus glands.

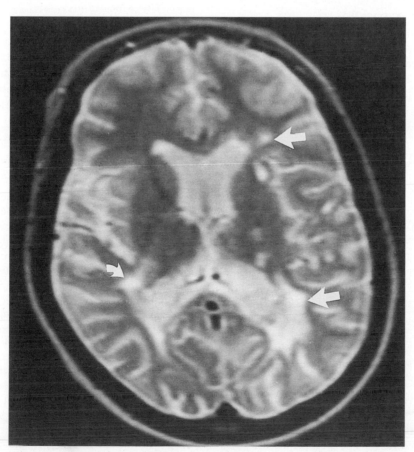

Figure 5-9.   Multiple periventricular and deep white matter foci of abnormal increased signal (*arrows*) on an axial T2-weighted magnetic resonance image in a patient with multiple sclerosis.

Symptoms appear at any age and are more prevalent in females during the first 30 years of life and thereafter are more prevalent in men. Onset is gradual, and muscles may be focally or generally involved. Weakness gets worse during the day and disappears after a sound sleep. The first signs of the disease often appear in constantly used muscles, such as the muscles of the eye and of respiration. Ptosis and diplopia are the most common early manifestations of the illness. Involvement of the cranial nerves also causes altered facial expression, regurgitation, choking, hypernasality, and a dropped jaw. Upper and proximal extremity weakness is greater than distal and lower extremity involvement. A myasthenic crisis may occur from a sudden increase in severity. Occasionally, acute onset consists of bulbar symptoms in which speech is involved along with generalized weakness that is rapidly fatal.

Diagnosis is predominantly made on clinical symptoms. Improvement after testing with an anticholinesterase drug confirms the diagnosis. Drug treatment is with neostigmine (Prostigmin) and pyridostigmine (Mestinon), the latter being longer lasting. These are known to inhibit acetylcholinesterase, allowing a higher concentration of the acetylcholine in the synaptic cleft. Overdoses of medication may result in cholinergic crises consisting of muscular fasciculation, salivation, and meiosis (contraction of the pupil). Thymectomy offers the best result in young women with disease of less than 5 years in duration. Myasthenic crisis is best treated by tracheostomy and controlled respiration. Plasmapheresis and steroids are also used in treatment. Prognosis is good in at least one-fourth of patients, in whom the disease is not progressive. Long periods of remission do occur, but some patients undergo a progressive course that may result in bulbar and respiratory paralysis.

Case Study

Patient One

A 60-year-old man went to see a neurologist with the complaint that he is easily tired. He claimed needing rest even after mild exertion. The neurologist who interviewed and examined the patient noted the following:

- A 6-month history of diplopia
- Some respiratory weakness with shallow breathing and limited vital capacity
- Near-normal strength after rest
- Progressive weakness after a brief period of physical activity
- The neurologist suspected myasthenia gravis. This diagnosis was confirmed by the results of an edrophonium (Tensilon) test, in which administration of this drug immediately improved the patient's physical strength.

Question: Can you relate this weakness after sustained physical activity to myasthenia gravis?

Discussion: In myasthenia gravis, an autoimmune disease, the motor end plate is damaged by antibodies, which are directed against acetylcholine receptors and restrict muscle contraction. Since normal-appearing muscles fatigue with persistent motor tasks, such patients are subjected to stress testing. See any book on motor speech disorder for the effect of this condition on speech. Anticholinergic drugs, such as edrophonium, increase muscle strength by slowing the enzymatic destruction of acetylcholine at the myoneural junction.

SUMMARY

The neuron is the fundamental unit of the nervous system. Its major characteristic is the ability to communicate within the nervous system, with other parts of the body, and with the environment. With billions of multisynaptic connections, the nerve cells serve higher mental functions that include memory, thinking, reasoning, calculation, and language. Neuroglial cells, which support and protect nerve cells, are important in tissue repair and participate in phagocytizing cellular debris. Nerve cells communicate with one another through nerve impulses that represent all neuronal activity. The nerve impulses have a chemical component that underlies the electric potential of the cells. A neurotransmitter is a chemical substance released at a synapse that transmits signals across neurons. There are two types of transmitters in the nervous system: **small molecules** and **large molecules** (peptides). Small-molecule neurotransmitters include **acetylcholine, dopamine, norepinephrine, serotonin, glutamate,** and **GABA.** They are known to have short-lasting effects. Large-molecule peptides produce long-lasting effects on postsynaptic nerve cells.

Technical Terms

acetylcholine	hyperplasia
acetylcholinesterase	hypertrophy
action potential	impulse
astrocytes	inhibitory postsynaptic
autoimmune	potentials
axon	locus ceruleus
axonal reaction	macrophage
chromatolysis	microglia
cytological	myelin
cytoplasm	necrosis
dendrites	nerve cell
depolarization	neurilemma
dopamine	Nissl bodies
endoneurium	node of Ranvier
epineurium	norepinephrine
excitatory postsynaptic	oligodendroglia
potentials	permeability
GABA	phagocyte
glial cells	polarization

Schwann cells   thymus
serotonin   wallerian degeneration
synapse

Review Questions

1. Define the following terms:

action potential	inhibitory postsynaptic potentials
astrocytes	macrophage
autoimmune	microglia
axon	myelin
axonal reaction	nerve cell
chromatolysis	neurilemma
cytological	Nissl bodies
cytoplasm	node of Ranvier
dendrites	oligodendroglia
depolarization	permeability
endoneurium	phagocyte
excitatory postsynaptic potential	polarization
	Schwann cells
glial cells	synapse
hyperplasia	wallerian degeneration
hypertrophy	

2. What structures make up a neuron or primary nerve cell? Describe their functions with a diagram of a typical nerve cell.
3. List major glial cells and describe their functions.
4. Explain how the following terms are related to impulse generation: action potential, depolarization, membrane excitability, polarized membrane, repolarized membrane, resting potential, subthreshold stimulus summation.
5. Describe the chemical and electrical events that are related to impulse transmission, beginning with resting potentials and ending with the generation of action potentials.
6. Describe the chemical properties associated with a resting membrane potential.
7. What is meant by depolarization of neuronal membranes?
8. Describe the function of the myelin sheath.
9. Describe the effects of inhibitory and excitatory postsynaptic potentials on a postsynaptic neuron.
10. Discuss how nerve and glial cells respond to injuries. Specifically, discuss the concepts of chromatolysis, wallerian degeneration, axonal reaction, and axonal regeneration.
11. Describe how axonal growth in the CNS is different from that in the PNS.
12. Name the primary neurotransmitters in the CNS and briefly discuss their functions.
13. Describe pathophysiology of multiple sclerosis and myasthenia gravis.
14. What degenerative change involves dissolution of the distal part of an axon and its myelin?

15. Match the following numbered functions to the associated lettered neuroglia cell type.

   i. provide structural support for brain cells
   ii. migrate to the site of lesion and seal the cavity or fill in the cavity with scar tissue
   iii. considered the scavengers of the CNS
   iv. form the myelin sheath in the CNS
   v. line the ventricles and contribute to the blood brain barrier
   vi. phagocyte cellular debris after a lesion
   vii. form the myelin sheath in the PNS
   viii. small numerous cells responsible to macrophage. (eating) the debris in the infarcted area of the brain
   ix. outline the infarcted area and contribute to the formation of the cystic cavity
   x. form the internal limiting membrane for the brain by fusing with the ventricular ependymal cells

   a. astrocytes
   b. oligodendrocytes
   c. microglia
   d. ependymal cells
   e. Schwann cells

16. Match the following neurotransmitters to the associated lettered function.

   i. acetylcholine
   ii. dopamine
   iii. norepinephrine
   iv. GABA

   a. It is the major chemical messenger in the PNS; it controls voluntary movements through its release by spinal or cranial motor fibers.
   b. Degeneration of the cells in the substantia nigra results in its reduced production and transmission.
   c. The neurons secreting it are thought to play a role in generating paradoxical sleep and maintaining attention.
   d. This neurotransmitter is implicated in Huntington's chorea, a degenerative disease characterized by involuntary movements.

6

Diencephalon: Thalamus and Associated Structures

Learning Objectives

After studying this chapter, students should be able to do the following:

- Identify major structures of the diencephalon and explain their functions
- Discuss the importance of the thalamus
- Describe the functions of major thalamic nuclei
- Provide an account of the locations of major thalamic nuclei
- Describe afferent and efferent projections of major thalamic nuclei
- Relate thalamic nuclei to their corresponding cortical areas
- Discuss sensorimotor and higher mental functions of the thalamus
- Explain thalamic syndrome

GROSS ANATOMY OF DIENCEPHALON

The **diencephalon**, the central core of structures concealed beneath the cortex, has well-marked boundaries. On the anteroposterior axis, the diencephalon extends from the **interventricular foramen** to the **posterior commissure**. The **cerebral cortex**, **lateral ventricle**, and **fibers of the corpus callosum** form the superior boundary, and the **third ventricle** marks the medial limit of the diencephalon. The **posterior limb of the internal capsule** is the lateral limit of the diencephalon; an arbitrary line drawn from the **mamillary bodies** of the hypothalamus to the **pineal gland** forms the ventral boundary of the diencephalon (Figs. 2-11, 2-18, and 6-1). The diencephalon is composed of four parts: **thalamus**, **epithalamus**, **subthalamus**, and **hypothalamus**.

The thalamus is the largest and the most prominent diencephalic nucleus. This is emphasized by the fact that all other diencephalic nuclei are functionally and spatially related to the thalamus. The thalamus serves as an **integrator** and **gateway** for information go-

ing to the forebrain. It consists of numerous nuclei connected with brain regions through **afferent** and **efferent** connections. The epithalamus, the oldest part of the diencephalon, includes the pineal gland and is concerned with diurnal and autonomic bodily functions. The subthalamus, a small region ventral to the thalamus, is important in motor functions through its connections with the **brainstem**, **basal ganglia**, and diencephalic structures. The hypothalamus is below the thalamus. Functionally, it is part of the **autonomic nervous system**, mediating endocrine and other metabolic states, such as body temperature, water balance, and sugar and fat metabolism. This chapter provides a simplified description of the thalamus related to its anatomy and functions.

THALAMUS

The thalamus, an ovoid nuclear mass, measures about 3 cm anteroposteriorly and 1.5 cm mediolaterally. It lies beneath the cortex in each hemisphere along the midsagittal line. The general location of the thalamus with respect to other surrounding structures can be seen on horizontal (Figs. 2-15 and 2-18), coronal (Figs. 2-19 and 6-1A), and midsagittal (Figs. 2-11 and 6-1B) sections of the brain. Removal of the overlying cortical mantle fully exposes the dorsal thalamus. The anatomical boundaries of the thalamus are identical to those of the diencephalon, except that the ventral limit of the thalamus is midsagittally marked by the hypothalamic sulcus (Figs. 2-11 and 6-1B). The thalamus serves three important functions. First, it channels sensory information to the cerebral cortex. Specific nuclei of the thalamus receive and channel sensations of pain, taste, temperature, audition, and vision to the primary sensory areas in the cerebral cortex. Second, it integrates sensorimotor information. Basal ganglia feedback is integrated with cere-

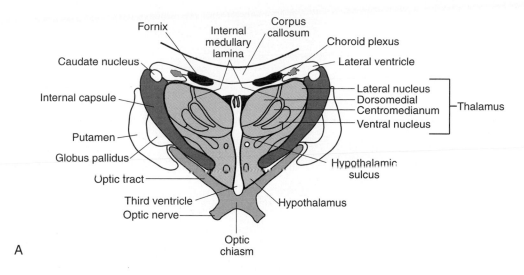

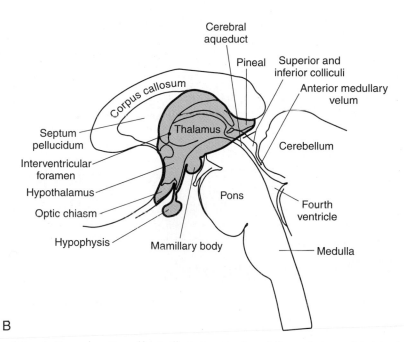

Figure 6-1.   A. Coronal section of brain illustrating location of diencephalon and its lateral and medial boundaries.
B. Midsagittal section illustrating general location of diencephalon (*thick line*) and its rostral, ventral, and caudal
boundaries.

bellar output before this integrated information is transmitted to the primary and premotor cortices (see Chapter 13). Third, it regulates functions of the associational cortex and is important in cortically mediated speech, language, and cognitive functions.

The thalamus is divided into many nuclei; each nucleus has bidirectional fiber connections to specific cortical areas. These thalamic connections form the thalamocortical functional units, which are involved in sensorimotor and cognitive functions. Some thalamic nuclei are known for their active participation in higher mental functions, whereas others, because of their anatomical connections are presumed to participate in

somatosensory functions, language, speech, and memory. Neuropathological observations and histochemical techniques illustrating retrograde degeneration of thalamic nuclei have helped develop detailed maps of the thalamic nuclei and their projections to the cortex.

Thalamic Structure

The thalamus consists of three tiers of nuclei: **medial** (mediodorsal), **lateral**, and **ventral** (Fig. 6-2). Each tier contains various nuclei:

Medial nuclear complex
    Dorsomedial nucleus

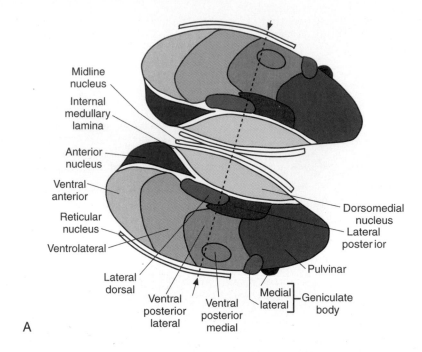

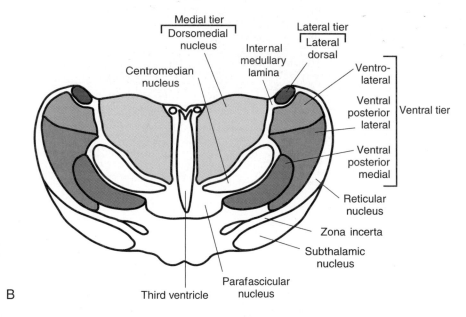

Figure 6-2.   Thalamic anatomy. **A.** Dorsolateral view of thalamus and its nuclei. **B.** Cross-section of thalamus showing three thalamic tiers (medial, lateral, and ventral) and their nuclei.

Midline nuclear complex
Lateral nuclear complex
    Lateral dorsal nucleus
    Lateral posterior nucleus
    Pulvinar
Ventral nuclear complex
    Ventral anterior nucleus
    Ventrolateral nucleus
    Ventral posterior nucleus (lateral and medial)
    Lateral geniculate body
    Medial geniculate body

Additional nuclei in the thalamus:

Anterior nucleus
Reticular nucleus
Intralaminar nuclei
    Centromedianus nucleus
    Parafascicular nucleus

The **internal medullary lamina**, a Y-shaped sheath of myelinated fibers, runs in a rostrocaudal fashion, dividing the thalamus into mediodorsal and lateral tiers (Fig. 6-1A). Rostrally, the two prongs of the internal medullary lamina surround the tubercle of the anterior nucleus; the stem of the internal medullary lamina splits posteriorly and contains the small intralaminar nuclei. The ventral tier of the thalamic nuclei is lateral and inferior to the lateral tier of the nuclei. The major thalamic nuclei follow.

Projections and Functions of Thalamic Nuclei

Each thalamic nucleus receives definitive information from thalamic or extrathalamic structures (Fig. 6-3A) and screens the information before transmitting it to functionally related areas of the cortex (Figs. 6-3B and 6-

4; Table 6-1). *Familiarity with the afferent and efferent projections is essential for understanding the importance of thalamic nuclei in sensorimotor, speech, language, and cognitive functions.*

ANTERIOR NUCLEUS

The anterior nucleus protrudes as an anterior tubercle in the floor of the lateral ventricle and is surrounded by the forks of the internal medullary lamina. The anterior nucleus is functionally related to the **limbic brain** (hippocampus, dentate gyrus, cingulate gyrus, and hypothalamus), and it in part contributes to

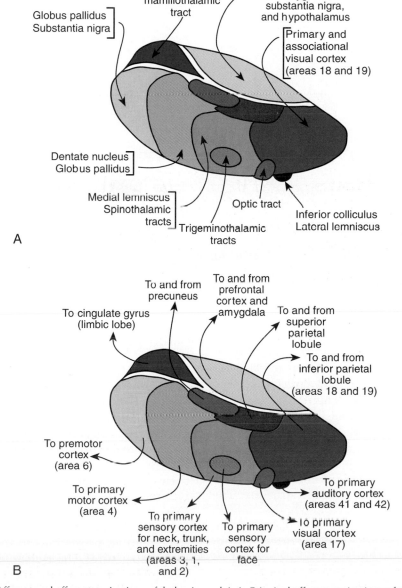

Figure 6-3. Afferent and efferent projections of thalamic nuclei. **A.** Principal afferent projections of major thalamic nuclei. **B.** Primary efferent thalamocortical projections of important thalamic nuclei.

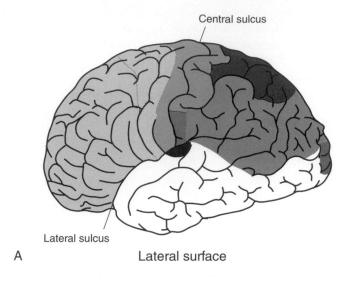

Central sulcus

Lateral sulcus

A   Lateral surface

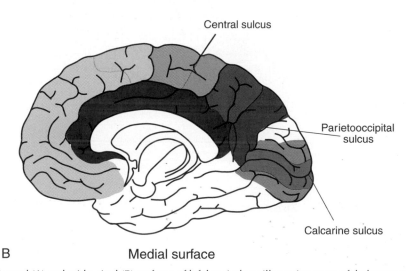

Central sulcus

Parietooccipital
sulcus

Calcarine sulcus

B   Medial surface

Figure 6-4. Lateral (**A**) and midsagittal (**B**) surfaces of left hemisphere illustrating areas of thalamocortical projections that correspond to thalamic sites in Figures 6-2 and 6-3.

digestive, respiratory, urogenital, and endocrine functions. **Afferent connection**: The anterior nucleus receives information from the ipsilateral and contralateral mamillary bodies of the hypothalamus through the **mamillothalamic tract**; the mamillary bodies in turn receive information from the reticular formation, hippocampus, and septum via the fornix. **Efferent projection**: The efferent cortical projection of the anterior nucleus passes through the anterior limb of the internal capsule to the **cingulate gyrus**, a limbic structure. The anterior nucleus mediates visceral and emotional information. Electrical stimulation and its ablation induce changes in blood pressure and emotional drives.

MEDIAL NUCLEAR COMPLEX

The **medial nuclear complex** consists of the **dorsomedial nucleus** and the **midline nuclear complex**.

Dorsomedial Nucleus

The dorsomedial nucleus, which is important in the development of emotion and personality, occupies the area between the periventricular gray matter of the third ventricle and the internal medullary lamina. This nucleus has extensive connections with other thalamic nuclei and the prefrontal cortex. **Afferent connection**: Information is primarily received from the prefrontal cortex, hippocampus, centromedianus nucleus, orbitofrontal cortex, and hypothalamus. **Efferent projection**: Projections are primarily bidirectional to the prefrontal and orbitofrontal cortices and limbic structures.

With its projections to the prefrontal cortex and limbic structures, the dorsomedial nucleus integrates visceral information with affect, emotions, thought processes, and judgment. The dorsomedial nucleus may also regulate moods that can be pleasant, unpleasant, euphoric, or depressive, depending on the nature of the sensory input and stored experiences. Clinically, the destruction of the dorsomedial nucleus has resulted in lowering the threshold for rage. Surgical lesions in the dorsomedial nucleus have been used to ameliorate anxiety-related disorders in humans. Lesions in the dorsomedial nucleus have been associated with memory loss in patients with Korsakoff's syndrome, a personality disorder caused by chronic alcoholism that is characterized by amnesia, disorientation, delirium, and hallucination.

Midline Nuclear Complex

The midline nuclear complex is a diffuse and less distinct cluster of nuclei above the hypothalamus in the periventricular walls of the third ventricle. The nuclei lie in the region of the massa intermedia fibers and bridge the gray matter across the third ventricle. **Afferent connection**: The midline nuclear complex receives information from the brainstem reticular formation. **Efferent projection**: With projection to the cingulate gyrus and the hypothalamus, it is known to serve important visceral functions.

LATERAL NUCLEAR COMPLEX

The **lateral nuclear complex** is a narrow cellular strip on the dorsolateral surface of the thalamus. It consists of three nuclei,: **lateral dorsal nucleus**, **lateral posterior nucleus**, and **pulvinar**, arranged in rostrocaudal fashion.

Lateral Dorsal Nucleus

Functions and connections of the lateral dorsal nucleus are poorly understood. The nucleus is immediately caudal to the anterior nucleus, and it has reciprocal connections with the medial parietal lobe (precuneus gyrus). It also receives afferents from the posterior cingulate gyrus. Its connections with the parietal and cingulate cortices suggest that the lateral dorsal nucleus is likely to contribute to visceral–sensory integration.

Table 6-1. Thalamic Nuclei: Afferent and Efferent Projections and Major Functions

Thalamic Nucleus	Afferents from	Efferents to	Major Functions
Medial nuclear complex			
Dorsomedial nucleus	Prefrontal cortex, substantia nigra, amygdala, hypothalamus	Prefrontal cortex, amygdala	Integrates visceral information with affect, emotions, thought processes, judgment
Midline nuclear complex	Brainstem reticular formation	Cingulate gyrus, hypothalamus	Regulates visceral functions
Lateral nuclear complex			
Lateral dorsal nucleus	Posterior cingulate gyrus (precuneus)	Precuneus region	Possibly serves visceral–sensory integration
Lateral posterior nucleus	Adjacent thalamic nuclei, superior parietal lobule	Superior parietal lobule	Participates in integrating, transcoding multiple sensory modalities underlying higher mental functions
Pulvinar	Primary, associational visual cortex; inferior parietal lobule	Inferior parietal lobule	Contributes to language functions: formulation, language processing, lexical properties, reading, writing
Ventral nuclear complex			
Ventral anterior nucleus	Globus pallidus, substantia nigra	Premotor cortex, primary motor cortex	Facilitates skilled movements; initiates voluntary movements
Ventrolateral nucleus	Dentate nucleus, globus pallidus (basal ganglia)	Primary motor cortex	Coordinates, integrates voluntary motor functions
Ventral posterior nucleus			
Lateral	Medial lemniscus, spinothalamic tracts	Primary sensory cortex	Relays somatosensory (protopathic and epicritic) sensation from neck, trunk, extremities
Medial	Trigeminothalamic tracts	Lower third of primary sensory cortex	Relays somatosensory (protopathic, epicritic) sensation from face
Lateral geniculate body	Optic tract	Primary visual cortex	Relays visual information
Medial geniculate body	Inferior colliculus, lateral lemniscus	Primary auditory cortex	Relays auditory information
Anterior nucleus	Mamillary body of hypothalamus via mamillothalamic tract	Cingulate gyrus (limbic lobe)	Mediates visceral, emotional information
Reticular nucleus	Cortexothalamus	Thalamic nuclei, including reticular formation	Presumably integrates, regulates thalamic neuronal activity
Intralaminar nuclei			
Centromedian nucleus	Globus pallidus, vestibular nucleus, superior colliculus, brainstem reticular formation, spinal cord (pain and sensory), motor, premotor, prefrontal cortices	Basal ganglia and thalamus	Modulates the excitability of the cortex (related to cognitive functions) and overall function of basal ganglia (related to sensorimotor functions)

Lateral Posterior Nucleus

The lateral posterior nucleus lies caudal to the lateral dorsal nucleus, and its functions are also inadequately understood. It receives information from the adjacent thalamic nuclei and is reciprocally connected to the **superior parietal lobule**. As a multisensory receiving area, the superior parietal lobule is concerned with the integration and transcoding of multiple sensory modalities underlying higher mental functions.

Pulvinar

The pulvinar, the most posterior portion of the thalamus and the largest thalamic nucleus, lies caudally in the lateral division. **Afferent connection**: The pulvinar receives its major projections from the primary and associational visual cortices, the superior colliculus, and the visual reflex center in the midbrain. The pulvinar is also connected with other thalamic nuclei. **Efferent projection**: The outgoing projections of the pulvinar terminate in the inferior parietal lobule, which is an association cortex. This cortical region includes important structures such as the angular and supramarginal gyri. With projections to this parietal region, the pulvinar makes important contributions to language formulation, language processing, lexical properties, reading, writing, and other important language functions.

VENTRAL NUCLEAR COMPLEX

The **ventral nuclear complex** consists of five primary nuclei: **ventral anterior nucleus**, **ventrolateral nucleus**, **ventral posterior nucleus**, **lateral geniculate body**, and **medial geniculate body**. Boundaries of these nuclei are not clearly demarcated, and they are known to have many overlapping fibers. This nuclear complex serves as the relay center for specific sensory and motor information.

Ventral Anterior Nucleus

The ventral anterior nucleus lies in the most rostral area of the ventral nuclear complex. **Afferent connection**: It receives input from the inner segment of the globus pallidus via the **ansa lenticularis** and the **fasciculus lenticularis** (see Chapter 13). Other afferent fibers to the ventral anterior nucleus come from the substantia nigra and the intralaminar and midline thalamic nuclei. **Efferent projection**: The outgoing projections of the ventral anterior nucleus extend to the premotor cortex (Brodmann area 6) and primary motor cortex (Brodmann area 4). The premotor cortex facilitates skilled and sequential movements, and the primary motor cortex is responsible for initiating voluntary movements.

Ventrolateral Nucleus

The ventrolateral nucleus lies in the medial portion of the ventral nuclear complex, and it is important in the regulation of volitional movements. **Afferent connection**: There are multiple sources that provide afferent inputs to the ventrolateral nucleus. As a motor relay nucleus, the ventrolateral nucleus receives fibers from the contralateral cerebellar hemisphere via the superior cerebellar peduncle. Additional inputs are received from the inner segment of the globus pallidus via the fibers of the ansa lenticularis and fasciculus lenticularis (see Chapter 13). **Efferent projection**: The ventrolateral nucleus projects to the primary motor cortex, which is responsible for initiating all voluntary movements. This nucleus is important in coordinating different aspects of motor functions because it integrates input from the basal ganglia (caudate nucleus, putamen, and globus pallidus) with feedback from the cerebellum before projecting the integrated information to the motor cortex. The projections of the ventrolateral nucleus directly contribute to voluntary motor tasks; a disruption of this projection results in motor abnormalities (dyskinesia).

Ventral Posterior Nucleus

The ventral posterior nucleus occupies the entire posterior half of the ventral nuclear mass, and it consists of two areas: the **ventral posterior lateral** and **ventral posterior medial nuclei**. Both these nuclei serve as thalamic relay centers for somatosensory (protopathic and epicritic) sensation from the body and face (see Chapter 7).

Ventral Posterior Lateral Nucleus. The ventral posterior lateral nucleus is the sensory relay nucleus that relays information from the body. **Afferent connection**: It receives sensations of pain, temperature, and discriminative touch from the body via the ventral and lateral spinothalamic tracts and the medial lemniscus. **Efferent projection**: The efferent fibers mediate the sensory information to the dorsal two-thirds of the primary somesthetic cortex in the postcentral gyrus (Brodmann areas 1–3), in which sensory information pertaining to all modalities is analyzed.

Ventral Posterior Medial Nucleus. The ventral posterior medial nucleus is lateral to the centromedianus nucleus and medial to the ventral posterior lateral nucleus. It serves as the thalamic sensory relay center for the sensation of taste, pain, temperature, and discriminative touch for the head and face. **Afferent connection**: The ventral posterior medial nucleus receives information from the secondary fibers of the trigeminal nerve. It also receives projections from the gustatory (taste) nucleus in the brainstem. **Efferent projection**: This nucleus projects sensory information to the lower third of the primary somesthetic cortex in the postcentral gyrus region, where sensory information reaches consciousness and is analyzed.

The projection fibers from the ventral posterior nucleus travel through the internal capsule and extend to the primary somesthetic cortex in the parietal lobe. Even though cortical participation is necessary for the refinement of these sensations and their interpretation in the context of previous experiences, some awareness of pain, temperature, and discriminative touch sensations has been demonstrated at the thalamic level.

Lateral Geniculate Body

The lateral geniculate body, beneath the pulvinar, is the thalamic relay center for the sensation of vision. **Afferent connection**: Afferents to the lateral geniculate body mediate the visual information from half of the visual field of each eye. These fibers originate from the ganglion cells in the temporal half of the retina from the ipsilateral eye and the medial half of the retina from the contralateral eye, and they carry a point-to-point projection of the retina to the lateral geniculate body. **Efferent projection**: The geniculocalcarine fibers from the lateral geniculate body terminate in the upper and lower lips of the calcarine fissure, which is the primary visual cortex, also Brodmann area 17 (see Chapter 8).

Medial Geniculate Body

The medial geniculate body is the circular area on the posterior surface of the thalamus beneath the pulvinar; it is the relay center for audition. **Afferent connection**: The afferent fibers to the medial geniculate body come from the organ of Corti in each ear via the fibers of the lateral lemniscus and brachium of the inferior colliculus. **Efferent projection**: The fibers leaving the medial geniculate body constitute auditory radiations (geniculo-Heschl's fibers) traveling through the internal capsule and terminating on the primary auditory cortex on the superior surface of the lateral fissure, the transverse Heschl's gyrus.

Additional Nuclei in the Thalamus

RETICULAR NUCLEUS

The reticular nucleus consists of a thin invisible layer of nerve cells between the **external medullary lamina** of the thalamus and the internal capsule. This nuclear complex consists of neurons that are similar to those in the brainstem reticular formation. Its axons project predominantly to thalamic nuclei, but some axons project to cells within the limits of the reticular nucleus. It receives collaterals from thalamocortical and corticothalamic projections. It is thought to integrate and regulate thalamic neuronal activity.

INTRALAMINAR NUCLEI

The **intralaminar nuclear complex** consists of several nuclei interspersed in the core of the internal medullary lamina (Fig. 6-2). The **centromedianus nucleus** and **parafascicular nucleus**, two important intralaminar nuclei, indirectly contribute to the diffuse reticular–brain activation system. **Afferent connection**:

The intralaminar complex receives afferents from the globus pallidus, vestibular nucleus, superior colliculus, and the brainstem reticular formation. The centromedianus and parafascicular nuclei also receive cortical afferents from the motor, premotor, and prefrontal cortical areas. The rostral intralaminar complex also receives input from the brainstem reticular formation and pain and other sensory inputs from the spinal cord. **Efferent projection**: The intralaminar nuclei predominantly project to the basal ganglia (putamen, caudate) and sparsely to the cortical areas.

The intralaminar system as a whole influences the excitability of the association cortex with both its intrathalamic projections and striate collaterals to the cortex. Thus, the thalamic intralaminar system is in a prime position to modulate the excitability and overall function of both the cortex and basal ganglia related to sensorimotor and cognitive functions. Intralaminar nuclei are also known to evoke a cortical recruiting response when directly stimulated with electrical impulses (Bhatnagar et al., 1989, 1990a, b). The frontal, parietal, cingulate, and orbital areas of the association cortex are predominantly involved.

FUNCTIONAL CLASSIFICATION OF THALAMIC NUCLEI

In accordance with the source of the afferent fibers, cortical projections, and type of the mediated information, these thalamic nuclei can be functionally classified as either specific or nonspecific. This classification scheme simplifies the thalamic anatomy and helps in learning these nuclei and their functions.

Specific Thalamic Nuclei

The specific sensory nuclei receive definitive information and project it to specific cortical areas. Based on the source and nature of the transmitted information, the specific nuclei are further divided into **primary sensory**, **secondary sensory**, and **association sensory nuclei**.

Primary sensory nuclei receive specific sensory information as follows: The **lateral geniculate body** receives visual input from both eyes and projects it to the visual cortex. The **medial geniculate body** receives tonotopic information from the contralateral ear and transmits it to the primary auditory cortex. The **ventral posterior lateral nucleus** receives sensations of pain, temperature, and discriminative touch from the body and relays them to the somatosensory cortex. The **ventral posterior medial nucleus** receives sensations of pain, touch, and temperature from the face and projects them to the somatosensory cortex.

Secondary sensory nuclei receive information from specific subcortical structures and project to well-defined cortical zones as follows: The **ventral anterior** nucleus receives information from the globus pallidus, substantia nigra, and intralaminar nuclei and projects it to the premotor cortex and intralaminar nuclei. The **ventrolateral nucleus** receives motor-specific information from cerebellum and globus pallidus and projects it to primary motor cortex. The **anterior nucleus** receives information from the mamillary bodies of the hypothalamus and sends it to the cingulate gyrus, a limbic structure. The **dorsomedial nucleus** relays substantia nigra, hypothalamic, and amygdala projections to the prefrontal cortex, which regulates intellectual functions.

Association sensory nuclei receive input from other adjacent thalamic nuclei and project to associational areas of the cortex. They include the following: **pulvinar**, with projections to the inferior parietal lobule, the area important for integration of crossed sensory modality and sensorimotor information, and **lateral posterior**, with projections to the superior parietal lobule.

Nonspecific Thalamic Nuclei

The nonspecific nuclei receive general–diffuse information from cortical areas, basal ganglia, and reticular information and project diffusely to the cortical areas, basal ganglia, and specific thalamic nuclei. For example, the intralaminar thalamic nuclei diffusely project to the cortex and control rhythmic electrical activity of the brain.

EPITHALAMUS

The epithalamus consists of two small structures: the **habenular nucleus** and **pineal gland** (Figs. 2-15 and 16-6). The cone-shaped pineal gland, an endocrine structure that is known to render an inhibitory influence over gonadal (sex gland) functions and contribute to diurnal rhythms, is attached to the caudal thalamus. The habenular nucleus receives fibers from the anterior hypothalamus, globus pallidus, posterior orbital cortex, and brainstem reticular formation. Impulses are predominantly projected to the midbrain reticular formation. This circuit is known to serve autonomic functions such as emotional drives and possibly sense of smell.

SUBTHALAMUS

Subthalamic structures, although anatomically included in the diencephalon, are functionally related to the **basal ganglia** and are discussed in Chapter 13 (Figs. 3-23, 13-3, and 13-6). The subthalamus refers collectively to several nuclei between the thalamus and the midbrain. The subthalamus primarily includes the **subthalamic nucleus** and secondarily the **prerubral** (**fields of Forel, or H fields**) area, and **zona incerta**.

The subthalamic nucleus is connected to the globus pallidus via bidirectional fibers, and it makes substantial contributions to motor functions. A lesion in this nucleus results in contralateral hemiballism, a motor disorder characterized by involuntary violent, flinging movements that persist during wakefulness but disappear during sleep (see Chapter 13).

The fields of Forel, or H fields (Fig. 13-5), are the prerubral region through which various motor fibers pass before terminating in the thalamus. The zona incerta lies in the subthalamus between the thalamic and lenticular fasciculi. It receives projections from the motor cortex. By projecting motor information to the superior colliculus and pretectal area, the zona incerta functions as a visuomotor coordinator.

HYPOTHALAMUS

The hypothalamus contains important nuclei and a tract that form the crossroads between the limbic system, brainstem, and thalamus. Below the thalamus, it forms the ventrolateral walls of the third ventricle. It includes the following structures: **optic chiasm, mamillary bodies, hypophysis (pituitary gland), infundibular stem (pituitary stalk)**, and **tuber cinereum** (see Chapter 16). The hypothalamus serves as the control center for the autonomic nervous system. It controls body hormones through neurophysis by means of neurosecretions. The neurosecretions control important metabolic activities of the body and provide for homeostatic states. It regulates body temperature, water and food intake, sugar metabolism, sexual behavior, and emotional states, such as feelings of well-being, anger, and aggression. Its lesion results in diabetes insipidus, which is characterized by increased urinary output and excessive thirst, disturbances of temperature control and food and water intake, and hormonal abnormalities.

COGNITIVE FUNCTIONS OF THALAMUS

The belief that the thalamus plays only a precognitive sensorimotor role is no longer accepted. In the past 30 years, evidence from neurolinguistic and neurosurgical research has shown that some language and speech functions are also asymmetrically lateralized, even at the thalamic level. In addition, the thalamus mediates overall alertness and tuning of cortical structures, and along with adjacent basal ganglia structures, it participates in speech and language processing. Penfield and Roberts (1959) first proposed that the thalamus, with its extensive projections, integrates speech and language functions. Recently, computed tomography scans have helped identify many cases of spontaneous thalamic lesions with subsequent aphasic disturbances. Using data from patients with hemorrhages in the dominant thalamus, investigators have found persisting aphasic symptoms such as verbal paraphasia, anomia, and jargon with otherwise intact comprehension and repetition. Evidence supporting thalamic participation in language functions has also come from intraoperative language and speech testing by the focal stimulation of thalamic nuclei, which was used for functional mapping during stereotactic operations. Stereotactic destructive lesions in the ventrolateral nucleus and pulvinar of the thalamus for the treatment of dyskinetic behaviors (Ojemann, 1983) further supported the belief that there are language-specific functions in the left dominant thalamus. Evaluation of language function in patients with lesions in the left ventrolateral nucleus and the pulvinar exhibited transient and lasting aphasia, including naming disturbances, speech-related disorders, and reduced word fluency. Recently it has been found that thalamic stimulation can facilitate verbal recall. In a series of studies (Bhatnagar and Andy, 1989; Bhatnagar et al., 1989, 1990a, b), facilitatory effects have been noted on verbal memory from stimulation of the left centromedianus, a neurolinguistically unexplored and previously unimplicated intralaminar thalamic nucleus. Some facilitatory effects on verbal memory were also found after stimulation of the right centromedianus nucleus of the thalamus. More recently, stutterlike syllabic reiterations were elicited by mechanical perturbation of the left thalamus intraoperatively, preparatory to a therapeutic lesion placed for chronic pain (Andy and Bhatnagar, 1991). Interestingly, stimulation in the similar area of the intralaminar thalamic nuclei in a few neurosurgical patients also led to the amelioration of acquired stuttering (Andy and Bhatnagar, 1992).

THALAMIC SYNDROME

Although the most discriminating analysis of somatosensory information and its integration with tactile, visual, and auditory information occurs in the sensory cortex at the parietal lobe, crude sensations of pain, touch, temperature, vibration, and taste can be appreciated at the thalamic level. Thalamic pathologies may alter the perception of somatic sensation. Consequently, thalamic syndrome (depending on location and extent of the lesion) is characterized by increased or decreased thresholds for sensations of touch, pain, and temperature on the contralateral half of the body. For some, contact with a wisp of cotton can be very painful. In other cases, threshold to pain is high, but once the pain threshold is reached, the sensation becomes exaggerated and painful. For example, the prick of a pin may provoke a burning sensation of pain, and pleasant musical tones may sound like uncomfortable discord. The pain associated with thalamic syndrome is usually poorly localized and intractable to analgesic agents. Paraesthesias, such as ant crawling sensation, also occur. Emotional responses, such as laughing and crying inappropriately, may accompany the thalamic syndrome. Thalamic syndrome most commonly results from the occlusion of the thalamogeniculate branch of the posterior cerebral artery.

Case Study

A 45-year-old man fell while taking a shower. His wife found him on the floor, fully conscious. Realizing that something was not right, she advised him to take a rest. Within a few hours, the patient became somewhat dysarthric: his speech was partially aphonic and slurred. He also developed weakness and pain in his right arm. At this point, his wife drove him to a hospital emergency room, where the attending physician noted the following signs:

Paresis in the right arm
Severe pain in the right shoulder and arm
Lowered pain threshold, as a slight touch to the arm caused excruciating pain
Dysarthric and dysphonic speech
Substantial word-finding difficulty
Good auditory comprehension

The presence of sensorimotor impairments without any sign of aphasia led the physician to suspect a subcortical lesion. Magnetic resonance imaging confirmed a left thalamic cerebrovascular accident (CVA).

Question: Can you account for these symptoms based on your understanding of the thalamic syndrome involving sensorimotor disorders, such as pain?

Discussion: A CVA in this patient affected the posterior region of the left thalamus, which affected the following:

- The weakness resulted from the interruption of adjacent motor fibers.
- Severe pain sensation resulted from the overreaction of the primitive pain mechanism secondary to the lesion.
- Involvement of the thalamocortical (parietal lobe) fibers accounted for the anomia, a sign typically seen in thalamic syndrome.

SUMMARY

The diencephalon, between the telencephalon and midbrain, consists of four major structures: thalamus, subthalamus, epithalamus, and hypothalamus. The thalamus is the largest and the most prominent diencephalic nucleus, so all other diencephalic structures are described in terms of their spatial relationship to it. It serves as the sensorimotor relay center that screens all sensory and motor information before channeling it to the cerebral cortex. The thalamus is divided into many functionally specific nuclei, and each of these nuclei makes direct anatomical projections to corresponding functional areas of the neocortex. The subthalamus is important in the organization of motor functions and is functionally related to the basal ganglia. The epithalamus, the oldest part of the diencephalon, consists of the habenular nucleus and pineal gland. The pineal gland, an endocrine organ, mediates its influence on sex glands and diurnal rhythm. The hypothalamus is a major diencephalic structure for controlling activities of the autonomic and endocrine systems.

Technical Terms

analgesia	nonspecific nuclei
diencephalon	specific nuclei
epithalamus	subthalamus
hypothalamus	thalamus

Review Questions

1. Define the following terms:

   analgesia   nonspecific nuclei
   diencephalon   specific nuclei
   epithalamus   subthalamus
   hypothalamus   thalamus

2. Outline the boundaries of the thalamus.

3. Discuss the primary functions of thalamus, epithalamus, subthalamus, and hypothalamus.

4. Label major thalamic nuclei and their afferent and efferent projections on Figure 6-5.

5. Discuss motor functions of ventrolateral and ventral anterior nuclei and describe the afferent and efferent connections of each nucleus.

6. Based on afferent and efferent connections, discuss functional importance of anterior nucleus and dorsomedial thalamic nucleus.

7. Discuss sensory functions of the ventral posterior lateral and ventral posterior medial nuclei and describe their afferent and efferent projections.

8. Discuss sensory functions of medial geniculate body and lateral geniculate body and describe their afferent and efferent connections.

9. Describe the sensorimotor symptoms associated with thalamic syndrome.

10. Discuss the cognitive functions of the thalamus.

11. Match the following numbered thalamic nuclei to the associated lettered area of the cortex, which they project to.

    i. ventrolateral nucleus   a. precentral gyrus
    ii. ventral anterior nucleus   b. premotor cortex
    iii. pulvinar   c. inferior parietal lobule
    iv. dorsomedial nucleus   d. prefrontal cortex

    i. lateral geniculate body   a. primary auditory cortex (Heschl's
    ii. medial geniculate body   gyrus)
    iii. ventral posterior lateral b. primary visual cortex (calcarine
    iv. ventral posterior medial   cortex)
    v. anterior nucleus   c. upper two-thirds of the postcentral gyrus
                                    d. lower one-third of the postcentral gyrus

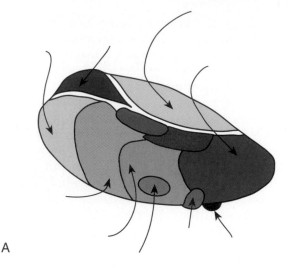

A

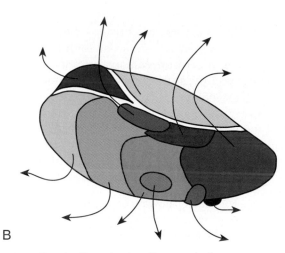

B

Figure 6-5.   Exercise figure for the afferent and efferent projections of the thalamus.

7

Somatosensory System

Learning Objectives

After studying this chapter, students should be able to do the following:

- List major modalities of sensation
- Relate receptor types to corresponding modalities of sensation
- Explain the three-neuron organization for somatic sensation in the face and body
- Describe the neural pathways for the epicritic and protopathic systems of the face and body
- Describe the neural pathways of proprioception
- Discuss common disorders of sensation
- Explain referred and phantom pain
- Relate various sensory disorders to plausible lesion sites
- Explain the rationale for assessing somatic sensation
- Discuss unconscious proprioception

SOMATOSENSATION

Somatosensation refers to pain, temperature, touch, and proprioception experienced as arising from the body. It begins with specialized receptors in the skin, muscles, joints, and blood vessels that convert sensory stimuli to neural signals and transmit them to the parietal lobe for conscious perception. Localized receptors in the skin and muscles feed into a single sensory nerve fiber, many of which combine to form a sensory fiber bundle. The afferent (sensory) fiber bundle joins the spinal efferent (motor) fiber bundle to form a spinal nerve (Fig. 2-33). Closer to the spinal cord, however, the afferent and efferent fiber bundles separate, forming dorsal and ventral spinal nerve fibers (Fig. 7-1). The afferent nerve fibers, having their cell bodies in the dorsal root ganglion (DRG), diverge sensory information by sending collaterals into dorsal horn nuclei. A few of the afferent collaterals terminate on spinal motor neurons for the activation of reflexes, whereas other collaterals travel to the

reticular formation and upper sensory centers on the opposite side. The ascending fibers carry information regarding pain, touch, temperature, and position sense and travel through the spinal cord, brainstem, and thalamus. The information is then projected to the primary sensory (postcentral gyrus) and the associational sensory (superior parietal lobule) cortices in the parietal lobe. In the sensory associational region, the lower-order tactile sensations are analyzed, elaborated upon, integrated with previous experiences, and raised to the highest conscious level for cognitive functions. The somatosensory system is discretely organized; each tract separately mediates its respective modalities of sensation, which maintains the point-to-point representation of its corresponding body surface (somatotopic organization). The higher cognitive functions of the parietal lobe are discussed in Chapter 19.

Knowledge of the **sensory receptors**, **ascending path** taken by sensory fibers, **points of fibers crossing**, and **cortical areas** related to underlying conscious perception provides the groundwork for understanding somatosensory organization. This knowledge not only helps one to examine the modalities of pain, touch, and temperature but also helps relate patterns of sensory deficits to lesion sites in the central pathways.

Types of Sensation

Physiologically, the somatic senses are divided into three primary types: **mechanoreceptive**, **thermoreceptive**, and **nociceptive** (Table 7-1). Mechanoreception relates to the mechanical displacement of the nerve endings and includes touch, pressure, vibration (tactile), and kinesthesia (limb position and movement). Touch is further divided into **fine discriminative** and **diffuse**, or **crude** (unlocalizable), types. Thermoreception includes the sensation of cold and heat. Nociception refers to pain related to tissue destruction.

153

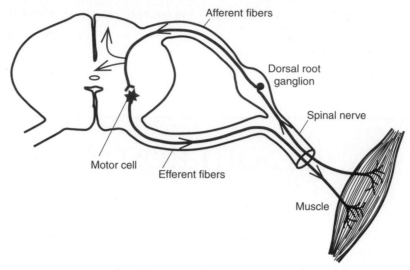

Figure 7-1. Cross-section of spinal cord illustrating afferent and efferent spinal fibers that join to form a spinal nerve.

Table 7-1. Types of Sensation

Somatic Senses	Mediated Modalities
Mechanoreception	Touch, pressure, vibration, and proprioception
Thermoreception	Cold and heat
Nociception	Pain

Specialized Receptors

Various structurally different receptors, including the somatosensory end organs, are located in the skin, limb joints, blood vessels, and muscles. The receptor type for each sensory modality is not easily identifiable. Primarily, the receptor type is identified by its maximum sensitivity to specific sensory stimuli, such as heat, pain, and touch, and its connection to nerve fibers that transmit these sensations. The main consideration in the function of any receptor is its adaptiveness to stimuli.

Quickly adapting receptors respond strongly when a stimulus is first applied. However, as the receptor adapts to the stimulus strength, the responses rapidly become weaker, eventually dying out. The nonadapting receptors do not respond so vigorously to the stimulus onset. Once activated, however, they continuously provide signals to the brain as long as the stimulus remains present. The basic types of sensory receptors in the body are **encapsulated endings**, **free nerve endings**, and **expanded tip endings** (Fig. 7-2; Table 7-2).

ENCAPSULATED ENDINGS

Receptors with encapsulated endings are the most sensitive and rapidly adapting mechanoreceptors. They mediate sensations of vibration and fine discriminative and deep touch. The encapsulated receptor consists of concentric layers of tissue around a central nerve ending. Any deformation of the external layer compresses

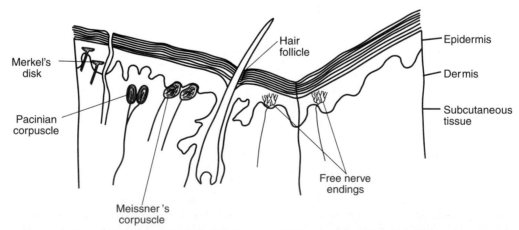

Figure 7-2. Common sensory receptors. Meissner's and Pacinian corpuscles are responsible for fine discriminative touch. Both types of receptors with encapsulated endings are sensitive to touch and are rapidly adapting receptors. Merkel's end organs, with expanded tips, mediate diffuse touch. Receptors with free nerve endings mediate pain and temperature.

Table 7-2.   Receptors for Somatic Sensation

Receptor Types	Suggested Mediated Modalities
Encapsulated endings	Tactile (discriminative and deep touch and vibration)
Pacinian corpuscle	
Meissner's corpuscle	
Free nerve endings	Pain, temperature (heat, cold); some tactile
Expanded tip endings	Tactile (touch, pressure); temperature
Merkel's receptors	
Ruffini's endings	

all fluid-filled inner layers, altering the contour of the capsule. The receptors in the encapsulated category are **Meissner's corpuscles** and **Pacinian corpuscles** (Fig. 7-2). Encapsulated receptors are commonly distributed in subcutaneous tissues, dermis (skin), fingertips, palm, lips, and external genitals.

FREE NERVE ENDINGS

The receptors with free nerve endings consist of fine fiber arborization and are distributed throughout the body, skin, cutaneous tissue, and visceral organs (Fig. 7-2). Free nerve ending receptors are nonadapting. They send signals at a slow rate for long periods and mediate the sensations of pain and temperature.

EXPANDED TIP ENDINGS

Merkel's receptors and **Ruffini's endings** are receptors with expanded tip endings; these mechanoreceptors are moderately adapting and transmit slowly (Fig. 7-2). They consist of nerve endings with knobs that mediate touch, temperature, and pressure; they are located in the dermis and joints.

Three-Neuron Organization of Somatosensory System

All somatosensory pathways are structurally organized in such a manner that a given sensory impulse enters the central nervous system, crosses the midline, and then ascends to the sensory cortex. This transmission of the sensory impulse is performed by three neurons and their fibers (Fig. 7-3). The **first-order neurons**, with their cell bodies in the DRG, collect sensory information from the periphery and transmit it to the second-order neurons in the CNS. The **second-order neurons**, depending on the modality of sensation, are either in the spinal cord or in the brainstem. The second-order fibers always cross the midline and ascend to the opposite thalamus, which contains the **third-order neurons**. The third-order fibers from the thalamus project to the primary sensory cortex.

INNERVATION PATTERN

The spinal organization of the sensory pathway is mixed, although predominantly ipsilateral to the side of the afferent input. Pathways mediating discriminative touch, which form relatively late in development, have the input axon proceeding up the **ipsilateral** side with the decussation delayed to the medullary level. However, the pathways, that mediate pain, temperature, and crude touch, decussate in the cord and proceed rostrally on the **contralateral** side. Consequently, a spinal lesion results in the loss of discriminative touch on the body ipsilateral to the lesion and loss of pain and temperature on the side contralateral to the lesion.

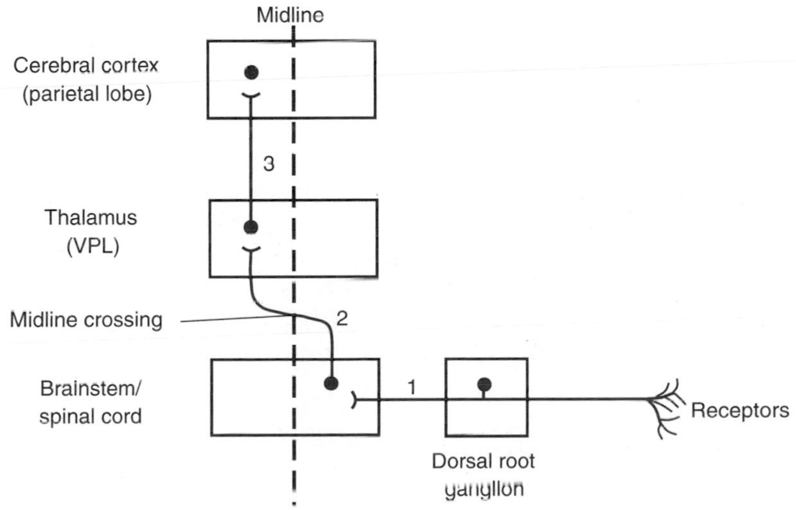

Figure 7-3. Three-neuron organization of somatosensory system. **First-order neurons** with their cell bodies in the dorsal root ganglion collect sensory information from body surface. First-order fibers transmit sensory information to second-order neurons in the central nervous system. Depending on the modality mediated, **second-order neurons** are in either spinal cord or brainstem. Second-order fibers, emanating from second-order neurons, cross the midline and terminate in the contralateral thalamus, which contains the **third-order neurons** for all modalities of somatic sensation. Third-order fibers from thalamic nuclei project to the primary sensory cortex in the parietal lobe.

ANATOMICAL DIVISION OF SOMATOSENSORY SYSTEM

Neuroanatomically, the somatosensory system is divided into the **dorsal column–medial lemniscal system** and the **anterolateral system** (Fig. 7-4). The dorsal column–medial lemniscal system, also called the **epicritic system**, is phylogenetically newer. The large myelinated fibers of the dorsal column system not only conduct impulses rapidly but also represent a precise map of the body surface. Epicritic sensation, which requires a high degree of intensity resolution, includes the sensations of fine discriminative touch, vibration, limb position, kinesthesia, and deep pressure. It is called the dorsal system because the fibers mediating these sensations travel in the dorsal spinal cord.

The anterolateral system is a phylogenetically older system made up of secondary sensory fibers that terminate in the thalamus. It is also called the **protopathic system**. The anterolateral system is further divided into the **lateral spinothalamic tract**, which mediates pain and temperature, and the **anterior spinothalamic tract**, which transmits diffuse (crude or nonlocalizable) touch. All of the ascending pathways are listed in Table 7-3.

Dorsal Column–Medial Lemniscal System

The dorsal column–medial lemniscal system mediates postural position sense, fine discriminative touch, and vibration. Position sense, which is mediated consciously and unconsciously, is divided into two types: **proprioception** and **kinesthesia**. Proprioception is awareness of limb position in space. It is important in the acquisition of skilled movements such as speech and writing, and it provides the cortex with a conscious

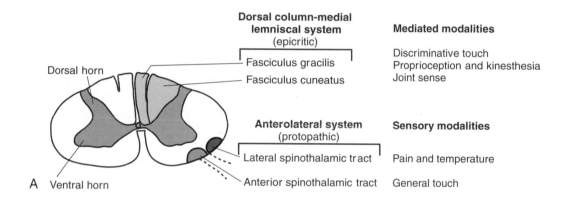

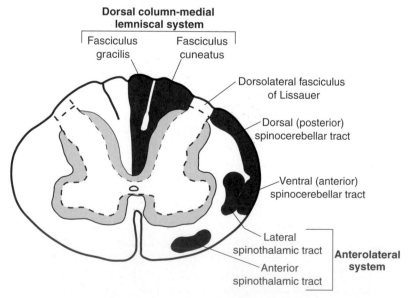

Figure 7-4. **A.** Anatomical division of somatosensory system. **B.** Locations of sensory pathways in spinal cord.

Table 7-3.   Primary Ascending Spinal Pathways

Spinal Pathways	Information Carried/Function
Fasciculus gracilis	Mediates discriminative touch (pressure, vibration, muscle and tendon stretch, joint movement) from lower half of body
Fasciculus cuneatus	Mediates discriminative touch (pressure, vibration, muscle and tendon stretch, joint movement) from upper half of body
Lateral spinothalamic tract	Transmits pain, temperature sensation
Anterior spinothalamic tract	As a backup sensory system, conveys diffuse touch
Dorsal spinocerebellar tract	Transmits unconscious proprioception from distal lower limbs, joints
Ventral spinocerebellar tract	Carries unconscious proprioception from muscles of lower extremities, proximal limbs, axial muscles
Cuneocerebellar tract	Mediates unconscious proprioception from upper limbs, joints

Table 7-4.   Components of Epicritic System, or Fine Discriminative Touch

Nerve Cell Order	Associated Fibers	Target Nucleus
First-order neuron (DRG)	With cell bodies in DRG, first-order central fibers enter spinal cord to form dorsal funiculus, ascend ipsilaterally to medulla	Nuclei gracilis and cuneatus in caudal medulla
Second-order neuron (nuclei gracilis and cuneatus)	Internal arcuate fibers, as second-order fibers, cross midline in medulla, ascend as medial lemniscus to thalamus	Ventral posterolateral thalamus
Third-order neuron (ventral posterolateral thalamus)	Thalamocortical projections, as third-order fibers, ascend from thalamus to cortex	Primary sensory cortex (body area)

awareness of the spatial position of body parts and the body during movements. Kinesthesia is awareness of limb movement. It is essential to the acquisition of skilled movements and provides information related to the direction and range of limb movements. Fine discriminative touch analyzes and identifies objects on tactual manipulation (**stereognosis**), recognizes figures and numbers written on the body (**graphesthesia**), discriminates between two or multiple points of touch, and includes the awareness of deep touch.

RECEPTORS

Meissner's corpuscles and Pacinian corpuscles, both of which are exceedingly sensitive and highly adaptive encapsulated end receptors, primarily serve epicritic sensation. They mediate discriminative touch and vibration. Additional receptors such as **muscle spindle organs** mediate kinesthesia, proprioception, and vibration.

NEURAL PATHWAYS

The dorsal column–medial lemniscal system consists of two fasciculi, the **fasciculus gracilis** and **fasciculus cuneatus** (Fig. 7-4, Table 7-4). Each fasciculus mediates discriminative touch from different body areas; however, both follow a standard **three-neuron sensory organization** (Fig. 7-5A). The **first-order fibers**, with their cell bodies in the DRG, collect sensory information from the body and enter the spinal cord. After entering the cord, the afferent axons divide into short and long branches. The short axons extend to the spinal dorsal gray horn and mediate reflexive activity. The long axonal fibers ascend **ipsilaterally** in the gracilis and cuneatus fasciculi and synapse on the **gracile** and **cuneate nuclei** in the medulla. The **internal arcuate fibers**, which

include the **second-order fibers** from the cuneate and gracile nuclei, cross the midline and form the **medial lemniscus**. The medial lemniscus, formed by the crossed dorsal column fibers, ascends and terminates on the third-order neurons in the thalamus. The projections from the **third-order neurons** in the thalamus travel to the sensory cortex in the parietal lobe (Table 7-4).

Fibers in the dorsal column–medial lemniscal system are arranged in a laminar fashion. Sacral fibers are most medial in the dorsal column. Lumbar fibers travel parallel to sacral fibers in the dorsal column and are laterally joined by fibers from the thoracic and cervical levels. Therefore, the fibers mediating sensation from the leg are medial, whereas the fibers from the arm are most lateral.

Fasciculus Gracilis

The fasciculus gracilis transmits epicritic sensations from the lower half of the body. This includes the afferent fibers entering the dorsal column approximately from the **sacral** to **midthoracic sections** of the spinal cord (Fig. 7-5B). After projecting short axons to the dorsal horn, the first-order fibers, with neurons in the DRG, ascend medially in the dorsal column of the spinal cord. Fibers of the fasciculus gracilis terminate in the nucleus gracilis, the second-order sensory neuron in the dorsal caudal medulla. From this point, fibers of the fasciculus gracilis merge with the fasciculus cuneatus.

Fasciculus Cuneatus

Fibers of the fasciculus cuneatus are lateral to the fasciculus gracilis in the dorsal column. Fasciculus cuneatus fibers carry epicritic sensations from the upper body and enter the spinal cord above the midthoracic level (Fig. 7-5B). These fibers ipsilaterally ascend the spinal cord dorsal column toward the brainstem and ter-

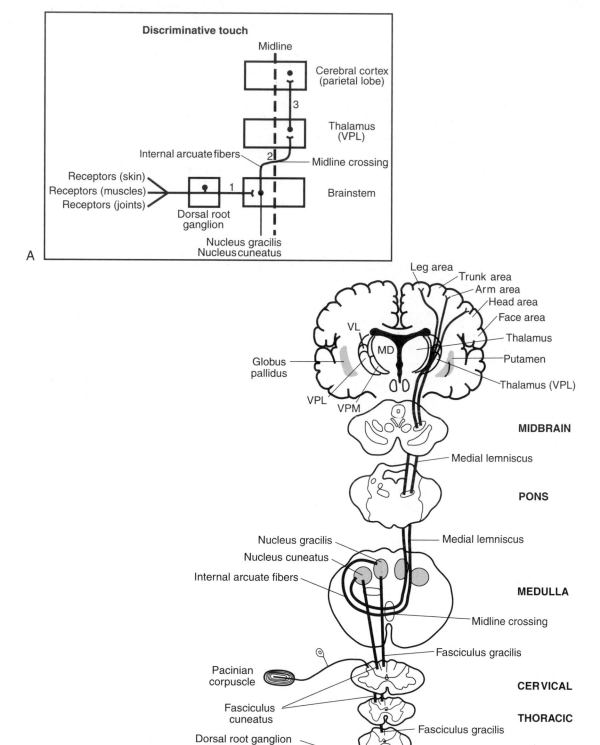

Figure 7-5. A. Three-neuron organization of dorsal column–medial lemniscal system. **B.** Dorsal white column. VL, ventrolateral; MD, mediodorsal (dorsomedial); VPL, ventral posterolateral; VPM, ventral posteromedial.

minate at the nucleus cuneatus, the second-order neuron, lateral to the nucleus gracilis in the dorsal caudal medulla.

The internal arcuate fibers, the second-order fibers from the nucleus cuneatus, travel ventromedially and cross the midline just above the pyramid in the medulla (Fig. 3-8). After the crossing (decussation), the internal arcuate fibers form the medial lemniscus, a fillet-shaped bundle of fibers. The medial lemniscus fibers ascend along the midline through the medulla (Figs. 3-9 to 3-11) and the pontine tegmentum (Fig. 3-14). Later they migrate dorsolaterally in the midbrain (Fig. 3-16) to enter the **ventral posterolateral nucleus** of the thalamus, the third-order sensory relay nucleus.

Awareness of sensation occurs at the cortical level; however, crude awareness of touch is also said to occur at the thalamic level. The third-order fibers from the ventral posterolateral nucleus of the thalamus pass through the posterior limb of the internal capsule. They terminate in the upper two-thirds of the postcentral gyrus, the **primary sensory cortex** in the parietal lobe. The primary sensory cortex, the site that analyzes the quality of sensory information, consists of Brodmann areas 3, 2, and 1. There is a specific somatotopic organization in the primary sensory cortex where the fibers from the lower extremity terminate along the superior medial aspect of the postcentral gyrus; the projections from the upper limbs terminate in the lateral region of the cortex (Fig. 7-6).

The elaboration and integration of the sensory information with previously stored experiences and with information from other sensory modalities is required for recognition of an object and interpretation of its significance. This analysis and integration of stimuli is ac-complished in the somesthetic association cortex (Brodmann areas 7, 39, and 40), which consists of the superior and part of the inferior parietal lobule and which lies at the crossroads of the temporoparieto-occipital regions. A lesion in the association cortex results in disorders of cross-modality integration, which include disturbances in somatosensory discrimination, tactile perception (graphesthesia and stereognosis), sensory agnosia, and impaired intersensory integration, in addition to cognitive impairments.

CLINICAL CONSIDERATIONS AND ASSESSMENT

Lesions interrupting the ascending fibers in the dorsal column system affect fine discriminative touch sensation and position sense (proprioception and kinesthesia). Inflammation of the peripheral nerve and dorsal root ganglion, degeneration (interruption) of spinal dorsal column fibers, neoplasm, and vascular infarcts in the cord are all common conditions that affect one's ability to process fine discriminative touch and related information.

Epicritic sensation is localizable and not painful, as opposed to nociceptive sensation (described next). The pattern of loss of epicritic sensation reveals the site at which the epicritic pathway has been interrupted. This can occur at the peripheral nerve, dorsal (posterior) spinal nerve root, or dorsal column (first-order sensory neuron); at the nuclei gracilis and cuneatus or medial lemniscus, before or after it crosses the midline of the brainstem (second-order sensory neuron); or at the ventral posterolateral (VPL) nucleus of the thalamus or its thalamocortical projection through the posterior limb of the internal capsule and corona radiata to the sensory cortex (third sensory neuron).

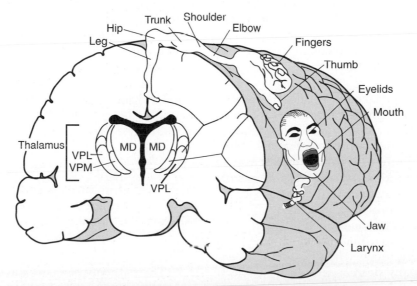

Figure 7-6.   Nucleus ventralis posterolateralis (VPL) of thalamus, the third-order sensory nucleus; projections from nucleus ventralis posterolateralis cross internal capsule and travel to primary sensory cortex in parietal lobe. VPM, ventral posteromedial; MD, mediodorsal (dorsomedial).

The pattern of deficit following a peripheral nerve injury differs from the pattern of a dorsal root or dorsal column injury; because peripheral nerves send their axons into the spinal cord over more than one dorsal root, a peripheral nerve injury causes more widespread loss of sensation than an injury to a single dorsal root. For example, the most commonly injured peripheral nerve is the median nerve, which supplies the thumb side of the hand (Table 2-5). After complete injury to the median nerve, the sensory loss includes the thumb, index finger, middle finger, and the side of the ring finger adjacent to the middle finger. (Usually, median nerve injury is not so severe—carpal tunnel syndrome—from compression of the nerve near the wrist.) By contrast, complete injury to the sixth cervical nerve root, one of the four adjacent cervical nerve roots that receive some axons from the median nerve, creates a loss of sensation in the thumb and part of the forearm but does not affect the other fingers supplied by the median nerve because they send their axons into the spinal cord via the seventh cervical nerve root, not the sixth.

Damage to the dorsal column of the spinal cord is rarely as selective as a peripheral nerve or nerve root injury; usually both dorsal columns are affected by injury or disease, and all modalities of epicritic sensation are lost or impaired below the level of the lesion. Occasionally one dorsal column is affected and the other is spared. Because axons in the dorsal column travel up toward the medulla on the same side on which they entered the spinal cord, the sensory deficit is always ipsilateral to the lesion. The key to clinically identifying the spinal cord as the site of injury is finding a level on the body below which sensation is abnormal— impaired, altered, or lost. For example, a lesion that completely interrupts the sensory pathways at the level of the 10th thoracic segment of the spinal cord creates a sensory deficit in all parts of the body below the umbilicus. If the entire spinal cord and not just its sensory pathways is damaged at a given level, motor functions are also lost below the level of the lesion. In the example of a T-10 injury, the patient is paraplegic.

The integrity of the dorsal column–medial lemniscal fibers is assessed by various sensory tests. Commonly employed tests are two-point tactile discrimination, vibratory sense, position sense, stereognosis, and graphesthesia. The **two-point discrimination test** examines a subject's ability to identify two close points of stimulation. Pencil tips or a special instrument, the esthesiometer, is used for stimulating two closely spaced points alternated with a single-point touch. The subject, with eyes closed, is asked to differentiate the one-point touch from the two-point touch. The distance between the two points is gradually decreased until the subject can no longer differentiate between two simultaneously touched points. In **stereognosis**, a subject with closed eyes is required to identify an object by feeling its con-

tour, weight, shape, and texture. In **graphesthesia**, a subject's ability to identify, with eyes closed, a number or letter written on the skin is tested. **Vibratory sense** is assessed with a tuning fork held against a bony surface. The subject must describe when and where the vibration was felt.

The **Romberg test** is used to evaluate proprioception. With eyes closed, a subject stands with feet together. Unsteadiness in this position indicates a lack of proprioception in the lower extremities. Kinesthetic awareness is tested by moving a subject's fingers and toes while he or she reports on the direction of joint movements. Kinesthetic proprioception concerning position sense is also tested by moving the subject's arm to 45° or more and then asking him or her to duplicate the shoulder angle with the other arm. Separate assessments of the upper and lower limbs can be used to evaluate the integrity of the fasciculi gracilis and cuneatus.

Anterolateral System

The anterolateral system, which mediates pain and temperature modalities, is named for the location of its fibers along the spinal white column. It follows the three-neuron organizational framework but differs from fibers in the dorsal column in respect to its **crossing point**. Fibers of the anterolateral system cross at various points in the spinal cord. The first-order fibers, with their cell bodies in the dorsal root ganglia, enter the spinal cord and travel one or two spinal segments up or down before synapsing on the second-order neurons in the spinal dorsal gray column: the **substantia gelatinosa** and **nucleus proprius**. The second-order fibers cross the midline of the spinal cord and travel to the **ventral posterolateral nucleus** of the thalamus, a third-order nucleus, which projects to the sensory cortex (Fig. 7-7A; Table 7-5).

The anterolateral system is divided into the **lateral** and **anterior spinothalamic tracts**. The lateral spinothalamic tract mediates the sensations of pain and temperature. The anterior spinothalamic tract mediates diffuse, or unlocalized (crude), touch.

LATERAL SPINOTHALAMIC TRACT

Receptors

End organs with free nerve endings are the primary mediators of pain and temperature sensations. Some encapsulated receptors also secondarily contribute to the modalities of pain and temperature.

Neural Pathway

The pathway carrying the sensations of pain and temperature (hot and cold) begins at the nociceptive receptors in the skin (Fig. 7-7B). The first-order fibers, with their nuclei in the dorsal root ganglia, carry sensations

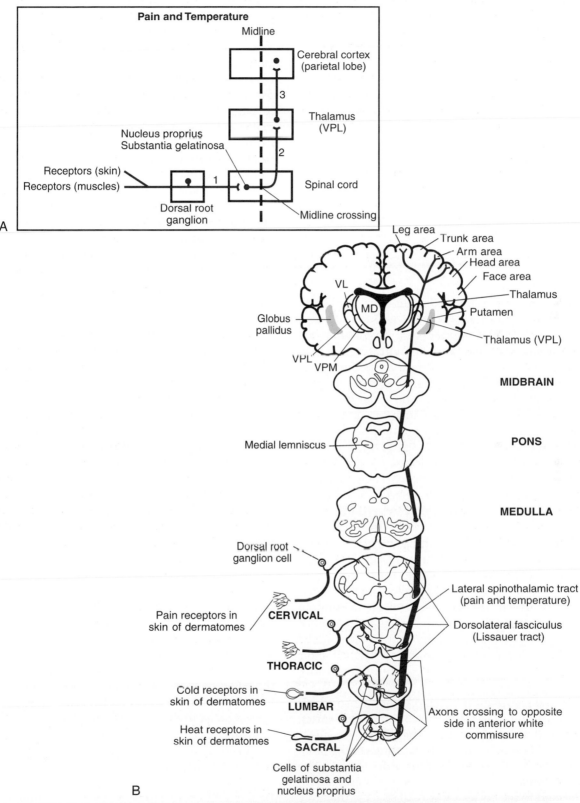

Figure 7-7. **A.** Three-neuron organization of anterolateral system. **B.** Lateral spinothalamic tract carrying pain and temperature sensation from body. VL, ventrolateral; MD, mediodorsal (dorsomedial); VPL, ventral posterolateral; VPM, ventral posteromedial.

Table 7-5. Components of Protopathic System: Pain, Temperature, and Touch

Nerve Cell Order	Associated Fibers	Target Nucleus
First-order nucleus (DRG)	With cell bodies in DRG, first-order fibers enter spinal cord	Nucleus proprius, substantia gelatinosa in spinal dorsal horn
Second-order nucleus (nucleus proprius, substantia gelatinosa)	Second-order fibers cross midline in spinal cord, form lateral and ventral spinothalamic tract, ascend to thalamus	Ventral posterolateral thalamus
Third-order nucleus (ventral posterolateral thalamus)	Thalamocortical projections, as third-order fibers, ascend from thalamus to cortex	Primary sensory cortex (body area)

from the receptors in the skin and enter the dorsolateral spinal cord. After entering the cord, these fibers travel up or down a few spinal segments in the **dorsolateral fasciculus (Lissauer's tract)** before penetrating the dorsal spinal gray matter. After penetration, the fibers terminate in the substantia gelatinosa and nucleus proprius. Collaterals from the substantia gelatinosa and nucleus proprius project via interneurons to motor neurons in the ventral gray horns and mediate withdrawal reflexes. The second-order fibers cross the midline in the ventral white commissure to ascend in the lateral spinothalamic tract (Fig. 7-7B). Fibers carrying pain and temperature sensation from the entire body travel in the lateral spinothalamic tract and ascend toward the brainstem on the way to the thalamus. After traveling through the medulla (Fig. 3-11) and ventrolateral pons (Fig. 3-14) and midbrain tegmentum (Fig. 3-16), the spinothalamic fibers terminate on the third-order neurons in the ventral posterolateral nucleus of the thalamus. **Thalamocortical fibers** travel through the internal capsule and corona radiata, then project to the upper two-thirds of the postcentral gyrus in the parietal lobe (Fig. 7-6). The primary sensory cortex is responsible for a finer analysis of sensation and determines its quality and source.

In fact, the stimulation of the primary sensory cortex does not result in the experience of pain. This cortex is involved in determining where the pain is (localization), but it is not involved in the hurtfulness of the pain. Pain may be characterized as sharp or dull (diffuse). The neuronal mechanism of sharp pain is well understood, as it is projected to the cortex by way of specific thalamic (VPL and ventroposterior medial [VPM]) nuclei (see Chapter 6). However, dull pain involves multisynaptic pathways. The lateral spinothalamic tract mediating nociceptive afferents from the body, viscera, or face gives

off many collaterals that terminate on the reticular nuclei in the brainstem; these project to the thalamus, hypothalamus, and hippocampus. The descending reticular (periaqueductal gray matter) projections are known to modulate pain perception. The reticular projections, along with other brainstem nuclei, project to the dorsal horns of the spinal cord to inhibit the pain-mediating pathways. By regulating the transmission of pain, the reticular projections participate in mediating many somatic and visceral responses to pain, such as changes in heart rate, alterations in the frequency and depth of respiration, nausea, and fainting.

An emotional response of hurtfulness of pain involves the limbic system. The nociceptive afferents from the body, viscera, or face reaching the thalamus also innervate the **intralaminar nuclei** (see Chapter 6) of the thalamus. These project into the limbic system, including the amygdaloid complex and associated old cortex. The experience including the affective aspect of pain—the hurtfulness of the pain—is undoubtedly associated with these projections.

Clinical Considerations and Assessments

An interruption of the ascending fibers at any point in the neuraxis alters the perception of pain and temperature. Damage to peripheral (spinal) nerves or the dorsal root ganglion or a pinched nerve root from a herniated disk usually results in pain perceived in the body area connected to the compromised neural structure. Damage to spinothalamic fibers also affects the transmission of pain and temperature to the sensorimotor cortex. Because pain and temperature fibers cross the midline in the spinal ventral gray matter, a lesion of the lateral ventral area of the cord results in loss of pain and temperature sensations from the opposite side of the body below the lesion. Similarly, a lesion at the brainstem level affects the contralateral half of the body. However, if the dorsal root ganglia, the nucleus proprius, or the substantia gelatinosa is damaged, sensation is affected on the ipsilateral half of the body. Knowing the point of fiber crossing is important in determining which cutaneous area will be affected as a result of a given lesion. This information is used to choose the site for the surgical management (**chordotomy**) of intractable pain. Patients' inability to perceive sensations in delineated body areas allow clinicians to relate the dermatomes involved with the level of the spinal cord damage. Once the affected **dermatomes** are determined, one can identify which afferent nerves or spinal dorsal roots are damaged.

Pain cannot always be solely attributed to its particular anatomical pathways. For example, **referred pain** occurs at one site but is sensed in another site. Pain sensation from viscera is poorly localized and serves as a good example of referred pain. The central nervous system does not contain special pathways devoted to visceral sensation; thus, visceral pain impulses follow the same pathways that are used by somatic pain afferents. Therefore, the brain is likely to interpret visceral pain impulses as somatic pain signals. For example, cardiac pain is referred to the chest and/or inner side of the arm. This is because the area of reference for pain coincides with the body parts served by somatic sensory nuclei from the same spinal segments that includes T1 to T-8. That means the sensory nuclei from the same spinal segment mediate sensation from different visceral and somatic areas (Table 7-6).

Phantom limb is another phenomenon related to pain. If a limb or substantial part of a limb is amputated, the patient may continue to have shooting pain and tingling and sometimes feel as if the fingers or toes are crossed or that the limb is bent behind the patient's back for many months after the surgery. The pain or discomfort is interpreted as originating from a phantom part of the limb. There are two explanations for the phantom pain: first, after section, the peripheral process of afferent neurons usually regrows. Often the growth tip encounters scar tissue, where it grows into a **hypersensitive tangle** or knot (neuroma). Irritation from pressure, from tightening scar tissue, or from a prosthesis often results in the generation of action potentials that upon projection to the forebrain are interpreted as pain in a no longer existing distal innervation zone. Second, it is difficult to forget a lifetime of learning the association between the distal, now missing part of the limb and the touch, pain, and position experiences associated with that part.

With its somewhat unlocalizable cortical representation, pain has proven to be a mysterious perception and is very challenging to treat. For example, the alleviation of pain by cutting the dorsal root (rhizotomy)or a tract (tractotomy) has usually been transient; the pain has most often returned, and with greater intensity. The ablation of the ventrobasal thalamus (a site associated with thalamic pain syndrome) generally decreases sensation from the contralateral side of the body, but it does not entirely suppress the pain. Intralaminar stimulation has, however, proven to be more beneficial (Bhatnagar, et al., 1990). Interestingly, direct stimulation of the exposed brain has resulted in an evoked sensation of tingling, pressure, and numbness, but it has never resulted in the evoked sensation of pain. This finding has al-

lowed neurosurgeons to operate on the brain of awake patients (Bhatnagar, et al., 2000).

Narcotics, **nonaddictive analgesics**, and **local anesthetics** are commonly used for pain relief. The best analgesic is morphine, an extract from the opium poppy. These agents suppress pain sensitivity by inhibiting receptor functioning, by blocking the transmission of pain impulses, or by blocking or slowing the central pain-processing mechanism. Local anesthetic agents are used to control pain by blocking its transmission peripherally or centrally.

The modality of pain is assessed by pricking the body surface with a pin or by pinching a skinfold. The subject is asked to describe the sensation. This is repeated until the area of deficit is mapped. There are three common types of altered responses to pain: **analgesia** (no sensation of pain), **hypalgesia** (decreased sensation to pain or higher pain threshold), and **hyperalgesia** or exaggerated response (increased pain sensation or lower pain threshold).

Thermal sensation is assessed by using hot and cold stimuli. Hot and cold stimuli are applied to various parts of the body and the subject is asked to differentiate them. Common pathological responses related to thermal sensation are **athermia** or **thermal anesthesia** (total absence of sensation), **hypothermia** or **thermal hypesthesia** (raised or elevated threshold of response to thermal stimuli), and **hyperthermia** or **thermal hyperesthesia** (lower threshold to temperature resulting in an exaggerated response).

ANTERIOR SPINOTHALAMIC TRACT

Information pertaining to two types of touch, discriminative and diffuse, travels in different neural pathways. Diffuse, or crude, touch refers to a global sensation that lacks a quantitative and qualitative description and does not determine a specific location. Diffuse touch is mediated through the anterior spinothalamic tract, which also includes collaterals from the dorsal column. Neuronal conduction for diffuse touch sensation follows the three-neuron organization system, similar to the organization of the system that mediates pain and temperature (Fig. 7-7A).

Receptors

The identity of nerve endings transducing diffuse touch is not fully resolved. All three types of receptive end organs (encapsulated endings, free nerve endings, and expanded tip endings) and the collaterals from the dorsal column contribute to this less well localized touch sensation.

Neural Pathway

The first-order sensory fibers transmit general touch sensations from the skin to the central nervous system. Upon entering the dorsolateral spinal cord, the

Table 7-6. Principal Dermatomes Commonly Cited for Referred Pain

Somatic Projection	Visceral Organ
C3–C4	Diaphragm
T1–T8	Heart
T10	Appendix
T10–T12	Testes, prostate
T10–T12	Ovaries, uterus

fibers disperse longitudinally in the dorsolateral fasciculus of Lissauer. They then travel up and down a few spinal segments before terminating in the nucleus proprius and substantia gelatinosa, the second-order nuclei in the dorsal horn. Some second-order fibers terminate in the adjacent gray matter, which serves spinal reflexes; however, most cross the midline in the ventral spinal gray matter and turn upward to form the anterior spinothalamic tract (Fig. 7-8). The anterior spinothalamic tract fibers ascend in this general location to the brainstem, where they move laterally, getting closer to the lateral spinothalamic tract (Figs. 3-11, 3-14, and 3-16). Before terminating in the ventral posterolateral nucleus of the thalamus, the anterior spinothalamic tract fibers give off many collaterals to the brainstem reticular formation. The third-order fibers from the thalamus travel through the internal capsule, then project into the upper two-thirds of the postcentral gyrus located in the parietal lobe. The anterolateral spinothalamic tract projects bilaterally to the sensory cortex.

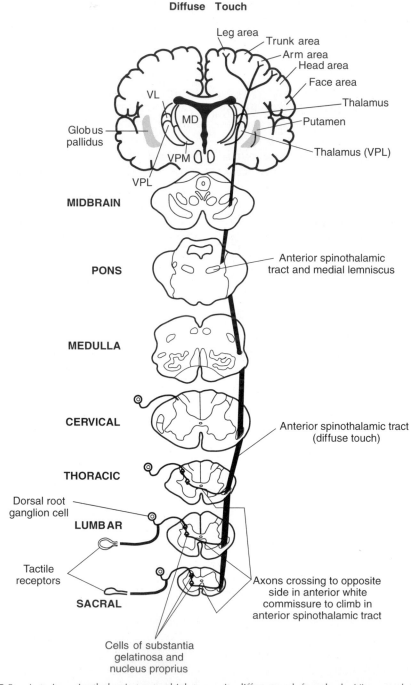

Figure 7-8. Anterior spinothalamic tract, which transmits diffuse touch from body. VL, ventrolateral; MD, mediodorsal (dorsomedial); VPM, ventral posteromedial; VPL, ventral posterolateral.

Clinical Considerations and Assessment

Diffuse touch serves as the backup sensory system for the dorsal–lemniscal column, and it projects to the cortex bilaterally. It can be assessed effectively only when the pathway for fine discriminative touch is not functioning. Because it is the secondary system, interruption of the anterior spinothalamic tract causes no obvious clinical deficit. Diffuse touch can be abolished only when the spinal cord is completely severed. Diffuse touch is tested using a piece of cotton or a wisp of wool. The stimulus is applied to various regions of the body while the patient is asked to report whether there is any sensation of touch. A subject relying on this backup system notices a touch but cannot determine its location or describe its quality.

TRIGEMINAL NERVE

The trigeminal nerve is the principal sensory nerve for the face and head. The **maxillary**, **ophthalmic**, and **mandibular** branches of the trigeminal nerve innervate different regions of the head, face, and intraoral structures. These branches cover the face and head area and mediate cutaneous sensations from the skin of the face, forehead, anterior half of the scalp, most of the dura mater, orbital cavities, and mucosal membrane in the nasal and oral cavities. Fibers of the trigeminal nerve are also joined by the small branches carrying general sensation from the **facial**, **glossopharyngeal**, and **vagus nerves**. Together, these nerves cover the remaining scalp, external ear, ear canal, tympanic membrane region, and pharyngeal and laryngeal areas.

The trigeminal system is comparable with the sensory system for the body. It contains different neural mechanisms for the epicritic system, which is responsible for fine discriminative touch, proprioception, and kinesthesia as well as the protopathic sensations of pain, temperature, and diffuse touch. In each system, different fibers serve epicritic and protopathic sensations from the head and face. The receptors serving the various sensations for the head and face are identical to the receptors previously discussed for the body.

Three-Neuron Organization of Trigeminal System

The trigeminal sensory system also follows the standard three-neuron organization; however, locations of the first- and second-order neurons for the trigeminal system are different (Fig. 7-9A). The peripherally located **semilunar (Gasserian) ganglion** of the trigeminal nerve serves as the first-order neuron. This is functionally identical to the DRG of the general sensory system. Afferent fibers, except for those associated with stretch receptors, have their cell bodies in the semilunar ganglion. There are two second-order trigeminal sensory nuclei in the brainstem, the **chief (principal) sensory nucleus** and the **trigeminal spinal tract nucleus**. The ascending first-order trigeminal sensory fibers synapse on the chief sensory nucleus, whereas the descending first-order fibers terminate in the nucleus of the trigeminal spinal tract. The second-order sensory fibers from these two central nuclei cross the midline and ascend to the **ventral posteromedial nucleus** of the thalamus. The third-order fibers from the ventral posteromedial nucleus travel through the internal capsule, then terminate in the lower third of the postcentral gyrus, which serves as the primary sensory cortex for the face.

Fine Discriminative Touch from Face

RECEPTORS

The encapsulated end organs are discussed in the section on the dorsal column–medial lemniscal system.

NEURAL PATHWAY

The encapsulated receptors, which are in the skin of the face and head, are the first to receive discriminative touch sensations. The first-order trigeminal (ophthalmic, maxillary, and mandibular) fibers, with their cell bodies in the semilunar ganglion, mediate fine discriminative sensation from the head, intraoral structures, and face. The central processes of the semilunar ganglion terminate in the cells of the chief (primary) sensory nucleus of the trigeminal nerve. The second-order trigeminothalamic fibers from the chief (primary) sensory trigeminal nucleus project to the thalamus. One fasciculus of fibers crosses the midline and ascends in the medial lemniscus (although it is considered to be part of the **ventral secondary ascending tract**) to the contralateral ventral posteromedial thalamic nucleus (VPM). The second fasciculus of fibers, which consists of a few uncrossed projections from the primary sensory nucleus, travels in the **dorsal secondary ascending tract** to the ipsilateral ventral posteromedial thalamic nucleus which play a role in reticular-cortical arousal. The ventral posteromedial nucleus of the thalamus relays sensation from the head and face. The third-order sensory fibers from the VPM travel through the internal capsule and project to the lower third of the postcentral gyrus, the primary sensory cortex for the face (Fig. 7-9; Table 7-7).

The neural mechanism for proprioceptive and kinesthetic sensations from the teeth, periodontium, palate, temporomandibular joint, and muscles of mastication is slightly different. It involves the **mesencephalic nucleus**, a trigeminal nucleus that is comparable with the dorsal root ganglion, but in the case of the trigeminal nerve, it is in the pons. This mediates sensation from stretch receptors and relays it to the trigeminal motor nucleus, controlling the mechanism of jaw reflex and the force of bite.

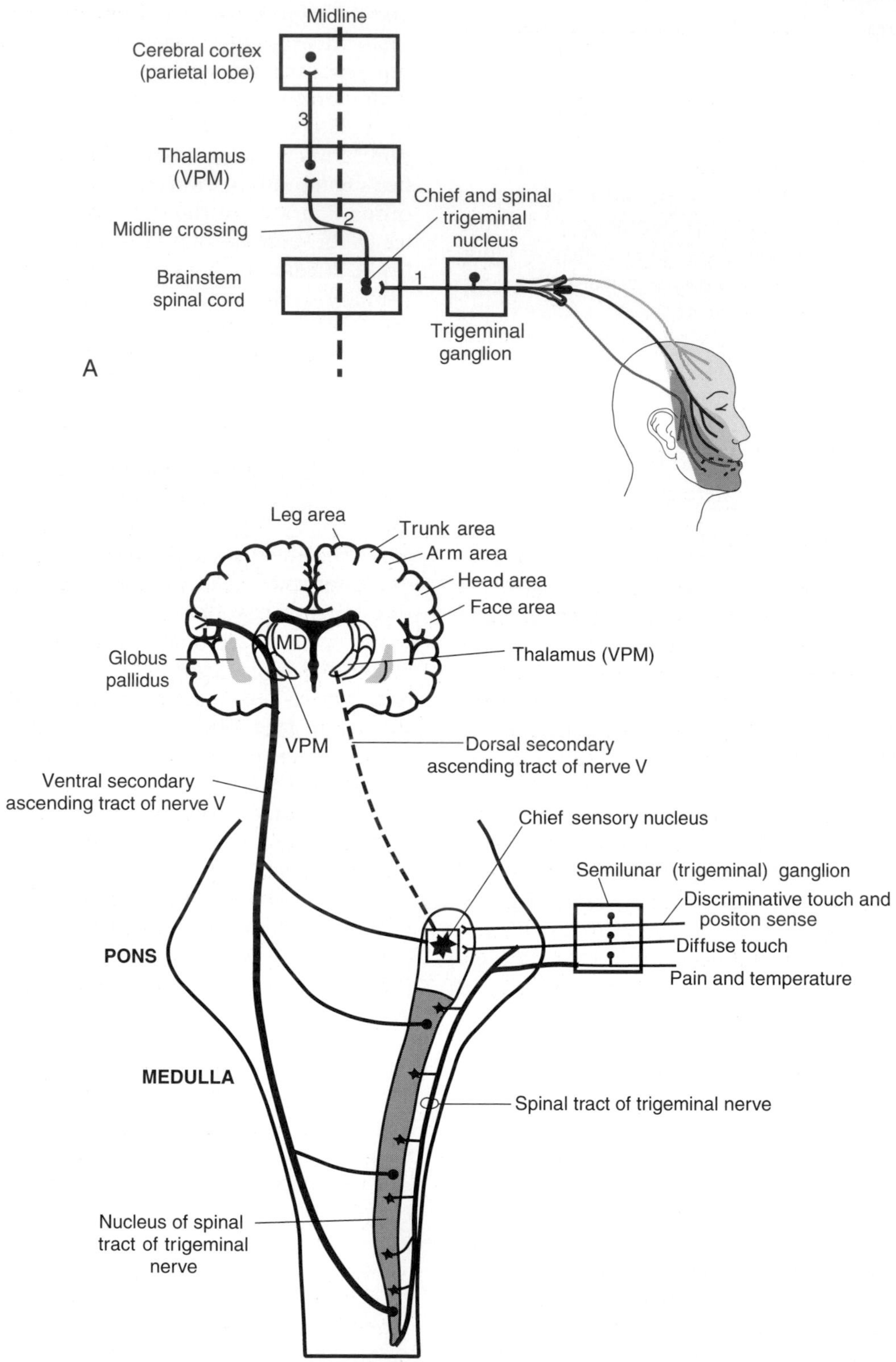

Figure 7-9. **A.** Three-neuron organization of epicritic and protopathic systems for trigeminal cranial nerve, the primary sensory nerve for face and head. **B.** Trigeminal fibers. First-order fibers with cell bodies in semilunar ganglion project to the trigeminal nuclear complex (chief sensory or spinal nuclei), a second-order neuron. Second-order projections from the spinal tract nucleus cross the midline and terminate in the ven- tral posteromedial (VPM) nucleus. Second-order fibers from the chief sensory nucleus project to the ipsilateral and contralateral ventral posteromedial nucleus of thalamus. Third-order sensory fibers from the thalamus travel through the internal capsule and terminate in the lower third of postcentral gyrus, the primary sensory area for the face. MD, mediodorsal (dorsomedial).

Table 7-7.   Trigeminal Epicritic Sensation (Fine and Discriminative Touch)

Nerve Cell Order	Associated Fibers	Target Nucleus
First-order neuron (trigeminal ganglion)	With cell bodies in trigeminal (Gasserian) ganglion, first-order fibers enter pons	Chief sensory nucleus
Second-order neuron (chief sensory nucleus)	Crossed, uncrossed second-order fibers from sensory nucleus ascend in ventral and dorsal secondary ascending tracts to thalamus	Ventral posteromedial thalamus
Third-order neuron (ventral posteromedial thalamus)	Thalamocortical projections, as third-order fibers, ascend to cortex	Primary sensory cortex (face area)

CLINICAL CONSIDERATIONS AND ASSESSMENT

Damage to both the semilunar ganglion (first-order neuron) and the chief sensory nucleus (second-order neuron) blocks the sensory projections involving fine discriminative touch and proprioception from half of the face, head, and intraoral cavity. However, damage to only one trigeminal branch (ophthalmic, maxillary, or mandibular) is likely to affect only a selected facial or intraoral area.

Discriminative sensation from the face and head can be tested by use of the procedure previously discussed for assessing the dorsal column–medial lemniscal system. The two-point discrimination test and the test for tactile recognition of objects or letters are commonly used to determine impairments of discriminative touch. Proprioception is assessed using passive jaw movement.

Pain and Temperature From Face

RECEPTORS

Free ending receptors are discussed in the section on the anterolateral system.

NEURAL PATHWAY

The central processes of the ophthalmic, maxillary, and mandibular trigeminal branches mediate pain and temperature from the nociceptive receptors in the facial and intraoral skin. The first-order trigeminal sensory fibers, with the cell bodies in the semilunar ganglion, enter the mid pons. They then turn downward (caudally), terminating in the spinal trigeminal nucleus. This tract extends to the fourth cervical level of the spinal cord. The spinal trigeminal tract also receives general somatic sensation from the facial, glossopharyngeal, and vagus nerves. Together these three nerves mediate pain and temperature sensations from the structures associated with the external ear and the mucosa of the pharynx, larynx, esophagus, and eustachian tube. The second-order trigeminal fibers from the spinal trigeminal nucleus cross to the opposite side of the medulla, then ascend in the ventral secondary ascending tract close to the medial lemniscus. The ventral secondary ascending fibers terminate in the contralateral ventral posteromedial nucleus of the thalamus. It is believed that there is some crude sensation of pain and temperature at the thalamic level. The third-order sensory fibers from the ventral posteromedial nucleus in the thalamus project to the lower third of the postcentral gyrus, the primary sensory cortex for the face and head (Fig. 7-9; Table 7-8).

CLINICAL CONSIDERATIONS AND ASSESSMENT

Inflammation of the semilunar ganglion causes excruciating pain in the ipsilateral half of the face. If the fibers in the ventral secondary ascending tract are damaged, the ability to sense pain in the contralateral half of the face is affected. **Tic douloureux** (trigeminal neuralgia) is a common trigeminal condition. It is characterized by episodes of intense pain. Other characteristics are that it is paroxysmal (sudden and stabbing) and often is initiated in a trigger zone. A trigger zone in the mouth requires the patient to twist the head in an attempt to avoid food or drink touching the zone. The worst-case scenario is involvement of the ophthalmic branch of cranial nerve V with the trigger zone on the conjunctiva, so that even blinking can trigger the pain. The excruciating pain cannot always be controlled by medication. Surgical treatment entails one of the following: decompression (pressure removal) of the semilunar ganglion, sectioning of the nerve root (rhizotomy), or transection of the fibers in the spinal trigeminal tract

Table 7-8.   Trigeminal Protopathic Sensation: Pain and Temperature

Nerve Cell Order	Associated Fibers	Target Nucleus
First-order neuron (trigeminal ganglion)	With cell bodies in trigeminal (Gasserian) ganglion, first-order central fibers enter pons	Spinal trigeminal nucleus
Second-order neuron (trigeminal spinal tract, nucleus)	Second-order fibers from spinal trigeminal nucleus cross midline and ascend in ventral secondary ascending tract to thalamus	Ventral posteromedial thalamus
Third-order neuron (ventral posteromedial thalamus)	Thalamocortical projections, as third-order fibers, ascend from thalamus to cortex	Primary sensory cortex (face area)

(tractotomy).

Pain and temperature are assessed by pricking with a pin or pinching a skinfold and using warm and cool objects as stimuli. The subject is asked to report the quality and location of the sensation to map its distribution. **Analgesia** (no sensation of pain), **hypalgesia** (decreased pain sensation or higher pain threshold), and **hyperalgesia** (increased pain sensation or lower pain threshold) are three common types of altered pain responses. Common pathological responses related to thermal sensation are **thermal anesthesia** or **athermia** (absence of thermal sensation), **thermal hypesthesia** or **hypothermia** (reduced sensitivity to temperature), and **thermal hyperesthesia** or **hyperthermia** (increased sensitivity to temperature).

Diffuse Touch From Face

RECEPTORS

All types of receptive end organs mediate diffuse touch.

NEURAL PATHWAY

Both dorsal and ventral **secondary trigeminal tract** fibers are involved in bilateral projections of diffuse touch from the face and head. The central processes of the ophthalmic, maxillary, and mandibular trigeminal branches mediate diffuse touch sensation. Fibers of these branches are divided into two groups. One turns caudally in the spinal trigeminal tract and synapses in the spinal trigeminal nucleus. The second terminates in the chief sensory nucleus of the trigeminal nerve. As they emerge from the spinal trigeminal nucleus, these second-order fibers are also joined by fibers of the glossopharyngeal and vagus nerves. These fibers cross the midline and course along the ventral secondary ascending tract to the ventral posteromedial nucleus of the thalamus. The crossed and uncrossed second-order fibers from the chief sensory nucleus of the trigeminal nerve travel in the dorsal secondary ascending tract. These fibers terminate in the ventral posteromedial nucleus of the thalamus. The third-order sensory fibers from the thalamus pass through the internal capsule and terminate in the lower third of the postcentral gyrus, the primary sensory cortex for the face and head (Figs. 7-6 and 7-9).

CLINICAL CONSIDERATIONS AND ASSESSMENT

Diffuse touch serves as the backup sensory system; it can be assessed effectively only when the pathway for fine discriminative touch is not functioning. However, damage to either trigeminal ascending tract (dorsal or ventral) causes partial to complete anesthesia in the face and head. Damage to the involved pathway or pathways can be determined by testing the modality of touch and its altered responses over the face.

UNCONSCIOUS PROPRIOCEPTION

Unconscious proprioception is the sensation of limb and joint position and range and direction of limb movements. Serving as the backup for conscious proprioception mediated by the dorsal column–medial lemniscal system, unconscious proprioception involving multiple afferent input to the cerebellum is important in the acquisition and maintenance of skilled motor activities, such as walking, speaking, writing, swallowing, and eye movement. The **spinocerebellar tracts** transmit unconscious proprioception and exteroceptive impulses from muscle spindles and limb joints to the cerebellum and help monitor and modify ongoing movement. The spinocerebellar pathways, unlike the other sensory pathways, follow a **two-order neuronal system** and do not directly project to the cortex. The system consists of three **second-order fiber tracts**: **ventral spinocerebellar**, **dorsal spinocerebellar**, and **cuneocerebellar**.

Innervation Pattern

Unconscious proprioceptive projections to the cerebellum are organized ipsilaterally to the input (as well as output). The developmentally newer and rapidly conducting (dorsal spinocerebellar and cuneocerebellar) pathway proceeds on the ipsilateral side to reach the same side of the cerebellum. The older ventral spinocerebellar projections cross back and remain ipsilateral.

RECEPTORS

Muscle spindles and Golgi tendon organs, which are located in muscles and from nerve endings in limb joints, mediate unconscious proprioception.

NEURAL PATHWAYS

Ventral Spinocerebellar Tract

The ventral spinocerebellar tract is a slowly conducting, multisynaptic pathway that mediates unconscious proprioception from the lower limbs (e.g., girdles, pelvis, and legs) and body axis bilaterally to the cerebellum. The first-order fibers terminate in undefined sensory cells in the dorsal gray column at the sacral and lumbar levels. Second-order fibers from these cells cross the midline to form the ventral spinocerebellar tract, which ascends in the ventrolateral white column of the cord (Fig. 7-4B). The tract fibers pass through the medulla, pons, and caudal midbrain, enter the cerebellum through the **superior cerebellar peduncle** (Fig. 7-10; Table 7-9), and terminate in the cerebellar **vermis**.

Dorsal Spinocerebellar Tract

The dorsal spinocerebellar tract mediates unconscious proprioception from the lower and middle regions of the body, including the legs, thighs, pelvis, abdomen,

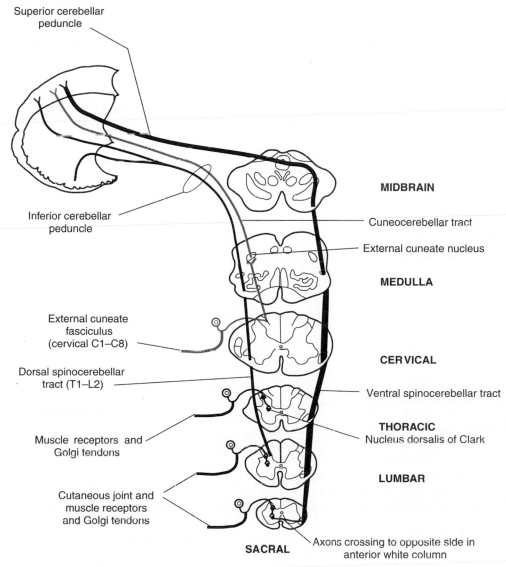

Superior cerebellar peduncle

Inferior cerebellar peduncle

External cuneate fasciculus (cervical C1–C8)

Dorsal spinocerebellar tract (T1–L2)

Muscle receptors and Golgi tendons

Cutaneous joint and muscle receptors and Golgi tendons

MIDBRAIN

Cuneocerebellar tract

External cuneate nucleus

MEDULLA

CERVICAL

Ventral spinocerebellar tract

THORACIC
Nucleus dorsalis of Clark

LUMBAR

Axons crossing to opposite side in anterior white column

SACRAL

Figure 7-10.   Spinocerebellar tracts: ventral spinocerebellar, dorsal spinocerebellar, and cuneocerebellar.

Table 7-9.   Spinocerebellar Projections

Pathway	Projection Fibers	Target Structure
Ventral spinocerebellar tract	With cell bodies in DRG, first-order fibers enter spinal cord, terminate on undefined sensory cells; second-order fibers cross midline and ascend to enter cerebellum via crossed fibers of superior cerebellar peduncle.	After two crossings, fibers carry unconscious proprioception from lower limbs to ipsilateral cerebellum
Dorsal spinocerebellar tract	With cell bodies in DRG, first-order fibers enter spinal cord and terminate on nucleus dorsalis of Clark; second-order fibers ascend ipsilaterally to enter cerebellum via inferior cerebellar peduncle	Uncrossed fibers mediate unconscious proprioception from distal lower limbs, joints, middle regions of body to ipsilateral cerebellum
Cuneocerebellar tract	With cell bodies in DRG, first-order fibers enter spinal cord, terminate on external cuneate nucleus; second-order fibers ascend ipsilaterally to enter cerebellum via inferior cerebellar peduncle	Uncrossed fibers mediate unconscious proprioception from distal upper limbs and joints to ipsilateral cerebellum

and thorax. There is substantial overlapping of innervation for the lower limbs because unconscious proprioception is also mediated by the ventral spinocerebellar fibers. The first-order afferent fibers from the muscle spindles, with their cell bodies in the dorsal root ganglion, transmit unconscious proprioception to the spinal cord, where they terminate on the **nucleus dorsalis of Clarke**, the second-order neuron. The nucleus dorsalis of Clarke is in the spinal dorsal gray column extending from the third lumbar segment to the eighth cervical segment. The first-order afferent fibers from below the third lumbar segment travel rostrally, synapsing on the nucleus dorsalis of Clarke. The second-order fibers are uncrossed; they ascend ipsilaterally in the dorsal spinocerebellar tract and eventually enter the ipsilateral cerebellar cortex via the **inferior cerebellar peduncle** (Fig. 7-10; Table 7-9).

There are two important properties of the dorsal spinocerebellar tract. First, the tract fibers remain uncrossed as they project to the ipsilateral cerebellum. Second, the tract alone mediates unconscious proprioception from the muscles in the middle body regions but mediates along with the ventral spinocerebellar tract from the lower limbs.

Cuneocerebellar Tract

A developmentally newer system, the cuneocerebellar fibers mediate unconscious proprioception from the upper limbs and neck. As there is no nucleus dorsalis of Clarke above the T-1 spinal segment, the uncrossed first-order spinocerebellar fibers from the upper limbs ascend to the medulla, terminating in the **external cuneate nucleus**, which is homologous to the nucleus dorsalis of Clarke. The second-order fibers form the cuneocerebellar tract enter the ipsilateral cerebellum via the inferior cerebellar peduncle (Fig. 7-10; Table 7-9).

CLINICAL CONSIDERATIONS AND ASSESSMENT

Because the spinocerebellar pathway serves as merely the backup for the dorsal–lemniscal system, it is not possible to determine clinically the extent to which kinesthetic and proprioceptive losses are solely due to the interruption of this tract. **Romberg test** is a clinical test for assessing cerebellar functions related to proprioception; it also reflects the functioning of conscious proprioception (dorsal–lemniscal system).

LESION LOCALIZATION
Rule 3: Spinal Central Gray Lesion
PRESENTING SYMPTOMS

Bilateral loss of pain and temperature sensation with preserved sense of touch in the same limbs (usually the two upper limbs) implies a lesion (cavitation or syringomyelia) in the spinal central gray.

RATIONALE

A cavitation in the central gray interrupts the decussating fibers of the anterior white commissure, which mediates pain and temperature sensation.

Case Studies

Patient One

A 35-year-old woman was in an automobile accident. She was taken to an emergency room. Upon a neurological examination, she exhibited the following signs:

- A complete loss of epicritic (two-point touch and proprioceptive) sensation in right lower limb
- Paralysis of the right lower limb with Babinski sign
- Loss of pain and temperature from the left lower limb

Computed tomography revealed a fractured thoracic vertebra with a fragment of bone in the spinal canal. The clinical findings indicated injury to the right half of the spinal cord at the T-12 level; this is also called the syndrome of spinal cord hemisection (Brown-Séquard syndrome) (Fig. 7-11).

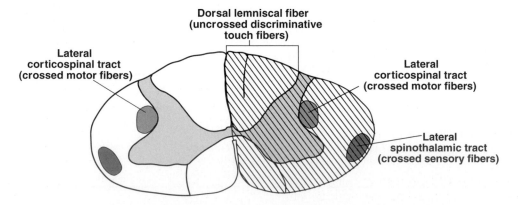

Figure 7-11. Anatomical involvement causing Brown-Séquard syndrome.

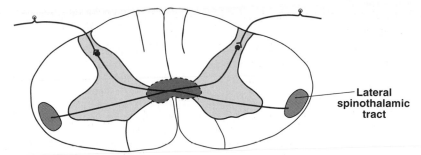

Figure 7-12. Anatomical involvement in syringomyelia.

Question: Can you account for these symptoms on the basis of your understanding of the crossing points for the dorsal–lemniscal system, corticospinal tract, and lateral spinothalamic tract?

Discussion: There are three important sensorimotor signs of spinal hemisection (Brown-Séquard syndrome): (a) spastic paralysis on the side ipsilateral to the lesion; (b) ipsilateral loss of proprioception, kinesthetic sense, and discriminative touch below the level of the lesion; and (c) contralateral loss of pain and temperature below the level of the lesion.

- The corticospinal fibers had already crossed the midline in the caudal medulla; consequently, a T-12 lesion caused motor impairments in the limbs ipsilateral to the lesion site. The positive Babinski sign implicates damage to the upper motor neuron fibers.
- Because the dorsal column fibers ipsilaterally ascend in the spinal cord and cross the midline in the caudal medulla, a proprioceptive loss from a T-12 lesion occurred on the body ipsilateral to the lesion.
- Pain and temperature fibers cross to the opposite side at every spinal level before forming the lateral spinothalamic tract. A T-12 lesion blocked transmission of pain and temperature from the contralateral body below the lesion site.

Patient Two

A 55-year-old cook consulted his doctor for lack of pain and thermal sensation in his hands and forearms. On examination, the physician found the following:

- A few burn marks on the palms and fingertips
- No response to pinpricks and thermal stimuli in the hands and forearms
- Some weakness and atrophy of muscles of the hand

Magnetic resonance imaging revealed syringomyelia, a cavity formation in C-6 to C-8 and T-1 regions of the cord (Fig. 7-12).

Question: Can you account for these symptoms on the basis of your understanding of pain and temperature fibers?

Discussion: Formation of the cavity in the spinal cord from C-6 to T-1 affected the following structures:

- Crossing of pain and temperature fibers from the arm and hand regions; consequently, the patient did not have sensation of noxious stimuli from the arms and hands.
- Nearby α-motor neurons in the gray matter of the anterior horns explain the weakness observed in his hands.

SUMMARY

Somatic sensation includes the physical experience of pain, temperature, touch, and proprioception. It begins with specialized receptors in the body and terminates in the parietal lobe. Receptors in the skin convert sensory stimuli to neural signals and transmit the stimuli on afferent nerve fibers to the primary sensory cortex

in the parietal lobe via the spinal cord, brainstem, and thalamus. This awareness is later transmitted to the sensory association cortex, where the information is analyzed, elaborated upon, integrated with previous experiences, and raised to the highest level of consciousness. The somatosensory system is discretely organized; the information collected by specialized receptors is transmitted on separate axonal tracts. Each tract mediates specific modalities of sensation. Within each tract a point-to-point somatotopic representation of the body surface (somatotopic organization) is maintained. This spatial organization of neurons, tracts, terminals, and nuclei is maintained up to the somesthetic cortex (body homunculus). Knowledge of sensory pathways, sensory receptors, points of fiber crossing, and cortical areas underlying conscious perception for different sensations provides a solid groundwork for understanding sensory organization. This knowledge enables one to relate patterns of sensory deficits with lesion sites and to solve clinical problems more effectively.

Technical Terms

adaptation	kinesthesia
analgesia	proprioception
anesthesia	protopathic
chordotomy	referred pain
encapsulated endings	sensory receptors
epicritic	spinocerebellar
expanded tip endings	spinothalamic
free nerve endings	stereognosis
graphesthesia	tactile

Review Questions

1. Define the following terms:

adaptation	protopathic
analgesia	referred pain
anesthesia	sensory receptors
chordotomy	spinocerebellar
epicritic	spinothalamic
graphesthesia	stereognosis
kinesthesia	tactile
proprioception	

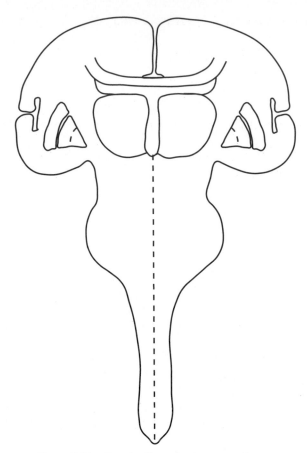

Figure 7-13.   Exercise figure for sensory pathway.

2. Discuss the three-neuron organization of the somatosensory system; specifically identify points of fiber decussation.

3. Illustrate the course of dorsal column–medial lemniscal fibers on Figure 7-13. Discuss what side of the body will lose discriminative touch (position sense, two-point touch, proprioception and kinesthesia) after a left pontine lesion involving the medial lemniscus. Explain why.

4. Trace the course of the lateral spinothalamic tracts on Figure 7-13 and discuss how a traumatic hemisection of the left lumbar (L-1) cord will affect sensory function (fine discrimination and pain). Will

these be lost on the side ipsilateral or contralateral to the lesion or on both sides of the body?

5. Describe Brown-Séquard's syndrome associated with the hemisection of the cord. Discuss the effect of the hemisection on the transmission of sensation (fine discrimination, pain, and temperature). What fiber tracts will be interrupted if damage to the left dorsal lemniscal system occurs at the lower thoracic level (T-2)? What body region will lose fine discriminative sensation? Will this loss involve only one half or both sides of the body?

6. Explain how syringomyelia, a condition involving cavitation of the spinal cord, can interrupt transmission of pain and temperature sensation while sparing affecting fine discriminative touch.

7. Explain how a patient with an infarction of the left mid pons involving the trigeminal nerve will have anesthesia of the left face.

8. Describe tic douloureux (trigeminal neuralgia); define altered pain sensation seen in the case of analgesia, hypalgesia, and hyperalgesia.

9. Differentiate between conscious and unconscious proprioception and describe pathways mediating both modalities of sensation.

10. Discuss the functions of the parietal association cortex in somatic sensation.

11. Explain why referred pain originates at one site but is sensed at another site.

12. Discuss the concept of phantom pain.

13. Describe Romberg testing.

14. What thalamic nucleus mediates projections from the trigeminal nuclear complex?

15. Discuss the function of the trigeminal chief sensory nucleus.

16. Upon examination of a patient, the neurologist made the following observations: epicritic sensations were completely lost on the left side of the body and were slightly diminished on the left side of the face; protopathic sensations were only crudely perceived on the left side of the body and face; spastic hemiplegia was noticeable on the left half of the body; the patient could wrinkle his forehead, but the left side of his mouth drooped. Explain how an infarct in the right internal capsule would produce such clinical symptoms.

17. Match the following numbered attributes to the associated lettered tract of the spinal cord.

    i. thermal sensitivity
    ii. crude or diffuse touch
    iii. pain sensation
    iv. unconscious proprioception
    v. vibratory sense
    vi. position sense
    vii. two-point discrimination

    a. lateral spinothalamic tract
    b. anterior spinothalamic tract
    c. spinocerebellar tracts
    d. dorsal lemniscal column

Learning Objectives

After studying this chapter, students should be able to do the following:

- Describe the anatomy of the eyeball and the function of each structure
- Describe the structures of the retina and their functions
- Explain structural and functional differences between cones and rods
- Provide an account of photochemistry in retinal photoreceptors
- Discuss the mechanism of color vision and its disorders
- Explain the neural mechanism of dark adaptation
- Describe optical properties of normal vision
- Discuss properties of the lens and its contribution to the formation of an image
- Define types of refraction error
- Explain the ways to correct refraction errors
- Discuss the central visual pathway
- Relate visual field defects with lesion sites
- Describe common visual reflexes
- Discuss the neural mechanism of visual reflexes

Not only is the visual system an important sensory modality, but its disturbances provide important clues to numerous neurological conditions. Visual perception involves a combination of four events: (*a*) the refraction of light rays by the lens and cornea; (*b*) the conversion of electromagnetic energy in light rays by the retinal photoreceptor cells into nerve impulses; (*c*) the transmission of impulses from the retinal photoreceptors to the thalamus and ultimately to the visual cortex in the occipital lobe; and (*d*) the perception of visual images in primary and secondary visual cortices. The organization of this chapter follows the order of neural events as they occur in visual processing, beginning with the anatomy of the eye. It ends with the primary visual cortex, which projects to the adjacent visual association region, where vi-

sual information is elaborated and synthesized with experiences and memory.

Distinguishing among three sets of easily confused terms is important: **optic nerve** and **optic tract**, **visual** and **retinal fields**, and **monocular** and **binocular vision**. The *optic nerve* includes the nerve fibers from the retina to the **optic chiasm**. The *optic tract* includes nerve fibers traveling between the chiasm and the **lateral geniculate body** of the thalamus. Thalamic projections to the visual cortex travel via the geniculocalcarine (optic radiation) fibers. The *visual field* is the area that can be seen. The *retinal field* is the focused representation of the visual field. The retinal image is the reverse of the visual field image; that is, up becomes down and left becomes right. The retinal field for each eye contains the portions of the visual field that are seen in common with the other eye (binocular) and a portion that is seen only by one eye (monocular). The *monocular visual field* is the lateral portion of the visual field that is perceived in only one eye (Fig. 8-1). By alternately closing the left and right eyes, one can produce a shift between right and left monocular vision. The *binocular visual field* is seen in both eyes as they simultaneously focus on a single object. Light rays from an object strike the corresponding identical retinal points in both eyes. Images from the two eyes merge into one image in the cortex. In double vision, this merging is interrupted; a slight deviation in the coordination of the eyes prevents light rays from striking corresponding (homonymous) retinal points.

EYEBALL

Anatomy of the Eyeball

The eyeball, a spherical structure, weighs about 7.5 g and is 2.4 cm (about an inch) long; more than five-sixths of its surface is concealed within the **orbital cav-**

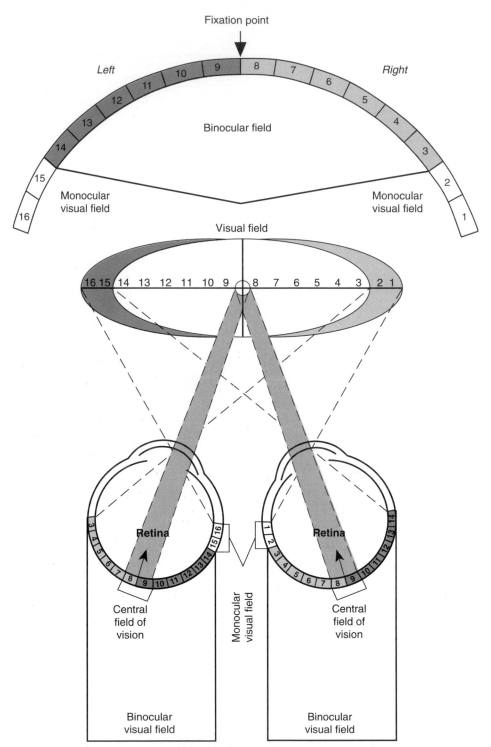

Figure 8-1. Binocular and monocular visual fields. *Shaded area*, binocular field; *open area*, monocular field.

ity. The eyeball is divided into a small **anterior** and a large round **posterior cavity** (Fig. 8-2*A*).

The anterior cavity contains structures that include the **ciliary body, suspensory ligaments, iris, cornea, and lens** (Fig. 8-2*B*). The principal function of these structures is to refract light rays to produce a sharply focused image on the retina. The anterior cavity is divided into **anterior** and **posterior chambers**. The anterior chamber includes the area between the cornea and iris,

and the posterior chamber includes the area between the iris and the suspensory ligament. The anterior chamber is filled with **aqueous humor**, a fluid similar to **cerebrospinal fluid** that is produced behind the iris by the **choroid plexus** of the **ciliary processes**. The aqueous humor flows through the pupil from the posterior chamber to the anterior chamber, and its production is balanced by its regular drainage into the venous system through the **canal of Schlemm**. Maintaining normal

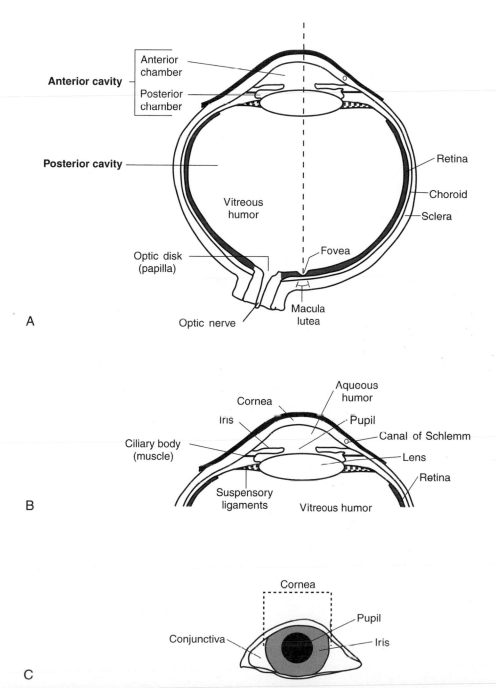

Figure 8-2. Structures of the eyeball. **A.** Cavities and chambers. **B.** Cross-section of the anterior cavity illustrating ciliary muscles and suspensory ligaments and their attachments to the lens. **C.** Anterior view of the iris around the pupil.

intraocular pressure and linking the lens and cornea with the circulatory system are two major functions of the aqueous humor. Any chronic increased intraocular pressure, wherein the production of aqueous humor exceeds its reabsorption, leads to **glaucoma**. Untreated glaucoma can cause blindness by restricting blood flow to the retina.

The posterior cavity is the area between the lens and the retina. It is filled with **vitreous humor**, a jellylike substance that in part maintains normal intraocular pressure, preventing the eyeball from collapsing. The aqueous humor of the anterior cavity undergoes constant replacement, but the vitreous humor is formed once in early life and is never replaced.

The eyeball consists of three ocular layers (Fig. 8-2): the outer **fibrous tunic** (**sclera**), the middle **vascular tunic** (**choroid**), and the inner **nervous tunic** (**retina**). The fibrous tunic, an extension of the meningeal **dura mater**, has two divisions: **sclera** and **cornea**. (The cornea is an ectodermal structure, though for convenience it is here considered a dural extension.) The sclera, (G. *skleros*, hard), the white of the eye, is a dense layer of opaque connective tissue that covers the round section of the eyeball. A larger part of the sclera is concealed within the orbital cavity. The cornea (L. *corneus*, horny), a nonvascular and transparent fibrous region of the eye, is in the exposed area of eyeball and covers the anterior chamber (Fig. 8-2B).

The middle vascular tunic consists of the **choroid**, **iris**, **ciliary** (muscle) **structure**, and **lens**. The choroid contains an elastic connective tissue membrane that lines the internal surface of the sclera. The choroid not only is the source of vascular supply to the sclera and outer retina, it also contains **melanocytes** (pigment-producing cells). Normally, the choroid pigment melanocytes make the eyeball opaque to stray light by preventing stray light from entering the optic globe through the sclera. In the pigment cell abnormalities related to **albinism** (many alleles, thus many grades of choroid pigment reduction), stray light penetrates to the retina and make vision in bright light difficult, even painful, thus causing photophobia (fear and avoidance of light).

The iris and ciliary muscle, which are the connective tissue of the choroid, are in the anterior chamber. The **radial** (dilator) and **circular** (constrictor) fibers of the iris surround the **pupil**, an opening in the center of the iris. Working like a diaphragm and controlled by the autonomic nervous system, the **iris** regulates pupil size, consequently controlling how much light enters the eye.

Ciliary muscle fibers, innervated by the parasympathetic projections of the third cranial nerve, form a ring or sphincter around the optic globe. They contract to narrow the diameter of the optic globe, reducing the tension on the suspensory ligaments (zonules of Zinn). This releases the tension on the lens capsule and allows the elastic lens to approach or assume its natural spherical or round shape. Denervated ciliary muscle results in a more highly refracting lens. The increased refraction of light entering the pupil is necessary to produce a sharp image in near vision.

The lens, which consists of multiple layers of protein fibers, is enclosed in a transparent capsule of connective tissue. It is held behind the pupil by suspensory ligaments that attach to the ciliary body. The lens is responsible for properly focusing images on the retina through the refraction of light rays. Abnormalities in the lens structure affect its refraction capacity, resulting in impaired focusing. The ciliary muscle and its processes regulate the changes undertaken by the lens to accommodate for near vision. A contraction of the circular iris fibers in response to parasympathetic activity decreases pupil size, reducing the amount of light entering the eye, whereas the constriction of radial fibers in response to sympathetic activity enlarges the pupil, allowing more light to enter.

The nervous tunic (retina) is the innermost layer of the eyeball. It consists of 10 layers of cells and lies in the posterior two-thirds of the eyeball. It contains the photoreceptor cells (rods and cones) that transduce light rays into neural impulses. Other retinal cells participate in transmission of visual impulses to the cortex.

Anatomy of Retina

The cellular layer known as the retina lies in the posterior portion of the eyeball. The retina is a specialized growth of the brain, a complex arrangement of 10 layers of cells, including nerve cells, neuronal processes, and supporting cells (Fig. 8-3). Only functions of the **rods** and **cones** (photoreceptors), the **bipolar cells**, and the **ganglion cells** are discussed in this chapter. The photoreceptor cones and rods form the most external cellular layer, whereas the **ganglion cells** constitute the proximal (internal) layer of cells in the retina. Light rays entering through the **cornea**, aqueous humor, pupil, lens, and vitreous humor first pass through the proximal layers of the **ganglionic**, **amacrine**, **horizontal**, **bipolar**, and other cellular components before striking the rods and cones. The electromagnetic energy in the light rays is absorbed by the photosensitive cells at the retinal level. Light rays that escape absorption at the retinal photosensor level are absorbed by the pigment cells of the surrounding choroid layer. This contributes to the sharpness of the focused image and also minimizes internal reflection.

The absorbed electromagnetic energy of the light rays activates the rods and cones, which transduce energy into local potentials. These potentials are transmitted to the bipolar cells, which by means of local potentials and the release of transmitters, affect the excitability of the ganglion cells. The ganglion cells are the first cells

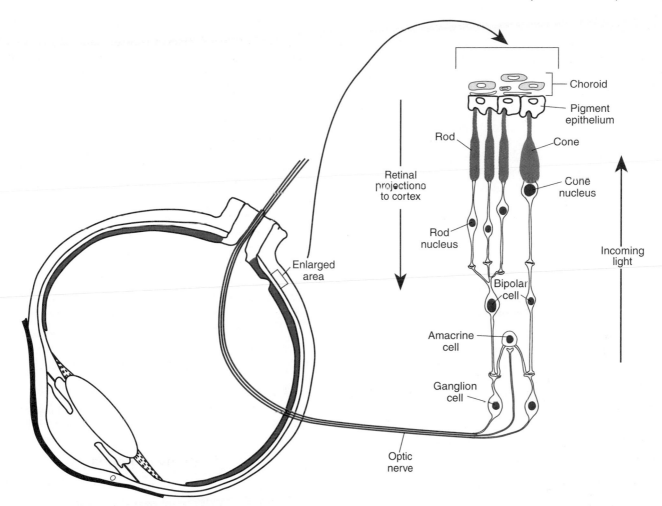

Figure 8-3.   Cellular organization of the retina with its three layers of cells: photoreceptors (rods and cones), bipolar cells, and ganglion cells. Light rays enter and pass through all of these layers to reach cones and rods, which are activated to generate action potentials. Action potentials from photosensors carrying visual code travel back to bipolar cells and ganglion cells. Ganglion cell projections form the optic nerve.

to generate action potentials. Ganglion cell axons converge at the **optic disk** (**papilla**, or optic nerve head) to form the **optic nerve**. Posteriorly, these axons pierce the eyeball, projecting to the **optic chiasm**, which also receives projections from the other eye.

The retinal photoreceptors, rods and cones, are functionally and structurally different. They are sensitive to light rays of different wavelengths, mediate vision under different light conditions, and contain different visual pigments.

DISTRIBUTION OF PHOTOSENSORS

By a rough estimate, there are approximately 130 million photoreceptors in the human retina. Of these, about 100 million are rods and 30 million are cones. Cone cells are predominantly in the central retina, which consists of the **macula lutea**, a small circular area lateral to the optic disk (Fig. 8-2A). Within the macula lutea is the **fovea centralis**. With a diameter of 700 μm and covering 2° of the retina from the center, the **fovea** exclu-

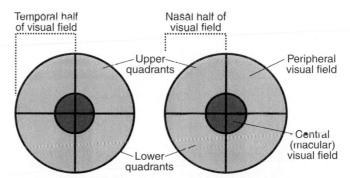

Figure 8-4.   Central and peripheral visual fields and their divisions into temporal and nasal half-fields and upper and lower quadrants.

sively contains cones and is the focal point of central vision (Fig. 8-4). The number of cones per unit gradually declines in regions farther from the fovea centralis, whereas the number of rods becomes greater in the peripheral retina.

FUNCTIONS OF PHOTOSENSORS

Cone and rod cells contain different visual pigments, are sensitive to light rays of different wavelengths, and operate efficiently under different light conditions. Cone cells have a high threshold for light and require bright daylight for function. They mediate sharp visual acuity, color vision, and tasks that require high temporal resolution. Hundreds of photons (elements of light) are needed to evoke responses from cone cells that are virtually nonfunctional in the dark. Conversely, rods, with a low threshold for light, function in dim light and mediate night vision. The presence of fewer photons can evoke a maximal response from the rods. For this reason, rods are nonfunctional in bright daylight. With sensitivity to selective components of the color spectrum, rods differentiate black, white, and shades of gray and detect movement. They also differentiate shapes but cannot resolve details or mediate color vision. By means of different degrees of resolution resulting from differential processing, rods and cones have specific patterns of connections to other nuclear layers of the retina. For example, because of poor spatial resolution, more than 20 rod cells converge on a single ganglion cell. Cone cells, which have a higher spatial resolution power, directly project to ganglion cells in a 1:1 ratio.

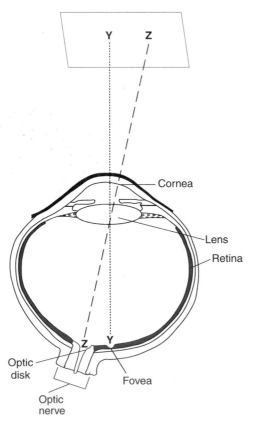

Figure 8-5. Blind spot. Fixation of the right eye on letter Y projects the adjacent letter Z onto the optic disk, which lacks receptors.

The macula lutea and the fovea centralis regulate **visual acuity**, **color discrimination**, and **sharp visual perception.** Visual images are focused in the macula for clarity and color analysis. In the fovea centralis, the inner layer of the bipolar and ganglion cells is pushed apart and displaced laterally, giving the appearance of a depressed pit. Because the fovea contains neither blood vessels nor many nerve fibers, it enables light rays to project directly on the photoreceptors (and serves the highest visual acuity and color perception).

The axons of the ganglion cells form the optic nerve, which travels the inner surface of the retina and converges at the optic disk (papilla) before exiting the retina through the optic disk (Fig. 8-5). As there are no photoreceptors present, there is no focusing of an image on the optic disk. This area is called the **blind spot**; it is approximately 15° medial to the center of the visual axis and can be tested by slowly moving an object in front of the retina. The object will briefly disappear as it is projected on the optic disk (e.g., letter Z in Fig. 8-5).

PHOTOCHEMISTRY OF RETINA

Photochemistry entails the absorption of electromagnetic energy in light rays by the visual pigments of rods and cones and its conversion into neural impulses. Photopigments are colored proteins in the outer segment membranes of rods and cones. They undergo structural changes upon absorbing light. Rods and cones transmit only local potentials to the bipolar cells, which in turn excite ganglion cells by means of neurotransmitters. The ganglion cells are the first cells to generate action potentials, which travel on their axons in the second cranial nerve.

The single type of visual pigment in rods is **rhodopsin**. All visual photopigments contain two elements: a glycoprotein known as **opsin**, and **retinal** (visual yellow), a light-absorbing molecule that is a derivative (aldehyde) of vitamin A. Exposure to dim light triggers a series of neuronal events related to the decomposition and regeneration of pigments. Rhodopsin breaks down into retinal and opsin. This chemical decomposition generates changes in the membrane potentials of the receptor cells. A series of biochemical events occurs in between to resynthesize the rhodopsin, which takes 7 to 30 minutes. This is also the time needed for adapting to darkness. The inability to see at night even after this normal period of dark adaptation is called **night blindness** (nyctalopia); it is usually caused by a deficiency of vitamin A. In daylight, rods are saturated by bright light and do not respond to light.

Similar to rods, the photopigment of cones consists of proteins called cone **opsin** and **retinal**, the light-absorbing molecules. The photochemical processing of cones is similar to that of rods, in which phototransduction involves the decomposition of the photopigment and its resynthesis. Because of sensitivity to different wavelengths (for color vision), cones contain three cone **opsins**, which promote maximum absorption of light from different parts of the light spectrum. The three types of opsin account for **trivalent color vision**. While vision in moderate daylight involves both rods and cones, cone cells help enjoy colors as well as the acuity and clarity of vision, whereas stars and the moon are seen with rods.

Three issues related to neural coding in the retina are **spectral sensitivity**, **color vision**, and **dark adaptation**.

Spectral Sensitivity

In addition to sensitivity to different light conditions, the other difference between rods and cones is that they are sensitive to different wavelengths of light. Consequently they have different **visibility curves**: the scotopic (rods) and photopic (cones) luminosity curves (Fig. 8-6). The scotopic (night vision) curve is obtained from eyes adapted to the dark. This rod-mediated visibility curve shows great sensitivity to light rays with wavelengths of 400 to 600 nm, with maximum sensitivity at 507 nm in the blue-green range. The same eye adapted to light has a photopic visibility curve that covers wavelengths of 425 to 700 nm, with maximum sensitivity to 555 nm in the yellow-green range.

Color Vision

Cone cells in the human eye are sensitive to wavelengths ranging from 400 to 700 nm. In this spectrum, the colors change from blue to red after passing through green, yellow, and orange. There are three types of cones in the retina with photosensitive pigments specialized for different wavelengths (**blue cones**, **green cones**, and **red cones**). Spectral differences in the cones make them respond best to lights of different wavelengths. Cones with sensitivity to blue have a maximum absorption at 445 nm. Cones with sensitivity for green respond with a maximum absorption at 535 nm. Cones responding with maximum absorption at 570 nm are sensitive to red. **Trichromatic** color vision results from the combination of the activities of the **red**, **green**, and **blue cones**.

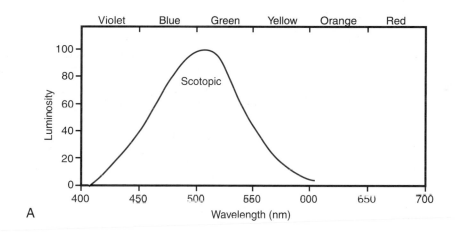

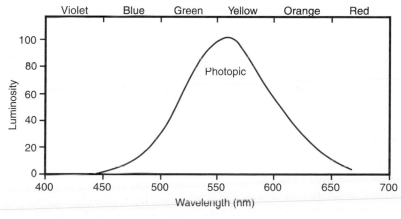

Figure 8-6.   Relative sensitivity of rods and cones to light of various wavelengths. **A.** Scotopic luminosity curve. **B.** Photopic luminosity curve.

Dark Adaptation

Dark adaptation is the normal night vision possible within a few minutes after entering a darkened room from a well-lit place. On entering, one at first sees very little; but with time, light sensitivity increases, enabling clearer vision. The normal period needed for adjustment to a dark room is between 7 and 30 minutes. This is the time needed for the rhodopsin to be reconstituted. The entire adaptation process is slow and complex and involves decomposition and regeneration of photopigments.

After a person moves from bright daylight to a dark room, the cones initially remain sensitive to light and continue to process colors by resynthesizing photopigments. Initially, both cones and rods increase their sensitivity to light; but in dim or no light, the cones, with their high threshold to light, gradually become nonfunctional and vision becomes **achromatic**. The rods, with their low threshold to light, begin functioning in dim light. As the rods start adjusting to dim light, colored lights become achromatic. The only color that does not become achromatic is red, because rods are insensitive to red light (Fig. 8-6A). The red wavelength is processed exclusively by the rod-free fovea centralis. Thus, one can be adapted to dark while continuing to process the red color.

For those who need to work simultaneously in dark and light areas, both dark adapted night vision and cone-mediated photopic vision can be maintained. Repeating 30-minute dark adaptation every time environments are changed can be avoided by wearing red goggles, since rod cells are not sensitive to red light.

OPTICAL MECHANISM

The eye functions as an optical instrument. Sharp focusing of an image depends on the adequate refraction of light rays, which ensures a properly focused image on the inner surface of the retina. Familiarity with the optical principle of **refraction** and **refractive properties** of the lens is essential to understanding the optical mechanism of the eye.

Refraction

Light rays travel in straight lines and slow down when entering a transparent medium from a medium of greater density. If the light rays strike the second surface with a different density at an angle, they bend. This is called **refraction**. The degree to which light rays bend depends on **two factors**: the **refractive index**[1] of the

medium into which the waves enter and the **angle** with which the rays strike the second surface. If traveling light waves strike a medium of a different density perpendicular to the wave front, the striking waves slow down, although they continue to travel along the same course without any deviation (refraction). However, if the waves strike an angled interface of a medium with a different refractive index (density), they bend.

Refractive power is measured in **diopter units**, and the total refractive power of the eye is 60 diopters. In the eye, refraction of light rays depends primarily on the **curvature** and **optical density** of the cornea and on the lens shape. The cornea alone contributes about 42 of the 60 diopters to the refraction. A simple example of refraction can be seen in a biconvex lens (Fig. 8-7A). In this lens, the top and bottom sections have an angulated shape, whereas the central section is rectangular. The angulated top section of the lens bends the striking waves downward, whereas the bottom angulated section of the lens bends the waves upward. The rectangular center portion of the lens (nonangulated and perpendicular to the wave front) permits light rays to pass through without deviation. All of these light rays converge at a common point to form the focused image, or **focal point**. Distance from the lens to the focal point is the **focal length**, while the point from which the rays originate is the **far point**. The power of a lens is defined in terms of the focal length. A lens with greater refracting power has a shorter focal length, and a lens with lower refractive power has a greater focal length. The lens is highly elastic. The action of the ciliary muscles can increase refractive power by 12 diopters. This elasticity of the lens (accommodation) decreases by age 45 and is virtually nonexistent by age 65.

Lens Types

Convex and **concave** are the two most common types of lenses (Fig. 8-7A). Each lens type contributes differently to refraction. A convex lens has a short focal length and adds greater convergence to bending light rays. Light rays striking the angled edges of the lens bend and converge to a common focus point beyond the lens, where they join the undeviating waves traveling through the center of the lens. The function of a convex lens is to reduce focal length. In contrast, a concave lens diverges parallel light rays and thus increases focal length by reducing the degree of refraction. Parallel running rays entering the central portion of a concave lens pass undeviatingly because the surface is perpendicular to the traveling beam. However, rays striking the inward-angled edges enter the lens ahead of the rays that strike the center of the lens. The inward-angled edge diverges rays away from the centrally entering rays of the lens. This divergence of rays increases the focal length.

---

[1] The refractive index of any transparent substance is the ratio of velocity of light in the air (300,000 km/second) to velocity of light in the second transparent substance. For example, a glass cube has a refractive index of 1.5 (air velocity 300,000 ÷ glass velocity 200,000 = 1.5).

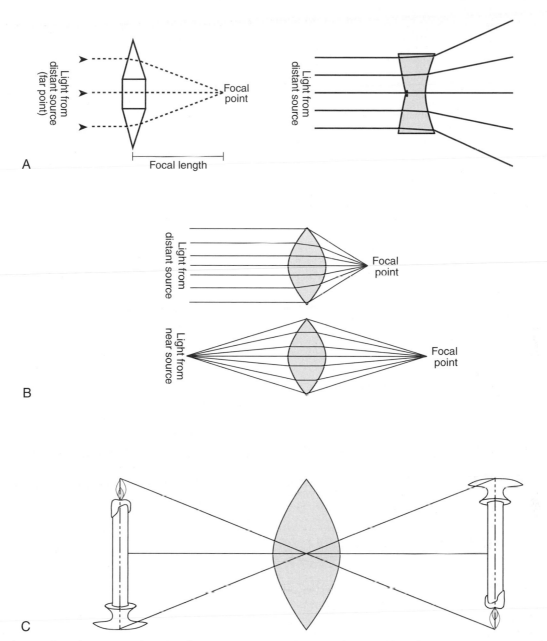

Figure 8-7. **A.** Refraction through convex and concave lenses. **B.** Two convex lenses possess similar refractive powers, but they have different focal lengths because rays entering the upper lens are parallel, whereas rays entering the second lens diverge. **C.** Eye as an optical mechanism in which the object focused on the retina is reversed in relation to the visual field.

Optics of the Eye

Focusing an image on the retinas of the two eyes entails four processes: **refraction** of light rays by the lens, **aperture** control of the pupil, **accommodation** of lens, and **convergence** of the eyes. Refraction of the rays leads to proper focusing of the image. The aperture of the pupil opening and the lens accommodation regulate the amount of light entering the eye and control the refractive power of the lens. Convergence refers to the voluntary control of the eye for tracking an object mov-

ing toward or away from the eyes and keeping it in focus.

For all practical purposes, a distance of 20 feet (6 m) between the lens and the object is considered usual for assessing vision. Light rays originating from an object placed 20 feet away are parallel to each other. They must be bent adequately to converge on the fovea centralis, the site of central vision. Light rays from an object closer than 20 feet are generally divergent (Fig. 8-7B). This divergence of rays is too great for the cornea and resting lens to focus the image on the retina. Therefore, greater refraction is required. This is made possible by lens accommodation, the modification of lens curvature by the action of the ciliary muscle. As the distance between the center of the lens and the fovea centralis is considered fixed at 17 mm, the lens and the refractive mechanism must assume different shapes to refract the parallel rays reflected from a **distant object** and the diverging rays from a **near object**.

Retinal Image Formation

Forming an image on the retina is guided by one optical principle: the retinal image is a completely reversed and inverted form of what is seen in the visual field. Light reflected from the top portion of an object is projected onto the **lower retina**. Rays from the bottom portion of an object strike the **upper retina**. The projected upside down image is also a mirror image of both left and right sides of an object (Fig. 8-7C). Even though the retinal image is upside down and reversed, objects seen are corrected by a learning process that begins at birth and is mediated by the associational visual cortex.

LENS SHAPE

The curvature of a lens determines its refractive power. A lens with greater outward spherical curvature has more refractive power than a flatter one and acutely bends light rays toward the focus point. A flattened lens has less refractive power. What makes the lens unique is its ability to change its curvature instantly to increase or decrease its refractive power. The action of ciliary muscles is responsible for this change in lens shape. Voluntary control of the lens shape is important, particularly when light rays are diverging from a near source. If the refractive power of the lens is unchanged, the diverging rays from this near object converge far behind the photosensors of the retina, resulting in an image that is out of focus. To keep the image of a near object in sharp focus, voluntary modification of the curvature of the lens occurs. This process is known as accommodation.

PUPILLARY APERTURE

The size of the pupillary aperture controls the amount of light entering the eyes and contributes to formation of clear retinal images. In bright light, pupil constriction is regulated by parasympathetic activity; it results in a narrow opening that allows only a small amount of light to enter. In dim light, the pupil sympathetically dilates to enlarge the opening, allowing maximum light to enter the eye. Reflexive pupil constriction also serves as a protective mechanism for the retina when the eye is suddenly exposed to intense light. The variable aperture of the pupil is controlled by the sympathetic and parasympathetic innervation of the dilator and constrictor muscle fibers of the iris.

CONVERGENCE

Convergence is turning of both eyes inward to keep in focus an object that is moving closer. This movement also contributes to binocular vision, which results when the images of an object are projected on corresponding points in both retinas. If an object moves closer to both eyes, both eyes move inward to keep the object in focus and to retain the projection of images on the same points in both retinas. A great degree of convergence is needed to see clearly objects extremely close to the eyes.

CENTRAL VISUAL PATHWAYS

The central visual mechanism includes the visual pathway from the retina of the eye to the primary visual cortex, on the midsagittal surface of the occipital lobe. Figure 8-8 summarizes the visual pathway. Two important characteristics of the central visual mechanism are (a) a point-to-point representation of the visual field from the retina through the geniculate body to the primary visual cortex and (b) the projection from each eye to both cerebral hemispheres (basis for binocular vision). Familiarity with the pathways carrying visual information and the crossing points of visual fibers will provide an understanding of the organization of the visual system (Table 8-1) needed to relate lesion sites with different visual field defects.

The optic nerve fibers from the retinal cells exit the orbital cavity through the **optic foramina** and enter the cranial cavity. Optic nerves from both eyes come together at the optic chiasm rostral to the hypothalamus (Figs. 2-8 and 2-11). The optic tract fibers from the optic chiasm travel caudally and laterally and terminate in the **lateral geniculate body**, the thalamic visual relay center. The geniculocalcarine fibers (optic radiation) loop laterally and caudally in the temporal lobe, travel to the occipital cortex, and terminate in the superior and inferior opercula (lips) of the **calcarine fissure**, the primary visual cortex, which is on the midsagittal surface of the occipital lobe (Table 8-2).

Retinal Representation of Visual Fields

Eyes do not function individually. The visual field overlaps; in fact, a large part of the visual field, the binocular area, is covered by both eyes (Fig. 8-1). Light rays from an object in the binocular visual field project to the corresponding portions of both retinas. However, for learning convenience and for keeping the path of visual projections to the cortex clear, visual fields for each eye are depicted separately (Fig. 8-8A).

The visual field, the area viewed by the eyes, has **central** and **peripheral** regions. The small area in the center of the visual field is the central visual field. This is projected onto the macula of the retina and is responsi-

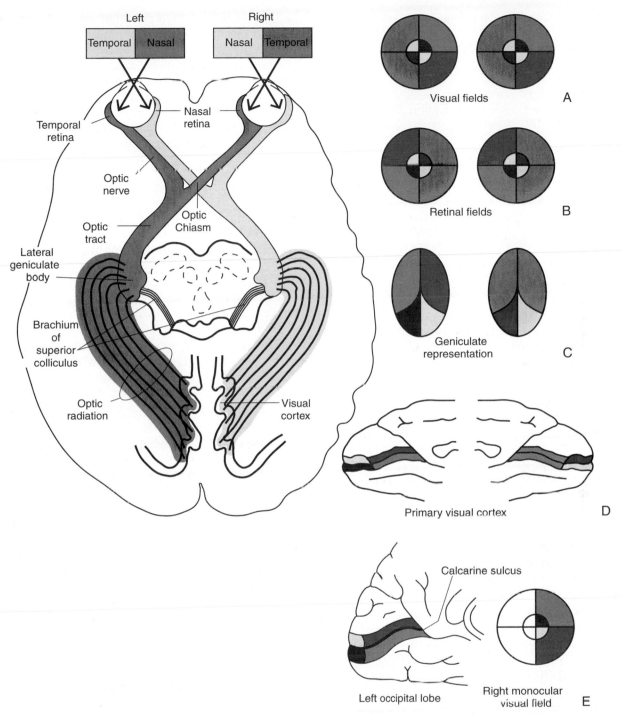

Figure 0-0. Visual pathways from retina to visual cortex in the occipital lobe and representation of visual fields as processed along the optic pathway. **A.** Visual fields. **B.** Retinal fields. **C.** Geniculate representation. **D.** Cortical representation. **E.** Right monocular visual field as mapped on the left primary visual cortex in the occipital lobe.

ble for the sharpest vision and color discrimination. The central field of vision is surrounded by a large peripheral visual field. The visual field for each eye is divided into two half-fields: **nasal** and **temporal** halves. Each of these half-fields is further divided into **upper** and **lower** quadrants (Fig. 8-4). **Retinal representation** of the visual

field for each eye is also divided into nasal and temporal halves, which contain upper and lower quadrants. The image in the visual field is projected to the retina in **reversed** and **inverted** form (Fig. 8-9B; Table 8-1). Light rays from the temporal half of the visual field project to the nasal half of the retina. Similarly, rays from the nasal

Table 8-1.   Rules Related to the Central Visual Mechanism

Rule One	Retinal image is reversed and inverted form of visual field image.
Rule Two	Nasal retinal fibers (representing temporal visual field) cross at optic chiasm and project to opposite cortex. Temporal retinal fibers (representing nasal visual field) remain uncrossed and project to ipsilateral cortex.
Rule Three	A. Geniculocalcarine fibers (representing lower visual field quadrant) pass dorsally through Meyer's loop and project to visual cortex. B. Geniculocalcarine fibers (representing upper visual field quadrant) pass ventrally and laterally through Meyer's loop and project to visual cortex.
Rule Four	Upper retinal fibers (representing lower visual field quadrant) terminate in upper visual cortex; lower retinal fibers (representing upper visual field quadrant) project to lower visual cortex.
Rule Five	Peripheral visual field is represented rostrally along calcarine fissure. Central visual field is represented caudally along calcarine fissure.

Table 8-2.   A Panoramic View of Visual Processes

Traveling light rays	Cornea
	Anterior cavity (aqueous humor)
	Lens
	Posterior cavity (vitreous humor)
	Retinal cells (ganglion, bipolar, rods, and cones)
Retinal processing	Changes in membrane potential in rods and cones
	Bipolar cells (local potential)
	Ganglion cells (action potential)
	Optic nerve
Cortical processing	Optic chiasm
	Optic tract
	Lateral geniculate body
	Geniculocalcarine fibers
	Visual cortex

half of the visual field fall on the temporal half of the retina. Light rays from the top of the object strike the lower retina, and rays from the bottom of the object strike the upper retina. Taking the projections for both eyes into consideration, light rays from an object in the right visual field fall on the nasal retina of the right eye and the temporal retina of the left eye. Light rays of an object from the left visual field strike the nasal half of the retina in the left eye and the temporal half of the retina in the right eye.

Retinal Representation to Optic Chiasm

Optic nerve fibers from the retinal ganglion cells enter the cranial cavity to reach the optic chiasm. Two rules account for the partial crossing of fibers at the chiasm. First, fibers from the nasal halves of the retinas (representing temporal visual fields for each eye) cross the midline to project to the opposite visual cortex. Sec-

ond, fibers from the temporal half of each retina (representing nasal halves of the visual fields) remain uncrossed and project to the ipsilateral visual cortex. This explains projection of the right visual field to the left hemisphere and projection of the left visual field to the right hemisphere (Fig. 8-8; Table 8-1).

Retinal Representation to Lateral Geniculate Body

Each optic tract (postchiasmic fibers) carries visual information from both eyes. The left optic tract mediates the right visual field for each eye. This means that the left optic tract contains the projections from the temporal half of the left retina (nasal visual field for the left eye) and the nasal half of the right retina (temporal visual field for the right eye). Similarly, the right optic tract transmits the left visual field for each eye and includes the projections from the nasal half of the left retina (temporal visual field for the left eye) and temporal half of the right retina (nasal visual field for the right eye). This arrangement of contralateral projections from each eye is consistent with contralateral sensory and motor organization. The optic tract projects to the lateral geniculate body of the thalamus.

Each lateral geniculate body receives a point-to-point projection from the homonymous (left or right) halves of the field of both eyes (Fig. 8-8C). The visual information is distributed on both sides of the geniculate body. Fibers from the upper retinal quadrants (representing lower visual field quadrants) terminate in the medial portion of the geniculate body, whereas fibers from the lower retinal quadrants (representing upper visual field quadrants) project to the lateral portion of the geniculate body.

Retinal Representation to Visual Cortex

Geniculocalcarine fibers, or **optic radiations**, constitute the last phase in the transmission of visual information to the visual cortex (Fig. 8-8D). Geniculocalcarine fibers enter the retrolenticular portion of the posterior internal capsule on their way to the primary visual cortex (Fig. 9-9). The geniculocalcarine fibers divide into the **dorsal** and **ventral** bundles of fibers. The dorsal bundle of fibers, traveling straight to the cells in the visual cortex above the calcarine fissure, carries information from the upper retinal quadrants (representing the lower visual field quadrants). The ventral bundle of fibers forms the temporal, or **Meyer's, loop**. These geniculocalcarine fibers first move rostrally and then make a lateral excursion around the inferior (temporal) horn of the lateral ventricle before traveling to the cells in the visual cortex below the calcarine fissure. These fibers mediate projections from the lower retinal quadrants (representing the upper visual field quadrants) (Table 8-1).

Visual Cortex

The primary visual cortex (Brodmann area 17) is bilateral; it lies on the midsagittal surface of the occipital lobe (Fig. 1-8) and is divided into two opercula, or lips, that are separated by the **calcarine fissure**. Each visual cortex receives information from both eyes. The lower lip of the visual cortex receives projections from the lower portion of the retina (representing the upper quadrant in the visual field). The upper lip of the visual cortex receives projections from the upper retina (representing the lower quadrant in the visual field). The central visual field, representing the macular region of the retina, occupies a comparatively large area in the caudal part near the occipital pole. The peripheral visual fields are represented in the anterior portions of the calcarine cortex (Fig. 8-8B and E) (Table 8-1).

Therefore, a lesion involving the visual cortex in one hemisphere results in cortical blindness in the opposite field of vision (hemianopia or hemianopsia). The extent of the blindness depends on the size of the lesion. The **visual association cortex** (Brodmann areas 18 and 19) wraps around the primary cortex on the medial and lateral surfaces and is reciprocally connected with the temporoparietal cortex. With afferents from the primary visual cortex, the visual association cortex synthesizes and elaborates visual information and is responsible for higher visual functions, such as recognition of an object, appreciation of its significance in the context of personal experiences, and visual memory. The association cortex is also important in the ability to read. A lesion in the association cortex may result in **visual agnosia**, in which one cannot recognize an object despite normal visual perception. Additional deficits that may arise are **color agnosia** and **prosopagnosia**, which are marked by impaired recognition of colors and faces. Higher visual cognitive functions are discussed in Chapter 19.

VISUAL REFLEXES

Visual reflexes are concerned with the changing of **pupil size** and **lens shape**. The ocular muscle fibers regulating these reflexes are innervated by parasympathetic fibers of the oculomotor nerve, which regulate pupillary constriction and lens accommodation, and sympathetic fibers, which regulate pupillary dilation (Fig. 8-10).

Pupillary Light Reflex

In the pupillary light reflex, the eyes react to bright light by constricting the pupils. The neural mechanism for these pupillary changes involves the **pretectal area**, the **Edinger-Westphal nucleus**, and fibers of the **oculomotor cranial nerve** (Fig. 8-9A). The ganglion cells in the retina, in response to illumination changes, send projections to the brain. These fibers leave the optic tract before the lateral geniculate body and synapse on cells in the pretectal area. The pretectal area is a group of nuclei in a small unspecified area between the superior colliculi. This area bilaterally projects to the Edinger-Westphal nucleus, the visceral nucleus of the oculomotor nerve. The preganglionic fibers from the Edinger-Westphal nucleus join the oculomotor fibers and innervate the ipsilateral **ciliary ganglion** in the orbit. The postganglionic fibers from the ciliary ganglion provide parasympathetic projections to the circular (constrictor) fibers of the iris. The constriction of the circular fibers narrows the pupillary aperture, a condition called **miosis** (Fig. 8-10A). Both pupils constrict in response to light entering one eye. The pupillary reaction in the eye exposed to light is the **direct response**, whereas the reflexive pupillary change in the other eye is the **consensual response**. In complete darkness, constriction of the radial (dilator) fibers of the iris results in pupil dilation, or **mydriasis** (Fig. 8-10B).

The pupil dilatory function involves both inhibition of the Edinger-Westphal nucleus and facilitation of sympathetic activity. Sympathetic projections exit at T-1 to T-3 and travel in the cervical sympathetic chain to the **superior cervical ganglion**, which sends postganglionic projections to the radial fibers of the iris muscle in the eyeball (Fig. 8-10B). Damage to the sympathetic system causes paralysis of the dilator fibers of the iris and results in permanent constriction of the pupil.

Cranial nerve III lesions alter the pupillary light reflex. Interrupted afferent projections from one eye affect the light reflex in both pupils. This is tested by checking to see if light projected into each eye elicits both direct and consensual responses. Presence of the consensual response without a direct pupil response suggests a lesion involving the projection from the Edinger-Westphal nucleus to the same eye. An interruption of the sympathetic fibers to the pupil results in a permanently constricted pupillary diameter (miosis). The resulting condition is part of **Horner's syndrome**, which is characterized by an ipsilaterally constricted pupil (miosis), drooping of the eyelid (ptosis), and loss of facial sweating (anhidrosis).

Accommodation Reflex

The accommodation (or near) reflex regulates the refractive power of the lens (Fig. 8-11A). The distance between the lens and retina remains the same as an object moves closer to the eyes. Keeping an object in focus requires increased refractive power of the lens, which occurs when the lens assumes a more nearly rounded (spherical) form. This reflexive modification of the lens curvature is controlled by the contraction of the ciliary muscles through the suspensory ligaments. The parasympathetic contraction (third cranial nerve) of the

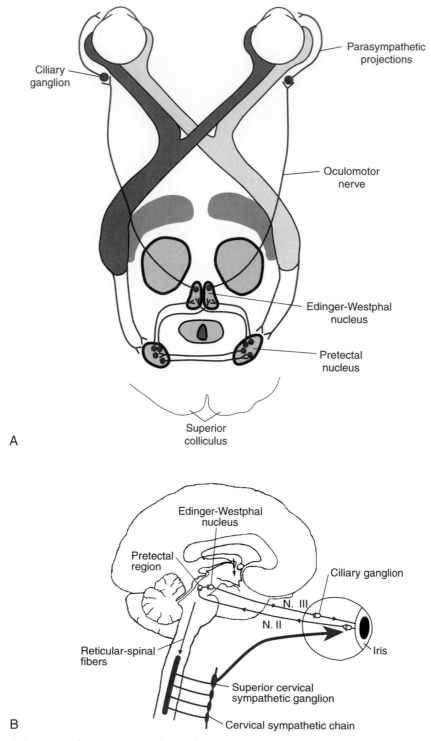

Figure 8-9. **A**. Parasympathetic innervation of the iris for pupil constriction in light reflex. **B**. Sympathetic innervation of the eyeball for pupil dilation in dark.

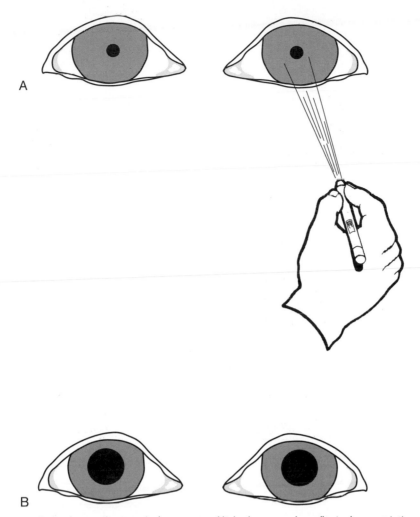

Figure 8-10. **A.** In light, the pupils controls the amount of light that enters by reflexively constricting, which results in a narrower opening. **B.** Pupils reflexively dilate in dark, allowing maximum light to enter the eye.

ciliary muscles pulls the ciliary processes forward and reduces tension in the suspensory ligaments. With no pulls from ligaments, the lens, because of its elasticity, assumes a more rounded form, thus acquiring greater refractive power. This is needed for clearly viewing objects that are close (less than 20 feet) to the eye (Fig. 8-11A). The relaxed state of ciliary muscles exerts tension on the suspensory ligaments that pull on the lens, flattening the lens. This reduces the refractive power, permitting far vision (Fig. 8-11B).

The neural mechanism of the accommodation reflex is slightly different from the light reflex. It involves the primary visual cortex in addition to the lateral geniculate body and the **mesencephalic reflex** center (Fig. 8-9A). As the image of an object moving closer begins to blur, the visual cortex sends projections to the superior colliculus, which mediates visual information to the pre-

tectal area. The pretectal nuclei send crossed and uncrossed fibers to the Edinger-Westphal nucleus, which projects preganglionic parasympathetic fibers in the oculomotor nerve to the ciliary ganglion. The postganglionic projections from the ciliary ganglion cause constriction of the ciliary muscle. Consequently, the lens, released from the tension of the suspensory ligaments, becomes more convex and acquires greater refractive power. The accommodation reflex has two additional components: eye convergence and pupillary constriction. Convergence of the eyes prevents double vision. Pupillary constriction (miosis) helps sharpen the image by reducing the pupillary aperture. The lens has its greatest accommodative power during youth. With advancing age, the lens gradually loses the flexibility to control refractive power (**presbyopia**, which usually sets in around age 45).

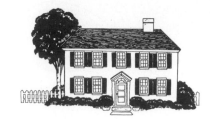

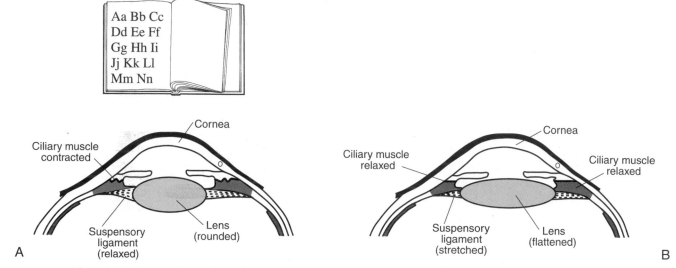

Figure 8-11. Lens accommodation for (**A**) near (less than 20 feet) objects and (**B**) distant (more than 20 feet) objects.

CLINICAL INFORMATION

Errors of Refraction

The refractive power of an eye is largely determined by the cornea and lens. In an **emmetropic** (normal) eye there is a normal relationship between axial length and the eye's refractive power, so that light rays from objects beyond 20 feet can converge on the fovea without any lens accommodation (Fig. 8-12*A*). Anytime the relationship between the refraction and focal length is not correct, the parallel light rays from distant objects converge either behind the retina or in front of it. Refractive problems cause blurred vision, visual fatigue, and possibly headaches. There are three common types of refractive errors: **hypermetropia** (farsightedness), **myopia** (nearsightedness), and **astigmatism**.

HYPERMETROPIA

The focal point in a **hypermetropic** or **hyperopic eye** falls behind the retina (Fig. 8-12*B*). Two factors contribute to this focusing error. First, the axial length of the eyeball is short. Second, the refractive power of the lens is inadequate. Hypermetropic subjects are farsighted (can see distant objects normally). This is because light

rays from distant objects are parallel (less divergent) and are adequately refracted for converging on the fovea. The problem is in focusing near objects. Young hypermetropic subjects may compensate for the refractive error by lens accommodation. Contracting the ciliary muscle removes tension from the suspensory ligaments and results in a convex lens with greater refractive power. However, after a limit, which is known as the **near point** of vision, the near objects can no longer be focused. Furthermore, continuous use of accommodation may cause hypertrophy of the ciliary muscle. Hypermetropic error may also be corrected by placing a convex lens in front of the eye, which adds greater refractive power needed for converging the light rays on the retina (Fig. 8-12*C*).

MYOPIA

The focal point in the myopic eye falls in front of the retina (Fig. 8-12*D*). Myopic subjects cannot see distant objects well. Two factors contribute to myopia. First, the eyeball has a long axis. Second, the lens has strong refractive power. Subjects with myopic eyes are nearsighted, as light rays from near objects are divergent and therefore require greater refraction and/or a longer axis for converging on the retina. Myopic errors of re-

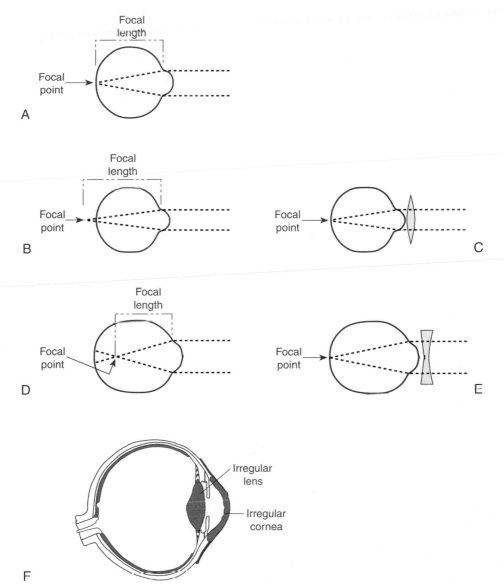

Figure 8-12.   Normally refractive eye, common refractive errors, and their corrections. **A.** In a normal (emmetropic) eye, light rays from a near or far object are adequately refracted so that rays converge directly on the retina, enabling formation of a clear image. **B.** In a farsighted (hypermetropic, or hyperopic) eye, an image is focused behind the retina. The resulting condition can be corrected with convex lenses (**C**). **D.** In a near-sighted (myopic) eye, an image is focused in front of the retina. This refractive condition can be corrected with concave lenses (**E**). **F.** Refractive errors of astigmatism, which result from irregular curvatures of the cornea, lens, or both. Consequently, horizontal and vertical points from various visual fields are focused at two different focal points on the retina, resulting in distorted vision.

fraction may be corrected by placing a concave lens before the eye. The concave lens diverges the light rays and adds focal length (Fig. 8-12*E*).

ASTIGMATISM

Astigmatism is a refractive error caused by irregular shape of the cornea, lens, or both (Fig. 8-12*F*). Horizontal corneal and/or lens diameters do not have the same refractive power as vertical diameters. Consequently, different portions of light rays passing through the lens focus at different points on the retina. Astig-

matic errors of refraction can be corrected by a combined cylindrical and spherical lens because it can bring all light rays into focus at the same retinal point.

Disorders of Color Vision

Various forms of color blindness are noted in clinical populations. Three major kinds of color vision anomalies are **protanomaly, deuteranomaly,** and **tritanomaly**. A protanopic subject lacks red cones and sees only green and blue. A deuteranopic person lacks green cones and sees only red and blue. A tritanopic person lacks blue cones and sees only red and green. The degree of impairment varies from complete color blindness to partial impairment. This deficit can be acquired, though it is primarily inherited. Inherited color blindness mostly occurs in males through an X-chromosome from the mother. Color blindness is usually absent in females because at least one of the two X-chromosomes is likely to have a normal gene for the cones.

Visual Acuity Assessment

Visual acuity refers to the ability to see details from a fixed distance. This is measured in **Snellen's chart** of letters and numbers (Fig. 8-13). The chart contains various sizes of letters with distances specified from which these letters can be read by those with normal vision. The chart is placed 20 feet from the subject, and each eye is tested. To the left of each line are a numerator and a denominator. The numerator represents the distance from which the visual acuity is measured (usually fixed at 20 feet). The denominator specifies the distance from which a person with normal vision can read the letter size in the line. For example, 20/80 visual acuity means that what should be readable from 80 feet can be read only from 20 feet; 20/20 exemplifies the normal acuity, whereas 20/400 is the worst visual acuity.

Visual Field Defects

A lesion at any point in the visual pathway results in the loss of a specific point in the visual field. The nature of the visual field loss depends on the point and extent of fiber interruption. The straightforward nature of the visual projections makes it easy to relate the locations of injury to specific patterns of field losses and vice versa. There are two types of field defects: homonymous and heteronymous. **Homonymous** refers to similar regions of visual field defects for each eye. This means either the right half of the visual fields for both eyes or the left half of the visual fields for both eyes is involved. **Heteronymous** refers to two different parts of the visual field being impaired. For example, the left half of the visual field for one eye may be affected, while the right half of the visual field for the other eye is affected; this is known as **bitemporal hemianopsia**. Injuries at selected points along the visual pathway result in predictable patterns of visual field defects (Fig. 8-14; Table 8-3).

MONOCULAR BLINDNESS

A complete severing of the optic nerve at any point between the eyeball and the optic chiasm results in total blindness in that eye. This occurs because none of the optic nerve fibers from the retina are spared (Fig. 8-14*A*). However, the actual implications of monocular blindness are slightly different because of binocular vision. If one eye is blind or closed, the other eye is still capable of covering the entire visual field except for a small, temporal crescent-shaped peripheral field for the blind eye. Thus, even after severance of the optic nerve, one is functionally blind only for this monocular portion of the field, although there may be additional problems with depth perception.

BITEMPORAL, OR HETERONYMOUS HEMIANOPSIA

Bitemporal hemianopsia is loss of vision in the temporal visual fields. It is associated with pathology of

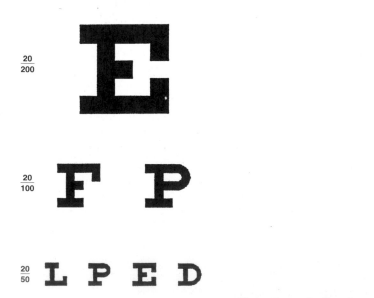

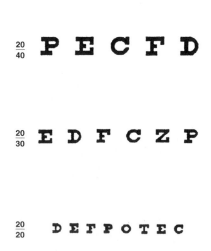

Figure 8-13. Snellen chart.

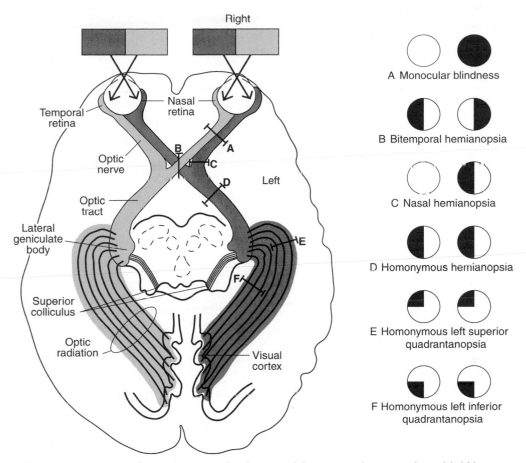

Figure 8-14.   Common lesion sites in visual pathways and the associated patterns of visual field losses.

Table 8-3.   Visual Field Loss and Associated Anatomical Sites

Lesion Site	Visual Field Loss
Optic nerve	Monocular blindness
Optic chiasm (usually secondary to pituitary gland tumor)	Bitemporal hemianopsia (tunnel vision)
Lateral edge of optic chiasm interrupting fibers from ipsilateral temporal retina	Nasal hemianopsia in one eye
Optic tract, post chiasmic or geniculocalcarine fibers	Homonymous hemianopsia
Temporal lobe pathology interrupting outer (ventral) geniculocalcarine tract fibers	Upper quadrantanopsia
Temporoparietal lobe pathology interrupting inner(dorsal) geniculocalcarine tract direct fibers	Lower quadrantanopsia

the optic chiasm (Fig. 8-14 *B*). A chiasmatic injury, usually induced by a tumor of the **pituitary gland**, interrupts fibers from both nasal retinas. It produces blindness in the temporal visual fields for both eyes, commonly called tunnel vision.

NASAL HEMIANOPSIA

Nasal hemianopsia refers to loss of vision in the nasal field of only one eye. The associated pathology encroaches on the lateral edge of the optic chiasm and selectively interrupts the fibers from the ipsilateral temporal portion of the retina. The result is nasal hemianopsia in the corresponding eye (Fig. 8-14C).

HOMONYMOUS HEMIANOPSIA

Homonymous hemianopsia is loss of vision in homonymous—either right or left—fields for both eyes. An interruption of fibers at any point in the course of the optic tract, geniculate body, or geniculocalcarine fibers results in homonymous (same field in both eyes) visual field losses (Fig. 8-14D). For example, a lesion in the right optic tract interrupts visual fibers from the retinas of both eyes, resulting in a left visual field defect for both eyes.

HOMONYMOUS LEFT SUPERIOR QUADRANTANOPSIA

Homonymous left superior quadrantanopsia is loss of vision in the superior left quadrants of the visual fields for both eyes. The geniculocalcarine fibers divide into the outer (ventral) and inner (dorsal) fascicles while traveling to the visual cortex. The outer fascicle of fibers carries information from the inferior retinal quadrants of the retina (representing the upper or superior quadrants in the visual fields); these fibers sweep around the inferior horn of the lateral ventricle in the temporal lobe in Meyer's loop. A temporal lobe lesion on the right side of the brain selectively interrupting these outer fibers of the geniculocalcarine tract causes blindness in the left upper quadrants of the visual fields of both eyes (Fig. 8-14*E*).

HOMONYMOUS LEFT INFERIOR QUADRANTANOPSIA

The inner fibers of the geniculocalcarine tract, carrying information from the superior or upper retinal quadrants, travel directly through the temporoparietal substance. Therefore, a right-sided temporoparietal lobe lesion interrupts the geniculocalcarine tract inner (dorsal) fibers; this interrupts the transmission of visual information from the right upper retinal quadrants, resulting in vision loss in the left lower visual field quadrants for both eyes (Fig. 8-14*F*).

Other Common Disorders of the Visual Mechanism

PRESBYOPIA

Presbyopia is the end result of the gradual reduction in ability to accommodate the lens for near vision, which usually begins around age 45. The lens loses its ability to assume the spherical curvature needed to view objects that are closer than 20 feet.

CATARACT

Cataract is primarily the age-induced painless production of nontransparent fibrous protein, which results in clouding of the lens or its capsule. The quality of the focused image depends on the degree of lens opaqueness. In severe cases, no image can be seen. The treatment of a cataract requires the surgical removal of the opaque lens.

GLAUCOMA

Glaucoma results from an increase in intraocular pressure and is often a cause of blindness. Consequent to inadequate draining of aqueous humor, the intraocular pressure increases. The pressure increase pushes the lens into the vitreous humor and irritates retinal neurons, which damages the retina. Progressively increasing tunnel vision is a symptom of this process, which is important, since glaucoma is medically treatable if corrected early.

INFLAMMATORY INFECTIONS

Conjunctivitis is an infectious inflammatory condition of the membrane that covers the inner surface of the eyelid and the outer surface of the globe. **Keratitis** is an infectious inflammation of the cornea. **Iridocyclitis** is an inflammatory reaction of the iris that affects the diaphragmatic functioning of the iris.

RETINITIS PIGMENTOSA

Retinitis pigmentosa is a progressive familial disease that begins in early childhood and involves the rod cells. Its clinical symptoms include peripheral pigmentary degeneration, vision loss in the peripheral visual field, and night blindness. In retinitis pigmentosa, the choroid layer of the retina gradually fails to remove the debris of broken outer segments of rods. Consequently, debris accumulates between the choroid layer and the sensory cells, preventing adequate nutritional supply to the rods and cones, which normally occurs by diffusion from choroid blood capillaries. Genetics (autosomal dominant inheritance) and vitamin A deficiencies are commonly suggested causes of this condition.

LESION LOCALIZATION

Rule 4: Visual Pathway Lesion

PRESENTING SYMPTOMS (A)

Blindness in one eye suggests an optic nerve lesion anterior to the optic chiasm.

RATIONALE

Each optic nerve contains fibers from both nasal and temporal regions of the retina of one eye.

PRESENTING SYMPTOMS (B)

Bitemporal hemianopsia (one does not see things laterally in the visual fields) results from a lesion compressing or otherwise interrupting crossing fibers (from the nasal retina of each eye) in the optic chiasm.

RATIONALE

Fibers mediating visual information from the temporal (outer) visual fields (perceived in the nasal part of the retina) cross the midline at the optic chiasm.

PRESENTING SYMPTOMS (C)

Homonymous hemianopsia is associated with a lesion of the optic tract anywhere between the optic chiasm and the occipital lobe.

RATIONALE

Fibers from the two eyes representing the same (homo) visual fields (e.g., the temporal visual field of the left eye and the nasal visual field of the right eye) travel together in the optic tract.

PRESENTING SYMPTOMS (D)

Visual agnosia, alexia (failure to comprehend written material), homonymous hemianopsia, and spared macular vision are all associated with a lesion of the visual cortex (Brodmann area 17) and visual association areas (Brodmann areas 18 and 19).

RATIONALE

Involvement of the visual cortex receiving optic tract fibers accounts for the contralateral hemianopsia. Involvement of the primary and associational visual cortices, which are supplied by the posterior cerebral artery, results in agnosia and alexia.

Case Studies

Patient One

A 65-year-old man gradually began having visual difficulty. He could see things well if they were right in front of him but did not see them if they were to his left or right. He was worried about developing tunnel vision like his diabetic neighbor, who had retinal degeneration. His ophthalmologist found nothing wrong with his retina and visual acuity. However, the examination revealed bitemporal hemianopsia. Magnetic resonance imaging revealed a tumor of the pituitary gland.

Question: Can you localize the possible lesion site affecting the retinogeniculate fibers?

Discussion: The pituitary gland tumor affected the retinogeniculate fibers from both nasal retinas at the level of the optic chiasm.

Patient Two

A 60-year-old right-handed architect was admitted to a hospital after a stroke. After the first 3 weeks of acute and intensive care, he exhibited severe sensory aphasia. He spoke fluently, but the verbal output contained many related and unrelated paraphasic errors and perseverations. Despite copious verbal output, there was little communication. He also had moderate reading and writing problems. An audiological examination revealed normal hearing, but the patient reported difficulty in understanding others. There were no sensory or motor deficits apparent. However, there was an upper right visual field defect. Magnetic resonance imaging revealed an infarct in the posterior left superior temporal gyrus involving the classical Wernicke's area (Brodmann area 22) and parts of the inferior parietal lobe.

Questions: Can you account for the right upper quadrantanopsia in this aphasic patient from a left temporal lobe lesion? Can you explain why he would have right hemianopsia, not left? Can you account for the affected fibers in terms of the retinal fields?

Discussion: The subcortical extension of the temporal lesion affected the left geniculocalcarine visual radiation fibers. These fibers carried information from the lower retinal quadrants representing the upper quadrants of the visual field.

Patient Three

A 65-year-old man with a history of hypertension had a minor stroke and lost consciousness for 5 minutes. He was taken to a hospital, where the attending physician noticed the following:

No sign of sensorimotor abnormality
Asymmetry in pupil size
Left pupil 2 to 3 mm larger in the dark

Question: Based on your understanding of the autonomic (sympathetic and parasympathetic) innervation of the eye, can you account for this clinical picture by relating symptoms to a brainstem lesion?

Discussion: The left pupil dilated larger than the right could result from either a right sympathetic or a left parasympathetic lesion. The crucial clinical point is the context in which the asymmetry is noticed: dark or light. The presence of pupillary asymmetry in the dark implies that the sympathetic system did not function well for the smaller (right) pupil. Thus, the patient had a right sympathetic lesion. However, if this pupillary asymmetry had been present in the light, it would indicate a left parasympathetic disruption.

SUMMARY

The visual system is concerned with image perception, which involves four events. (*a*) Lens and cornea of the eye refract light rays. (*b*) Retinal photoreceptor cells convert the electromagnetic energy of light rays into changes in membrane potential. (*c*) Integrating processing by other retinal neurons, the retinal ganglion transmit generated action potentials to the thalamus with relay to the visual cortex. (*d*) Visual images are perceived in the primary visual cortex and interpreted in the associational visual cortex. Optical disturbances affect image formation, whereas lesions interrupting visual fibers result in different visual field losses.

Technical Terms

aqueous humor	miosis
astigmatism	monocular vision
binocular vision	mydriasis
bitemporal hemianopia	myopia
blind spot	near point
cones	optic disk
far point	photopsin
focal length	refraction
focal point	retina
fovea	rhodopsin
homonymous hemianopia	rods
hyperopia	scotopic vision
iris	visual acuity
luminosity curve	visual field
macula lutea	vitreous humor

Review Questions

1. Define the following terms:

aqueous humor	cones
astigmatism	far point
binocular vision	focal length
bitemporal hemianopia	focal point
blind spot	fovea

homonymous hemianopia	refraction
hyperopia	retina
iris	rhodopsin
macula lutea	rods
monocular vision	scotopic vision
myopia	visual acuity
optic disk	visual field
photopsin	vitreous humor

2. With a diagram illustrate the visual pathway identifying the optic nerve, optic chiasm, optic tract, lateral geniculate body, and visual cortex. Specifically discuss the visual field representation on the retina, optic chiasm, and visual cortex.

3. Illustrate the visual field defects (monocular blindness, bitemporal hemianopsia, nasal hemianopsia, homonymous hemianopsia, upper left quadrantanopsia, and lower left quadrantanopsia) associated with various lesion sites with a diagram.

4. Explain the events related to light refraction, lens accommodation, pupil constriction, and inverted image formation. Outline how convex or concave lenses differentially contribute to refraction.

5. Describe the refractive abnormality displayed by patients with myopia and hypermetropia. Discuss the ways they are corrected with special lenses.

6. Describe the mechanisms of light reflex and lens accommodation. Outline the neural pathways involved.

7. How does the iris participate in regulating pupil opening?

8. Describe the role the ciliary muscle plays in lens accommodation.

9. Describe how rods and cones are stimulated. How do they contribute to vision? How do they differ in color sensitivity and retinal distributions?

10. Describe night blindness and what causes it.

11. Describe how visual acuity is recorded.

13. A patient exhibits acuity of 20/20 for the right eye and 20/80 for the left eye. What do these numbers tell? Which eye has better visual acuity?

14. What lesion site is commonly associated with bitemporal hemianopsia?

15. People with Wernicke's aphasia commonly exhibit no vision in the right half of both visual fields. Name this defect and the implicated lesion site.

16. A lesion in the lower nasal portion of the retina would produce blindness in which portion of the visual field?

17. To avoid double vision, the eyes are aligned so that images fall on corresponding (homonymous) points. A point that is homonymous with one in the right upper nasal retina is found in which quadrant of the left retina?

18. Match the following numbered structures to the associated lettered function or definition that best describes that structure.

i. sclera	a. drains aqueous humor from the posterior to the anterior chamber
ii. canal of Schlemm	b. layer of connective tissue that covers the eyeball
iii. rods	c. transparent covering of the anterior chamber
iv. cornea	d. supplies blood to the retina
v. choroid	e. regulates pupil size and the amount of light entering the eye
vi. iris	f. reduces tension on the lens
vii. lens	g. refracts light to properly focus images on the retina
viii. ciliary body	h. central retinal field
ix. fovea centralis	i. focal point of central vision
x. macula lutea	j. mediate visual acuity and color vision
xi. cones	k. mediate night vision

Learning Objectives

After studying this chapter, students should be able to do the following:

- Describe the basic properties of sound
- Define the decibel unit used for measuring sound
- Discuss the structures and functions of the outer, middle, and inner ear
- Discuss the mechanism for localizing sound
- Describe the functions and anatomy of the central auditory mechanism
- Explain distinctive characteristics of the auditory system
- Discuss the effects of cortical and subcortical lesions on hearing
- Differentiate between conductive and sensorineural hearing losses
- Describe the common audiometric tests and discuss their clinical importance
- Explain the neuronal pathways mediating various auditory reflexes
- Explain the functions of the descending auditory pathway

Hearing is essential to the acquisition of spoken language. It serves as a foundation for verbal communication, the most common form of social interaction. Hearing impairment restricts effective communication. The process of audition (hearing) begins when sound waves strike the tympanic membrane. The resulting vibration of the tympanic membrane converts the pressure waves into mechanical energy, causing the middle ear bones (ossicles) to move back and forth. This mechanical energy is further transformed into a hydraulic form of energy in the cochlear fluid of the inner ear. The patterned hydraulic waves in the inner ear stimulate the sensory hair cells in the cochlea, which generate nerve impulses. These impulses are transmitted by the fibers of cranial nerve VIII to the cochlear nuclei in the brainstem, which project these nerve impulses to multiple synaptic points

in the brainstem and the thalamus. The combined signals from both ears are analyzed for sound localization in the brainstem according to their intensity and frequency. Auditory impulses finally travel to the primary auditory cortex, on the superior surface of the temporal lobe in the gyrus of Heschl, which is responsible for perception. The perceived auditory impulses further travel to Wernicke's (associational language) area in the left hemisphere, where the auditory signals are analyzed and interpreted into language-specific meaningful messages and the comprehension of spoken language takes place.

This chapter provides a functional description of the anatomy and physiology of hearing from the ear to the primary auditory cortex. It begins with a brief description of the properties of sound, followed by a functional description of the anatomy of the ear. Finally, it describes the central auditory pathways that include auditory projections from the cochlear nuclei in the pons and medulla oblongata to the primary auditory cortex in the temporal lobe.

SOUND, PROPERTIES, AND MEASUREMENTS

Sound is created when a force sets an object into vibration so that molecular vibration in the medium propagates a pressure wave. It is the movement of the molecules in the medium that transmits sound. Sound is characterized by two major attributes: **frequency** and **intensity**. **Time**, either the elapsed period or the sound onset phase, is also a property of sound.

Frequency refers to the speed of vibration or the number of complete cycles that a particle executes; it is expressed in cycles per second, or **Hertz (Hz)**. Frequency determines the pitch of the sound or tone; the human ear can detect sounds within a range of 20 to

20,000 Hz. The most important frequencies for under-standing speech are in the range of 250 to 8000 Hz. Low-frequency sound waves are perceived as having a low pitch, whereas high frequency sound waves are perceived as having a high pitch. However, the relationship between frequency and pitch is not always linear.

Intensity of sound is represented by the amplitude of the sound waves. It refers to the strength of molecular movement and is correlated with perceived loudness. The strength of molecular movement is measured in terms of its sound pressure in dynes per square centimeter, or μPa. Because the range of sound pressures to which the human ear is sensitive is quite large, it has been measured in **decibels** (**dB**). The decibel is defined as the log of the ratio between the **measured sound pressure** (Px) and a well-defined **reference sound pressure** (Pr). The formula for calculating the **sound pressure level** (SPL) in decibels of a given sound is as follows:

$$dB\ SPL = 20 \log Px/Pr$$

Conventionally, the reference sound pressure is 0.0002 dyne/cm^2, or 20 μPa, which corresponds to the sound pressure required to make a 1000-Hz sound just audible to the human ear. If Px is the same as Pr, intensity of the sound in dB SPL is 0:

$$dB\ SPL = 20 \log Px/Pr$$

$$dB\ SPL = 20 \log 1$$

Because log 1 = 0

$$dB\ SPL = 20 \times 0$$

$$dB\ SPL = 0$$

Zero decibels does not mean absence of sound but rather that the measured sound pressure is the same as the reference sound pressure. If the measured sound pressure is 100 times the reference sound pressure, the intensity of the measured sound pressure in dB SPL would be 40 dB, because the log of 100 is 2.

For an illustration of the dB SPL for the ratios of different Px:Pr, see Table 9-1. The human ear is sensitive to the intensity range of 0 to 140 dB SPL. Sounds of more than 140 dB cause pain. Prolonged and repeated exposure to sounds above 90 to 100 dB SPL may cause permanent structural damage to the hair cells in the cochlea (Table 9-2).

Changes in intensity are perceived as changes in loudness. As intensity increases, there is a perceived increase in loudness. However, there is not always a 1:1 relationship between loudness and intensity. This is because the human ear is not equally sensitive to all sound frequencies. More intensity is required at some frequencies for a listener to just detect the presence of that sound

Table 9-1. Ratio Values and Corresponding Decibels of Pressures

Ratio	Log[a]	Pressure (dB)
1:1	0.00000	0.0
2:1	0.30103	6.0
3:1	0.47712	9.5
5:1	0.69897	14.0
9:1	0.95424	19.1
10:1	1.00000	20.0
17:1	1.23045	24.6
20:1	1.30103	26.0
30:1	1.47712	29.5
40:1	1.60206	32.0
50:1	1.69897	34.0
60:1	1.77815	35.6
70:1	1.84510	36.9
80:1	1.90309	38.0
90:1	1.95424	39.0
100:1	2.00000	40.0
1,000:1	3.00000	60.0
10,000:1	4.00000	80.0
100,000:1	5.00000	100.0
1,000,000:1	6.00000	120.0

[a] Multiply log by 20 to calculate the decibel value.

Table 9-2. Sound Pressure Levels (dB SPL) Representing Common Daily Activities

Daily Activities	Sound Pressure Levels (dB)
Plane at takeoff or rock music	120–140
Approaching train	100
Average traffic noise	70–80
Conversational speech	60–70
Average home environment	50
Quiet office	40
Soft whisper 4 feet away	20–30
Audible sound	0

than at other frequencies (Fig. 9-1). For example, the average normal-hearing listener needs 45.5 dB SPL to hear a 125-Hz sound but requires only 8.5 dB SPL at 2000 Hz.

The best known reference for decibel is termed the **hearing level** (**HL**), which indicates sound intensity in

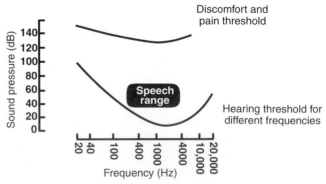

Figure 9-1. Thresholds of hearing sensitivity for various frequencies.

relation to average normal hearing. A 0-dB HL denotes the intensity level that is barely heard by the human ear.

ANATOMY AND PHYSIOLOGY

External Ear

The external ear includes three structures (Fig. 9-2): the cartilaginous **pinna**, the **external auditory meatus**, and the **tympanic membrane**. The external ear in humans is not as well developed as it is in dogs and cats. In humans, the pinna contributes to detecting the direction of sound by channeling collected sound waves into the **external auditory meatus**. The tympanic membrane is attached to the external auditory meatus at the end and separates it from the middle ear. The canal serves as the resonator, allowing peak resonance for the frequencies that are important for most human voices.

Middle Ear

The middle ear is an air-filled cavity between the tympanic membrane and the cochlea of the inner ear. It contains three interconnected small bones (ossicles) that are suspended by ligaments and serve as a mechanical lever system. The ossicles of the middle ear (the **malleus, incus**, and **stapes**) connect the **tympanic membrane** to the **oval window** of the cochlea of the inner ear. The malleus, the first bone, is attached at approximately the midpoint of the tympanic membrane. The incus, the second bone, is between the malleus and the stapes. The footplate of the stapes, the third bone, sits in the oval window of the cochlea. The **eustachian tube**, which runs from the middle ear to the nasopharynx, ventilates the middle ear by equalizing middle ear pressure with the atmospheric pressure in the external ear.

The primary functions of the middle ear are (*a*) to transmit sound pressure variations by converting acoustic energy into mechanical energy, (*b*) to equalize pressure, and (*c*) to reflexively control the energy transmission to the inner ear by regulating movements in the ossicular chain.

TRANSMISSION OF SOUND PRESSURE VARIATIONS

The transmission of vibrations from the tympanic membrane through the ossicles to the oval window entails a decrease in amplitude but an increase in force. This amplification in the force of movement results from two mechanical properties: the area ratio of the tympanic membrane to the oval window and the lever action of the ossicles. The area of the oval window (3.5 mm^2) is only about 14% of the effective area of the tympanic membrane (50 mm^2). Also, the lever action of the ossicles provides a mechanical advantage of 1.3 times. Because pressure equals force per unit area, the discrepancy in the size of the tympanic membrane and the oval window, along with the lever action of the ossicles, allows the middle ear to increase sound pressure by approximately 18 (14 × 1.3) times on the cochlear fluid. This amount of amplification is required to overcome the greater impedance of the cochlear fluid compared with air.

The mass, weight, and stiffness of the middle ear structures pose a clear restriction on their speed of motion, which limits the range of sound frequencies that can be efficiently transmitted through the middle ear.

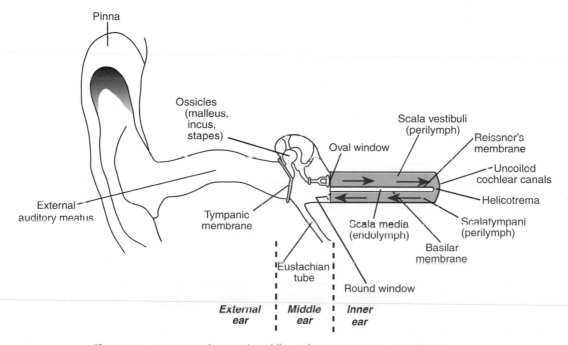

Figure 9-2.   Anatomy of external, middle, and inner compartments of human ear.

We hear only the sound frequencies that are not dampened by such motion limitations imposed by the mass and stiffness of the middle ear system.

PRESSURE EQUALIZATION

The eustachian tube connects the middle ear cavity to the nasopharynx. Opening during swallowing, sneezing, and other reflexive activities, the eustachian tube equalizes the pressure in the middle ear with the atmospheric pressure on the other side of the tympanic membrane. This pressure equalization is needed to ensure efficient transmission of sound from the tympanic membrane to the oval window. Any infection of the membranous lining of the eustachian tube, or a middle ear infection, may restrict the opening of the eustachian tube to the nasopharynx. The air trapped in the middle ear is absorbed and negative pressure results, which has a damping impact on ossicular movements.

REFLEXIVE CONTROL OF OSSICLE MOVEMENT

Energy transmission through the middle ear and movement of the ossicles are influenced by two muscles in the middle ear cavity: the **tensor tympani** and the **stapedius**. The primary function of these muscles is to reflexively protect the auditory mechanism from structural damage by controlling ossicular motion when a person is exposed to high-intensity sounds. The stapedius muscle, controlled by the facial nerve, restricts ossicular movements by pulling the stapes outward. The tensor tympani muscle, which is regulated by the trigeminal nerve, also participates in restricting ossicular movements. Combined, both muscles reflexively stiffen the ossicular system and attenuate the transmission of energy for high-intensity sounds from the external ear to the inner ear (attenuation reflex). The usual latency time of this reflex is 50 to 150 msec. However, this muscle contraction is inadequate to protect the ear in the case of prolonged noise exposure, such as loud music or industrial noise, since sound is attenuated by only 10 dB. Furthermore, this attenuation is largely caused by the action of the stapedius muscle and is known to affect low-frequency sounds only. The overall extent of noise attenuation by the tensor tympani is known to be small.

Inner Ear

The inner ear consists of a dual-functional mechanism for serving the special sensory modalities **audition** and **equilibrium** (discussed in Chapter 10). Both of these functions are served by interconnected fluid-filled membranous labyrinth ducts (Fig. 9-3). The inner ear consists of the **bony labyrinth** and the **membranous labyrinth**. The bony labyrinth is a series of cavities in the petrous portion of the temporal bone. The interconnecting canals and cavities of the bony labyrinth contain the three semicircular ducts and the cochlea. The membranous labyrinth of the **saccule**, **utricle**, and **semicircular ducts** mediates equilibrium (see Chapter 10), whereas the **cochlear portion** of the labyrinth serves hearing.

COCHLEAR STRUCTURE

The cochlea is a snail-shaped structure coiled two and one-half times around the **modiolus**, the central bony core of the cochlea (Fig. 9-3). To provide lengthwise orientation to the cochlear anatomy, it is uncoiled in Figures 9-2 and 9-5 and sectioned in Figure 9-4. The

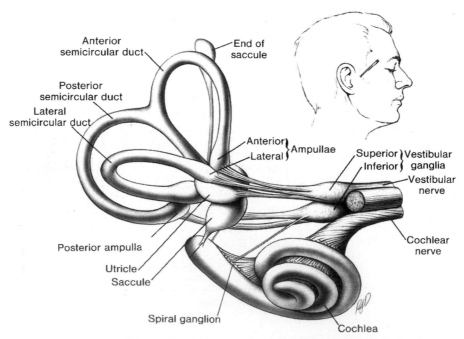

Figure 9-3. Labyrinthine and circuitous cochlea and cochlear and vestibular nerves.

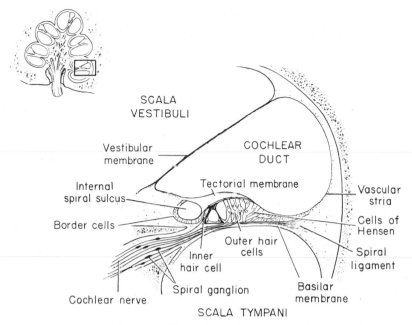

Figure 9-4.   Cochlear duct on a radial section of the cochlea. The location of the depicted region is shown in the inset (*upper left*). The section illustrates the cavities of scalae vestibuli, media, and tympani and the structures of the cochlear duct.

cochlea consists of three fluid-filled scalae (cavities): the **scala vestibuli**, **scala media**, and **scala tympani**. On lengthwise examination, the scala vestibuli is the uppermost compartment, which follows the inner contour of the cochlea and joins the scala tympani though a small aperture, the **helicotrema**. The scala tympani lies at the bottom and follows the outer contour of the cochlea. The scala media, which ends near the cochlear apex, is between the scala tympani and scala vestibuli.

The scalae vestibuli and tympani are filled with **perilymph**, a fluid similar in composition to cerebrospinal fluid. The scala media is filled with **endolymph**, which is similar to extracellular fluid. **Reissner's (vestibular) membrane** separates the scala media from the scala vestibuli, whereas the **basilar membrane** separates the scala media from the ventrally located scala tympani. The scala media (cochlear duct) contains a sensory structure called the **organ of Corti**, which contains sensory hair cells, the primary receptor cells. These sensory cells in humans are arranged into three to five rows of **outer hair cells** and one row of **inner hair cells**, which lie along the length of the basilar membrane. The cilia (apical ends) of the outer hair cells project to the overlying gelatinous **tectorial membrane**, which extends over the organ of Corti. The bases of the inner hair cells are connected to the cochlear nerve endings.

COCHLEAR FUNCTION

The cochlea is concerned with transferring sound vibrations into neural impulses. It absorbs the mechanical energy produced by the movements of the stapes and transduces this mechanical energy into hydraulic

energy, which passes though the perilymph in the scala vestibuli and the scala tympani. Since the basilar membrane is structurally flexible, it responds to the pressure in cochlear perilymph by its displacement. As the basilar membrane is displaced at its base, the deformation moves toward the apex of the cochlea as a traveling wave. As the pressure wave moves, its velocity slows but the amplitude increases toward the apex, reaching maximum at some point. This location of peak is frequency dependent in such a manner that high frequencies peak near the base and low frequencies peak near the cochlear apex (Table 9-3). Different sound frequencies produce different traveling wave patterns, with a peak amplitude at different regions of the cochlea. Each sound frequency produces an invariant wave pattern that implicates the specific regions of the basilar membrane with maximum vibrations. The peak amplitude of the traveling wave for high-frequency sound occurs near the base of the basilar membrane. As the frequency of the stimulus decreases, the peak amplitude of the traveling wave moves toward the helicotrema. A signal consisting of many frequencies causes a sound wave to travel with multiple peaks along the basilar membrane. The hair cells are the most stimulated at the point of the

Table 9-3.   Cochlear Locations Tuned to Specific Frequencies

Frequency	Site of Maximum Amplitude
High	Near oval window
Medium	Middle
Low	Near helicotrema

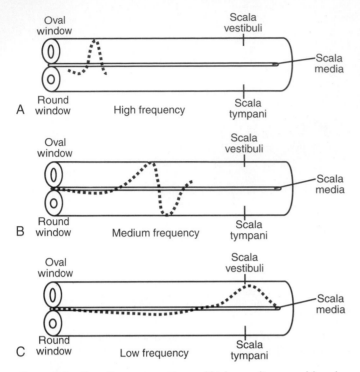

Figure 9-5. Traveling wave patterns of high-, medium-, and low-frequency sounds and corresponding basilar membrane displacements.

maximum oscillations (Fig. 9-5), which suggests that the cochlear frequency selectivity is related to the mechanical properties of the basilar membrane. However, the frequency selectivity may also relate to structural and electrical properties of hair cells.

Displacement of the basilar membrane produces mechanical displacement of the cilia of the hair cells relative to the tectorial membrane. The shearing effect on the apical ends of the hair cells depolarizes the dendritic ends of these cells and generates action potentials, which travel to the brainstem through the fibers of cranial nerve VIII.

ELECTRICAL TRANSDUCTION

The chemical properties of action potentials, discussed in Chapter 5, include the ionic properties of the hair cells and transmission of the charged particles through the cell membranes. There is a notable ionic gradient difference between the endolymph and the perilymph. Cilia or stereocilia, the receptors of the hair cells, are immersed in endolymph, which has an environment with high concentration of potassium, whereas the hair cell body is surrounded by sodium-rich fluid of perilymph. This creates an inward gradient for potassium entry into the cells. The mechanical deformation of the receptive ends during the wave motion in the cochlea opens ion-specific channels, allowing the inward movement of potassium into cell bodies through the cilia in the scala media. This sodium influx, along with the opening of the calcium channels, causes cell depolarization. An action potential is generated and transmitted while the cell body is repolarized and returns to a resting potential.

Retrocochlear Auditory Mechanism

The retrocochlear portion of the auditory system (Fig. 9-6) transmits auditory signals from the hair cells in the organ of Corti to the brainstem **cochlear nuclei**. The hair cells project nerve impulses to the peripheral axons of the unipolar **spiral ganglia** (first-order neuron). The central processes of these cells form the acoustic branch of cranial nerve VIII and pass through the **internal auditory meatus**, a canal in the petrous portion of the temporal bone, before synapsing upon the cochlear nuclei at the pontomedullary junction (Figs. 9-4 and 9-6). There are approximately 30,000 spiral ganglia cells located in the **modiolus**.

Central Auditory Pathways

The physiology of the sensory system includes a three-neuron pathway (see Chapter 7). However, the

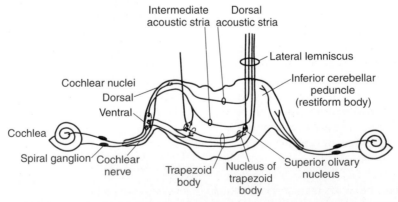

Figure 9-6. Retrocochlear neural mechanism. Peripheral processes of spiral ganglions project to hair cells in cochlea; their central processes transmit impulses to cochlear nuclear complex at pontomedullary junction.

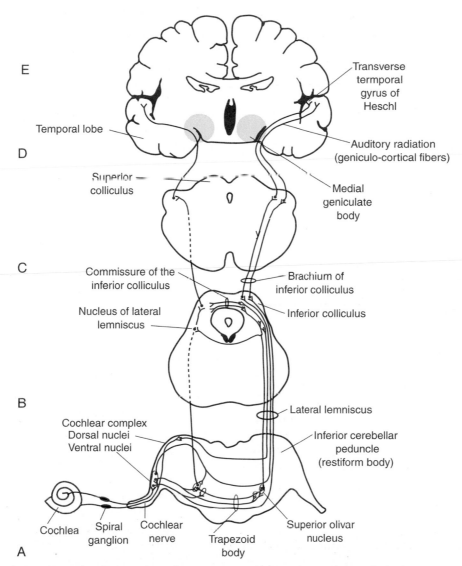

E

Transverse
termporal
gyrus of
Heschl

Temporal lobe

D

Auditory radiation
(geniculo-cortical fibers)

Superior
colliculus

Medial
geniculate
body

C

Commissure of the
inferior colliculus

Brachium of
inferior colliculus

Nucleus of lateral
lemniscus

Inferior colliculus

B

Lateral lemniscus

Cochlear complex
Dorsal nuclei
Ventral nuclei

Inferior cerebellar
peduncle
(restiform body)

Cochlea   Spiral   Cochlear
            ganglion   nerve

Trapezoid
body

Superior olivar
nucleus

A

Figure 9-7. Auditory pathways. Central auditory pathway begins as secondary fibers arising from cochlear nuclear complex and forming crossed and uncrossed stria. These fibers synapse on the superior olivary nucleus and ascend through the brainstem to the auditory cortex. **A.** Medulla **B.** Pons. **C.** Inferior colliculus level. **D.** Medial geniculate body of thalamus. **E.** Transverse gyrus of Heschl.

three-neuronal organization is not fully applicable to the auditory system. The auditory cortical projections are perhaps the most complex to describe because of their multiple synaptic relays at various levels between the cochlear nuclei (second-order neurons) and the thalamus (third-order neurons).

The **central auditory pathway** (Fig. 9-7) extends from the **cochlear nuclear complex** to the **primary auditory cortex.** The acoustic cranial nerve (myelinated) fibers enter the brainstem laterally at the pontomedullary junction and synapse upon the cochlear nuclear complex. Structures in the central auditory pathway are the **cochlear nuclei,** the **superior olivary nuclei,** the **lateral lemniscus,** the **inferior colliculus,** the **brachium of inferior colliculus,** the **medial geniculate body,** the **auditory**

radiations (geniculocortical fibers), and the **primary auditory cortex** in the **transverse gyros of Heschl.**

COCHLEAR NUCLEUS

Fibers of the acoustic cranial nerve enter the brainstem at the pontomedullary junction dorsolateral to the inferior cerebellar peduncle (restiform body). They terminate in the cochlear nuclear complex (second-order neuron), which is divided into **dorsal** and **ventral nuclei** (Figs. 3-11, 9-6, and 9-7). The dorsal cochlear nucleus lies dorsolateral to the restiform body, whereas the ventral cochlear nucleus is ventrolateral to the restiform body. The entering fibers of the acoustic (eighth) cranial nerve also divide into dorsal and ventral branches and synapse onto the respective cochlear nuclei.

An important principle governing the functional representation at the cochlear nuclear complex and through the auditory pathway is the discrete tonotopic organization. There is a one-to-one relationship between the tonal representation of the hair cells in the organ of Corti and the cells in the cochlear nuclear complex. The fibers from the apex of the cochlea, which carry low frequencies, terminate at the superficial layers of the cochlear nucleus, whereas fibers from the base of the cochlea, which carry high frequencies, penetrate deeper in the nucleus and thereby preserve the tonal correspondence. This discrete tonotopic representation is retained throughout the ascending fibers of the central auditory pathway and all its nuclei up to the auditory cortex.

COCHLEAR PROJECTIONS

The cochlear nuclear complex sends multiple projections to both the ipsilateral and contralateral ascending auditory pathways. The exact nature of these projections is not as clear as it seems to be in the diagrams of the brainstem. Although most auditory fibers cross the midline to project to opposite cortical areas, a small number of fibers do not cross the midline but instead ascend ipsilaterally. The cochlear projections that cross the midline travel in three bundles: the **dorsal acoustic stria,** the **intermediate stria**, and the **trapezoid body**. Again, there is a function for each of these channels in terms of mediating a specific attribute of the signal; however, our knowledge of those attributes is incomplete. The cells along the crossing fibers of the trapezoid body form the nucleus of the trapezoid body. The fibers of the dorsal acoustic stria cross the midline and terminate in the contralateral lateral lemniscus without sending projections to any of the olivary nuclei. The collaterals from the fibers of the intermediate acoustic stria may project to the ipsilateral and/or contralateral superior olivary complex, and the main body of fibers joins the contralateral lateral lemniscus. The fibers of the trapezoid body, by far the most important and largest stria, cross the midline to terminate in the superior olivary nucleus, which is located laterally in the dorsal pons. The auditory fibers that are ipsilateral either send projections to the ipsilateral superior olivary nucleus or bypass it on their way to the ipsilateral lateral lemniscus.

SUPERIOR OLIVARY NUCLEUS

The **superior olivary nucleus,** a collection of nuclei in the pons, is known to receive auditory inputs from both the ipsilateral and contralateral cochlear nuclei. It contains binaural cells (lateral superior olive and medial superior olive) that are uniquely equipped to calculate differences in time and intensity of auditory stimuli from both ears. The superior olivary nuclei contain two large dendrites extending from the opposite sites of the soma. The medial dendrite receives projections from the contralateral cochlear nuclei, whereas the lateral dendrite receives from the ipsilateral cochlear nuclei. This structural arrangement allows the superior olivary nucleus to compare information from both ears. By integrating time and intensity differences received from both ears, the superior olivary nucleus contributes to the spatial localization of the sound. This ability to localize sound is remarkable, as the path difference between the ears is only 5 inches or so.

LATERAL LEMNISCUS

The **lateral lemniscus**, the primary ascending auditory pathway, extends from the superior olivary nucleus to the inferior colliculus of the midbrain (Fig 3-14). Its fibers climb laterally in the pontine tegmentum. The cell bodies along the fibers form the nucleus of the lateral lemniscus. The lateral lemniscus receives crossed and uncrossed projections from the dorsal and intermediate striae; thus it retains bilateral representation with added representation from the opposite ear. This explains why pathology of the central auditory pathway at any level does not lead to deafness in one ear. The fibers of the lateral lemniscus ascend in the brainstem toward the inferior colliculus in the midbrain (Figs. 3-15 and 9-7). On their way to the midbrain, the fibers of the lateral lemniscus pass dorsolaterally in the tegmentum of the pons, potentially making numerous connections.

INFERIOR COLLICULUS

The fibers of the lateral lemniscus ascend through the pons to the **inferior colliculus** in the midbrain (Fig. 3-15). Only some of the lateral lemniscus fibers are actually known to synapse upon the inferior colliculus; the remaining fibers pass without synaptic relays to it. Both inferior colliculi are connected through the **commissural fibers** of the inferior colliculus, permitting further crossing and integration of monaural and binaural auditory input. This integration has additional implications for the localization of a sound source. The inferior colliculus is also concerned with auditory–visual reflexes. Besides mediating auditory reflexes, the inferior colliculus serves as the way station for auditory transmissions. The primary output of the inferior colliculus is to the thalamus, as its projections travel through the **brachium** of the inferior colliculus to the medial geniculate body (Figs. 2-21, 3-16, 9-7, and 9-8). Part of the auditory information from the inferior colliculus is projected to the adjacent **superior colliculus** (the midbrain structure that mediates visual reflexes), the **reticular formation**, and the **cerebellum**. At these sites, the information about the angular location of the sound source received is integrated with visual and other sensory inputs. This integrated information is projected on various pathways to coordinate reflexive movements of the eye, head, and body toward the sound source.

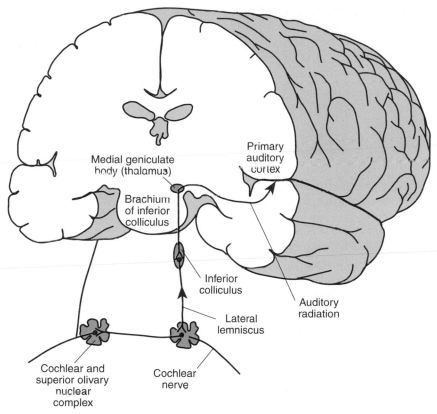

Figure 9-8.   Auditory pathways from cochlear nucleus to primary cortex through synaptic connections with inferior colliculus and medial geniculate bodies. Course of geniculocortical fibers illustrates lateral transition of these fibers through internal capsule to gyrus of Heschl.

MEDIAL GENICULATE BODY

The **medial geniculate body** is the thalamic relay center for the transmission of auditory information. It is in the laterocaudal portion of the thalamus, and it receives its input from the ipsilateral inferior colliculus in the midbrain (Figs. 3-16, 9-7, and 9-8). There is no known crossing of impulses directly at the level of the medial geniculate body. Nonetheless, the possibility remains for some information to cross to the other side through thalamic commissural fibers. The projections of the medial geniculate body (auditory radiations or geniculocortical) pass ventrally (sublenticular) and caudally (retrolenticular) to the lenticular portion of the internal capsule (Fig. 9-9). They terminate in the ipsilateral primary auditory cortex, the gyrus of Heschl, in the superior temporal lobe (Fig. 9-8).

PRIMARY AND AUDITORY ASSOCIATION CORTEX

The **primary auditory cortex** (Brodmann area 41) is in the **transversely oriented gyri of Heschl**, which are buried in the lateral sylvian sulcus on the dorsal surface of the superior (first) temporal gyrus. This area is surrounded by the **auditory association area** (Brodmann area 42), which extends onto the lateral surface of the temporal lobe. Both of these regions receive projections from the medial geniculate body. The auditory areas of the hemispheres are interconnected by commissural fibers. The auditory cortical region is surrounded by the area of the **planum temporale** (temporal planum) and is hidden by the overlying operculum of the temporal, parietal, and frontal lobes (Fig. 9-10). In most individuals, the left planum temporal area is larger than in the right brain, a fact that has been related to the cerebral dominance.

Receiving impulses through crossed and uncrossed fibers from both ears, the primary auditory cortex is known to retain the cochlear tonotopic representation. The geniculocortical fibers mediating higher frequencies terminate in the posteromedial region of the gyrus of Heschl, and the fibers transmitting lower frequencies synapse in the anterolateral region. The area between these two regions receives fibers carrying the middle range of frequencies. Research on cats seems to suggest that the primary auditory cortex is not absolutely essential for frequency discrimination; rather it has vital importance in auditory discriminations that are based on the timing patterns of auditory events, such as human speech perception. Patients with unilateral cortical lesion usually exhibit nearly normal hearing thresholds. However, they are found to exhibit impaired ability to perceive and discriminate speech. Both hearing and speech perception are known to be impaired after bilateral cortical lesions.

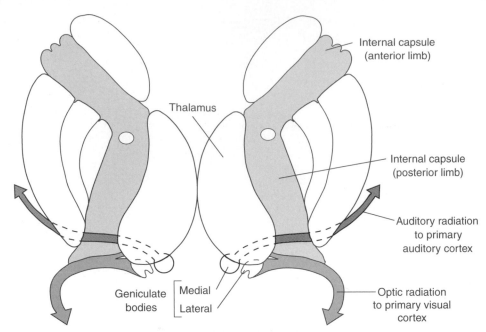

Figure 9-9. Horizontal schematic of auditory projections from medial geniculate bodies to primary auditory cortex. It depicts transition of geniculo-cortical fibers below posterior limb of internal capsule.

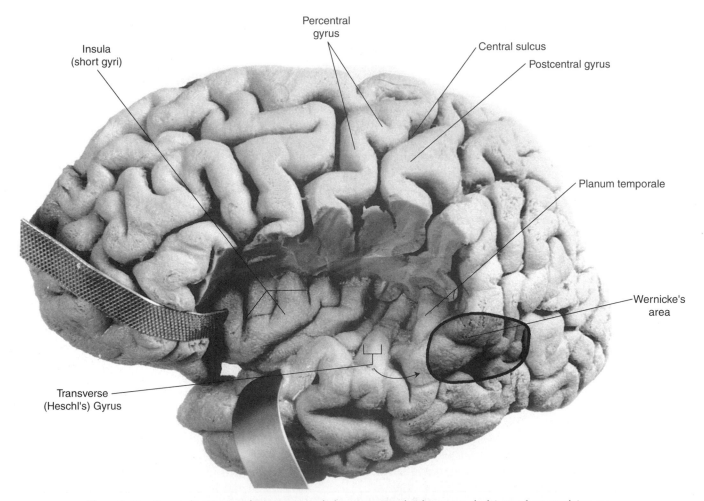

Figure 9-10. Exposed primary auditory cortex and planum temporale after removal of tissues from overlying operculi of frontal and parietal lobes; also the projections from the primary auditory cortex to Wernicke's area (association language cortex).

The primary auditory cortex is the site of auditory sensation and perception. An extensive axonal bundle connects the primary auditory cortex to Wernicke's area (Brodmann area 22), the **language associational cortex**. This association cortex includes part of the planum temporale and posterosuperior first temporal gyrus; it is concerned with recognizing language stimuli, interpreting their meanings with respect to previous auditory memories and linguistic experiences, and comprehending spoken language. Wernicke's area (Fig. 9-10), as part of the larger language interpretative cortex, also receives visual and somesthetic information and contributes to language formulation. See Chapter 19 for a discussion of the integrative functions of the temporal lobe.

AUDITORY REFLEXES

Auditory reflexes coordinate head and eye movements toward sound and influence vestibular functions. This reflex mechanism primarily involves three anatomical pathways. The **first pathway** includes the projections from the inferior colliculus to the superior colliculus and tectum, integrating auditory and visual systems and controlling extraocular movements. The **second pathway** from the superior olivary nucleus to the **medial longitudinal fasciculus** projects to the abducens, oculomotor, and trochlear nerves. Impulses traveling on these two pathways regulate ocular movements in response to auditory stimuli. The **third pathway** includes the auditory projections to the vestibular nuclear complex and cerebellum and participates in equilibrium.

DISTINCTIVE PROPERTIES OF AUDITORY SYSTEM

There are four distinctive auditory system characteristics: (*a*) bilateral auditory representation, (*b*) sound source localization, (*c*) tonotopic representation, and (*d*) descending auditory projections for tuning of the receptors.

Bilateral Auditory Representation

Bilateral auditory representation at the cortex is credited to the multiple crossings of auditory information through ascending interconnections at the levels of the cochlear nuclei, the lateral lemniscus, and the inferior colliculus. The primary auditory cortex in each hemisphere receives input from both ears; however, the major input to the primary auditory cortex is from the opposite ear, with fewer projections from the ipsilateral ear. A lesion at any point along the central auditory pathway extending from the pons to the auditory cortex does not result in complete deafness in the opposite ear; it causes only a mild loss of hearing, if any. However, a bilateral cortical ablation or lesion involving the primary and association auditory cortex (Brodmann areas 41 and 42) results in profound loss of auditory discriminative and speech perceptive skills.

Sound Source Localization

The interaural difference of the time and intensities of auditory impulses is important in localizing the source of a sound. Interaural time delay is the temporal difference when a given sound reaches the two ears at different times. The ear nearest the source receives the information first. The time difference between the ears can be estimated by dividing the difference in path length by the sound speed. Intensity difference is the differentially perceived loudness of a sound. This loudness difference is used to determine a sound's location, as the sound is less intense at the ear farther from the sound source.

The sound-localizing mechanism begins at the level of the superior olivary nucleus. It is the first nucleus to receive crossed and uncrossed projections from both ears, and it uses the time delay and intensity difference to determine the exact location and direction of sound sources.

Tonotopic Representation

Discrete tonal representation at the cochlear level is maintained throughout the central auditory pathway. Despite the multiple interconnections and crossings in the ascending pathways, the tonal representation from the hair cells in the cochlea is retained throughout the auditory system. Tones are even represented in the primary auditory cortex, where a single neuron responds best to certain sound frequencies.

Descending Auditory Projections

Parallel to the afferent auditory projections to the auditory cortex, descending fibers are known to exist along the pathway from the primary auditory cortex to the cochlear hair cells that conduct impulses in the reverse direction. These descending fibers provide feedback circuits to refine the perception of pitch and loudness and to sharpen the reception of specific frequencies through the process of lateral inhibition. The recurring connections of the descending fibers begin from the primary auditory cortex and make synaptic relays to the thalamus, brainstem (inferior colliculus), and superior olivary nucleus before terminating in the cochlear hair cells. The descending connections, consisting of corticogeniculate, corticocollicular, colliculo-olivary, and colliculo-cochleonuclear fibers, not only sharpen the signals by improving the signal-to-noise ratio but also enhance cues for sound localization and contribute to the quality of the perceived sound by suppressing competing signals.

CLINICAL INFORMATION

Hearing Impairments

Clinically, hearing impairment is divided into two major types: **conductive** and **sensorineural**. Pathologies of the outer and middle ear, which affect sound transmission to the cochlea, cause a **conductive hearing loss**. Lesions affecting the sensory receptors in the organ of Corti and/or the fibers of the auditory nerve cause a **sensorineural hearing loss**. **Mixed hearing loss** includes both conductive and sensorineural impairments. Retrocochlear lesions produce **nerve deafness**, whereas hearing loss associated with brainstem lesion is called **central deafness**.

CONDUCTIVE HEARING LOSS

If the movement of the ossicles is restricted for some reason, the impinging energy is less efficiently transmitted through the middle ear, affecting the transmission of all frequencies. The effects of conductive pathologies are less severe, usually resulting in a partial loss of hearing. **Serous otitis media**, a noncontagious middle ear infection, is the most common cause of conductive hearing loss in children. Middle ear fluid accumulation secondary to eustachian tube malfunction in serous otitis media causes a variable and fluctuating hearing impairment. If it is not treated, it may cause long-term problems in speech and language development for children. Since the process of serous fluid accumulation is slow, the loss of hearing is not easily detected by parents and family members. Impacted cerumen can also cause a middle ear hearing loss.

In adults, the most common cause of hearing loss due to middle ear pathology is otosclerosis, a dominant autosomal condition in which a pathological growth of bone near the oval window impedes the movement of stapes. In this case, surgical removal of the stapes and insertion of a Teflon prosthesis can restore hearing in most cases.

SENSORINEURAL HEARING LOSS

Sensorineural loss of hearing is associated with pathology in the cochlear nuclei and/or the auditory nerve. Damage to the sensory hair cells and their fibers can result in hearing losses that range from mild to complete loss of hearing in the affected ear. Exposure to noise is the most common cause of sensorineural hearing loss. Other causes include **Ménière's disease**, **vestibular** and **acoustic schwannomas**, **presbycusis**, and **degenerative conditions**.

Noise exposure, a prolonged and repeated exposure to intense noise, can destroy hair cells. Prolonged exposure to occupational noise (industrial environment, loud rock music, engine noise) is a commonly recognized risk. **Ménière's disease** is a chronic condition associated with edema of the membranous labyrinth marked by progressive hearing loss, ringing in the ears, and dizziness. **Vestibular** or **acoustic schwannoma** is a tumor of Schwann cells that occurs at the cerebellopontine angle. Because of the involvement of cranial nerve VIII, it results in unilateral deafness and tinnitus. Other symptoms associated with this vestibular or acoustic schwannoma are unsteady gait, vertigo, and dizziness. In later stages, the un-

treated tumor can involve the intracranial roots of the trigeminal and facial cranial nerves and cerebellar structures. This involvement produces loss of pain and temperature sensation from the ipsilateral face, facial weakness, loss of taste from the anterior part of tongue, and cerebellar symptoms, such as unstable gait and ataxia. **Presbycusis** is an age–induced hearing impairment. This progressive hearing loss primarily affects the high frequencies and results from the degeneration of hair cells in the first turn of the cochlear duct.

MIXED HEARING LOSS

In mixed hearing loss, patients exhibit lowered sensitivity to both air- and bone-conducted stimuli. A typical audiogram also reveals an air–bone gap, with bone conduction being better.

EFFECTS OF CORTICAL LESION

Hearing loss, a common sequela of cochlear lesion, can also result from bilateral cortical or brainstem lesions. However, nearly normal auditory function is retained after a unilateral cortical or brainstem lesion because the afferents from both ears project to the bilateral cortical areas. The only sensory deficit arising from a unilateral (primary auditory) cortical lesion may be impairment in the ability to localize a sound source, though the ability to identify the direction and intensity of sound is usually spared.

Involvement of the language association cortex results in aphasic deficits. Anatomical changes affecting Wernicke's area produce a full-blown **paragrammatic syndrome** (Wernicke's aphasia), which is characterized by impaired comprehension of spoken language, reduced ability to read and write, and impaired lexical retrieval. Words can be spoken fluently, although speech remains largely meaningless. **Pure word deafness** is another language syndrome that is associated with cortical lesion. This uncommon disorder is manifested by a severe loss of language comprehension, even though speech production, reading, and writing are only minimally affected. Higher language functions that are mediated by Wernicke's area spared, while Wernicke's area is deprived of all auditory input. A bilateral temporal lesion is the most likely cause, as it involves the fibers radiating from the gyrus of Heschl and isolates Wernicke's area both from the adjacent auditory cortex and from the transcallosal pathway from the right cortex (see Chapter 19).

Evaluation of Hearing Disorders

There are many technical and complex tests of hearing. Specialized training in audiology is required for administering them and interpreting their results. Only the most common of these tests are discussed here.

The differential diagnosis of hearing loss is determined by testing the subject's hearing threshold for air- and bone-conducted sounds. Commonly used tests include the **tuning fork assessment, tympanometry, pure tone audiometry,** and **brainstem auditory evoked potential audiometry**.

TUNING FORK

Tuning forks are often used to informally differentiate a conductive hearing loss from a sensorineural hearing loss. **Rinne** and **Weber** are two commonly used tests.

Rinne Test

In the Rinne test, the stem of a vibrating tuning fork (512 Hz) is placed on the mastoid process and the subject listens to the tone by bone conduction. When the intensity of the stimulus decreases and the fork is no longer heard by the subject, the fork is placed in front of the ear so the subject can attempt to hear it by air conduction. A subject with normal hearing or a sensorineural hearing loss should again hear the tone (positive Rinne), since hearing through air conduction is more sensitive than through bone conduction. The subject with a conductive hearing loss will not hear the tone again (negative Rinne).

Weber Test

In the Weber test a vibrating tuning fork is placed on the scalp at the vertex and the patient is asked to localize the sound, specifically if he or she hears the tone and whether it is more pronounced in one ear. In subjects with normal hearing or bilaterally symmetrical hearing loss, the sound is sensed in the midline. In the case of a unilateral conductive hearing loss, the sound is heard mainly in the affected ear. However, it is heard mainly in the better ear in the case of a unilateral sensorineural loss.

TYMPANOMETRY

The mobility of the tympanic membrane can be affected by middle ear conditions that restrict its movement. Tympanometry is used to assess the compliance of the tympanic membrane and middle ear under conditions of changing air pressure (relative to atmospheric pressure) in the external auditory meatus. In tympanometry, the middle ear impedance is measured by bouncing the sound wave patterns off the membrane. Different echo patterns help detect middle ear pathology (e.g., pressure changes in fluid, immobility of ossicle, and eustachian tube dysfunctioning), which is likely to change middle ear mechanics in various ways.

PURE TONE AUDIOMETRY

Pure tone audiometry is used to establish the threshold of hearing across the frequency range that is most important for human communication. A pure tone audiometer generates pure tones at various frequencies and intensities. The calibration of the audiometer takes into consideration the differential sensitivity of the human ear to various frequencies by making 0 dB HL at each frequency equal to the lowest intensity level in dB SPL required by the average normal listener to hear that frequency. Hearing threshold is expressed in terms of the lowest intensity level required for an individual to

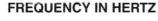

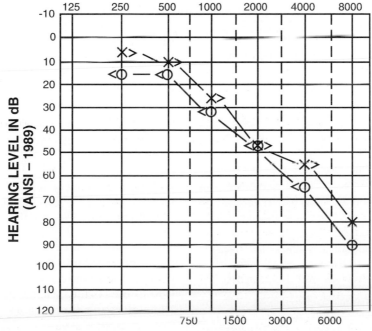

Figure 9-11.   Audiogram illustrating bilateral sensorineural loss with air conduction and bone conduction thresholds averaging at the same dB level.

respond at a given frequency. In audiometry, hearing is tested by determining the air and bone conduction thresholds. The results of testing are plotted on an audiogram, a graphic representation of the subject's bone and air conduction responses to each frequency (Fig. 9-11).

Hearing loss refers to the increase in intensity above normal sensitivity required to reach threshold. For example, a 50-dB loss at 1000 Hz means that the subject requires 50 dB of sound pressure above normal sensitivity to obtain threshold. In the case of a conductive hearing loss, the threshold for bone conduction is better than the air conduction threshold. This threshold difference is the air–bone gap. In a sensorineural loss, hearing sensitivity from bone conduction is equal to the decreased sensitivity of air conduction (Fig. 9-11).

BRAINSTEM AUDITORY EVOKED POTENTIALS

Brainstem auditory evoked potential audiometry is test of synchronous neural firings from the brainstem auditory pathway within 10 msec after stimulus onset. Within this period, five negative peaks identified from the vertex indicate the electrical activity produced in the auditory pathway (Fig. 20-11). Each of these response classes indicates a different anatomical point in the auditory pathway (Table 20-2). By taking into consideration the altered latency or absence of the peaks, one can locate a cranial nerve VIII or brainstem lesion site. This is a very reliable and clinically powerful test, as it does not require the patient's participation and can be performed on infants and uncooperative patients (see evoked potentials in Chapter 20).

Case Studies

Patient One

A 65-year-old university professor complained of difficulty hearing with her left ear accompanied by ringing, nausea, and dizziness. She was taken to a hospital. On testing, she exhibited the following signs:

Hearing loss in left ear
Tendency to fall to her left side
Loss of pain and temperature sensation on left side of face and right side of body
Difficulty swallowing

Magnetic resonance imaging of the brain revealed a small infarct in the dorsolateral medulla on the left side.

Question: How could a dorsal medullary lesion cause problems with hearing and equilibrium and account for the sensory loss and difficulty swallowing?

Discussion: The cochlear and vestibular branches of cranial nerve VIII enter the brainstem at the junction of the medulla and pons. Occlusion in the posterior inferior cerebellar artery affected the second-order (vestibular and cochlear) nuclei of cranial nerve VIII, descending tract of the trigeminal nerve, lateral spinothalamic tract, and motor nucleus of the vagus nerve. The involvement of the left cochlear nucleus affected the hearing threshold in the left ear. The involvement of the left vestibular nucleus accounted for her falling to the left. The involvement of the

trigeminal system resulted in analgesia and thermal anesthesia on the left side of the face. The interruption of the crossed fibers of lateral spinothalamic tract resulted in the loss of pain and temperature sensations from the right side of the body. The involvement of the adjacent vagus nucleus and fibers resulted in swallowing problems.

Patient Two

A 50-year-old man lost hearing in his right ear and had right-sided imbalance. At first, he compensated by using his left ear when using the telephone. He decided to see his physician, as his equilibrium-related difficulty worsened. He began hearing a high-pitched ringing in the right ear and noticed right facial weakness. The examining physician observed the following symptoms:

Right-sided facial weakness
Mild unsteadiness while walking
Right ear hearing loss of 45 dB, which increased to 65 dB for higher frequencies, established by pure tone audiometry
Marked reduction in right ear speech discrimination

Positive Rinne findings and poor speech discrimination in the right ear ruled out a conductive hearing loss. Magnetic resonance imaging confirmed right acoustic schwannoma at the cerebellopontine angle. Surgical removal of the tumor relieved the pressure and largely restored the impaired functions.

Question: Based on your understanding of auditory and vestibular pathways, can you account for this clinical picture by relating the symptoms to the involved pathways?

Discussion: A Schwann cell tumor (schwannoma) at the cerebellopontine angle compressed both branches of cranial nerve VIII roots. This resulted in right ear hearing loss and a right-sided equilibrium problem. The neoplasm also compressed the facial cranial nerve root, creating Bell's palsy, or facial paralysis secondary to facial nerve injury. Unsteadiness while walking resulted from the involvement of the vestibular nerve.

SUMMARY

Audition begins in the external ear, when collected sound waves strike the tympanic membrane. The resulting vibration of the tympanic membrane converts sound waves into mechanical energy, causing the middle ear bones to move back and forth. This mechanical energy is further transformed to a hydraulic form of energy in the cochlear fluid of the inner ear, which activates the sensory hair cells in the cochlea and transforms the hydraulic energy to electrical nerve impulses. The nerve impulses are transmitted by cranial nerve VIII fibers to the cochlear nuclei in the brainstem. The cochlear cells project these nerve impulses to multiple synaptic points in the brainstem and the thalamus before transmitting the nerve impulses to the primary auditory cortex in the temporal lobe. The auditory impulses travel from the primary and secondary auditory cortex to Wernicke's (associational language) area, where the auditory signals are analyzed and interpreted into meaningful language-specific messages.

Clinically, there are two major types of hearing impairment: **conductive** and **sensorineural**. Pathologies of the outer and middle ear, which affect sound transmission to the cochlea, cause **conductive hearing loss**. Lesions affecting the sensory receptors in the organ of Corti and/or the fibers of the auditory nerve cause a **sensorineural hearing loss**. There are many methods of assessing hearing, which are used for a differential diagnosis of hearing loss. It is necessary to have specialized training in audiology before administering them and interpreting their results.

ACKNOWLEDGMENT

I thank my colleague Edward W. Korabic, Ph.D. for his assistance and comments.

Technical Terms

audiogram	lateral lemniscus
audiometry	medial geniculate body
auditory association cortex	primary auditory cortex
conductive hearing loss	sensorineural hearing loss
decibel	superior olivary nucleus
hearing loss	trapezoid body
inferior colliculus	

Review Questions

1. Define the following terms:

audiogram	intensity
audiometry	lateral lemniscus
auditory association cortex	medial geniculate body
cochlea	middle ear
conductive hearing loss	primary auditory cortex
decibel	sensorineural loss
eustachian tube	superior olivary nucleus
frequency	trapezoid body
inferior colliculus	vertex

2. Explain the relationship between amplitude and loudness and between frequency and pitch.
3. Determine the decibel values for sound pressure 10 times, 100 times, and 1000 times the reference sound pressure. Explain how to calculate these values.
4. Label the oval window, round window, cochlea, vestibular membrane, basilar membrane, scala vestibuli, scala media, scala tympani, helicotrema, and organ of Corti, with a diagram of a longitudinal section of the cochlea.
5. Illustrate the course of the auditory pathway with a diagram, identifying major structures from the inner ear to the auditory cortex. Arrange these structures into three groups: brainstem, diencephalon, and forebrain.
6. Describe the primary function of the superior olivary nucleus.
7. What auditory fibers form the trapezoidal bodies?
8. Why does a unilateral lesion of the gyrus of Heschl, medial geniculate body, or lateral lemniscus not cause a complete hearing loss in the ear contralateral to the lesion site?
9. Discuss how a lesion in the upper brainstem (midbrain) level would affect hearing sensitivity.
10. Describe pathophysiologies that underlie conductive and sensorineural hearing loss.
11. Match the following numbered terms to the associated lettered explanations.
    i. conductive hearing loss
    ii. sensorineural hearing loss
    iii. Rinne tuning fork test
    iv. Weber tuning fork test

    a. A tuning fork is placed on the scalp at the vertex and the patient is asked whether he or she hears the tone and whether it is more pronounced in one ear.
    b. The butt of a tuning fork is placed against the mastoid process, and the subject listens to the sound by bone conduction.
    c. Pathologies that affect the sensory receptors in the organ of Corti and/or the auditory nerve fibers.
    d. Pathologies that affect the sound transmission to the cochlea.

Vestibular System

Learning Objectives

After studying this chapter, students should be able to do the following:

- Discuss the importance of the vestibular system in equilibrium
- Describe the anatomy of the vestibular system
- List the primary projections of the vestibular complex
- Explain the physiology of equilibrium
- Describe the mechanism of nystagmus
- Discuss how the vestibular system controls movements
- Explain methods used for assessing the vestibular mechanism
- Describe common dysfunctions of the vestibular system

The vestibular system regulates the position of the head and neck in space; monitors righting motor reflexes; coordinates eye, head, and body movements; and controls eye fixation during body and head movements. It is done subconsciously by integrating information received from receptors in the semicircular ducts of both inner ears. The vestibular system is closely associated with the visual and proprioceptive systems. It constantly integrates the incoming visual information and proprioceptive cues from the entire body, which contribute to the execution of complex, skilled, and coordinated activities, such as dancing, skating, and acrobatics. A person born with congenital atresia (absence) of the vestibular apparatus is usually well oriented when his or her eyes are open but is disoriented in the dark.

ANATOMY OF VESTIBULAR SYSTEM

The major components of the vestibular system are the **semicircular ducts**, **vestibule (saccule** and **utricle)**, and **vestibular nuclei** (Figs. 10-1 to 10-4). Other functionally associated structures are the **medial longitudinal fasciculus**, **brainstem reticular formation**, **midbrain tectal** and **tegmental areas**, and **cerebellar nuclei**. The sensory receptors (hair cells) in the semicircular

ducts respond to rotations of the head and changes in body position. They project impulses to the brainstem vestibular nuclei, which in turn transmit the information to the medial longitudinal fasciculus, cerebellum, and brainstem reticular network to coordinate eye, head, and neck movements.

Semicircular Ducts and Vestibular Sacs

The inner ear consists of two parts: a **bony labyrinth** and a **membranous labyrinth**. The bony labyrinth is made of a series of cavities in the petrous portion of the temporal bone. Inside the bony labyrinth is the membranous labyrinth, which consists of fluid-filled membranous tubes. **Perilymph** fills the space between bony and membranous labyrinths, whereas endolymph fills the membranous ducts. The three semicircular ducts in the inner ear are connected to the **vestibule** (**utricle** and **saccule**). The semicircular ducts are at right angles to one another like the sides of a cube and are named according to their relative positions: **anterior**, **posterior**, and **lateral** (Fig. 10-2). These spatially different positions enable the receptors in the ducts to detect changes in the planes of all body movements. Each semicircular duct contains an enlarged end area called the **ampulla**, which contains **cristae**. The cristae are made of sensory hair cells (**cilia**) covered by a gelatinous, mass-filled capsule called the **cupula**, which extends upward to the ampullary roof (Fig. 10-3B). The hair cells are sensitive to head angular movement. When the head turns, the endolymph in the semicircular duct flows toward the cupula. This builds pressure on one side, bending the cupula and distorting the cilia. Distortion of the cilia generates sensory impulses, which are projected to the vestibular nuclei in the brainstem.

Inside the vestibule are two membranous sacs, the utricle and saccule. The utricle and saccule, the en-

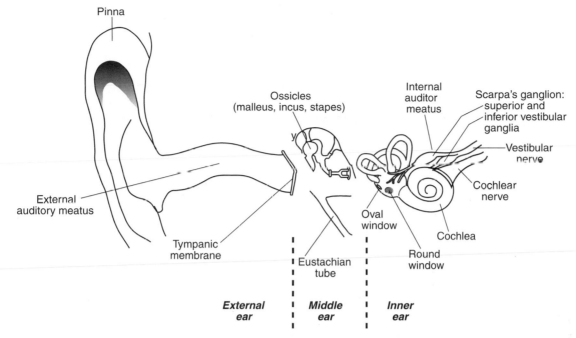

Figure 10-1. Anatomical relationship among external, middle, and inner parts of the ear on a frontal plane.

dolymph-containing dilations, are a continuation of the membranous tubes of the semicircular ducts. Both ends of the semicircular canals are connected to the utricle. The maculae of the utricle and saccule (saclike dilations) also contain sensory receptors (hair cells). A thin layer of gelatinous mass, the **otolithic membrane**, covers these hair cells (Fig. 10-3C). The otolithic membrane contains calcium crystals, which add mass to the membrane. The maculae lie in the horizontal plane when the head is held horizontal, so that the otolithic membrane sits directly on the hair cells. In this case, if the head is tilted or linearly accelerated, the gravitational pull of the otolithic membrane bends the cilia and changes membrane potentials of the receptor cells, resulting in action potentials (impulses). The vestibular labyrinths and the receptors of both sides interact in harmony when the vestibular system is functioning normally. The vestibular receptors, like cochlear terminals, do not exhibit significant adaptations. Thus, the endings in the utricular and saccular maculae signal steady-state gravitational information as well as some dynamic changes (changes in inertia during linear acceleration and deceleration movements of head).

Vestibular Nerve and Nuclei

The vestibular nerve is formed by the fibers of the first-order sensory neurons in the vestibular ganglion (Scarpa's ganglion). The peripheral processes of **Scarpa's ganglion** contact the hair cells in the utricle, saccule, and semicircular canals, and its central projections form the **vestibular nerve** (Figs. 10-3 and 10-4). The vestibular ganglion of Scarpa consists of superior and

inferior ganglia; each of these receives specific vestibular fibers. These ganglia lie in the cavity of the petrous bone (the bony labyrinth), and their central processes exit the petrous bone through the **internal auditory meatus** to reach the junction of the medulla and pons.

The vestibular nerve fibers, which carry information concerning body equilibrium to the vestibular nuclei in the brainstem, join the auditory afferents to form cranial nerve VIII before they emerge from the internal auditory meatus to enter the pontocerebellar junction of the brainstem. Beside the vestibular and cochlear fibers, also in the internal auditory meatus are the fibers of facial nerve. Thus, a lesion at this point has significant implications for a series of symptoms that include vertigo, tinnitus, sensorineural hearing loss, and facial (Bell's) palsy.

Upon entering the brainstem, the vestibular and auditory nerve fibers of the eighth cranial nerve separate on their way to project to different groups of nuclei. Vestibular fibers terminate in the **vestibular nuclear complex** in the lateral-dorsal area of the medulla. The vestibular nuclear complex consists of the **superior vestibular nucleus, lateral vestibular nucleus, medial vestibular nucleus**, and **inferior vestibular nucleus** (Fig. 10-4). The auditory nerve fibers project to the cochlear nuclei that lie lateral-dorsal at the pontomedullary junction.

Primary Vestibular Projections

Vestibular nerve fibers enter the brainstem at the pontomedullary junction, and most of them terminate in the vestibular nuclear complex. The vestibular complex

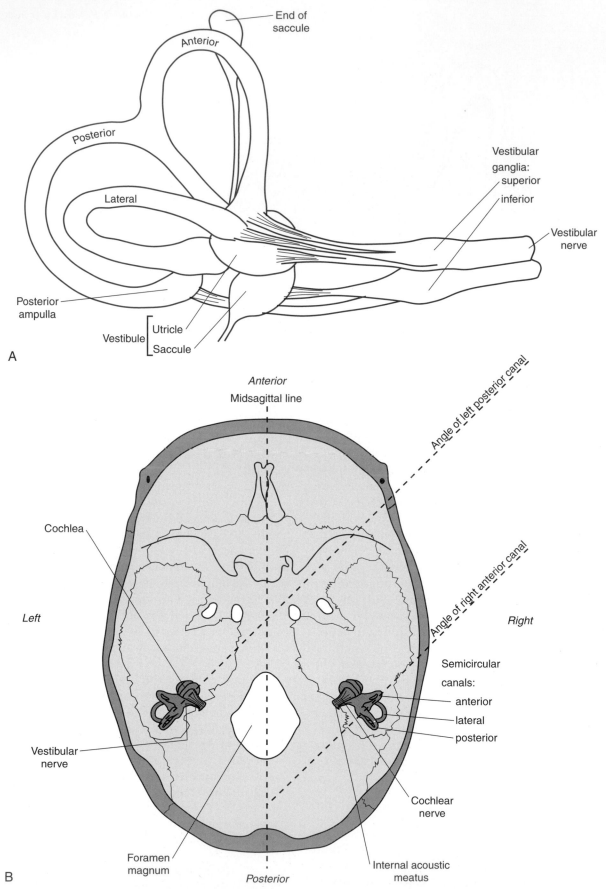

Figure 10-2. **A.** Structures important for equilibrium: semicircular canals, utricle, saccule, vestibular ganglia, and vestibular nerve. **B.** Orientation of anterior, horizontal, and posterior semicircular canals in base of skull. Note that plane of vertical orientation for anterior and posterior canals forms similar angles in relation to midsagittal line.

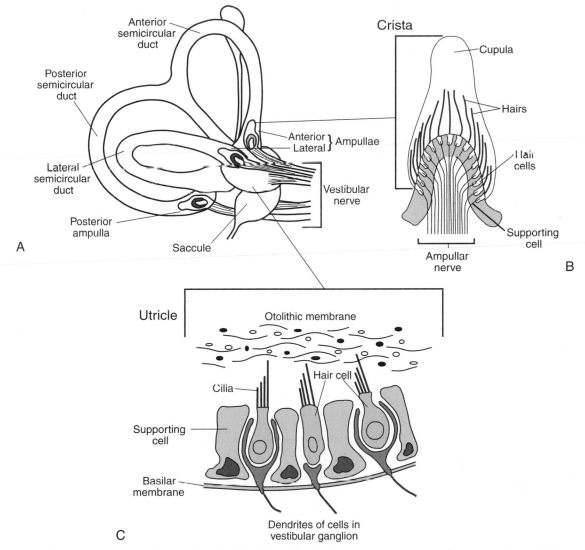

Figure 10-3. **A.** Semicircular canals and enlarged ampullae that house cristae. **B.** Hair cells, nerve, and cupula in ampulla. **C.** Hair cells and otolithic membrane arrangement of maculae of saccule and utricle.

then distributes multiple secondary projections to the **cerebellum, spinal cord, nuclei of extraocular nerves (oculomotor, trochlear, abducens)**, and other parts of the **brainstem** (Fig. 10-4). Of the fibers that bypass the vestibular nuclei, many instead enter the cerebellum through the **inferior cerebellar peduncle**.

PROJECTIONS TO CEREBELLUM

The major projections from the vestibular nuclei go to the older cerebellar structures, which include the **flocculonodular lobe, vermis**, and **fastigial nucleus**. Most of these projections arise from the medial and inferior vestibular nuclei. The cerebellar cortex also projects back to the vestibular nuclei and thus plays an important role in integrating additional information from the vestibular nuclei to the vestibulospinal tract for equilibrium maintenance. With constant and updated vestibular feedback coupled with cerebellovestibular projec-

tions and spinocerebellar proprioceptive input, the cerebellum not only participates in monitoring body and head positions, but also regulates the necessary muscular adjustments needed for body equilibrium.

PROJECTIONS TO MEDIAL LONGITUDINAL FASCICULUS

The fibers of the medial longitudinal fasciculus are in the midline of the pons, medulla, and midbrain. The medial longitudinal fasciculus fibers, with feedback from the vestibular nuclei, project impulses to the **oculomotor** (cranial nerve III), **trochlear** (cranial nerve IV), **abducens** (cranial nerve VI), and **spinal accessory** (cranial nerve XI) motor nuclei. These projections coordinate eye and head movements through the innervation of ocular and neck muscles. Crossed and uncrossed projections from the medial longitudinal fasciculus activate appropriate extraocular muscles for regulating conju-

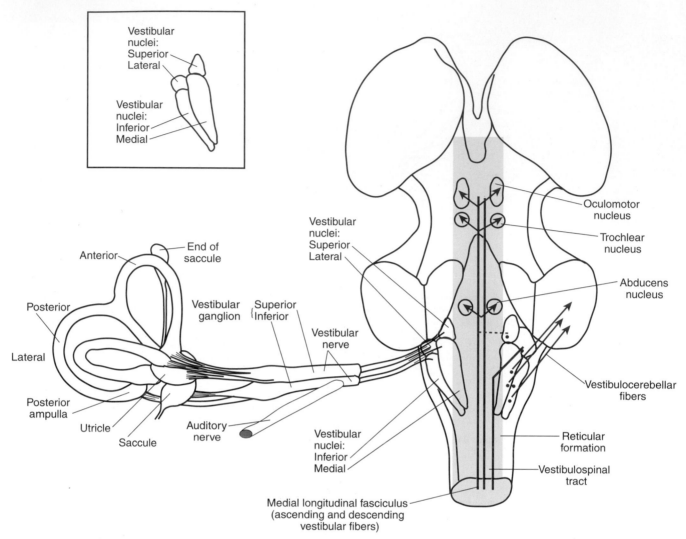

Figure 10-4. Semicircular canals, vestibular ganglia, and their projections to vestibular nuclei in brainstem.

gate eye movements and regulating visual fixation. The world would appear out of focus if not for these important vestibulo-ocular connections. Lesions of the medial longitudinal fasciculus (usually the result of multiple sclerosis or a stroke) produce dysconjugate eye movements.

PROJECTIONS TO SPINAL CORD

Fibers originating from the lateral vestibular nucleus descend through the medulla, enter the ventral column of the spinal cord, and terminate at different spinal levels as they supply various axial muscles. The primary function of the vestibulospinal projections is to maintain the extensor tone that is needed to counteract the pull of gravity. This is done as the vestibulospinal projections activate the antigravity muscles. Sensory fibers from the spinal cord terminate in the caudal dorsal part of the vestibular nucleus, completing the feed-

back circuit between the brainstem and spinal cord, a circuit that is necessary for equilibrium maintenance.

ADDITIONAL VESTIBULAR PROJECTIONS

Additional vestibular fibers send projections to the brainstem reticular formation and thalamus. These projections mediate several important functions, including the maintenance of body equilibrium essential to all motor functions and regulation of visceral activities, such as nausea and vomiting.

PHYSIOLOGY OF EQUILIBRIUM

Two physiological mechanisms control equilibrium: they are **dynamic** and **static**. **Dynamic** (kinetic) **equilibrium** regulates the maintenance of body and head positions during rotational and angular movements that involve acceleration and deceleration. **Static**

equilibrium regulates straight-line movements of the head in space and also regulates both head and body positions during rest.

Dynamic Equilibrium

The hair cells of the cristae in the semicircular ducts regulate dynamic equilibrium. The angular and rotational head movements serve as the stimuli for the receptor cells in the semicircular ducts. Particularly, each group of receptors responds to movement that is oriented in the plane of the duct. When receptors in the duct of one side are excited, receptors in the corresponding semicircular duct of the opposite side are simultaneously inhibited. On rotation of the head, the moving endolymph in the canal deforms the cristae. Deformation of hair cells generates nerve impulses, which travel to the brainstem.

The unipolar neurons in the vestibular ganglion that innervate the cristae are constantly active, firing even without a stimulus. This neuronal firing either increases or decreases when cristae are deformed by rotational and angular movements. The frequency of firing increases when the crista bends toward the utricle. The firing rate decreases when the crista bends away from the utricle.

Sensation of Rotation

Three important events in body rotation represent three phases of the movements of endolymph in semicircular canals; they are best demonstrated with a rotating chair. Each phase relates to the specific state of endolymph inertia and produces a different rotatory sensation.

STAGE 1

When a person rotates to the right (clockwise), the endolymph in the horizontal canal tends to move in the opposite direction (counterclockwise) to the head movement (Fig. 10-5A). This occurs because of the stationary state of the fluid (inertia). The cristae project into the endolymph and move to the left (counterclockwise) with the endolymph. The directional bending and movement of the cristae influence the impulses that are transmitted to the brainstem vestibular nuclei. The brainstem vestibular nuclei interpret this rotation sensation to be clockwise, which is opposite to that of the endolymph movement.

STAGE 2

After 20 seconds of moderate rotation, the endolymph loses its inertia, gathers momentum, and starts moving in the direction of the rotation of the body (Fig. 10-5B). The endolymph and cristae have acquired a new state of inertia related to the turning body, and the hair cells are no longer distorted. Because the endolymph at this stage is rotating at the same speed and direction as the body, the sensation of rotation at this point is minimal with eyes closed.

STAGE 3

When the rotation of the chair suddenly stops (Fig. 10-5C), the body stops, but the endolymph continues moving clockwise. This results in a counterclockwise sensation of rotation. This directional change occurs because the fluid-containing horizontal ducts have stopped rotating, but the fluid, having attained rotational inertia, continues to move. The cristae bend clockwise with the clockwise movement of the endolymph, and this activates the sensation of rotating in the direction opposite to that sensed in stage one.

Static Equilibrium

Static equilibrium, which depends on the utricle and saccule, monitors and maintains a balanced position

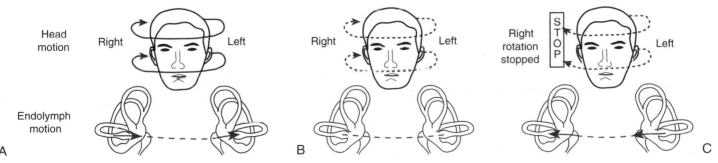

Figure 10-5. Three stages of endolymph movement as related to sensation and direction of body rotation with eyes closed. These head rotations involve endolymph in horizontal (lateral) semicircular canals. *Arrows*, direction of motion. **A.** Beginning rotation. Counterclockwise movement of endolymph induces a clockwise sensation of rotation. **B.** Constant rotation. After a period of head turning, endolymph and bony canals rotate at same rate, and sensory cells in ampullae are not stimulated, so there is no longer any sensation of rotation. **C.** Halted rotation. Clockwise rotation suddenly stops. Endolymph continues to flow clockwise because of its inertia and induces a sensation of counterclockwise rotation.

of the head and body in space against gravity during rest and during straight-line head movements. The mechanism for these sensory receptors is similar to that of the semicircular ducts. The deformation of the apical ends of the receptors, by the movements of the **otolithic membrane**, generates nerve impulses that are transmitted to the brainstem. Gravity acting on the otolithic membrane causes the macula to respond quickly to any tilting movement of the head; prolonged fluctuating activation of the maculae produces motion sickness.

The vestibular ducts supplement the control of static equilibrium through predictive functions. An example of such a function is detection of a slight change in head position while a person is running that prevents a fall. In contrast, the utricle cannot detect loss of balance until it actually occurs. Being off balance must be detected quickly if the person is to initiate appropriate adjustments.

Nystagmus

The function of the vestibular reflexes is to maintain a stable, conjugate visual fixation point. If the head rotates in any plane slowly, the vestibular reflexes produce the exact opposite conjugate eye rotation, maintaining the fixation point. These slow rotatory eye movements and the reflex wiring involve the vestibular nuclei and the archicerebellum. If the slow rotation reaches the limit of eye rotation, a rapid correction (saccadic movement) brings the conjugate fixation to a new point in the environment. Then the slow compensatory counterrotation begins again, maintaining the new fixation point followed by a rapid corrective movement. This saccadic network is also used by the visual system in shifting the fixation point in the **visual startle reflex** and by the auditory system in the **auditory startle reflex**.

The rhythmic movements of the eyeballs in nystagmus, the most common vestibular reflex, is a normal compensatory reflex. It consists of two phases: (*a*) a slow phase in which the eye slowly drifts away from the central field of gaze toward the periphery and (*b*) a fast phase in which the eye, with a sudden jerk, returns to the central field of gaze. Nystagmus is identified according to the direction of its quick phase. Left nystagmus occurs when the quick component is to the left.

These are normal compensatory reflexes. If the head rotation continues, the sequence of slow-fast-slow reflexes continues. The absence of nystagmus with continued head turn is abnormal, and so is its emergence without any head rotation. A new method of assessing nystagmus is nystagmography (ENG), which is based on electro-oculography and involves the placement of skin electrodes at outer canthi to register horizantal or vertical nystagmic movements.

Induced Vestibular Eye Movements, or Nystagmus

The influence of the vestibular system on eye movements is best illustrated by rotating a person in a rotating chair. The rotation induces ocular nystagmus, a rhythmic eye movement with slow and fast components (Fig. 10-6). During clockwise rotation of the vestibular ducts (with counterclockwise flow of endolymph in the horizontal semicircular canals), the eyes move slowly counterclockwise. The fast component of nystagmus is clockwise in the direction of rotation (Fig. 10-6*A*). During a counterclockwise rotation (Fig. 10-6*B*), the fast component of nystagmus is counterclockwise.

Nystagmus can originate in the occipital lobe or in the vestibular apparatus. **Opticokinetic nystagmus** is vision dependent and not vestibular instigated. It can be

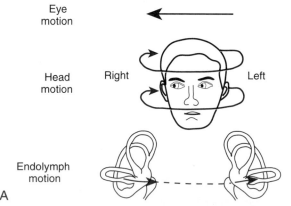
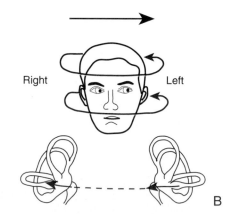

Figure 10-6. Nystagmic movements. **A.** Right nystagmus. In the beginning of a slow clockwise head rotation, inertia induces counterclockwise flow of endolymph in the lateral semicircular canal. Resulting vestibulo-ocular reflex causes a quick jerk of the eyes clockwise. **B.** Left nystagmus. In the beginning of counterclockwise head rotation, inertia induces clockwise flow of endolymph in the lateral semicircular canal. Resulting vestibulo-ocular reflex causes a quick jerk of the eyes counterclockwise.

activated by visual fixation on a moving pattern. Vestibular nystagmus is independent of visual input. However, visual input can be used to suppress vestibular nystagmus.

Professional figure skaters and ballet dancers have developed the capacity to control eye movements independent of vestibular feedback. Neither shows any reactive nystagmic movements during and after body rotations. To prevent reactive nystagmus, ballet dancers and figure skaters learn to use visual feedback to suppress vestibular input by quick head rotations laterally over the shoulders. This facilitates continued eye fixation on the same object while the body continues to turn more slowly. Untrained persons do not have this compensatory mechanism and fall after only a few body rotations.

CLINICAL INFORMATION

Disturbances of Vestibular System

MOTION SICKNESS

Motion sickness, the most common disorder of the vestibular system, is characterized by vertigo, the subjective sensation of body rotation. It is also associated with dizziness, or light-headedness, nausea, and vomiting. In some instances the symptoms are disabling. This is true especially after repeated up and down movements, such as in an airplane in rough weather or on a boat in high waves. Fortunately, most people adapt to these circumstances, and those who do not can be treated with an antihistamine, such as dimenhydrinate (Dramamine).

VERTIGO

Vertigo, the sensation of spinning through space (**subjective vertigo**) or of the environment spinning around one (**objective vertigo**) can be very disabling. It is mostly associated with impaired function of the vestibular apparatus and is commonly found in people who suffer from **Ménière's disease**, a condition of obscure etiology characterized by abnormally high endolymphatic pressure in the vestibular apparatus. Ménière's disease also involves the organ of hearing and includes tinnitus (ringing, humming in the ear), hearing loss, and eventual deafness. Either acute or chronic labyrinthitis may also cause vertigo.

LABYRINTH DYSFUNCTION

Labyrinthitis (irritation of intercommunicating semicircular ducts and vestibule of the vestibular apparatus) is a common labyrinth dysfunction and often a cause of vertigo. Impairment of the labyrinth on one side (unilateral) causes a short period of vertigo, disequilibrium, nystagmus, and some nausea and vomiting. The patient tends to fall toward the side of lesion. This is likely to result from impaired downward pressure on one foot secondary to unopposed vestibulospinal activity on the normal side. The disequilibrium that occurs after bilateral destruction of the labyrinth is generally transient, although it sometimes persists and recurs for many months. Incidentally, vestibular impairment in animals has been found to be more incapacitating than in humans. One reason may be that animals rely less on visual input for equilibrium than do humans.

CLINICAL DIAGNOSTIC TESTS

The **acceleration–rotation chair** and **caloric stimulation** are commonly used to evaluate vestibular functions.

Acceleration-Rotation Chair

The integrity of vestibular projections to cranial nerve nuclei that regulate extraocular muscles and to motor nuclei of the spinal cord can be examined by stimulation of the labyrinth in a rotating subject. The rotation test, also called the **Bárány test**, is performed on a subject seated in a rotating chair with his or her head tilted forward 30°. The head tilt accommodates the semicircular canals being tested in the horizontal plane. After turning clockwise for 20 seconds, the chair is suddenly stopped (Fig. 10-5C). Because of inertia, the endolymph moves in the direction of rotation (clockwise) and its pressure causes the cupula to bend in the same (clockwise) direction. The movement of the endolymph induces nystagmus (quick phase) in the direction opposite (counterclockwise) to the motion of endolymph. This postrotatory effect is used to evaluate vestibular functions.

Caloric Stimulation

The vestibular end organ can also be assessed by caloric stimulation of the semicircular ducts. This involves the irrigation of both ear canals with water of different temperatures to induce nystagmus. Caloric stimulation of the vestibular end organ causes contralateral conjugate deviation of the eyes. Cold water causes nystagmus to the side opposite the canal tested, whereas warm water causes nystagmus to the same side.

The ice water is a crude test often used in emergencies to differentiate frontal lobe from brainstem lesions in unconscious patients after head injury. In the ice water test the external canal is filled with cold water for 20 seconds. A frontal lobe lesion is suspected if the induced nystagmus to the side opposite the tested canal lasts about 30 to 45 seconds.

Case Study

A 50-year-old woman had sudden episodes of ringing in the ears, dizziness, vomiting, and vertigo. Every time she got up, she felt unsteady.

She was taken to a hospital and on testing exhibited the following:
- No vestibular response in the left ear on caloric testing
- Head posture tilted to the left
- Severe vertigo
- Deafness in the left ear
- Loss of pain and temperature sensation on the left side of face

Magnetic resonance imaging of the brain revealed an infarct in the dorsal lateral region of the left medulla and caudal region of the left pons.

Question: How could this infarct account for the vestibular problems and other secondary signs?

Discussion: This infarct in the left dorsolateral medullopontine region, an area supplied by the branches of cerebellar arteries (an unnecessary detail at this time), affected the following structures:
- Damage to the vestibular nuclear complex was confirmed by the absence of nystagmus on caloric testing of the left ear.
- Damage to the left vestibular complex interrupted vestibular projections to the cervicospinal cord, which regulates head posture. Interruption of these fibers caused the head to tilt to the left.
- Damage to vestibulospinal projections also interrupted vestibular projections to the extensor muscles of the limbs on the ipsilateral side. Consequently, the patient was falling to the left.
- Destruction of the vestibular nucleus caused the sensation of vertigo.
- Damage to the cochlear nerve and cochlear nucleus caused impaired hearing in the left ear.
- Because the auditory fibers cross in the brainstem, it is likely that there was also diminished hearing in the right ear.
- The lesion also affected the spinal nucleus of the trigeminal tract, which is within the infarct region. This affected the mediation of pain and temperature from the left side of the face.

SUMMARY

The vestibular system is a reflexive sensorimotor system that controls equilibrium. With sensory receptors in the semicircular canals of the inner ear, nuclei in the brainstem, and direct connections to other brainstem systems, the vestibular apparatus helps humans maintain a balanced upright posture, coordinate head and body movements, and control eye fixation on a point in space, even during body and head movements. The vestibular system is closely associated with the visual and proprioceptive systems; it constantly integrates incoming visual and proprioceptive cues that contribute to the execution of highly complex, skilled, and coordinated activities like dancing, skating, and acrobatics. The functional importance of the vestibular system becomes evident in patients whose body balance is impaired by Ménière's disease or tumors of cranial nerve VIII.

Technical Terms

cristae	medial longitudinal fasciculus
cupula	nystagmus
endolymph	semicircular canals
equilibrium	static labyrinth
inertia	vertigo
labyrinth	vestibule
macula	

Review Questions

1. Define the following terms:

cristae	medial longitudinal fasciculus
cupula	nystagmus
endolymph	semicircular canals
equilibrium	static labyrinth
inertia	vertigo
labyrinth	vestibule
macula	

2. Describe the function of the vestibular system.
3. Describe functions of the semicircular ducts, vestibular sacs, vestibular nerve and nuclei, and medial longitudinal fasciculus.
4. Describe rotational sensations in a rotation chair related to the three phases of endolymph movement.
5. Describe nystagmus and explain how rotation (Bárány chair) induces ocular nystagmus.
6. Explain why the following statement is true or false: During a clockwise rotation of the vestibular canals (with counterclockwise flow of endolymph in the horizontal semicircular canals), the eyes move slowly in a counterclockwise direction. The quick component of nystagmus is clockwise, in the direction of rotation.
7. A young man, after a traumatic head injury, complained of vertigo, nausea, and tinnitus in the left ear. He also exhibited a nystagmus to the right. Discuss the possible site of lesion.
8. Discuss the mechanism and rationale of caloric testing.
9. How is the medial longitudinal fasciculus involved in the process of conjugate eye movement?
10. What are the symptoms of vestibular neuritis?
11. A 28-year-old woman was seen for a complaint of dizziness, nausea, and vomiting. On examination she exhibited a tendency to fall to the right, left nystagmus, deafness in the right ear, analgesia on the left body, hoarseness, and swallowing difficulty. Discuss the structures in which a lesion (semicircular canals, brainstem, cochlea, or tumor at the cerebellopontine angle) might account for this syndrome.
12. Describe how ballet dancers and professional skaters control vestibular activity so that they do not exhibit rotational nystagmus.
13. Describe the symptoms and discuss the pathophysiology of Ménière's disease.

11

Motor System 1: Spinal Cord

Learning Objectives

After studying this chapter, students should be able to do the following:

- Discuss the anatomy of the spinal cord
- Describe the functions of the major spinal structures
- Discuss the importance of lower motor neurons and the motor unit
- List the major ascending and descending spinal tracts
- Describe the functions of the major sensorimotor tracts
- Explain the role of muscle spindles in reflexive motor functions
- Discuss the importance of the Golgi tendon organ
- Describe the physiology of basic spinal reflexes
- Discuss lower motor neuron syndrome
- Explain the common pathological conditions affecting spinal cord functions
- Describe sensorimotor symptoms associated with spinal cord injuries

Motor activity is a hierarchically organized function under additional control by reflex mechanisms and neural networks in a rostral segment of the CNS (Fig. 11-1). These arbitrarily identified anatomical levels, from the lowest to the highest, are the **spinal cord, cerebellum, brainstem, basal ganglia**, and **motor cortex**. Each ascending level in the hierarchy makes a specific contribution to the final motor activity, which is also influenced in part by the activity of higher motor centers. For example, the midbrain systems modulate reflexes organized at medullary or spinal levels. The forebrain systems dominate the midbrain and spinal motor activity. Motor responses begin in the spinal cord as simple reflexes, whereas the higher motor centers participate in the regulation of skilled and patterned movements. Neuronal impulses from higher levels also initiate, inhibit, or facilitate motor functions at the brainstem and spinal cord, thus partially regulating all motor behavior.

This higher cortical control provides a type of parallel processing with rostral domination of hierarchical motor organization and simultaneous control of the segmental output itself. Since substantial time is involved in the conduction of afferent information, local (spinal) reflexes often are activated first, and motor mechanisms at higher hierarchic levels are activated much later. The best example of reflexive movement is unexpectedly stepping on a tack. This triggers a leg withdrawal reflex, which is already in progress before the forebrain can inhibit or modify the reflex. However, the higher motor systems can inhibit such a withdrawal reflex if the stimulus is expected and another response has been learned. For example, if someone has to pick up a hot cup, the withdrawal reflex can be inhibited while the hot cup is being moved to a supporting surface, even though the fingers are being burned.

The hierarchically defined motor functions and the nature of the specific contributions by each level are discussed in Chapters 11 to 14.

The spinal cord is a major element in the regulation of sensorimotor functions. Many stereotyped motor responses (reflexes), which are largely independent of voluntary motor control, are generated in the spinal cord and can be triggered by cortical and/or environmental stimuli. The spinal cord also relays sensory information to the cerebrum, which is vital to learning skilled and coordinated motor activity.

SPINAL PREPARATION

Spinal cord functions are most easily demonstrated by a **spinal preparation**, which entails separating the cord from the regulating influence of the brain by cutting the cord. This separation allows for examination of spinal reflexes independent of the inhibitory or facilitatory influence exerted by higher centers of motor

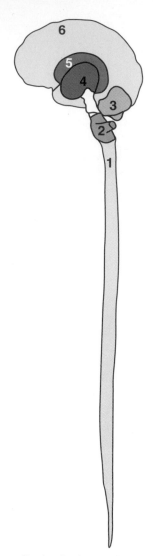

Figure 11-1. Six ascending levels of motor organization: *1*, spinal cord; *2*, brainstem; *3*, cerebellum; *4*, diencephalon; *5*, basal ganglia; *6*, cerebral cortex.

control. Immediately after the spinal cut is made, the flexor and extensor reflexes become completely inactive, but they gradually reemerge.

INNERVATION PATTERN

The general motor function in the spinal cord and brainstem is organized ipsilateral to its output and reflex input. The spinal alpha-motor neurons and their axons (final common pathway) extend to innervate the muscles ipsilaterally. Consequently, lower motor neuron (LMN) signs in the brainstem and spinal cord are ipsilateral to the damage of the cell body or its axon.

GROSS ANATOMY OF SPINAL CORD

The spinal cord extends from the base of the skull to the lower back and is approximately 43.5 cm long and 1 cm in diameter. It is divided into five regions: **cervical,**

thoracic, **lumbar**, **sacral**, and **coccygeal**. Thirty-one pairs of **spinal nerves** emerge from the spinal cord (Fig. 11-2). These nerves have mixed function; they carry sensory information from peripheral receptors to the central nervous system (CNS) and transmit motor information from the CNS to the muscles. The nerves are named after the region of the spinal cord to which they are attached and are numbered in sequence. There are eight pairs of cervical spinal nerves (C-1 to C-8); 12 pairs of thoracic spinal nerves (T-1 to T-12); five pairs of lumbar spinal nerves (L-1 to L-5); five pairs of sacral spinal nerves (S-1 to S-5); and usually one pair of coccygeal spinal nerves.

During fetal and early postnatal growth, the vertebral column grows faster than the spinal cord. Therefore, in adults, the spinal cord diminishes toward the lumbar region and ends as the **conus medullaris** at the second lumbar vertebra. The nerve root fibers from L-3 to S-5 spinal segments lengthen downward to reach the corresponding skeletal level before exiting the vertebral-spinal canal. These stretched nerve roots are collectively called the **cauda equina**. The stretched spinal cord remnant of the cauda equina is attached to the coccyx and is called the **filum terminale** (Fig. 11-2). The fact that the spinal cord does not extend into the fluid-filled subarachnoid space of the lumbosacral area has important clinical implications. This dural sac, at levels below the first lumbar vertebra (though much lower in the case of children because of less disparity between the length of the cord and vertebral canal), is used for extracting cerebrospinal fluid for diagnostic purposes (spinal tap or puncture) and for administering therapeutic and anesthetic drugs without risking damage to the spinal cord (see Chapter 20).

Internal Anatomy

Seen in cross-section, the spinal cord consists of an outer ring of **white matter** and a butterfly-shaped central **gray area** (Fig. 11-3). The white matter contains ascending and descending fibers, whereas the gray matter contains nerve cell bodies and small unmyelinated network of fibers (neuropils). There are four **gray horns,** two dorsal and two ventral, and four **roots** of fibers, two dorsal and two ventral. The dorsal horns contain the secondary sensory nerve cells that receive sensory information from the body through the **dorsal root ganglia** fibers. The ventral horns contain motor nerve cells, which project through the anterior roots to activate muscles, glands, and joints. The gray columns on each side of the cord are connected through the **commissures** made up of crossing fibers. The dorsal root consists of the fibers that transmit impulses to the CNS. Before the dorsal root fibers join the spinal cord, they form an enlarged area called the dorsal root ganglia (DRG), which contains sensory nerve cell bodies. The axonal processes

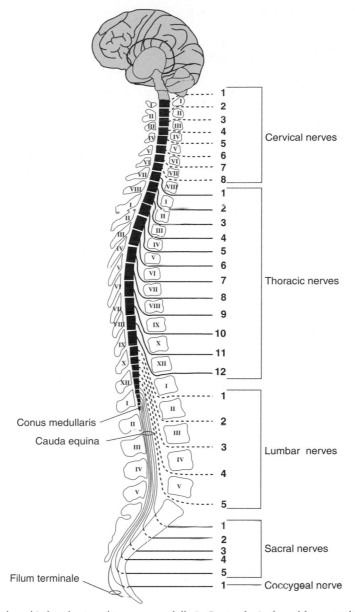

Figure 11-2. Spinal cord is foreshortened to conus medullaris. Roots of spinal cord form cauda equina in lumbar and sacral areas.

Cervical nerves
1 2 3 4 5 6 7 8

Thoracic nerves
1 2 3 4 5 6 7 8 9 10 11 12

Conus medullaris
Cauda equina

Lumbar nerves
1 2 3 4 5

Sacral nerves
1 2 3 4 5

Filum terminale

Coccygeal nerve
1

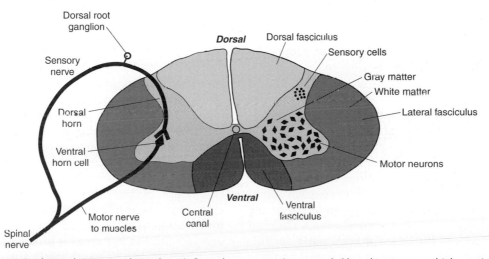

Figure 11-3. Internal anatomy of spinal cord. Central gray matter is surrounded by white matter, which consists of three fasciculi (funiculi): dorsal, lateral, and ventral.

Dorsal root ganglion

Sensory nerve

Dorsal horn

Ventral horn cell

Spinal nerve

Motor nerve to muscles

Central canal

Ventral

Ventral fasciculus

Dorsal

Dorsal fasciculus

Sensory cells

Gray matter

White matter

Lateral fasciculus

Motor neurons

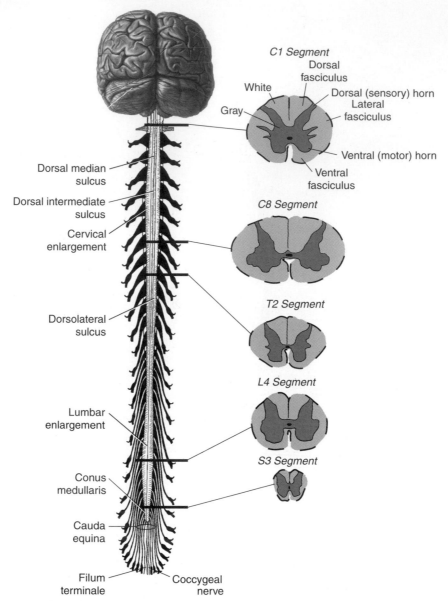

Figure 11-4. Dorsal spinal cord and its internal anatomy in five cross-sections. Increase in cord size at cervical and lumbar levels corresponds to nerve supply for upper and lower extremities, respectively.

of the motor neurons form the **ventral nerve root** fibers and send motor impulses from the CNS to the muscles. After traveling through the pia mater, subarachnoid space, arachnoid membrane, dura mater, and intervertebral foramina, the fibers from both the dorsal and anterior roots merge to form a **spinal nerve**.

In their distributions, the spinal nerves form **rami** and **plexuses** (see Chapter 2). After a spinal nerve exits the intervertebral foramina, it divides into the dorsal and ventral rami. The dorsal ramus fibers of each spinal nerve are concerned with the muscles and skin in the posterior part of the body. The ventral ramus fibers of the spinal nerve supply the anterior body parts, including the upper and lower limbs. The ventral rami of spinal nerves, except the nerves from T-2 to T-11, form a

network of nerve fibers called plexuses before projecting to target muscles and body parts (Fig. 2-33B). Rami of the nerves from T-2 to T-11 directly innervate body parts. The nerve fibers that emerge from a plexus are named after the body regions they innervate. Examples are the **cervical, brachial, lumbar, sacral,** and **coccygeal plexuses**. With each ramus containing both sensory and motor fibers, a lesion involving a ramus or spinal nerve results in both paralysis and loss of sensation for a specific region of the body.

The size and shape of the spinal cord are not uniform along its entire length (Fig. 11-4). The cord in the cervical and lumbar areas is broad and flattened in contrast to its shape in the thoracic areas. Widening at the cervical and lumbar segments of the cord results from

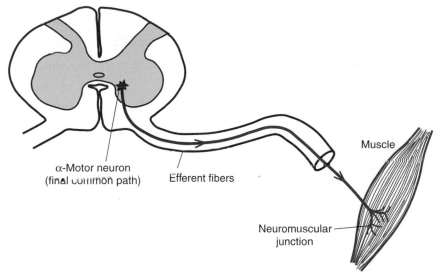

Figure 11-5.   Components that form final common pathway and motor unit. Motor unit is composed of motor neuron, efferent fibers, neuromuscular junction, and muscle.

the concentration of nerve cells and their fibers, which is necessitated by the sensory and motor control of the upper and lower extremity muscles. The upper extremities, especially the hands, possess more specialized sensory and motor functions than the legs, trunk, and viscera and therefore require a greater concentration of peripheral nerve fibers. Thus, the size of the gray column at the cervical level is larger than at the lumbar level.

Segmental Organization

The spinal cord is anatomically and functionally organized in transverse segments extending from the cervical to the sacral region. This organization of the spinal cord indicates segmental sensorimotor innervation of the body (**dermatomes** and **myotomes**) with various distributional shapes and sizes (Fig. 2-35). Dermatomes (innervation zone of the neurons in a single DRG) and myotomes (muscle or muscles innervated by all lower motor neuron axons exiting the cord via a single ventral root) may overlap each other, but because of muscle migration during development, they are not always the same.

Motor Unit

The **lower motor neuron (LMN)** and the **motor unit** (Fig. 11-5) are two important components of spinal motor control. The LMN cell body provides the output pathway to peripheral function via its axon, which travels through the ventral root and peripheral nerves to innervate a skeletal muscle, where it forms multiple axon branches to activate many muscle fibers. The LMN is also the **final common pathway**, because the efferent impulses from the motor cortex pass through this motor neuron before they can produce a muscle movement. The motor unit consists of four components: **motor cell body**, **efferent fibers**, **motor end plate** (branching off the axonal fiber in myoneural/neuromuscular junctions), and **innervated muscle fibers**. A motor unit can fire repeatedly, resulting in sustained shortening of the muscle fiber elements. Damage to the LMN cell or the beginning axon eliminates the entire function of a motor unit. Damage to one of the terminal axon branches weakens the unit projections. Generalized skeletal muscle disease (e.g., muscular dystrophy) or reduced nerve–muscle transmission (e.g., myasthenia gravis) weakens or eliminates the unit's force generation and produces muscle degeneration.

Motor units can be small or large, and a muscle can contain many motor units, depending on the nature of its motor control. For example, the small hand flexor muscle used for delicate and coordinated motor control can have 10 to 30 muscle fibers per motor unit, whereas large muscles like the quadriceps can have as many as 3,000 muscle fibers per motor unit.

TRACTS OF SPINAL CORD

The white matter of the spinal cord consists of three major bundles of longitudinal axons (fasciculi): the **dorsal**, **lateral**, and **ventral columns** (Fig. 11-3). In most instances, each fasciculus contains bundles of ascending and descending fibers. The tracts are difficult to pinpoint on a cross-section of the spinal cord; however, their approximate locations can be determined from clinical evidence. The dorsal fasciculus consists largely of ascending (sensory) fibers, whereas the lateral and anterior fasciculi contain both descending (motor) and ascending (sensory) fiber bundles (Table 11-1). General locations of the various sensorimotor spinal tracts are illustrated in Fig. 11-6.

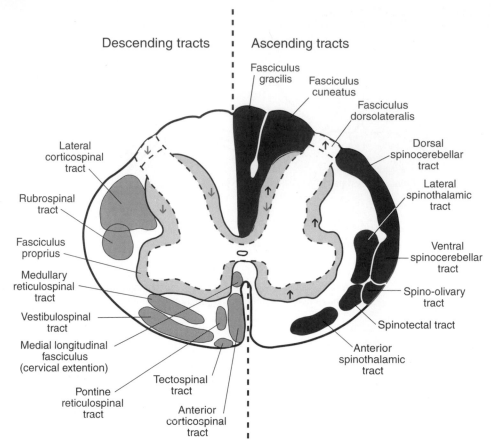

Descending tracts | Ascending tracts

Figure 11-6. Ascending (red) and descending (gray) spinal pathways. Fasciculus proprius and fasciculus dorsolateralis are known to contain both ascending and descending fibers.

Descending Tracts

CORTICOSPINAL TRACTS

Fibers of the corticospinal motor tract arise from pyramidal cells (the largest are Betz cells) in the cortex. Most of these cells are in the **precentral gyrus (primary motor cortex, Brodmann area 4)**; however, some of these cells are in other areas of the brain, including the **premotor cortex**, **primary somesthetic cortex**, and **supplementary motor cortex**. On their way to the spinal cord, the corticospinal fibers cross the midline at the caudal end of the medulla and form the lateral corticospinal tract in the spinal cord. There are two corticospinal tracts, **lateral corticospinal tract** and **anterior corticospinal tract** (Fig. 11-7; see Chapter 14).

Lateral Corticospinal Tract

Lateral corticospinal fibers provide a mechanism by which the cerebral cortex intervenes in the control of skeletal muscles during delicate, skilled manipulation of the distal parts of the limbs, including the fingers and to some extent the toes and forearms. This tract contains myelinated fibers and is the largest of the motor tracts. After emerging from the pyramidal cells (including the giant Betz cells) in the motor cortex, the corticospinal fibers cross the midline at the lower end of the medulla and enter with the spinal cord. Approximately 90% of the corticospinal fibers are known to cross (decussate) the midline to form the lateral corticospinal tract. Its fibers synapse on the ventral horn α-motor neurons and regulate muscle activity. A lesion to fibers of this tract causes profound weakness and loss of all individual digital manipulation skills. This condition called paresis, or upper motor neuron (UMN) paralysis, can be **monoplegia** (paralysis of one extremity) or **hemiplegia** (paralysis of arm and leg on one side of the body).

Anterior Corticospinal Tract

The anterior corticospinal tract contains the 8 to 10% of corticospinal fibers that do not cross the midline at the medulla oblongata. Instead, these fibers continue descending ipsilaterally. These uncrossed fibers are confined to the cervical levels and eventually cross the midline before synapsing on the ventral horn α-motor neuron and internuncial cells. These axons provide a mechanism through which the cerebral cortex regulates precision in the movements of axial and girdle muscles.

Table 11-1. Ascending and Descending Spinal Pathways

Spinal Pathways	Function
Ascending tracts	
Fasciculus gracilis	Transmits discriminative touch from the lower half of body
Fasciculus cuneatus	Transmits discriminative touch from the upper half of body
Dorsal spinocerebellar tract	Mediates unconscious proprioception from distal lower limbs
Ventral spinocerebellar tract	Mediates unconscious proprioception from muscles of lower extremities and proximal limbs
Cuneocerebellar tract	Mediates unconscious proprioceptive information from upper limbs
Lateral spinothalamic tract	Transmits sensations of pain and temperature
Anterior spinothalamic tract	As a backup sensory system, mediates diffuse touch
Spino-olivary tract	Mediates proprioceptive information from limbs
Spinoreticular tract	Provides sensory input to reflex networks of the brainstem.
Spinotectal tract	Mediates sensory input to eye and head orientation reflex networks of superior colliculus
Descending tracts	
Lateral corticospinal tract	Carries motor commands for muscle control during digital tasks
Anterior corticospinal tract	Marks uncrossed motor fibers responsible for motor precision of axial and girdle muscles
Tectospinal tract	Uses visual and auditory impulses to regulate postural body movements
Rubrospinal tract	Transmits cerebellar projections to spinal cord for regulating muscle tone to support body against gravity
Vestibulospinal tract	Projects vestibular input to muscles for regulating reflexive adjustments of body posture
Reticular descending tracts	Relays brainstem reflex modulation to spinal reflex mechanism; regulates muscle preparedness

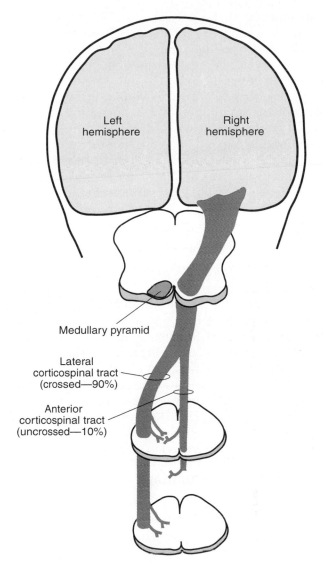

Figure 11-7. Corticospinal fibers predominantly project to contralateral half of body.

EXTRAPYRAMIDAL TRACTS

Several **extrapyramidal motor, reticular**, and **autonomic tracts** transmit information essential for smoothly coordinated motor function and upright, balanced posture. This indicates that the motor system is not exclusively a corticospinal system. Rather, its functional organization is highly complex, involving many additional pathways. Some of the more notable extrapyramidal paths are the following:

The **tectospinal tract** regulates neck and body twisting movements with extensor support for the visual and auditory startle reflexes. For example, in response to a sudden bright, moving light entering the visual field from one side or a loud sound to one side, a powerful reflexive behavior involves a sudden turning

of the head, neck, and body toward the stimulus. Originating from the superior colliculus, the tectospinal fibers cross the midline in the midbrain and descend to terminate in the ventral horn motor nuclei of the cervical and lower regions of the cord.

The **rubrospinal tract** originates from cell bodies of the red nucleus, which receive their afferents from the contralateral cerebellum and ipsilateral primary motor (Brodmann area 4) and supplementary motor (Brodmann area 6) cortices. This tract transmits impulses from the red nucleus to the spinal LMN to regulate muscle tone for limb extension in support of the body against gravity.

The **vestibulospinal tract** projects the vestibular impulses to the spinal LMNs. By regulating extensor muscle tone, these fibers control the reflexive adjustment of the body and limbs to keep the head stable. Originating from the nerve cells in the vestibular nucleus and incorporating projections from the inner ear and cerebellum, the vestibulospinal fibers extend throughout the length of the cord, giving off collaterals to α- and γ-motor nuclei. More than a dozen reticulospinal tracts deep in the white spinal columns transmit important autonomic and reticular information that is essential for survival.

Originating from the pons (**pontine reticulospinal tract**) and medulla (**medullary reticulospinal tract**), the reticular projections regulate coordinated motor functions. Reticular stimulation has been found to facilitate or inhibit voluntary and reflexive movements by altering muscle tone through the γ-motor system.

AUTONOMIC PATHWAYS

The hypothalamus is the central integrator and distributor of important autonomic projections to the brainstem and spinal visceral nuclei, and it regulates motor functions of the sympathetic and parasympathetic systems (see Chapter 16). Brainstem reticular nuclei, including the **locus ceruleus**, also relay projections that regulate spinal autonomic motor functions. These projections are primarily excitatory. Cells in the brainstem project to the cervical and thoracic segments, and they are primarily excitatory to **phrenic motor neurons** and thoracic motor neurons participating in inspiration, vomiting, and coughing reflexes (see Chapter 16).

Ascending Tracts

The ascending fibers of the spinal cord transmit sensory information from various body parts (Fig. 11-6). The sensory impulses are pain, thermal sense, touch, proprioception, and kinesthesia (see Chapter 7). Projections from the sensory cortex refine cortical motor efferents to the spinal cord.

FASCICULUS GRACILIS

The fasciculus gracilis is composed of axons arising from the spinal dorsal root ganglia in the sacral, lumbar, and lower six thoracic levels (Fig. 11-6; see Chapter 7). The fibers of the fasciculus gracilis mediate the sensations of discriminative touch, joint movement, and vibrations from the lower half of the body.

FASCICULUS CUNEATUS

Consisting of large fibers, the fasciculus cuneatus mediates the sensations of fine discriminative touch, joint movement, and vibration from the upper half of the body. Its fibers enter the cord from the upper six thoracic and all cervical levels (Fig 11-6; see Chapter 7.5). The fasciculus cuneatus fibers, along with the fasciculus gracilis, terminate in the medullary relay nuclei of cuneatus and gracilis. Secondary fibers from these nuclei (internal arcuate fibers) decussate to form the medial lemniscus, which ascends to the **ventral posterolateral nucleus** of the thalamus and then to the primary sensory cortex.

ANTERIOR SPINOTHALAMIC TRACT

The anterior spinothalamic tract is a backup sensory system. Its fibers mediate the sensation of crude and nonlocalizable touch (Figs. 7-8 and 11-6). After emerging from the cells in the spinal gray, these fibers cross the midline through the anterior commissure within several segments of the cord before ascending in the anterior spinothalamic tract. They terminate in the ventral posterolateral nucleus of the thalamus, and from there they project to the primary sensory cortex.

LATERAL SPINOTHALAMIC TRACT

The fibers of the lateral spinothalamic tract (Figs. 11-6 and 11-7) transmit pain and temperature sensation. Fibers of this tract, like those of the anterior spinothalamic tract, arise from the spinal dorsal horn nuclei and ascend in the lateral fasciculus to the thalamus and then to the cortex.

VENTRAL SPINOCEREBELLAR TRACT

The fibers of the ventral spinocerebellar tract mediate unconscious proprioception from the muscles of the lower extremities and proximal limbs, and they coordinate the movement and posture of the lower extremities (Figs. 11-6 and 7-10).

DORSAL SPINOCEREBELLAR TRACT

The uncrossed fibers of the dorsal spinocerebellar tract emerge from the large cells of the **nucleus dorsalis of Clarke** at the medial base of the dorsal horns from L-3 to T-1. These fibers mediate unconscious proprioception from the distal regions of the lower limbs (Figs. 11-6 and 7-10).

CUNEOCEREBELLAR TRACT

The cuneocerebellar fibers mediate unconscious proprioceptive information from the upper limbs to the cerebellum (see Chapter 7); these are concerned with fine and delicate control of the upper limbs (Fig. 7-10).

MOTOR NUCLEI OF SPINAL CORD

The spinal gray matter contains thousands of motor nerve cells, which are either **anterior motor neurons** or **interneurons** (**internuncial cells**). The anterior motor neurons include α- and γ-motor neurons (Fig. 11-8). The efferent fibers of α- and γ-motor nerve cells form the ventral roots of spinal nerves that innervate skeletal muscles. These are called **LMN** to distinguish them from the corticospinal neurons of the motor and sensory cortex, which are called **upper motor neurons** (**UMN**). The interneurons function as association cells interconnecting cell bodies within sensory and motor neuron pools.

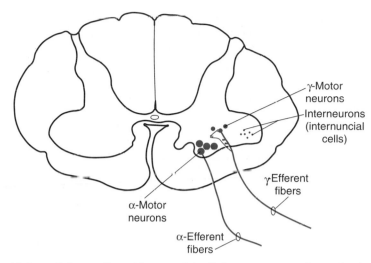

Figure 11-8. α-Cells, γ-cells, and internuncial cells in anterior gray column of spinal cord.

The dendritic and axonal projections of the internuncial cells connect adjacent spinal cord cells.

The cervical spinal cord gray matter also contains two specialized motor nuclei. One supplies the **phrenic nerve**, which innervates the diaphragm and participates in respiration (see Chapter 16). The other motor nucleus contributes to the spinal roots of the **spinal accessory cranial nerve**, which regulates head and shoulder movements (see Chapter 15).

The α- and γ-motor neurons receive motor impulses directly from the motor centers in the forebrain, brainstem, and cerebellum. The supraspinal projections to α- and γ-motor neurons, which initiate voluntary motor activities, are represented by balanced inhibitory $(-)$ and excitatory $(+)$ cortical outputs to the spinal motor neurons.

α-Motor Neurons

The α motor neurons are the major motor neurons of the spinal cord. Their axons, with a diameter of 9 to 16 μm, rapidly conduct impulses. They pass through the ventral spinal root before innervating the extrafusal fibers of the skeletal muscles responsible for voluntary and reflexive movements of the head, trunk, and extremities. On the average, one α-neuron fiber innervates more than 200 muscle fibers. These motor neurons are also the final common pathway, because all efferent impulses from the CNS must pass through these cells before activating muscles.

γ-Motor Neurons

The γ-motor neurons, which lie alongside the α-cells in the spinal ventral horns, are smaller and half as numerous. With axonal processes smaller in diameter, they are slow impulse conductors.

The primary role of γ-LMN neurons is to modulate the length of the spindle fibers and thus modulate the excitability of the annulospiral (Ia) endings. This regulates the stretch reflex muscle tone and allows the CNS to regulate its own state of excitability. The γ-motor neurons are controlled by synaptic input from the brainstem reticular formation and the vestibular system. The γ-efferent fibers leave through the ventral nerve root and contract the end (contractile) portions of the intrafusal muscle fibers, stretching the central parts of the muscle spindles. On being stretched, the muscle spindles send a volley of afferent projections to the α-motor neurons, causing the reflexive contraction of the extrafusal fibers of the muscle.

Interneurons

As functionally specialized cells, the interneurons are diffusely present throughout the spinal cord and brain. There are approximately 30 times as many interneurons as motor neurons. The interneuron cells serve as filters, integrating all sensory and motor functions of the CNS. They are commonly identified as reticular cells at the level of the brainstem. Most interneurons are inhibitory cells. The **Renshaw cell**, which is in the anterior horn of the spinal cord, is an inhibitory interneuron that receives axonal collaterals from nearby motor neurons; it inhibits the activity of the same or related adjacent motor neurons. This recurrent inhibition by the Renshaw cell facilitates and sharpens the activity of the projecting motor neuron from which it receives the collaterals.

MOTOR FUNCTIONS OF SPINAL CORD

The basic motor function of the spinal cord is a reflexive motor response. A reflex response is a stereotyped movement to sensory stimulation. The neuronal circuitry for reflexes is present at each segmental level throughout the spinal cord. It consists primarily of

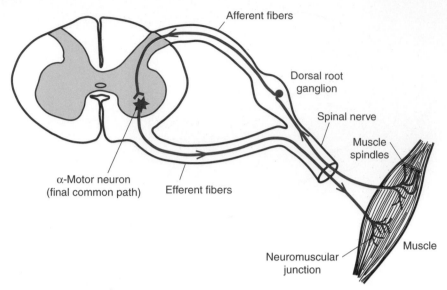

Figure 11-9. Neuronal circuitry for a spinal reflex.

muscle spindles, afferent fibers, α-motor neurons, efferent fibers, and muscle tissue (Fig. 11-9).

For the most part, reflex functions of the spinal cord are independent of voluntary control, although they are indirectly influenced by descending impulses from the motor cortex and brainstem motor centers. The input from higher motor centers participates in providing a homeostatic state of motor control resulting in smooth motor movements. If released from higher levels of motor control, as in the case of a lesion, the spinal cord reflexes become hyperactive.

Muscle Spindles and Their Role in Motor Activity

There are two types of specialized receptors in muscles: muscle spindles and Golgi tendon organs (Fig. 11-10). **Muscle spindles** detect the degree and rate of change in muscle length and also help maintain muscle tone. **Golgi tendon organs** monitor the degree of muscle tension during muscle contraction and reflexively inhibit muscle contraction, permitting the muscle to stretch to prevent injury caused by excessive contraction.

MUSCLE SPINDLES

The muscle spindle, a complex sensorimotor organ, is small, consisting of three to five specialized intrafusal fibers that lie parallel to the surrounding extrafusal (striate) muscle fibers. The center of an intrafusal fiber is wrapped by a fast-conducting **annulospiral (primary) sensory ending**. If stretched, it generates an afferent response in the afferent fiber from the spindle. The afferent impulses travel to α-motor neurons in the spinal cord via fast-conducting type Ia nerve fibers with a velocity of approximately 100 m/second, causing the muscle to contract (Fig. 11-10A).

Muscles consist of extrafusal and intrafusal fibers. **Extrafusal fibers** make up the large mass of the skeletal (striated) muscle. They are attached to bone by fibrous tissue extensions called tendons and are controlled by α-motor neurons. Striated muscles are composed of **myosin filaments**, which are responsible for the contractility (shortening) of the muscle. **Intrafusal fibers**, which contain muscle spindles, are attached to the extrafusal fibers and are controlled by γ-motor neurons. Both ends of the intrafusal fibers contract, but the central region, which is devoid of myosin filaments, does not contract.

The γ-motor neurons control both ends of the intrafusal fibers. A contraction of both ends of the intrafusal fibers causes the central portion of the intrafusal fiber to stretch passively. A similar stretch of the spindles can occur if the entire muscle (skeletal) mass is stretched. Whenever the central portion of the intrafusal fiber stretches, the annulospiral primary sensory endings become depolarized and discharge impulses. These impulses travel in two types of sensory nerve fibers: **type Ia** (fast) fibers and **type II** (slow) fibers. Type Ia (primary) fibers innervate the central region of the spindles, whereas the type II (secondary) fibers innervate areas of the intrafusal fibers on each side of the primary ending (Fig. 11-10A).

As the spindles stretch, a surge of sensory input is directed to the α-motor neurons, which in turn reflexively contract the muscle mass to decrease muscle length progressively. The contraction of the entire muscle halts the stretch of the spindles. With diminished spindle stretching, sensory input from the intrafusal fibers to the α-motor neurons stops.

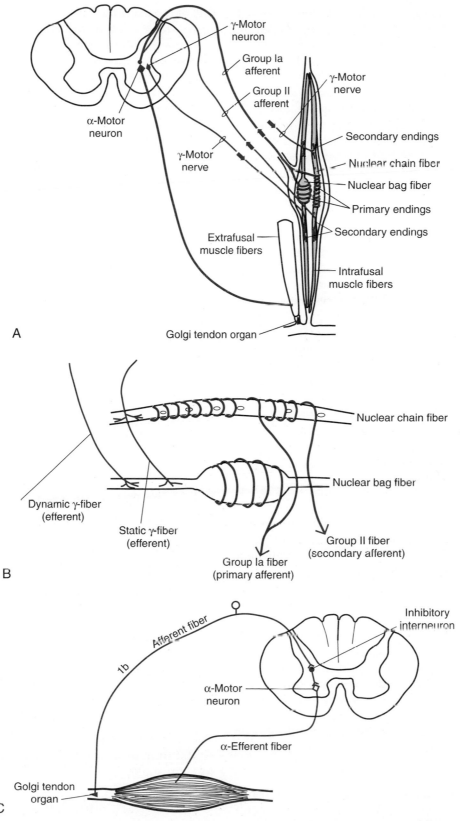

Figure 11-10. **A.** Extrafusal and intrafusal muscle fibers in relation to muscle stretch (muscle spindle) and tension (Golgi tendon) receptors. **B.** Nuclear bag and nuclear chain fibers. **C.** Golgi tendon organs, which mediate autogenic inhibition.

Stretching the central portion of the intrafusal fibers can induce a stretch reflex. This can be elicited by either contracting the ends of the intrafusal fibers by γ-nerve impulses or lengthening the surrounding striate muscle. The latter is illustrated by the classic knee jerk (stretch or myotatic) reflex. Beginning with a subject's leg relaxed, a tap of the patellar tendon at the knee with a reflex hammer immediately stretches both the extrafusal and intrafusal fibers of the quadriceps muscle. After a brief delay, the stretch is followed by a reflexive contraction of the same muscle. The response entails a spinal cord reflex triggered by sensory impulses in the annulospiral nerve endings of the intrafusal fibers that were stretched by the knee tap.

The intrafusal fibers are divided into **nuclear bag** and **nuclear chain fibers** (Fig. 11-10*B*). Nuclear bag fibers are long and have many nuclei in their center. The nuclear chain fibers are smaller and have fewer nuclei. Primary sensory endings (type Ia) innervate the central part of both the nuclear bag and nuclear chain fibers. Secondary sensory endings (type II) innervate the nuclear chain fibers only at sites beyond each end of the primary sensory endings. The intrafusal nuclear bag fibers mediate **dynamic sensory responses**, while nuclear chain fibers mediate **static responses**.

DYNAMIC RESPONSES

The dynamic responses are mediated through primary (type Ia) sensory endings that terminate on the nuclear bag fibers of the muscle spindle. With a stretch of the muscle mass and/or the muscle spindle, there is a simultaneous distortion of the primary (type Ia) sensory nerve endings. This causes a surge of dynamic sensory input to the α-motor neurons of the spinal cord. The α-motor impulses from the anterior horn cells activate a contraction of the muscle mass, shortening the muscle. Sensory input from the type Ia nuclear bag fibers stops when intrafusal fibers cease stretching.

STATIC RESPONSES

Static responses are generated in the secondary sensory endings of the nuclear chain fibers. Intrafusal fibers respond to stretch, a response proportional to the intensity of the stretch. The static sensory input from the intrafusal chain fibers maintains the muscle at the stretched position longer, lasting several minutes or hours.

GOLGI TENDON ORGANS

Golgi tendon organs are the second type of sensory muscle receptors (Fig. 11-10*C*). They innervate the tough tissues that attach muscles to bones. The Golgi afferent impulses regulate muscle tension and prevent damage from excessive muscle contraction. Whenever the muscle stretch or contraction is excessive, type Ib projections from the Golgi tendon organs have an effect opposite to

that of type Ia projections from muscle spindles. The excessive tension in the muscles stimulates the tendon organ type Ib fibers, which activate the intervening interneurons of the spinal cord. The interneurons in turn inhibit the spinal motor nuclei to the muscle. This accounts for autogenic inhibition. The Golgi-mediated reflex is protective, preventing the generation of a too-sudden or excessive force that could damage the muscle or its insertion.

Movement Initiation

Muscle contractions can be initiated and modified through either the γ- or α-motor systems. Increased activity of one system is accompanied by increased discharges in the other system. This causes the muscle to assume a new, appropriate length. A situation in which both α- and γ-motor neurons are at subthreshold, with the muscle at its resting length, is reviewed in Figure 11-11*A*. In this resting state, the spindles are adequately stretched. Any further stretching of the spindles depolarizes them and triggers a volley of action potentials to the α-motor neurons.

One way to alter this resting state and initiate a muscle contraction is through the stimulation of α-motor neurons. Activating them causes the extrafusal muscle fibers to contract. With contraction of the extrafusal fibers of the muscle, the intrafusal fibers become slack, and consequently the spindles lose their sensitivity to muscle length. To correct this impaired spindle sensitivity, the **rubrospinal**, **vestibulospinal**, and **reticulospinal tracts** reflexively discharge the γ-motor neurons and contract the end portions of the intrafusal fibers, straightening the spindles. As a result, the spindles regain their sensitivity to muscle length (Fig. 11-11*A*).

The other way to alter the resting state and initiate a muscle contraction is to contract the ends of the intrafusal fibers by way of the γ-motor neurons (Fig. 11-11*B*). The γ-mediated contraction of the ends of intrafusal fibers increases sensitivity of the spindles and their afferent fibers. The annulospiral endings send a volley of action potentials to the α-motor neurons on type Ia fibers, shortening the extrafusal fibers. Once the muscle has contracted enough to decrease the stress on the center of the intrafusal fibers, the rate of the type Ia firing decreases, and the extrafusal fibers cease contracting. The new desired muscle length permits maintenance of equilibrium in which the activity in type Ia fibers is below threshold.

SPINAL REFLEXES

Stretch, or Myotatic, Reflex

The muscle stretch reflex, the simplest of all, is perhaps the most discussed motor act involving a single synapse in the spinal cord. The classic example of this

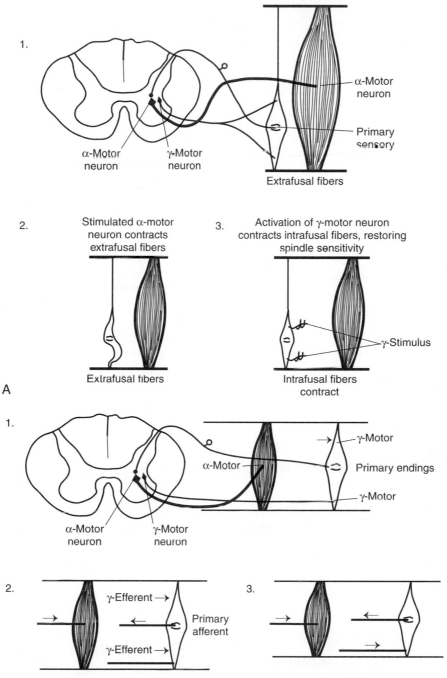

Figure 11-11. The α- and γ-motor neurons in movement initiation and maintenance of sensitivity to stretch in muscle spindles. **A.** α-Mediated voluntary contraction of extrafusal muscle fibers leaves intrafusal fibers and their spindles without sensitivity to stretch. This condition is corrected by reticular and vestibulospinal projections to γ-motor neurons, which contract intrafusal fibers and restore spindle stretch sensitivity. **B.** In γ-initiated movement, γ-cells activate intrafusal fiber ends, deforming annulospiral endings of spindle afferent fibers, which synaptically activate alpha motor neurons causing contraction of extrafusal muscle cells.

monosynaptic, or two-neuron, reflex is the knee jerk, which is initiated by tapping the patellar tendon of the quadriceps femoris muscle with a reflex hammer (Fig. 11-12). A tap of the tendon (input) leads to a brief stretch of the muscle, which stimulates the sensory endings of spindles. The muscle spindles send afferent projections to α-motor neurons, and activation of the α-motor neu-rons causes a quick contraction (muscle jerk) of the same muscle (output).

The common element in all stretch reflexes is that the stretched muscle contracts after a brief delay. The principal receptors are the muscle receptors that respond to stretching of the muscle affected (e.g., by tapping of the patellar tendon). Sensory inputs from the

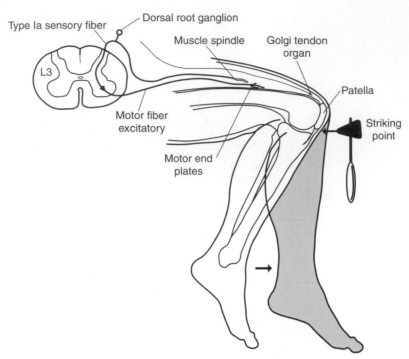

Figure 11-12. Neuronal circuitry for stretch (patellar tendon) reflex. Tapping the patellar tendon briefly stretches extrafusal fibers of quadriceps muscle and raises tension of its muscle spindles. Spindles respond to muscle stretching by sending a volley of impulses directly to α-motor neurons in the L-3 segment of the spinal cord. L-3 efferent fibers cause extrafusal fibers of quadriceps to contract. This muscle contraction eliminates tension on spindles.

stretched muscle spindles monosynaptically activate the α-motor neurons at the L-3 level. The α-motor efferent fibers to the muscle complete the reflex arc. The efferent fibers from the α-motor neurons cause contraction of the extrafusal muscle fibers. The reflexive contraction of the muscle restores it to a resting position, decreasing the sensory spindle impulses. Tendon jerk reflexes can be elicited at several spinal segments involving different nerve roots. For example, the biceps muscle involves C-5 and C-6 segments; the triceps muscle is regulated by C-6 and C-7 segments; the knee jerk reflex involves L-2 to L-4 segments; and the ankle jerk reflex involves spinal segment S-1.

Withdrawal, or Flexor, Reflex

As a protective response to pain or painful stimuli, flexion of the arms or legs is based on a series of nerve synapses and is therefore a polysynaptic reflex. A withdrawal reflex involving one or several body parts is commonly seen when one touches a hot pan or steps on a nail or glass. The number of body parts that respond is proportional to the strength of the painful stimulus.

The neural mechanism of the limb withdrawal reflex (Fig. 11-13) involves pain receptors in the skin, afferent pain fibers, substantia gelatinosa, interneurons, and α-motor neurons. The afferent pain and temperature fibers from the skin enter the spinal cord through the dorsal root and terminate in the **substantia gelatinosa** with collaterals to interneurons in the dorsal gray horns. Interneurons distribute signals to

the appropriate α-motor neurons, initiating the limb withdrawal response; the number of motor neurons recruited by pain fibers depends on the strength of the stimulus. The reflex continues for several seconds after the stimulus ceases. A withdrawal reflex generally begins even before one is aware of the painful stimulus because the afferent information triggers a spinal response before the ascending signal of pain reaches the forebrain.

Reciprocal innervation of motor neurons is a neuronal arrangement: the stimulation of one group of neurons causes inhibition of an associated group of neurons. This neuronal arrangement is essential to smooth motor function. For example, in arm flexion, the interneurons activating the motor neurons for the biceps simultaneously inhibit the motor neurons for the paired triceps. This antagonistic effect—wherein one muscle contracts while the paired muscle extends because it is inhibited from simultaneous contraction—exemplifies reciprocal inhibition (Fig. 11-13). Anatomically, this involves interneurons that are inhibitory to α-motor neurons of the antagonistic muscle.

Crossed, or Intrasegmental, Extensor Reflex

The crossed extensor reflex is a complex movement pattern in which withdrawal of the limb (flexor response) on one side is accompanied by the extension of the opposite limb approximately 0.5 second after the flexor response (Fig. 11-14). This multisynaptic reflex system, which moves limbs on the opposite side of the

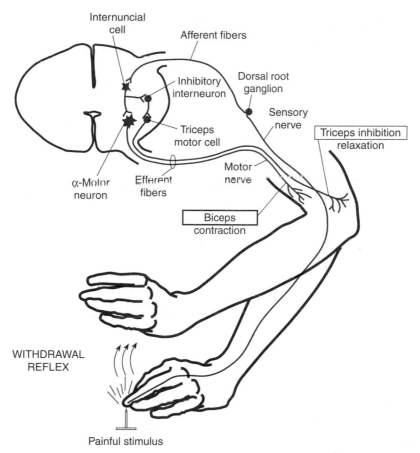

Figure 11-13. Neuronal circuitry for withdrawal (flexor) reflex. A painful stimulus to hand results in a reflexive flexing of upper limb, causing withdrawal of hand from painful stimulus. Circuitry involves diverging interneuronal elements. This circuitry not only withdraws limb but also inhibits antagonistic muscle from contracting through reciprocal inhibition.

body, is considered a genetically programmed protective behavior for survival, as it moves the entire body away from the painful stimulus. Its neural mechanism involves the crossing of sensory information to the opposite side through polysynaptic circuits of interneurons recruiting the opposite limbs. The crossed limb extension follows the flexing action of the limb ipsilateral to the stimulus. Reverberating polysynaptic circuits in interneuronal pools thus sustain the complex withdrawal behavior for long periods, even after the reflex triggering stimulus has ceased. This is necessary to keep the body protected until the brain takes over body control.

NEUROTRANSMITTERS

Four important excitatory neurotransmitters are released by the activity of brainstem projections to the spinal cord: **epinephrine, norepinephrine, serotonin,** and **acetylcholine.** The pontine reticular **nucleus ceruleus** and the **lateral medullary reticular formation** transmit epinephrine and norepinephrine to the spinal cord (see Fig. 13-1 for locations of the reticular formation and its nuclei). Their influence is thought to be inhibitory, enhancing the signal-to-noise ratio in the spinal sensorimotor conduction system. These neurotransmitters are slow-acting and have a long-lasting effect.

The caudal reticular **raphe nuclei** at most levels of the brainstem send serotonin projections to the lower brainstem and spinal cord. The projections to the spinal cord synapse in the ventral and dorsal horns and in the sympathetic lateral columns. In addition, they synapse on spinal **enkephalin interneurons** and provide some control over pain transmission.

Acetylcholine is the major chemical messenger of the peripheral nervous system. Released by the efferent spinal fibers in the myoneural junction, acetylcholine regulates voluntary or reflexive motor movements. A diminished effect of acetylcholine occurs in **myasthenia gravis** and similar disorders associated with muscle weakness. Weakness can be caused by either excessive action of the **enzyme acetylcholinesterase** or inadequate release of acetylcholine at the myoneural junction. Acetylcholine also regulates autonomic functions. Except for the sympathetic postganglionic cells, acetylcholine is the primary neurotransmitter of the autonomic nervous system, which controls major visceral functions (Table 16-1).

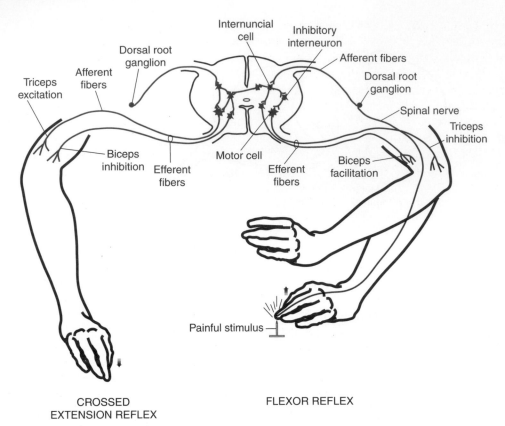

CROSSED
EXTENSION REFLEX

FLEXOR REFLEX

Figure 11-14.   Neuronal circuitry for crossed extensor reflex marked by the contraction of muscle on one side accompanied by extension of opposing muscle or muscles. This reflex involves interneurons that diverge sensory information. This crossed sensory information activates motor neurons to extend agonistic muscle, whereas interneurons inhibit motor nucleus for antagonistic muscle, ensuring smooth extension of limb.

CLINICAL CONSIDERATIONS

Trauma, tumors, infections, impaired blood circulation, and degenerative conditions are common causes of spinal cord lesions. The testing of sensory and motor functions is the most reliable clinical method for determining the integrity of the spinal cord. The contraction of striate muscles during reflexes provides a clinician with important information about the complex internal mechanism of the entire motor system. Muscle reflexes are clinically examined on both sides of the body to determine whether muscular movements are symmetrical and the quality of movements is normal. Absent or reduced (**hypoactive**) or increased (**hyperactive**) quality of muscle reflexes indicates pathology in the nervous system. Spinal reflex functions are controlled via balanced excitatory (+) and inhibitory (−) supraspinal projections to the motor neurons. The corticospinal system is predominantly excitatory to motor neurons in the spinal cord. Loss of this system reduces recruitment of motor neurons and thus produces weakness. This muscle paresis is gradually converted over several weeks into spasticity, which includes hyperexcitability of many stretch reflexes (upper motor neuron syndrome). In contrast to brisk (hyperactive) reflexes with interrupted supraspinal fibers, lesions involving spinal motor neurons and/or their efferent spinal fibers lead to reduced or absent muscle reflexes (hyporeflexia or areflexia, respectively). **Myelography, angiography, computed tomography**, or **magnetic resonance imaging** is used to determine the precise nature of the lesion.

There are two types of spinal cord disorders: segmental and longitudinal (pathway specific). **Segmental disturbance** implicates a spinal level of lesion; below this level of the lesion, sensory and motor functions are impaired. The severity of the deficit depends on the site and extent of the lesion. **Longitudinal disturbance** selectively affects specific nerve cells and their axons. The longitudinal involvement of axonal bundles may impair both sensory and motor systems.

Lower Motor Neuron Syndrome

LMN refers to a motor neuron and its axon in the brainstem or spinal cord. The LMN cell body provides the output pathway to peripheral function via its axon, which traverses the ventral root and peripheral nerves to innervate a skeletal muscle. LMN lesions of either the cell body in the spinal cord ventral horn (e.g., polio myelitis, amyotrophic lateral sclerosis, vascular damage, spinal cord tumor) or of lesions to the LMN axon in the ventral root or peripheral nerve results in **denervation** of the innervated **skeletal muscle fibers** and loss of muscle power (weakness) and precise control. Small lesions can result in the loss of one or several motor units. Large lesions or peripheral nerve destruction can result in complete muscle weakness and total flaccidity. Such a lesion results in **LMN syndrome** (Fig. 11-15), in which muscle fibers are disconnected from motor efferents and descending cortical impulses and reflexive sensory input cannot reach the target muscle fibers. Deprived of their trophic efferents, the affected muscle fibers gradually degenerate. Clinical signs of LMN, which include **flaccid paralysis, absent reflexes, muscular fibrillation**, and eventual severe **atrophy** (wasting) of the muscle involved, are unilateral to the lesion.

With no projections of motor impulses from the motor neuron, the muscle fibers are completely paralyzed for both reflexes and voluntary motor movements; this paralysis is characterized by flaccid muscle tone. Denervated muscle fibers pass through several stages: a brief period of hyperexcitability and spontaneous firing (**fibrillation**), followed by silence of firing and **atrophy** (shrinking of muscle). Fibrillation is the contraction of individual denervated muscle cells, which contract under the influence of acetylcholine circulating in the blood. If they are not reinnervated within 6 months or so, the skeletal muscle cells die and are permanently replaced by scar tissue. However, this is more severe than reduced muscle mass from disuse, which is often seen in **UMN syndrome**.

Destroyed LMN cell bodies are not replaced. However, destroyed LMN axons (peripheral nervous system) may regenerate, and if they are properly directed past scar tissue and through their former peripheral nerve path, they can reinnervate to their former muscle fiber targets. Skilled peripheral nerve surgery, inhibition of scar tissue formation, and efforts to maintain denervated muscle fibers until reinnervation occurs are all necessary for the success of reinnervation.

Common Spinal Syndromes

COMPLETE SPINAL TRANSECTION

Vertebral dislocations, myelitis (inflammation of the spinal cord), and tumors can cause spinal transection. Immediately after the transection, all sensory and motor functions are lost bilaterally below the lesion (see rule 5 in Chapter 1) but are spared above the lesion (Fig. 11-16). Thus, the body regions affected depend on the spinal level of the lesion. Spinal shock abolishes sensorimotor functions and persists for weeks. After a while, the reflex activity gradually returns at levels below the lesion. However, with the interruption of the corticospinal tract, after several weeks the patient exhibits UMN syndrome, which includes loss of delicate manipulative capabilities in the forearm and fingers, hyperactive stretch reflexes, Babinski's sign, and clonic movements, in which a passively moved limb undergoes rapid and repeated contraction and relaxation. With spastic legs, the patient eventually assumes an extended posture, which is characterized by extended lower limbs. If the lesion is above the level of innervation of the upper limbs, they often also assume a flexed posture.

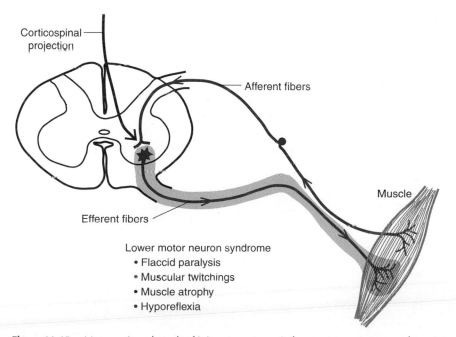

Figure 11-15.   Motor unit and result of injury to motor unit (lower motor neuron syndrome).

BROWN-SÉQUARD'S SYNDROME: SPINAL HEMISECTION

Lateral hemisection of the spinal cord produces the following three clinical conditions (Fig. 11-17); understanding them requires knowledge of the locations and crossing points of the sensorimotor pathways.

1. **Signs of a lesion in the corticospinal tract on the ipsilateral half of body.** In the case of a right-sided lesion at C-4, there is spastic paralysis in the right arm and leg (UMN symptoms). Also, Babinski's and

Hoffman's signs are present. In Babinski's sign, there is abnormal extension of the big toe in response to a scraping stimulus to the sole of the foot (Fig. 14-5). In Hoffmann's sign, the thumb and other fingers flex from the flicking of the nail or distal phalanx.

2. **Ipsilateral sensory loss.** Destruction of the dorsal lemniscal column, which contains tactile and proprioceptive axons ascending ipsilaterally to relay to the contralateral forebrain, results in loss of vibratory and discriminative sensation in the ipsilateral half of

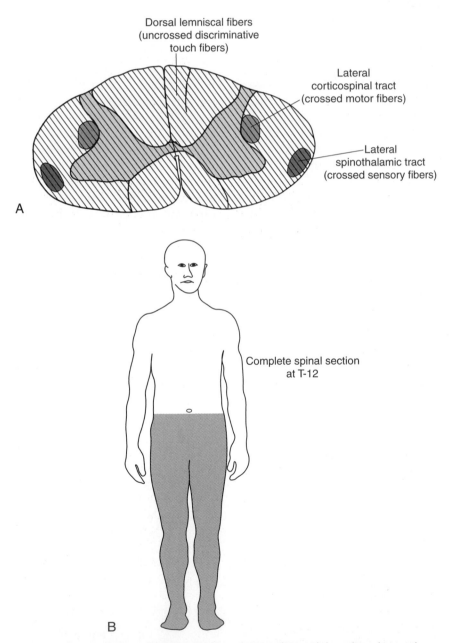

Figure 11-16. Complete transection of thoracic spinal cord (**A**) resulting in bilateral paralysis and sensory loss below the level of lesion with spared functions above the level of lesion (**B**).

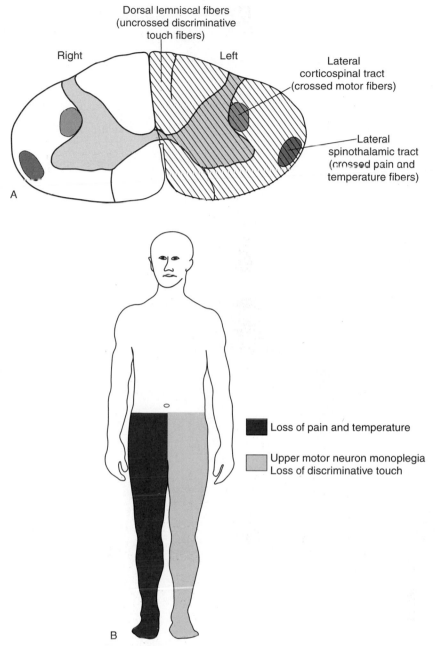

Figure 11-17.   A spinal cord hemisection at T-12 (**A**) resulting in typical sensorimotor deficit pattern characterized by ipsilateral paralysis, ipsilateral sensory loss (discriminative sensation), and contralateral pain and temperature loss (**B**).

the body. The ascending dorsal lemniscal fibers cross the midline in the caudal medulla (see Chapter 7).

3. **Contralateral pain and temperature sensation loss.** With fibers of the lateral spinal thalamic tract crossing immediately after entering the spinal cord, an interruption at the right C-4 level affects pain and temperature from the left (contralateral) side of the body below the level of the lesion (see Chapter 7).

SYRINGOMYELIA

Syringomyelia is a developmental condition marked by a cyst or cavity within the central portion of the spinal cord. It is characterized by two clinical symptoms: loss of pain and temperature sensation and impaired motor control. With the central (gray) region being the site of degeneration, the crossing of sensory (pain and touch) fibers is interrupted. This interruption

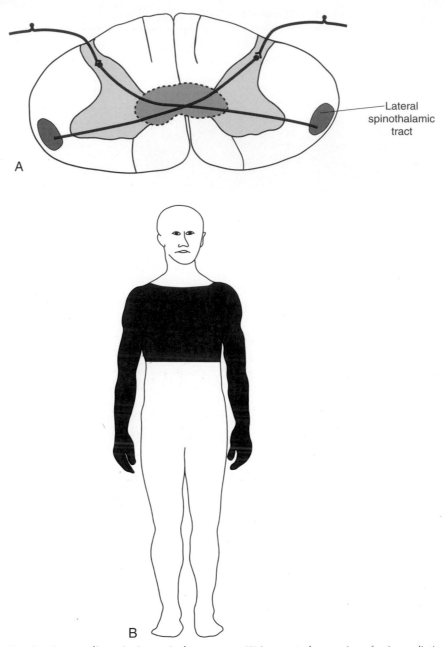

Figure 11-18. A syringomyelic cavity in cervical gray matter (**A**) interrupts the crossing of pain-mediating spinotha-lamic fibers, causing a bilateral loss of pain and temperature and possibly bilateral flaccid paralysis of muscles of upper limbs (**B**).

of crossing fibers results in a bilateral pattern of pain and temperature loss (Fig. 11-18*A*). If the cyst extends into the spinal motor nuclei in the involved segments, bilat-eral signs of LMN syndrome in the involved muscles in-clude flaccid paralysis, hyporeflexia, and hypotonia.

The sensorimotor symptoms depend on the level of the spinal cord implicated. For example, a cavitation in the central spinal area at C-4 to C-6 produces bilateral loss of pain and temperature for the arms, forearms, thumbs, and index fingers. A large cavitation involving C-3 through T-4 , in addition to the loss of pain and tem-perature, affects shoulders and chest (Fig. 11-18*B*).

SUBACUTE COMBINED DEGENERATION

Subacute combined degeneration is associated with pernicious anemia, which results from malabsorp-tion of vitamin $B_{12.}$ The bilateral subacute degeneration of the cord mostly involves the fibers in the dorsal lem-niscal column and corticospinal tract. Involvement of the dorsal column fibers results in bilateral loss of posi-tion and vibratory sense, while the interruption of the corticospinal fibers produces a weakness of limbs bilat-erally. The presence of paresthesia (numbness and tin-gling) indicates peripheral nerve involvement. As the disease progresses to the cerebral cortex, higher mental functions are affected.

LESION LOCALIZATION
Rule 5: Complete Spinal Cord Lesion
PRESENTING SYMPTOMS

Paralysis and sensory loss bilaterally below the level of the lesion with spared functions above this level indicate a complete spinal cord trans-sectional injury.

RATIONALE

The spinal cord contains all ascending (sensory) and descending (motor) fibers. A complete lesion affects the transmission of these functions below the lesion point and spares such functions above the lesion point. Impaired bowel and bladder control and autonomic reflexes are commonly seen in a spinal cord injury.

Rule 6: Spinal Hemisection: Brown-Séquard's Syndrome
PRESENTING SYMPTOMS

Ipsilateral loss of position and vibratory sensation below the level of the lesion, ipsilateral body paralysis, and contralateral loss of pain and temperature indicate spinal hemisection.

RATIONALE

1. Transection of the fasciculus gracilis and fasciculus cuneatus results in the loss of position and vibration sense along with discriminative touch on the side of the lesion.
2. Involvement of fibers of the corticospinal tract below its decussation produces spastic hemiplegia on the side of lesion.
3. Because the fibers mediating pain and temperature cross the midline after entering the spinal cord, interruption of them results in loss of pain and temperature sensation on the opposite side.
4. Impaired bowel and bladder control is commonly seen in spinal cord injury.

Rule 7: Peripheral or Central Lesion
PRESENTING SYMPTOMS

Paralysis and sensory (pain and temperature) loss affecting the same single limb suggests a lesion either in the peripheral nerve or in the cortex.

RATIONALE

The descending and ascending sensory fibers supplying a single limb are together only in the peripheral (nerve, plexus) area or in the somatosensory cortical area.

Case Studies

Patient One

A 3-year-old girl woke up with pain in her right leg. She had no control of her right leg and could not walk. She was taken to a hospital and examination revealed the following:

- No voluntary movement in the right leg
- Diminished tone in the leg muscles
- Knee jerk and Achilles reflexes absent

Computed tomography findings were normal. Clinical testing revealed that the LMNs from L-1 to L-5 were involved.

Question: How does involvement of LMNs from L-1 to L-5 affect control of the leg?

Discussion: An acute viral infection (poliomyelitis) affected LMNs and thereby caused weakness of the leg.

Patient Two

A 30-year-old window washer fell from her ladder and injured her back at the T-11 to T-12 level. With bilateral flaccid paralysis of the legs, she was rushed to a hospital, where she was observed for a few days. In an examination completed a few days later, she demonstrated the following symptoms:

- Spastic paralysis in the left leg
- Positive Babinski sign in the left leg
- Loss of position sense (proprioception) and discriminative touch in the left leg
- Loss of pain and temperature in the right foot

Magnetic resonance imaging revealed a crushed appearance of the cord at T-11 to T-12 on the left.

Question: Can you relate this clinical picture to T-11 to T-12 pathology based on your understanding of the sensorimotor fibers?

Discussion: This is an example of Brown-Sequárd's syndrome, which is associated with spinal hemisection and is characterized by three signs:

- Paralysis on the side of the lesion
- Loss of fine discriminative touch and position sense on the side of the lesion
- Impaired sensation of pain and temperature on the side opposite to the lesion

Immediate flaccid paralysis followed by spastic paralysis indicates a spinal shock secondary to an UMN lesion, which was confirmed by positive Babinski sign in the left foot. The loss of position sense and discriminative touch from the left toes and leg indicates the involvement of the dorsal–lemniscal column fibers; the loss of pain from the right leg suggests interruption of the left spinothalamic pathway. Mediating pain and temperature sensation from the right side of the body, this pathway crosses in the spinal cord at the level of entry. In this case, the initial loss of functions indicated injury to both sides of the spinal cord, but permanent injury was restricted to the left side only.

Patient Three

A gymnast lost control of her body while exercising and fell flat, hurting her back. Unconscious for several minutes, she was rushed to a nearby hospital. After she awoke, she was unable to move. A neurological examination revealed the following:

- Flaccid paralysis of both lower limbs
- No deep tendon reflexes in either leg
- Loss of touch, pain, and temperature sensation below the midthoracic (T-6 to T-7) region
- No bladder or bowel control

Magnetic resonance imaging revealed a complete spinal section at the midthoracic level. The patient's clinical picture changed within a week and she began to exhibit these signs:

- Hyperreflexia in both lower limbs
- Spastic paralysis of both lower limbs
- Impaired control of bowel and bladder functions
- Some return of touch and pressure sensation in the lower limbs

Question: Based on your understanding of spinothalamic and corticospinal pathways, can you account for this clinical picture by relating symptoms to a complete midthoracic spinal section?

Discussion: A complete midthoracic transection of the cord affected the motor control of the lower limbs. The absence of muscle reflexes for a few days immediately after the injury is called spinal shock. The return of hyperactive reflexes and spasticity, indicating an UMN lesion, reflects the loss of descending inhibitory influences. In UMN involvement, Babinski's sign is also expected. The loss of consciousness in this case was attributed to a cortical concussion, since it is not a feature of spinal cord injury.

SUMMARY

Motor function is hierarchically organized at six arbitrarily identified neuraxial levels, with the spinal cord being the lowest. Motor nuclei of the spinal cord are the final common pathways for both spinal reflex and cortical projections to muscle fibers. Consequently, the spinal cord is crucial in reflex muscle contractions and voluntary movements. The environmentally triggered reflex responses regulated by the spinal cord include stretch (myotatic) reflex, withdrawal (flexor) reflex, and crossed extensor reflex. Even though these reflexes are independent of voluntary motor control, intact cortical projections to the spinal cord are important in the regulation of these reflexes. Constantly relayed sensory information, which is vital to coordinated motor activity, is integrated at every level of the nervous system. Spinal lesions, which interrupt both cortical and spinal reflex projections to limb muscles, result in LMN syndrome. The clinical picture of this syndrome is characterized by flaccid paralysis, absent reflexes, and atrophy of muscle fibers.

Technical Terms

α-**motor neuron**	**atrophy**
afferent	**axon**
crossed extension reflex	**motor unit**
efferent	**muscle spindles**
extrafusal fibers	**myoneural junction**
γ-**motor neuron**	**reciprocal inhibition**
Golgi tendon organ	**reflex**
hyporeflexia	**skeletal muscle**
interneuron	**stretch reflex**
intrafusal fibers	**withdrawal reflex**
lower motor neuron	

Review Questions

1. Define the following terms:

α-motor neuron	lower motor neuron
atrophy	motor unit
crossed extensor reflex	muscle spindles
extrafusal fibers	myoneural junction
γ-motor neurons	reciprocal inhibition
Golgi tendon organ	reflex
hyporeflexia	skeletal muscle
interneurons	stretch reflex
intrafusal fibers	withdrawal reflex

2. Discuss the significance of cervical and lumbar enlargements.
3. Describe the structures and functions of a spinal segment.
4. Discuss the concepts of the final common pathway and motor unit.
5. Discuss the functions of α- and γ-motor neurons and interneurons.
6. Discuss how the spinal cord serves as a reflex center. Illustrate the reflex pathway with a diagram.
7. Describe the mechanisms of stretch reflex, withdrawal reflex, and crossed extensor reflex with a labeled diagram.
8. Describe the function of muscle spindles and Golgi tendon organs.
9. Describe the following terms related to a reflex: reciprocal inhibition, monosynaptic, polysynaptic, ipsilateral, and contralateral.
10. Compare the activation of α-motor neurons directly through the motor cortex and indirectly via γ-motor neurons.
11. Describe LMN syndrome and provide a rationale for its clinical symptoms.
12. Explain why an LMN lesion is likely to affect isolated muscles instead of half of the body.
13. Explain the pathophysiology of muscular flaccidity following an LMN lesion.
14. List the components of a motor unit and describe their functions.
15. Discuss the rationale for ipsilateral loss of discriminative touch and body paralysis with contralateral loss of pain and temperature in Brown-Séquard's syndrome.
16. Describe the clinical symptoms resulting from a complete spinal section.

12

Motor System 2: Cerebellum

Learning Objectives

After studying this chapter, students should be able to do the following:
- Discuss the importance of the cerebellum in motor activity
- Describe the major anatomical structures of the cerebellum
- Describe the function of each principal cerebellar structure
- Explain major cerebellar afferent and efferent projections and discuss their functions
- Discuss the neuronal circuitry of a cerebellar functional unit
- Describe the major symptoms of cerebellar dysfunction
- Outline common diseases of the cerebellum

The molar level planning of a movement sequence involves the **premotor cortex** and the **supplementary motor cortex**. The fine details of this plan are managed by the **motor cortex**. However, ongoing modifications in the motor plan require participation of the cerebellum, a structure that functions as an error control device and coordinates all relevant input and output systems during movement, particularly rapid, alternating, and sequential movements. The more precise the activity, especially rapid movements, the more cerebellar function, either normal or abnormal, becomes evident. The need for the cerebellum would be minimal if there were no sequential and rapid movements.

In its regulation of movement, the cerebellum constantly monitors all motor output to muscles by receiving input from all parts of the somatosensory cortex and some from brainstem reflex networks. Spinocerebellar tracts bring to the cerebellum information on body and limb position (proprioception) and joint movement (kinesthesia). The cerebellum then compares the efferent commands for intended movements with the sensory information received in terms of anticipated and ongoing motor programs. It considers targeted movement in relation to body position, muscle preparedness, muscle

tone, body equilibrium, distance, and duration. If any sensorimotor discrepancy is detected during the comparison between body position and motor impulse, the cerebellum sends corrective outputs in two directions. **Ascending feedback**, related to what is going on and what modifications have been made in terms of limb preparation, travels to the motor cortex via the ventrolateral thalamus. **Descending feedback** (via the **rubrospinal tract** and **reticulospinal tract**) to the lower motor neurons (LMNs) modulates muscle tone reflexes at each moment in time during the ongoing movement. The ascending and descending functions occur simultaneously, even though the ongoing modifications involve the descending output function. The ascending output is informational; it is used by the thalamus and cortex the next time the movement is made. In the case of sensorimotor discrepancy, the cerebellum can increase or decrease the rate of movement and stop movements at any time.

The cerebellum contributes specifically to **muscle synergy**, **muscle tone**, **movement range** and **strength**, and **maintenance of body equilibrium** by contributing both built-in and learned modifications to the motor plan. Muscle synergy refers to the **coordination** and **smoothness** in **time** and **space** of the ongoing movement, essential for fine and skilled movements. Transitions and alterations in trajectory are smoothed out by anticipatory checking of momentum and damping of oscillations. The cerebellum monitors the range, strength, and velocity of movements in reaching targets. Thus, it is vital to the control of very rapid muscular activities, such as speaking, running, typing, playing the piano, and dancing; these activities require the highest level of constantly changing muscle synergy and movement velocity. In the case of cerebellar malfunctioning, a cortically controlled movement results in hitting the target, but the trajectory is jerky and it requires corrections. Muscle tonal regulation involves maintaining constant tension in healthy muscles and ensuring that the muscles are prepared. Equilibrium likewise ensures that the stable posture needed for executing motor movements is maintained. The cerebellum is not concerned with the conscious appreciation of sensations and cognitive processing. It participates in motor learning, motor memory, and movement execution by automatically regulating and integrating information with sensorimotor mechanisms without reaching conscious awareness.

INNERVATION PATTERN

The relevant cerebellar sensorimotor organization is **ipsilateral** to both **the input source** (muscle spindles) and **the output target** (LMN). This is in contrast to the forebrain motor mechanism, whose organization is contralateral (see Chapter 14). The developmentally older **ventral spinocerebellar system** (see Chapter 7) and newer **dorsal spinocerebellar system** send input to the ipsilateral side to reach the cerebellum. Consequently, the effect of cerebellar lesion is evident on the body **ipsilateral** to the lesion site. The only reasonable explanation for this ipsilateral organization is that the cerebellum is wired for extremely fast functional feedback from incoming signals that might indicate immediate need for modification in the ongoing movement.

CEREBELLAR ANATOMY

The cerebellum is dorsal to the junction of the pons and medulla (Figs. 2-9 and 2-30) and occupies most of the posterior fossa under the **tentorium cerebelli**. The cerebellum consists of the **cerebellar cortex**, two **hemispheres**, **internal white substance**, four **pairs of nuclei** embedded within the cerebellar white matter, and three **cerebellar peduncles**. The cerebellar surface is folded into small folia to accommodate its large size (Fig. 2-27). Each cerebellar hemisphere is divided into three transverse lobes: **floccular nodular**, **anterior**, and **posterior** (Figs. 2-28, 2-29, and 12-1A). Longitudinally, the cerebellum is divided into **median** (vermal), **paramedian** (paravermal), and **lateral hemispheres** (Fig. 12-1B).

Four large nuclei are embedded in the white matter of each cerebellar hemisphere. Listed from lateral to medial, they are the **dentate nucleus**, **emboliform (lentiform) nucleus**, **globose nucleus**, and **fastigial nucleus** (Fig. 12-2). The dentate, the largest of the group, has a convoluted appearance in cross-section. Most fibers traveling through the **superior cerebellar peduncle** originate from the dentate nucleus; this pathway participates in the coordination of limb movements, along with the motor cortex and **basal ganglia**. Emboliform and globose nuclei also regulate the movements

of ipsilateral extremities. The fastigial nucleus is concerned with body posture.

Similar to the cerebral cortex, the cerebellum has a well-defined sensory and motor representation of the body. The cerebellum has two sensory body representations: tactile stimulation activates potentials ipsilaterally in the anterior lobule and bilaterally in the paramedian lobules (Fig. 12-3), and activation of a specific sensorimotor area in the cerebral cortex evokes a similar response from the same somatotopic region in the cerebellum. Motor representation tends to overlap the area covered by sensory mapping.

Transverse and Longitudinal Cerebellar Regions

The cerebellum contains three transverse regions (Table 12-1 and Fig. 12-1A): **archicerebellum** (floccular nodular lobe), **paleocerebellum** (anterior lobe), and **neocerebellum** (posterior lobe).

The archicerebellum (or **vestibulocerebellum**), the oldest part of the cerebellum, includes the **nodulus** and paired **flocculi**. Functionally concerned with equilibrium, this lobe is closely related to the **vestibular component** of cranial nerve VIII, and it primarily receives vestibular projections. The flocculi- and nodulus-containing lobe regulates muscle tone via the **vestibulospinal tract** (see Chapter 11).

The paleocerebellum is the cerebellar region rostral to the primary fissure. It is equated with the **anterior lobe**, which includes the **superior vermis**, the **paravermal zone**, and parts of the cerebellar hemispheres that receive data from general sensory receptors via the **spinocerebellar tract**. The paleocerebellum receives impulses from proprioceptive stretch receptors (spindles) in the muscles of the arms, legs, trunk, and face. It is most concerned with muscle tone and walking posture. The cerebellar projections through the reticulospinal, rubrospinal (red nucleus to spinal cord), and vestibulospinal tracts modify muscle tone (see Chapter 11).

The neocerebellum, developmentally newer and the largest portion of the cerebellum, includes the remaining lateral region of the cerebellar hemisphere. Located between the primary and posterolateral fissures, it forms the posterior lobe. The neocerebellum receives afferent projections from the contralateral sensorimotor cortex. The afferent fibers make up most of the crossed middle cerebellar peduncle. After the necessary sensorimotor integrated processing, the neocerebellum projects to the contralateral motor cortex and spinal cord by way of the **dentate nucleus** and **red nucleus**. The neocerebellum is concerned with the coordination of the cortically directed fine, or skilled, movements, including speaking, writing, and dancing.

There are three **longitudinal cerebellar regions** (Fig. 12-1B). The most medial region is the vermis, which is treelike; it is divided into the rostral, medial,

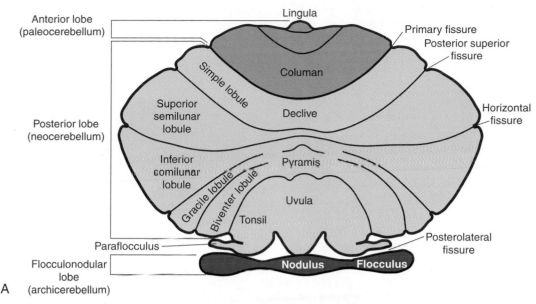

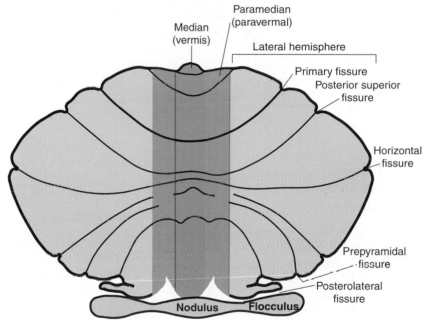

Figure 12-1. **A.** Cerebellar lobes. Cerebellar region caudal to posterolateral fissures is archicerebellum (flocculonodular) lobe. Area rostral to primary fissure is the anterior lobe. Area between primary and posterolateral fissures is the posterior lobe (neocerebellum). **B.** Cerebellum divided longitudinally into vermal, paravermal, and lateral cortices.

and posterior regions (Fig. 2-27). The vermis contributes to body posture by regulating axial muscles. On either side of the vermis is the paravermal region, which regulates movements of ipsilateral extremities. The remainder of the cerebellar hemispheres form the lateral zone, which along with the **red nucleus** and **thalamus** regulates skilled movements of the ipsilateral extremities.

Important structures in the rostral vermis are the **lingula** (tongue), **central lobule**, and **culmen** (ridge). The medial vermis structures are the **declive, folium,** and **tuber.** The posterior vermis contains the **pyramis, uvula,** and **nodulus.**

Cerebellar Connections

The **inferior peduncle, middle peduncle,** and **superior cerebellar peduncles** connect the cerebellum to the brainstem (Figs 2-29, 2-30, and 12-4). All afferent and efferent fibers traveling to and from the cerebellum pass through these three bundles (Table 12-2). Fibers that travel through the inferior and middle cerebellar peduncles are afferent; they mediate almost all sensorimotor input to the cerebellum. Fibers of the superior cerebellar peduncle are largely efferent; they transmit output from the cerebellum to the brainstem and on to the thalamus, motor cortex, and spinal cord.

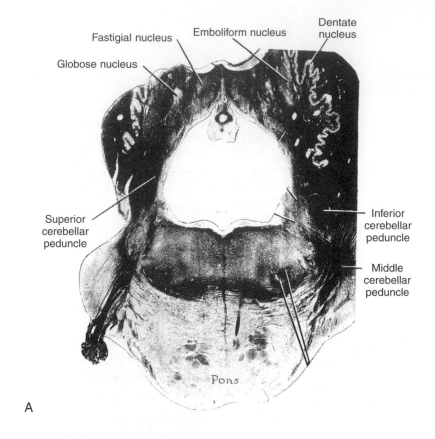

A

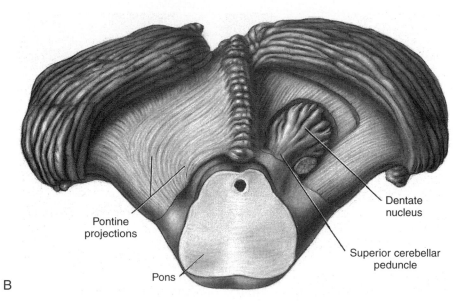

B

Figure 12-2.   **A.** A section of the pontine tegmentum and cerebellum illustrating deep cerebellar nuclei: dentate, emboliform, fastigial, and globose. **B.** Dissected dentate nucleus with a portion of cerebellum.

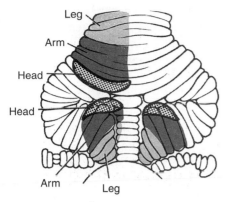

Figure 12-3. Somatotopic localization of sensorimotor functions in the cerebellar cortex of a monkey. Sensorimotor representation of body is ipsilateral in anterior lobe, bilateral in posterior cerebellum.

Table 12-1.   Cerebellar Lobes and Their Functions

Cerebellar Lobe	Functions
Archicerebellum (floccular nodular lobe)	Equilibrium
Paleocerebellum (anterior lobe)	Muscle tone, equilibrium, body posture
Neocerebellum (posterior lobe)	Limb coordination

AFFERENT PATHWAYS

Afferents to the cerebellum originate from the spinal cord, brainstem, and motor cortex (Fig. 12-4). The ratio of afferent to efferent cerebellar fibers, approximately 40:1, underscores the significance of cerebellar

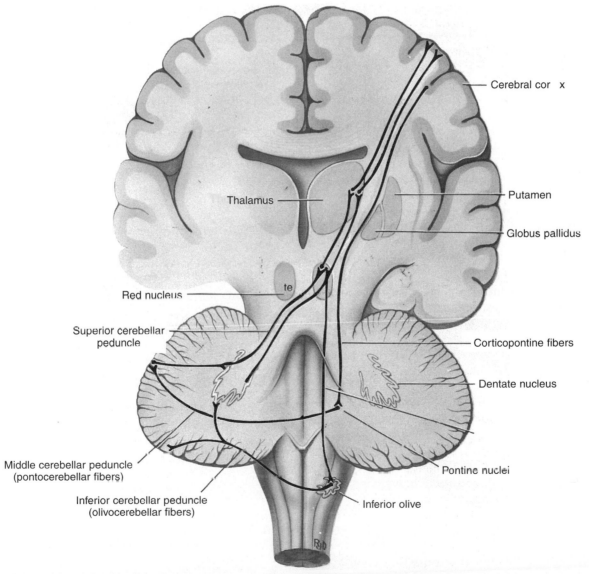

Figure 12-4. Principal afferent and efferent cerebellar projections traveling through inferior, middle, and superior cerebellar peduncles. Olivocerebellar fibers traveling through the inferior cerebellar peduncle transmit brainstem and spinal projections to the cerebellum. Traveling through the middle cerebellar peduncle, the corticopontine and ponto cerebellar fibers form the major cerebellar afferent system. Efferent fibers of the superior cerebellar peduncle decussate in the mesencephalon at the inferior colliculus level before ascending to contralateral motor cortex and descending to brainstem reticular nuclei and spinal cord.

Table 12-2.   Afferent and Efferent Cerebellar Connections

Cerebellar Peduncle	Afferent fibers	Efferent fibers	Function
Inferior	Vestibular, spinal cord, reticular formation, olivary nucleus, stretch receptors of upper limbs		Mediates sensorimotor information from spinal cord and brainstem
Middle	Cortex by way of pontine nuclei		Relays sensorimotor information from opposite cerebral cortex
Superior		Projections from dentate, emboliform, globose cerebellar nuclei	Transmits cerebellar outputs to brainstem, then to thalamus, motor cortex, spinal cord

sensory input to the regulation of synergy in motor functions.

The inferior cerebellar peduncle is an important afferent pathway through which ascending inputs from the distal portions of the limbs gain a rapid entry to the ipsilateral cerebellum. Important pathways that enter through the inferior cerebellar peduncle are the **vestibulocerebellar, dorsal spinocerebellar, reticulocerebellar, olivocerebellar,** and **cuneocerebellar tracts**.

The vestibulocerebellar fibers carry vestibular information from the cristae of the semicircular ducts and vestibule to the cerebellum. Most vestibular fibers are bidirectional and form an ipsilateral communication system between the vestibular system and cerebellum (flocculonodular lobes and the fastigial nuclei). These afferents keep the cerebellum informed of the vestibular output from the inner ear, which is essential for maintaining upright posture. They also permit the coordination of ongoing body movement during movement of the head. Fibers of the dorsal spinocerebellar tract carry unconscious proprioception from muscle spindles, Golgi tendon organs, and tactile receptors in the muscles and joints (Fig. 7-10). These ipsilateral fibers keep the cerebellum informed of momentary changes in tension, range, and strength of muscle movement and provide error signal feedback during ongoing movement (see Chapter 7). The brainstem reticular nuclei—with afferents from the cerebral cortex, spinal cord, vestibular complex, and the red nucleus—project bilaterally to the paleocerebellum through the reticulocerebellar tract. Also included in the inferior cerebellar peduncle is a specialized motor cortex originating system, the **cortico-olivary system**. The cortico-olivary fibers terminate ipsilateral to the motor cortex in the **inferior olivary nucleus**. This nucleus is a major source of climbing fibers that provide direct feedback to the **cerebellum**. The olivocerebellar fibers decussate to enter the contralateral inferior cerebellar peduncle, terminating ipsilateral to the spinal cord input, which is consistent with other inputs. Additional afferents, fibers of the **cuneocerebellar tract**, mediate proprioception from the stretch receptors of the upper limbs and neck to the ipsilateral cerebellum.

Afferent fibers entering the cerebellum via the middle cerebellar peduncle contain afferents from the cerebral cortex that synapse in the pons. Pontine nuclei project to the opposite side of the cerebellum via the crossed fibers of the middle cerebral peduncle. Forming the largest of the afferent fibers to the cerebellum, the middle cerebellar fibers enter the cerebellum as the mossy fibers. The cortical projections terminate in the ipsilateral pontine nuclei. The pontine nuclei, with inputs from the tectum, also mediate visual and auditory information, which provide directional context for ongoing movement. Fibers from the pontine nuclei cross the midline, enter the contralateral middle cerebellar peduncle, and terminate in the opposite cerebellar hemisphere (Fig. 12-4). Thus, the right side of the motor cortex provides input to the left side of the cerebellum, which is also the side that receives ascending input from the left side of the body (see the discussion of the innervation pattern).

EFFERENT PATHWAYS

The cerebellar efferents arise from three deep cerebellar nuclei, the dentate, the emboliform, and the globose, and course through the superior cerebellar peduncle (Fig. 12-4). While the superior cerebellar peduncle also contains some afferents to the cerebellum from the axial muscles, joints, and proximate parts of the limbs, it is largely efferent. Carrying cerebellar efferents to the brainstem, thalamus, and motor cortex, the fibers of the superior cerebellar peduncle decussate at the level of the **inferior colliculus** (Figs. 3-15 and 12-4); some of the crossed fibers terminate in the contralateral **red nucleus**, whereas most continue and project to the thalamus on their way to the motor cortex. The cerebellar efferent fibers from the red nucleus project to the following neuraxial structures:

Spinal Cord

Some cerebellar projections from the red nucleus descend to the spinal cord in the rubrospinal tract and continuously modulate muscle tone reflexes during ongoing movement (see Chapter 11).

Basal Ganglia and Motor Cortex

Cerebellar efferent fibers traveling to the contralateral cortex via the red nucleus and the ventrolateral (VL) nucleus of the thalamus inform the motor cortex of the

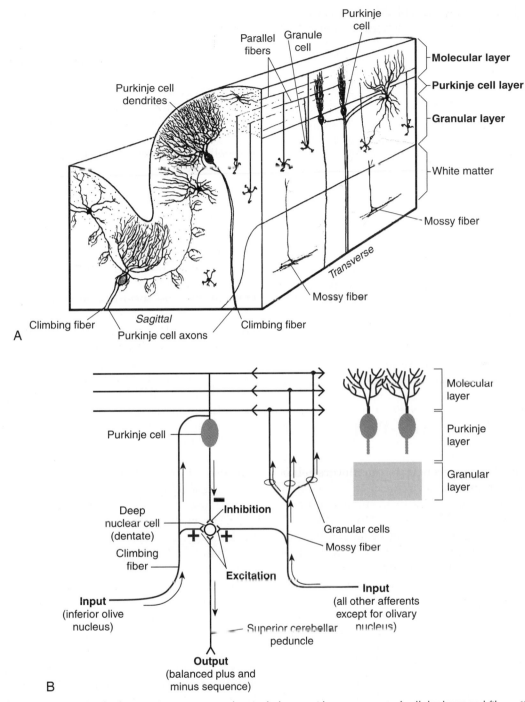

Figure 12-5. A. Cerebral cortex in transverse and sagittal planes, with arrangement of cellular layer and fibers. B. A cerebellar functional unit.

corrections to be made during ongoing movements. The corrective cerebellar output to the cortex is integrated with the basal ganglia feedback to the motor cortex in the ventrolateral thalamus (see Chapters 6 and 13; Fig. 13-3).

Reticular Formation

Much cerebellar output is directed to the brainstem reticular formation, which projects to the cranial nerve nuclei for speech and to the spinal motor neurons.

Reticulospinal and rubrospinal projections regulate the ongoing control of muscle tone reflex during movement.

Vestibular Nuclei

The cerebellum is connected to the vestibular complex via bidirectional fibers. Originating from the fastigial nucleus, cerebellar projections exit through the inferior cerebellar peduncle and terminate in the vestibular complex. These efferents not only coordinate ongoing motor activity during movement of the head, they also project to other levels of the brainstem and upper spinal cord.

CEREBELLAR CORTEX

Structure

The cerebellar cortex is uniform in all areas and consists of three cellular layers: **molecular**, **Purkinje**, and **granular** (Fig. 12-5*A*). The molecular cell layer, the most external layer, is primarily composed of parallel running axons and dendrites that interconnect with other cellular layers, particularly the Purkinje cells. The middle layer is the Purkinje cell layer, which consists of a thin row of large nerve cells. Purkinje cell axons penetrate the granular cell layer, and most of these fibers terminate in deep cerebellar nuclei. Importantly, all impulses leaving the cerebellar cortex must pass through a Purkinje axon. The granular cell layer, the innermost cellular layer, is made up of small, closely packed granule cells. Granular cells have short dendrites that synapse onto the mossy fiber axons. The granular cells also project to the molecular layer and provide extensive axonal parallel fibers that synapse on the dendritic spines of the Purkinje cells.

Neuronal Circuitry of a Cerebellar Functional Unit[a]

The microcircuitry of the cerebellum follows a uniform functional and anatomical pattern in all areas of the **archicerebellum**, **paleocerebellum**, and **neocerebellum**. All input axons, with branches to both the deep nuclei and the cerebellar cortex, mediate excitatory information to the outer cellular layer, where they excite a stripe of Purkinje cell dendrites. Axons of the Purkinje cells project to inhibit the activity of the deep cerebellar nuclei, which serve as the final cerebellar output. The cerebellum is made of millions of such units, each with identical neuronal circuitry. The neuronal circuitry processes all afferent information and forms the cerebellar outputs essential for regulating muscle synergy and tone.

The neuronal circuitry of a functional unit (Fig. 12-5*B*) consists of **cerebellocortical cellular layers**, **deep nuclei**, and **afferent** and **efferent** fibers. There are millions of functional units in the cerebellar cortex, and each cerebellar unit includes a Purkinje cell. The Purkinje cells constantly inhibit the deep cerebellar nuclei that form the cerebellar outputs.

All afferents to the cerebellum travel via **climbing fibers** or **mossy fibers**. Climbing fibers are fewer and

are most directly related to cerebellar Purkinje cells. These include all olivocerebellar projections (inferior cerebellar peduncle) to the cerebellar cortex. The cortico-olivary cerebellar projections of the climbing fibers are highly developed in primates and humans, as they provide the motor and premotor cortex with means of determining the activity status of the cerebellar region at any moment, an important aspect for regulating muscle synergy. After sending **excitatory collaterals** to deep cerebellar nuclei (Fig. 12-5*B*), the climbing fibers travel to the cerebellar cortex, where they synapse on the dendrites of the Purkinje cells, which immediately fire their inhibitory message to the deep cerebellar nuclei. This important afferent system is known for the direct excitability of the Purkinje cells.

Mossy fibers, which make up all other sources of afferent projections to the cerebellum, are most directly related to the sensory input systems concerned with the correlations and modulations that precede cerebellar output. First, the mossy fibers, like climbing fibers, branch to supply excitatory input to both the deep nuclei and the cortex. In the cortex, information is relayed to the outer cortical layer by granule cells whose excitatory axons enter the outer cortical layer and split, sending long axons (parallel fibers) in opposite (medial and lateral) directions for long distances along the folia. The outer cortical layer also receives dendritic projections from Purkinje cells. This explains why climbing fibers directly activate the Purkinje cells, whereas mossy fibers indirectly interact with Purkinje cells. The climbing fibers cause a highly specific output, whereas the mossy fibers cause a less specific but tonic type of response.

The cortical parallel fibers excite a large strip of Purkinje cell dendrites. Each parallel fiber excites many Purkinje cells. Therefore, one Purkinje cell receives input from thousands of parallel fibers. Mediating summated excitatory input, axons of Purkinje cells project to the deep cerebellar nuclei, where they are inhibitory. The deep cerebellar nuclei are also bombarded by the prior excitatory inputs from both climbing and mossy afferent fibers. The deep nuclei fire, depending on the relative timing and strength of these ascending and descending inputs, to provide cerebellar output. The cerebellar cortex also contains an elaborate series of inhibitory feedback circuits consisting of small cells, such as basket cells, Golgi cells, and spindle cells. These regulate the general excitability of the cortex and prevent it from a general cerebellar seizure state.

Under normal physiological conditions, the cerebellar output to the cortex, basal ganglia, reticular formation, and spinal cord is excitatory (+), continuously balanced by afferent excitation and Purkinje inhibition (−). For skilled and digital activities that require rapid and alternating movements, the timing is most important in the sequence of excitatory and inhibitory neuronal events. If there is any alteration in the sequence of

---

[a] "Neuronal Circuitry of a Cerebellar Functional Unit" is based on Guyton AC. Organ Physiology: Structure and Functions of the Nervous System. Philadelphia: Saunders, 1976.

excitatory (+) and inhibitory (−) events and/or the timing interval between the neuronal event changes, the cerebellum sends faulty output signals to the brainstem and cortex. This in turn alters muscle synergy, tone, and equilibrium and affects the integrity of the neuronal circuitry of the motor cortex, reticular formation, and spinal cord. Consequently, motor functions become incoordinated. Rapid motor patterns that depend on muscle synergy and normal tone are most strongly affected by altered timing and sequencing of facilitation and inhibition. Cerebellar signals to the brainstem are rapid and transient. Deep cerebellar nuclei constantly fire signals, sending them to the motor cortex. Any decrease in cerebellar output alters the balanced nature of the cerebellar output essential for well-coordinated activity.

CLINICAL CONSIDERATIONS

Substantial evidence suggests that the neocerebellar cortical region is essential for the learning of precision in sequential movements. It is not clear, though, whether the synaptic connectivity in the cerebellum, somewhere else, or both is necessary. Smaller unilateral cerebellar lesions can be compensated by retraining. However, unless they occur in young children, massive and bilateral cerebellar lesions result in lack of adaptation and cause long-term effects.

Remember that vision cannot compensate for cerebellar abnormality, a fact that helps differentiate between the disturbances of the cerebellum and the dorsal–lemniscal ascending system (see Chapter 7). For example, the **Romberg test** is used to evaluate proprioception. A subject stands with arms extended in front, feet together, and eyes closed. If the patient's arm drifts downward and/or the subject begins to tilt on that side because of unsteadiness, the cause may be cerebellar (input or output), vestibular, or proprioceptive abnormality. However, if the subject's eyes are open and the arm drifts or unsteadiness occurs, the abnormality is in the cerebellum, not in the dorsal–lemniscal column, since vision cannot compensate for cerebellar malfunctioning. Further distinction between vestibular and cerebellar abnormality requires additional clinical skills, since lesions involving both systems produce unsteadiness and a tendency to fall to one side. The caloric test in each ear and vertigo testing can help in determining the underlying cause.

Signs of Cerebellar Dysfunction

Minor damage to cerebellar systems produces subtle alterations that are difficult to evaluate clinically. Major damage to the cerebellum and its input or output systems invariably results in conspicuous motor impairments. The motor impairments are marked by a reduced smoothness and accuracy of movement, which include **dyssynergia** and **motion** or **action tremor**. Patients with cerebellar pathology cannot control body parts that otherwise seem normal with regard to strength and somatosensation. Cerebellar dysfunction is most pronounced in skilled activities that require rapid, alternating movements. Furthermore, the relevant cerebellar organization is ipsilateral to both the input source and output target. As a result, cerebellar lesions produce ipsilateral motor disturbances.

Cerebellar dysfunction is tested by **tandem walking**, the **finger-to-nose test**, **alternating movements**, **hopping**, **limb rebounding**, and **diadochokinetic movements**. As with many other cerebral degenerative conditions, there is no treatment for degenerative cerebellar lesions. Common cerebellar impairments include the following.

ATAXIA

Skilled movement entails approaching the target with smoothness in time and space. This smoothness of movement requires continuous correction for momentum of the moving parts; the cerebellum is essential for this correction. **Ataxia** is lack of order and coordination in muscle activities; coordinated motor activities are decomposed into segments. For example, while walking and turning, a patient stops before making a turn and then turns in slow motion (**bradykinesia**). The subject then resumes walking awkwardly and slowly. There is mild muscular weakness (**asthenia**). Ataxic signs always occur ipsilateral to the side of cerebellar damage. **Asynergia**, an impairment in the direction and force of a given movement, is a local condition usually involving paired muscles.

DYSDIADOCHOKINESIA

Dysdiadochokinesia is a failure in the sequential progression of motor activities displayed by clumsiness in rapid and alternating movements. The ability to alternate movements is best tested by asking a subject to repeat a sequence of alternating movements that include tapping or articulating the phonemic sequence /pa ta ka/ or performing rotating movements.

DYSARTHRIA

Impaired ability to make the needed modifications and alterations in ongoing movement produces a drastic effect on skilled movements, such as speech. This results in **dysarthric** speech. Ataxic dysarthria is commonly seen in bilateral cerebellar disturbances. Speech in ataxic dysarthria is slow, slurred, and disjointed; each word or syllable is spoken individually, known as scanning speech.

DYSMETRIA

Dysmetria denotes an error in the judgment of a movement's range or the distance to the target. Motor movements either falling short of the target (undershooting) or extending past it (overshooting) are dysmetric errors. Dysmetria results from the failure to incorporate the range and distance of stationary and moving targets.

INTENTION TREMOR

Intention tremor results from impaired ability to dampen accessory movements during a skilled movement sequence. Evident during a movement, the tremor becomes more severe as the target is approached—as demand for the function of the cerebellum becomes more important. Perhaps a better term for this clinical phenomenon is **motion tremor**, as the tremor disappears during rest. Intention tremor is different from the **resting tremor** of Parkinson's disease. In Parkinson's disease, during rest the patient exhibits a pill-rolling tremor that disappears during volitional movements (see Chapter 13).

HYPOTONIA

Tone is the slight tension that is constantly present in the muscle and easily detected during passive manipulation of the limbs. The functional cerebellum is trained via the γ-efferent influence on the stretch reflex to optimize continuously the motor tone of each muscle contributing to a movement. This includes opposing muscle groups that contract simultaneously to provide joint stability. In **hypotonia**, normal muscle tension (resistance to passive stretch) is decreased and the muscle becomes floppy. Hypotonia ipsilateral to the side of cerebellar dysfunction is a common sign of cerebellar pathology and is often accompanied by asthenia, a condition in which the muscles are likely to tire quickly.

REBOUNDING

Rebounding reflects impaired motor tone adjustment and a loss of rapid and precise corrective response, as the patient loses the ability to predict, stop, or dampen movement. For example, if a flexed arm is held back and suddenly let go, a person with cerebellar pathology cannot detect the sudden limb release. The hand movement does not stop, and the patient strikes his or her own face.

DISEQUILIBRIUM

Impaired vestibular processing in the cerebellum results in **disequilibrium** that predominantly affects the legs. Affected people walk as if they are drunk. The gait is unsteady, and the body wavers toward the side of the lesion.

Common Cerebellar Pathologies

CEREBROVASCULAR ACCIDENT

Thromboembolic or **hemorrhagic** involvement of the vertebrobasilar artery system interrupts blood circulation to the cerebellum. The **vertebrobasilar artery** may affect the circulation of one or all of the three cerebellar arteries: **anteroinferior**, **superior**, and **posteroinferior** (see Chapter 17).

TOXICITY

Toxicity consequent to chronic alcoholism may cause progressive subacute cerebellar degeneration. It occurs past middle age and is characterized by gross cerebellar atrophy and the loss of all cellular elements in the anterior lobe, most crucially the Purkinje cells. The most significant symptom is a wavering (wide-based, shuffling) gait similar to that of an intoxicated person. In half of cases, the disturbance is limited to the lower extremities. In other cases, there is incoordination, dysmetria, and dyskinesia in the upper extremities as well. Speech may be monotonous, slurred, or explosive, which disappears as the blood alcohol level attenuates with time. However, the remaining cerebellar deficits, once established, may not improve even with proper nutrition and vitamin treatment.

PROGRESSIVE CEREBELLAR DEGENERATION

Many types of ataxias are due to cerebellar degeneration, including hereditary ataxia. **Friedreich's ataxia**, the most common, is an autosomal recessive hereditary degenerative condition characterized by combined sensory and motor dysfunctions. Most commonly affected are the cerebellar afferent pathways, including the olivocerebellar or spinocerebellar pathways, and efferent pathways, including the dentatorubral pathways. This condition usually appears between ages 10 and 20 and is characterized by ataxia (incoordination and unsteadiness in walking), dysarthria, tremor, weakness, loss of proprioception, nystagmus, dysmetria, and scanning speech. There is no medical treatment for Friedreich's ataxia.

Case Studies

Patient One

A 17-year-old began to have weakness in his legs. His movements were clumsy when he was playing and running. He was taken to the family physician, who noted the following signs:

- Broad-based gait
- Unsteadiness in walking
- Weakness in the lower limbs and loss of delicate movements
- Release of primitive reflexes, such as positive Babinski and others
- Loss of proprioception and discriminative touch from both lower limbs
- Positive Romberg sign (the patient could not stand straight with his eyes closed).

Magnetic resonance imaging revealed pathological changes in the spinal cord involving the dorsal and lateral funiculi at the lumbar level. Friedreich's ataxia was suspected.

Question: Can you account for these symptoms based on your understanding of the sensorimotor pathways?

Discussion: The observed degenerative changes had the following effects:

- Involvement of the corticospinal tract fibers not only resulted in weakness but also in the appearance of other pyramidal signs: loss of delicate movements and release of primitive reflexes.

- Because damage to the spinocerebellar fibers prevented transmission of unconscious proprioception to the cerebellum, incoordination and unsteadiness resulted.
- Damage to the fasciculus gracilis due to spinal degenerative changes resulted in loss of discriminative sensation from the legs.

Patient Two

An 18-year-old man had headaches, nausea, and vomiting for several months. He was first treated with aspirin. He returned to the hospital as his condition worsened and exhibited the following:

- Drowsiness
- Ataxia
- Spells of falling down
- Marked dysarthric speech

A cerebellar tumor was confirmed on magnetic resonance imaging.

Question: Can you account for these symptoms based on your understanding of the sensorimotor pathways?

Discussion: The gradual progression of the symptoms indicated a neoplastic (tumor) growth. The presence of a mass affected all cerebellar functions, including coordination, equilibrium, and motor speech. Surgical excision of the tumor relieved all symptoms, and the patient's clarity of speech improved remarkably.

SUMMARY

The cerebellum does not initiate motor movements, nor does it alter sensation. It functions as a servomechanism, constantly monitoring all body motor activities and comparing intended movements (planned by the motor and premotor cortex) against the updated sensory information it receives. By calculating discrepancies between sensory and motor states, it regulates the quality of motor movements generated elsewhere in the motor cortex, brainstem, or spinal cord. With its ability to make alterations for greater precision and smoothness during ongoing movement, the cerebellum is essential for learning skilled movements. The cerebellum contributes to muscle synergy, tone, and equilibrium. Signs of cerebellar dysfunction include paresis, hypotonia, ataxia, asymmetry, intention tremor, dysdiadochokinesia, dysarthria, and disequilibrium. Subjects with cerebellar pathology lack the ability to control and regulate motor functions. Small lesions of the cerebellar cortex may cause minimal impairments that can be compensated for. However, massive cerebellar damage involving the deep nuclei or the superior cerebellar peduncle can cause permanent and lasting deficits unless it occurs at a very young age. Cerebellar impairments do not affect reasoning, thinking, memory, or language.

Technical Terms

archicerebellum
asthenia   dysdiadochokinesia
asynergia   hypotonia
ataxia   mossy fibers
climbing fibers   neocerebellum
deep cerebellar nuclei   paleocerebellum
diadochokinesia   Purkinje cells
dysarthria

Review Questions

1. Define the following terms:
   archicerebellum   dysdiadochokinesia
   asthenia   hypotonia
   asynergia   mossy fibers
   ataxia   neocerebellum
   climbing fibers   paleocerebellum
   diadochokinesia   Purkinje cells
   dysarthria
2. Describe the anatomy of the cerebellum in terms of its hemisphere, lobes, and pathways.
3. Describe the transverse and longitudinal cerebellar divisions, and discuss their functions.
4. From what peripheral end organs does the cerebellum receive its input of unconscious proprioception?
5. Describe the role of the cerebellum in motor activity, outlining the anatomical connections through which the cerebellum influences motor activity. Also define muscle synergy, muscle tone, movement range and strength, and body equilibrium.
6. Describe the anatomy and function of a cerebellar functional unit with a labeled diagram.
7. List and define the common signs of cerebellar dysfunction.
8. Explain why the effects of a unilateral cerebellar lesion manifest on the body ipsilateral to the lesion.
9. Describe the rationale of Romberg sign.
10. Describe how a cerebellar lesion is likely to affect motor speech.
11. Match the following definitions to the associated lettered pattern:
    i. incoordination in general   a. ataxia
    ii. overshooting or undershoot-   b. dysmetria
        ing when approaching a   c. asthenia
        moving target   d. dysdiadochokinesia
    iii. incoordination in rapid alter-
        nating movements
    iv. muscle weakness

13

Motor System 3: Brainstem and Basal Ganglia

Learning Objectives

After studying this chapter, students should be able to do the following:

- Discuss the role of the reticular formation in motor functions
- Describe reticular influence on spinal motor functions
- Discuss the pathophysiology of decerebrate rigidity
- Describe the role of the basal ganglia in motor functions
- Discuss structurally and functionally related structures of the basal ganglia
- Explain the neuronal circuitry for common basal ganglia circuits (loops) along with their afferent and efferent projections
- Describe the inhibitory or excitatory influence of afferent and efferent projections of basal ganglia circuits
- List clinical signs of basal ganglia impairments
- Describe major movement disorders associated with basal ganglia lesions
- Discuss primary neurotransmitters of the basal ganglia, their projections, and their functions
- Discuss common disorders of the basal ganglia, such as Parkinson's disease, Wilson's disease, and Huntington's chorea

As discussed before, the motor system is built upon a set of intersegmental levels in the central nervous system. These levels constitute a ladder of hierarchical control such that the brainstem modulates reflexes and motor activity at the medullary and spinal levels and the forebrain modulates all of the lower levels. The hierarchical vertical motor system, which also serves speech and other motor activities, is regulated by motor inputs from various sources. Direct motor pathways originate in the motor cortex and descend in the **pyramidal tract** (corticobulbar and corticospinal) to the motor neurons in the brainstem and spinal cord. In addition to cortical input, the brainstem and spinal motor neurons receive indirect projections from various extrapyramidal sources that include the **basal ganglia, cerebellum,** and **brainstem reticular formation**. These inputs refine the cortical motor directives to the lower motor neurons (LMN) in the medulla and spinal cord.

BRAINSTEM MOTOR MECHANISM

Located between the diencephalon and the spinal cord, the brainstem plays a significant role in modulating the output function of a reflex network, tonal function, and sensorimotor activity. The brainstem receives pyramidal, extrapyramidal, and spinal inputs and is the primary contributor to **muscle tone** and **postural control**. The brainstem sensorimotor mechanism is composed of the **red nucleus**, the **cranial nerve nuclei**, and most important, the **reticular formation**.

Brainstem Anatomy

The red nucleus and cranial nerve nuclei, two major brainstem structures, are discussed in chapters 12 and 15. This chapter focuses on the motor functions of the reticular formation. Structurally, the reticular formation is composed of a diffuse core of neurons and a few specific clusters of sensory and motor neurons that extend from the caudal diencephalon to the upper cervical segments (Fig. 13-1A). Reticular neurons have an extensive network of overlapping dendrites and axons and receive inputs from the motor cortex, basal ganglia, and cerebellum before projecting to the spinal and cranial motor neurons. Interspersed within the reticular core are the cranial nerve nuclei that regulate motor and visceral functions, including speech activity. Functionally, the reticular cells, along with the cranial nerve cells, form the pivotal point for many functions of the brainstem and lower motor levels. The brainstem reticular formation is important in **cortical arousal**, **tonal modulation** of **spinal** and **cranial motor functions**, and **pain processing**. With multiple and extensive projections, the

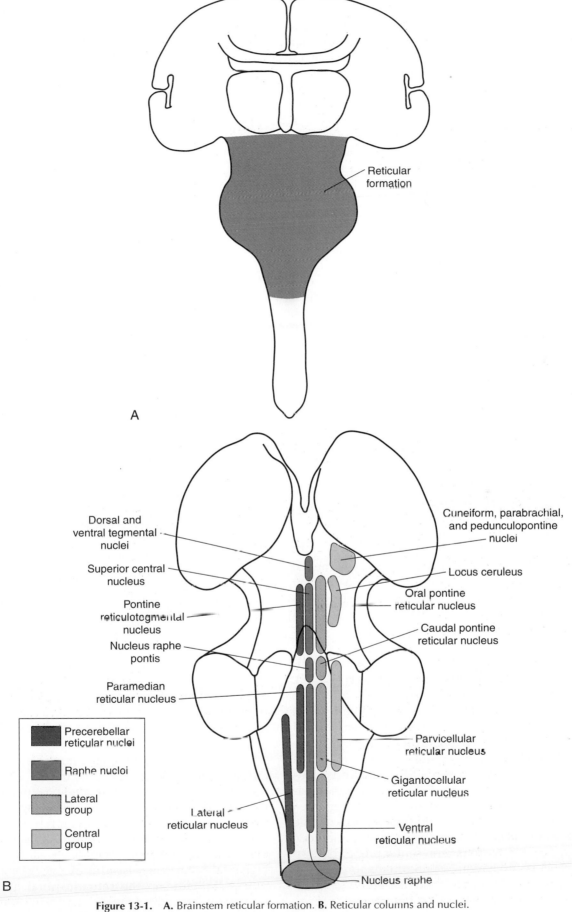

Figure 13-1. **A.** Brainstem reticular formation. **B.** Reticular columns and nuclei.

reticular formation also regulates many vital, integrated activities such as **vomiting, coughing, cardiovascular functions, swallowing,** and **respiration**, the last two being the most important for speech functions (see Chapter 16). Functionally, the reticular nuclei interact with various neuraxial structures and sensorimotor information and regulate virtually all sensorimotor activities. Arranged in four columns (Fig. 13-1B) are the specific reticular nuclei: the **reticularis gigantocellular, pontis oralis and caudalis, lateral reticular, ventral reticular, paramedial reticular, raphe, ceruleus,** and **interstitial nuclei.**

Anatomically, the most outstanding features of the reticular formation are its extensive afferent and efferent projections. These projections interact with virtually all ascending and descending pathways, thus influencing all neurally coded information at every level of the nervous system. It receives extensive input from the spinal cord, brainstem, cerebral hemispheres, cranial nerves, basal ganglia, and hypothalamus. It projects to nearly every level of the nervous system.

Reticular Motor Functions

The reticular formation controls both stereotyped and vital activities that can function independently from cortical inputs. These activities are performed unconsciously by the brainstem, as displayed by **anencephalic children**, who are born without the neocortex but can still eat, suck, expel unpleasant food, cry, yawn, swallow, vomit, breathe, sleep, awaken, and turn the eyes and head toward an object.

MUSCLE TONE REGULATION

Spinal motor output, reflexive activity, and muscle tone are under the constant control of the descending brainstem reticular networks. Muscle tone results from the action and modulation of the stretch reflex, which in a gravitational environment provides the basis for postural (antigravity) support. To control muscle tone, the brainstem reticular formation is divided into the **reticular facilitatory** and **reticular inhibitory areas** (Fig. 13-2), which directly affect the excitability of the α-LMNs. The upper and lateral part of the brainstem (midbrain, pons, and medulla) form the reticular facilitatory area. A small area in the lower and medial region of the medulla forms the reticular inhibitory area. Stimulation of the facilitatory area induces an excitation of LMNs and leads to increased tone in the muscles of the extremities. Conversely, stimulation of the inhibitory reticular area controls motor neuron activity and thus reduces muscle tone. Under normal conditions, the reticular projections to the spinal motor neurons represent a proper balance between reticular excitation (+) and inhibition (−). Lesions in the brainstem alter the reticular outputs, changing muscle tone and causing motor impairments.

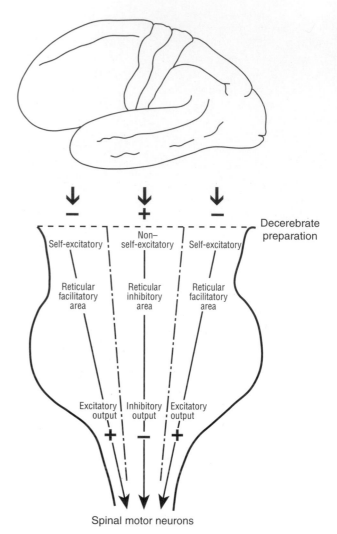

Figure 13-2. Intrinsically self-sustained reticular facilitatory areas and a non–self-sustained reticular inhibitory area.

Physiologically, the **reticular facilitatory area** is **intrinsically excitatory**; it requires no other source to drive it. Its intrinsic excitation and constant firing are controlled by the inhibitory signals that descend from the motor cortex and basal ganglia. In contrast, the **reticular inhibitory area** is **not intrinsically excitable**; it requires another source to drive it. Efferent commands from the basal ganglia and motor cortex activate this inhibitory area, whose stimulation results in the inhibition of muscle tone.

A lesion above the vestibular nucleus disconnects the cortex and basal ganglia from the brainstem reticular formation and causes an extended posture, **decerebrate rigidity**, marked by extensor posturing of all limbs. Functionally, this lesion releases the reticular facilitatory area from higher inhibitory control and simultaneously inactivates the reticular inhibitory area. Released from higher inhibitory impulses, the excessive facilitatory impulses traveling in the **reticulospinal** and **vestibulospinal tracts** induce muscle rigidity. A transection of the brainstem just below the vestibular nucleus releases the spinal cord from the tonic reticular and vestibular impulses. This leads to flaccid paralysis and hypotonia. This extreme form of hypotonia results from a complete shutdown of efferent activity from α-LMNs, as for example during the early stages of spinal shock. Together the reticular formation and vestibular complex also support the body against gravity and maintain equilibrium.

RECIPROCAL EXCITATION AND INHIBITION

Stimulation in the medial reticular formation also causes the flexor muscles of the same side of the body to contract and the extensor muscles to relax. Stimulation in the lateral reticular formation causes the extensor muscles to contract and the flexor muscles to relax. These reactions are accompanied by crossed extensor and flexor movements.

Summary of Brainstem Reticular Motor Mechanism

The reticular formation contains a network of neurons in the brainstem, including sensory and motor nuclei in addition to specialized reticular cells. The reticular formation uses integrated sensory and motor input to regulate spinal motor activity and influence muscle tone.

BASAL GANGLIA

The basal ganglia, like other structures, modify motor movements, including speech, that begin in the cortex. Current understanding of motor functions of the basal ganglia is based on observations of motor disorders resulting from lesions in them. Under normal physiological conditions, the basal ganglia are considered to help **regulate muscle tone**, **adjust associated automatic motor movements** (arm swinging during locomotion, follow-through during throwing, facial expressions, and basic emotional vocalization) and **suppress movements** extraneous to other motor activity. Basal ganglia also participate in learned reflex control, which relates to automatic aspects of skilled motor activity after overlearning and adds grace to motor movements. The motor cortex is very much involved in the early acquisition of all learned and skilled movements, many aspects of which later, with practice, become motor automatisms and require some regulating role by the basal ganglia.

The basal ganglia nuclei do not directly control the spinal motor neuron activity. Instead, they participate in motor activity by projecting their ascending input primarily to the cortical motor areas on the same side by way of the thalamus and secondarily project descending input to the contralateral brainstem reticular reflex network. There are no **LMNs** or **upper motor neurons (UMNs)** in the basal ganglia (see Chapters 11 and 14);

therefore, basal ganglia lesions do not produce paralysis; rather, they result in loss of inhibitory control and inappropriate release of patterned behaviors like chorea, dystonia, athetosis, tics, and tremor in addition to paucity of associated movements.

Basal ganglia output to the UMN is generally **inhibitory**, permitting the specific motor patterns by precise release from inhibition. Cortical influence on the basal ganglia is excitatory and discrete. Neuronal circuitry of the basal ganglia generally reduces the excitability of the corticothalamocortical circuit. Cortical activity selectively releases this basal ganglia inhibition, resulting in increased UMN output. In general, the circuitry of the basal ganglia provides species-specific learned motor control and built-in reflex control patterns as a component of highly skilled movement sequences.

The following **movement disorders** have commonly been observed from basal ganglia lesions: **involuntary motor movements** (chorea, dystonia, athetosis, ballism, and tremor), **bradykinesia** (slow movement due to a decrease in spontaneity), **hypokinesia** (movement marked with limited excursion), **altered posture**, and **changes in muscle tone**. All of these affect motor speech quality and thus are also causes of dysarthria. Basal ganglia impairments implicate one or more neurotransmitters. **Parkinson's disease** and **Huntington's chorea** are basal ganglia diseases that result from the deficient synthesis of different neurotransmitters. Both of these diseases are characterized by involuntary movements, motor speech disorders, and cognitive impairments.

Innervation Pattern

The motor organization in the basal ganglia is **contralateral** to sensory input and motor output. The basal ganglia communicate to the motor cortex on the **same side** but influence the activity of the brainstem and spinal nuclei on the **opposite side**. Consequently, the effect of a basal ganglia lesion is evident on the side of body contralateral to the lesion.

Anatomy

The basal ganglia consist of three primary subcortical nuclear masses: the **caudate nucleus**, the **putamen**, and the **globus pallidus** (Figs. 2-15 and 2-16). Various names are used to group the basal ganglia structures: **lenticular nucleus, neostriatum, striatum, corpus striatum, pallidum, and paleostriatum** (Table 2-2). Also, the **substantia nigra** and the **subthalamic** nucleus are brainstem structures that are functionally connected to the basal ganglia (Figs 3-17 and 3-18). These primary and secondary structures participate as a whole in motor functions with the motor cortex, cerebellum, and reticular formation.

The caudate nucleus is a C-shaped structure with

an elongated mass, a large head, and a narrow tail (Fig. 2-17). The head of the caudate is embedded in the lateral wall of the anterior horn of the lateral ventricles. The tail of the caudate nucleus extends along the wall of the lateral ventricle and continues along the surface of the inferior horn in the temporal lobe until it terminates in the **amygdaloid nucleus**. The putamen is lateral to the globus pallidus and is anteriorly connected with the head of the caudate nucleus; this is because of a common embryological source of development. Lateral to the putamen are the external capsule, the claustrum, and the insular cortex. The globus pallidus, which consists of medial and lateral components, is between the posterior limbs of the internal capsule and the putamen (Figs. 2-15 and 2-16).

The basal ganglia nuclei primarily synthesize five major neurotransmitters, **dopamine, γ-aminobutyric acid (GABA), acetylcholine, substance P,** and **enkephalin.**

Melanin-containing nerve cells in the **substantia nigra** secrete dopamine, an inhibitory neurotransmitter released through synaptic terminals in the striatum (caudate nucleus and putamen). Some cells in the striatum secrete acetylcholine, a local facilitatory and inhibitory neurotransmitter, which in part also regulates functions in adjacent structures, such as the thalamus and globus pallidus. Most of the striatal cells synthesize substance P and GABA, both of which inhibit the substantia nigra. GABA projections within the striatum and serotonin projections from the midbrain to the striatum further participate in the metabolic activity of the basal ganglia.

Basal Ganglia Circuitry

The anatomy and physiology of the basal ganglia can be understood better if they are viewed as a set of in-

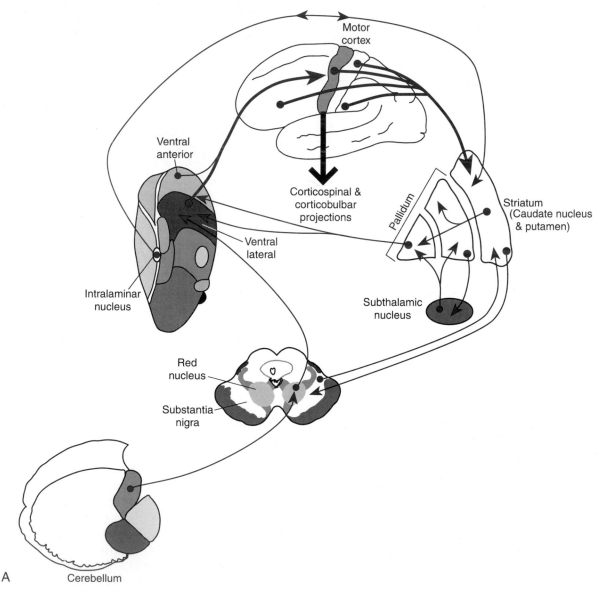

Figure 13-3. A. Inhibitory and disinhibitory projections of the basal ganglia. *(Figure continues)*

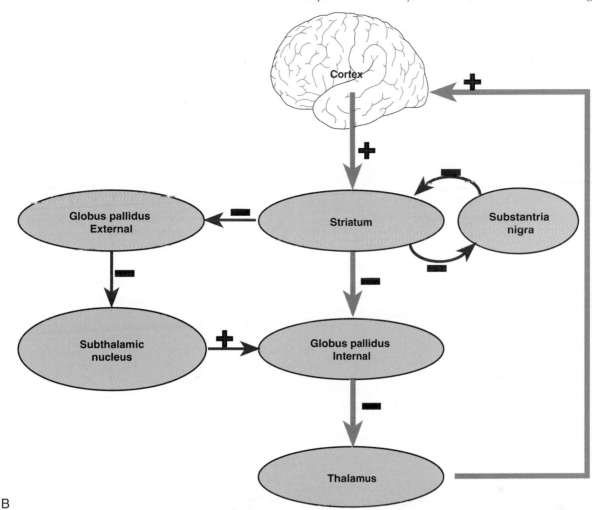

B

Figure 13-3. B. *(continued)* Afferent and efferent fibers forming basal ganglia loops. Major basal ganglia loops: *1,* Cortex → striatum → globus pallidus → thalamus (ventral lateral and ventral anterior) → cortex. *2,* Striatum → substantia nigra → striatum. *3,* Globus pallidus → subthala-mic nucleus → globus pallidus. *4,* Thalamus (intralaminar nuclei) → striatum. *5,* Cerebellum → red nucleus → thalamus (ventral lateral and ventral anterior) → cortex.

hibitory or facilitatory **interconnected loops** (Fig. 13-3). All of the afferents to the basal ganglia enter the striatum (caudate and putamen), while the basal ganglia efferents leave through the globus pallidus. The basal ganglia have major projections to the cortex via the thalamus. The basal ganglia also have direct descending projections to the contralateral reticular reflex networks.

Physiology of Basal Ganglia Circuitry

The physiology of the basal ganglia is discussed in terms of its ascending feedback to the cortex. Basal ganglia influence the activity of the motor cortex by either **inhibiting** or **disinhibiting** (release from inhibition) components of its circuitry and their projections using neurotransmitters like dopamine, GABA, acetylcholine, and substance P. This circuitry modulation regulates the net inhibitory output of the basal ganglia to the thalamus, which contains intrinsically facilitatory output to the motor cortex.

In a normal physiological state, the neostriatum (caudate and putamen) receive facilitatory (+) afferents from the **premotor cortex**, **motor cortex**, and **supplementary motor cortex** as well as the thalamic intralaminar centromedianus nucleus. Neostriatal influence on the globus pallidus (external and internal) and the substantia nigra is inhibitory (−); it is transmitted through its cholinergic, GABA, and substance P projections. The dopaminergic projections from the substantia nigra inhibit most of the striatal neurons, although facilitating some. The globus pallidus (external), which receives inhibitory (−) cholinergic projections from the striatum, is inhibitory (−) to the subthalamic nucleus, which in turn disinhibits (+) the internal globus pallidus. The globus pallidus, integrating all the extrinsic and intrinsic impulses of the basal ganglia circuitry, is inhibitory (−) to the thalamus, which integrates inhibitory (−) basal ganglia output with corrective and facilitatory (+) cerebellar output and sends intrinsically facilitatory projections to the cerebral cortex (Fig. 13-3*A*).

Anatomy of Basal Ganglia Circuitry

Four major anatomical loops, or circuits, of the basal ganglia are known; these circuits also influence motor speech functions that are important to students of communicative disorders. Each circuit makes a specific inhibitory or facilitatory contribution to cortical motor function (UMN pathway). **The first** is the largest and most central loop. It transmits motor impulses from the somatosensory cortex to the striatum, globus pallidus, and thalamus before coursing back to the neocortex. The remaining three loops are small; they act as subloops of the first basal ganglia loop. These subloops influence the motor cortex via the globus pallidus and thalamus. **The second loop** is concerned with the conduction of bidirectional projections of the striatum, connecting it to the substantia nigra. **The third loop** transmits bidirectional projections connecting the globus pallidus to the subthalamic nucleus. **The fourth loop** transmits bidirectional projections connecting thalamic intralaminar nuclei and the striatum. In addition, there is a secondary loop that connects the cerebellum with the contralateral motor cortex by way of the red nucleus and the ventrolateral thalamus. All neuronal loops receive their primary inputs from multiple cortical and subcortical areas and participate in motor activity by projecting their outputs to the neocortex and brainstem. Each of these anatomical loops has been observed to make a specific contribution in motor activity. A detailed description of the afferent and efferent projections of the basal ganglia loops follows (Fig. 13-3B).

STRIATUM

The striatum, made up of the caudate nucleus and putamen, inhibits the functions of the globus pallidus and substantia nigra.

Afferents

The striatum receives input (Figs. 13-3 and 13-4) from the cortex (corticostriate fibers), thalamus (thalamostriate fibers), and substantia nigra (nigrostriate fibers). The corticostriate fibers project from all parts of the primary and associational (premotor and supplementary) motor cortical areas to the caudate nucleus and the putamen.

The corticostriate connections are reciprocal, and there is no greater representation of the cortex in one area of the striatum than another. Projections from the sensorimotor cortex enter the caudate nucleus through the internal capsule and enter the putamen through the external capsule. There is a notable overlapping of fibers from various parts of the cortex to the striatum, with greatest projections from the prefrontal and other associational areas.

The second source of input to the striatum is the intralaminar thalamic nuclei. Facilitatory projections from

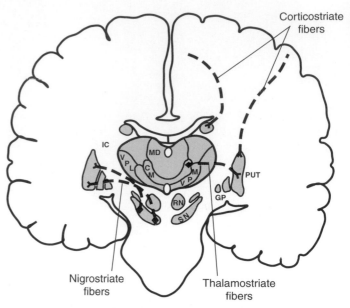

Figure 13-4. Three major striatal afferent systems: corticostriate fibers, thalamostriate fibers, and nigrostriate fibers. *CM*, centromedian; *GP*, globus pallidus; *IC*, internal capsule; *MD*, dorsomedial; *PUT*, putamen; *RN*, red nucleus; *SN*, substantia nigra; *VPL*, ventroposterolateral; *VPM*, ventroposteromedial.

the intralaminar (**intralaminar centromedian** and **parafascicular nuclei)** nuclei mediate ascending somesthetic (proprioceptive), reticular, vestibular, and auditory information to the neostriatum. This provides important feedback with respect to cortical arousal and physiological preparedness in fine-tuning basal ganglia pathways.

The third source of input to the striatum is from the substantia nigra. Nigrostriate fibers from the **pars compacta region** of the substantia nigra have axonal terminals filled with dopamine, which inhibit some striatal functions. Substantia nigra lesions, which deplete dopamine production, are thought to cause the motor impairments associated with Parkinson's disease.

Efferents

The striate efferent fibers radiate from the putamen (Fig. 13-3) to the globus pallidus (striatopallidal fibers); their influence is inhibitory to the globus pallidus. Striatopallidal fibers, which originate from the GABA-ergic and acetylcholinergic neurons in the striatum, terminate in either the external or internal segments of the globus pallidus. The second striatal efferent projection is to the substantia nigra. Striatonigral fibers, also inhibitory, terminate in the **pars reticulata** region of the substantia nigra. The striatonigral fibers, which include fibers from both the caudate nucleus and putamen, transmit GABA and substance P through their terminals. The striatonigral and nigrostriatal fibers, both inhibitory, are reciprocal in organization.

GLOBUS PALLIDUS

The globus pallidus consists of external and internal components (Fig. 13-3).

Afferents

Afferents entering the globus pallidus arise primarily from the striatum (inhibitory) and the subthalamic nucleus (facilitatory). Most striatal output to the thalamus travels via the globus pallidus.

Efferents

As the output nucleus of the basal ganglia, the globus pallidus projects to the thalamus via the **pallidothalamic fiber bundle** and **pallidosubthalamic fiber bundle**.

The major basal ganglia outputs, which are inhibitory, arise from the internal segment of the globus pallidus and terminate in the **ventrolateral** and **ventroanterior nuclei** of the thalamus (see Chapter 6). These pallidal projections are transmitted through two fasciculi, the **ansa lenticularis** and the **lenticular fasciculus**. Three anatomical structures that pertain to the pallidothalamic fibers can often be confusing: **field H of Forel** (prerubral area), **field H_1 of Forel**, and **field H_2 of Forel**. These three fields of H are where the pallidothalamic fibers cross the internal capsule, turn laterally to move upward, and enter the thalamus (Fig. 13-5). Fibers of the ansa lenticularis loop around the internal capsule and enter field H of Forel (prerubral field) in the subthalamic region. They turn rostrally and laterally, forming part of the thalamic fasciculus, in field H_1 of Forel. Conversely, the lenticular fasciculus fibers pass through the internal capsule and appear as field H_2 of Forel. The lenticular fasciculus fibers join the ansa lenticularis fibers at field H_1 of Forel to form the thalamic fasciculus. The thalamic fasciculus fibers terminate in the ventrolateral nucleus of thalamus, which projects to the motor cortex. The ventrolateral and anterior thalamic nuclei also receive cerebellocortical projections from the dentate nucleus of the cerebellum. Thus, at the thalamic level, the cerebellocortical projections intermingle with the basal ganglia projections to the cortex.

The fibers from the external region of the globus pallidus also send inhibitory projections to the subthalamic nucleus (Figs. 13-3 and 13-6). In addition, descending basal ganglia output travel to the contralateral reticular reflex network in the midbrain tegmentum. Interruption of these projections to the reticular network has been associated with disorders of associated movements, such as arm swinging during locomotion and follow-through during throwing.

SUBTHALAMUS

The subthalamus is ventral to the thalamus and between the internal capsule and hypothalamus. It contains the **subthalamic nucleus,** the **zona incerta**, and the tegmental fields of Forel (field H of Forel). The subthalamic nucleus lies in the inner surface of the internal capsule and above the medial part of the substantia nigra (Figs. 3-18 and 3-23). Its dysfunction is associated

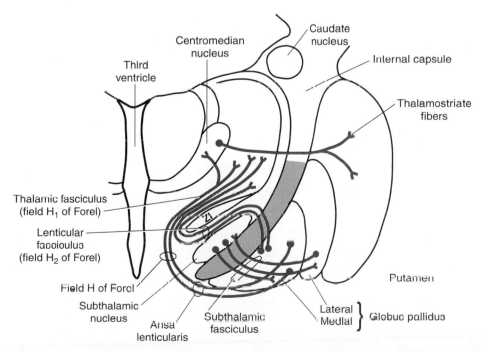

Figure 13-5. Origin and course of pallidothalamic (ansa lenticularis and lenticular fasciculus) projections. Fibers of ansa lenticularis travel around internal capsule and enter the prerubral field (field H of Forel). Fibers of lenticular fasciculus leave inner globus pallidus and course through field H_2 of Forel and join fibers of ansa lenticularis to form thalamic fasciculus (field H_1 of Forel). Thalamic fasciculus terminates in ventrolateral and ventral anterior nuclei of thalamus.

with ballism, with signs appearing on the side opposite to the lesion.

Afferents

The basal ganglia afferents to the subthalamic nucleus emerge from the external segment of the globus pallidus (Figs. 13-3 and 13-6). Additional projections come from the precentral motor cortex and the prefrontal area.

Efferents

Subthalamic efferents include facilitatory projections, primarily to the globus pallidus (Figs. 13-3 and 13-6) and secondarily to the substantia nigra. With its efferent projections, the subthalamic nucleus can modulate all output from the striatal system.

SUBSTANTIA NIGRA

The substantia nigra, a mesencephalic horizontal band of neurons, consists of the **pars compacta** and **pars reticulata** regions. The pars compacta region is packed with dark-pigmented neuromelanin-containing cells that produce dopamine or its precursors and inhibit striatal functions.

Afferents

The major input to the substantia nigra comes from the striatum via the striatonigral fibers that inhibit its functioning (Fig. 13-3).

Efferents

The substantia nigra projects back to the striatum through its terminals that contain dopamine, which inhibits most of the striatal functioning (Figs. 13-3 and 13-4). Its afferent and efferent projections involve different neurotransmitters.

Basal Ganglia Neurotransmitters

The function of the basal ganglia depends on balanced interaction involving several major neurotransmitters: **dopamine, acetylcholine, GABA, enkephalin,** and **substance P**. All of these neurotransmitters are **inhibitory** and are vital to regulation of motor movements. Dopaminergic neurons from the substantia nigra project to the caudate nucleus and render inhibitory influence on cholinergic (acetylcholine) striatal neurons. In turn, the cholinergic striatal neurons, which are primarily inhibitory, synapse on striatal GABA neurons. GABA fibers, which are also inhibitory, project intrinsically to the basal ganglia and the substantia nigra, completing the circuitry between the substantia nigra and the basal ganglia. Terminals with substance P, another basal ganglia inhibitory neurotransmitter, project to the substantia nigra from the basal ganglia. Impairment within a neurotransmitter system results in specific **movement disorders**, such as Parkinson's disease and Huntington's chorea. The role of Enkephalin in movement is not clear. Enkephalin projections in the basal ganglia and in surrounding structures like thalamus pri-

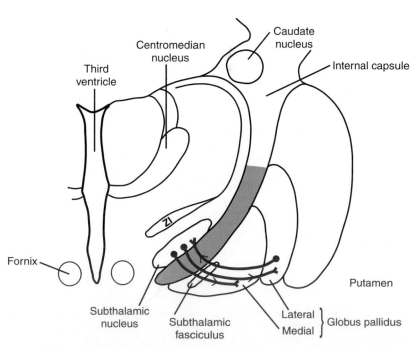

Figure 13-6.   Pallidal projections to subthalamic nucleus and efferent projection from subthalamic nucleus.

marily participate in controlling pain. One way it is done is by suppressing the activity of substance P, a neurotransmitter stimulating pain perception.

Clinical Consideration of Basal Ganglia

The basal ganglia serve an important role in **motor activity** and help regulate mood and personality. The involvement of various neurotransmitters differentially affects the quality of motor functions. Basal ganglia disease results in loss of inhibitory control and inappropriate release of patterned behavior, which includes **dyskinesia** (involuntary movements, such as tremor at rest, chorea, athetosis, dystonia, and ballism), **bradykinesia** (slow movement), **hypokinesia** (movements with limited range), **disturbance of posture**, and **altered muscle tone** (Table 13-1).

The involuntary movements of dyskinesia interrupt the motor activities of the speech musculature (dysarthria) and the limbs. At this time, only limited chemical and surgical treatment is available for basal ganglia disorders; the goal of such treatments is to restore the inhibitory function of the basal ganglia. While supplementing dopamine secretion with L-dopa has been used with limited success, adrenal medulla transplant with subcortical stimulation appears to be an additional avenue of treatment and is undergoing active investigation.

ATHETOSIS

Athetosis refers to the slow, involuntary writhing of predominantly axial and speech muscles accompanied by varying degrees of hypertonia. Athetosis of the buccofacial muscles affects motor speech and results in dysarthria. These movements occur in a sequence, so that they blend together to form a continuous action. A typical example of athetosis is torsion of the hand, arm, neck, shoulder, and pelvic girdle. Athetotic movements commonly occur after a lesion involving the globus pal-

lidus, its descending projections to the reticular network, or both.

BALLISM

Ballism is characterized by violent, forceful flinging movements of the arms and legs. It may also involve the neck musculature. Ballism, the most violent form of dyskinesia, usually involves one side of the body (hemiballism) and is associated with lesions in the subthalamic nucleus contralateral to the side with the dyskinesia.

CHOREA

Chorea is a series of rhythmic involuntary movements that appear to be graceful. The choreic movements occur predominantly in the distal extremities and muscles of the face, tongue, and pharynx. Chorea affects swallowing and speech and induces hypotonia in muscles. There are two common extrapyramidal diseases that characterize chorea: **Sydenham's chorea** and **Huntington's chorea**. Sydenham's chorea begins in childhood. It is a postinfectious condition appearing several months after a streptococcal infection with subsequent rheumatic fever. The clinical characteristics, which are purposeless involuntary contractions of muscles in the distal limbs, hypotonia, and emotional lability, become apparent between ages 5 and 13 years. Improvement occurs over weeks or months, and exacerbations of the disease can occur without recurrence of infection.

Huntington's chorea, a more common clinical condition, is inherited through an autosomal dominant gene. Its symptoms usually appear in the third decade of life. Huntington's chorea is a progressive condition characterized by choreic movements, cognitive deficits (dementia), dysarthric speech, and personality and mood changes. It is associated with degenerative changes in the caudate nucleus and frontal and parietal lobes. With no cure or treatment, it invariably leads to death.

TREMORS

Tremor, the most common form of dyskinesia, consists of constantly alternating motor activity in one or more parts of the body. The tremor, which results from the alternate contraction of opposing muscles, occurs in a rhythmic sequence of four to six contractions per second. Clinically, tremors are divided between **resting** and **intentional**, or **action**, **types**. Resting tremor, associated with Parkinson's disease, results from substantia nigra lesions. Intentional, or action, tremor is evident during voluntary movements and ceases during resting states. Intentional tremor is associated with cerebellar lesions.

Electrically, tremor may be considered a low-threshold discharging system. This is supported by clinical observations demonstrating the elimination of ab-

Table 13-1.   Involuntary Movement Disorders and Associated Lesion Sites

Clinical Lesion Site	Involuntary Movements
Diffuse lesions in globus pallidus and corpus striatum	Athetosis: slow twisting movements in muscles of upper extremities
Degenerative changes or infarction in subthalamic nucleus	Ballism: wild flinging movements that usually involve one side of body
Striatal lesions primarily involving caudate nucleus	Chorea: rhythmic, quick involuntary movements of muscles in distal extremities
Diffuse basal ganglia pathology	Dyskinesia: accessory movements associated with a desired motor act
Degenerative changes in substantia nigra	Tremor: rhythmic pill-rolling movements of fingers at rest accompanied by akinesia and rigidity

normal discharges, either by a lesion or through therapeutic electrical stimulation. Common symptoms associated with tremor include a masked face, infrequent blinking, slow movement, disturbed equilibrium, stooped posture, impaired speech, and impaired swallowing. Dyskinetic movements disappear in sleep during the suppression of the brainstem reticular activating system. Anxiety exaggerates dyskinetic movements.

Associated Movement Disorders

Loss of basal ganglia inhibition through direct descending projections to the reticular network at least in part affects automatic aspects of the associated movements, which include arm swinging during locomotion, follow-through in club swinging, facial expressions, and emotional vocalization.

Basal Ganglia Diseases

PARKINSON'S DISEASE

James Parkinson, a British physician, first described Parkinson's disease, the best-understood basal ganglia disease, in 1817. He described it as a "progressive condition marked with involuntary tremulous motion with lessened muscular power . . . with a propensity to bend the trunk forward and to pass from a walking to a running phase." However, sensation and intelligence were not found to be impaired. Originally called paralysis agitans, Parkinson's disease has these cardinal symptoms: tremor at rest, **cogwheel muscular rigidity** (muscles respond with cogwheel-like jerks to the use of constant force in bending the limb), **bradykinesia** (slowed execution of body movements), **akinesia** (slow beginning or inability to initiate a movement), **shuffling gate**, **expressionless face**, **flexed posture**, and **dysarthria**. Diagnosis is made on clinical grounds, usually in the sixth decade, with a peak at 75 to 84 years of age. The frequency of Parkinson's disease is approximately 160 cases per 100,000 in the United States, and it affects men and women in equal proportions.

Parkinsonian symptoms relate to pathological changes in the dopamine-producing nerve cells in the pars compacta region of the substantia nigra. Degeneration or depigmentation of these cells causes a dopamine deficiency. Patients with Parkinson's disease lose nigral dopaminergic neurons that normally manufacture dopamine and send it to the striatum. Because dopamine acts as an inhibitory neurotransmitter, the insufficient production of dopamine is interpreted as a state of disinhibition. Consequently, striatal abnormal discharges are released to generate the parkinsonian dyskinesia.

Dopamine deficiency is overcome by giving the patient large quantities of L-dopa, a biosynthetic precursor of dopamine. This drug stimulates the synthesis of dopamine in surviving cells of the substantia nigra and avails to the striatum. It was first thought that L-dopa would ameliorate the symptoms, arrest the disease, and even revert some of the degenerative changes. However, L-dopa was found only to control some symptoms for a few years. It does not arrest or revert the degeneration of the dopaminergic nigral cells. In Parkinsonism, as many as 90% of the dopaminergic neurons are degenerated or partially degenerated. The few remaining cells may compensate if large amounts of L-dopa can bypass the rate-limiting enzyme for dopamine. If not, dopa decarboxylase, which is not specific for dopaminergic neurons, may synthesize dopamine from nondopaminergic cells such as serotonergic cells, which are known to project to the basal ganglia.

Tardive dyskinesia is one of the complications associated with excessive L-dopa treatment of Parkinson's disease. It is characterized by facial and lingual involuntary movements. Once it emerges, this dyskinesia does not vanish with discontinuation of the L-dopa treatment. Dyskinesia of facial and lingual movements, similar to that seen in patients with Parkinson's disease who have had long-term L-dopa therapy, can also occur in patients who receive antipsychotic drugs such as trifluoperazine and haloperidol. The mechanism of action is not well understood; however, dopaminergic cells are blocked by these drugs, altering the balance between the intrastriatal dopaminergic, cholinergic, and GABA-ergic systems.

HUNTINGTON'S CHOREA

Huntington's chorea is another well-understood disease of the basal ganglia. George Huntington, an American physician, first described it in 1872. Huntington, his father, and his grandfather observed the same symptoms in members of successive generations of the same families. Huntington's disease has the following four characteristics: *hereditary transmission*, *onset in adult age*, *chorea*, and *cognitive deficits* (dementia). Huntington's chorea is inherited as an autosomal dominant disease in which each offspring of a carrier parent has a 50% chance of inheriting and developing the disorder (see Chapter 20). Signs of the disease that first appear around the third decade include **forgetfulness**, **personality changes**, and **clumsiness in motor movements**. The **choreiform movements** gradually increase. The cognitive deficits lead to the subcortical type of dementia. Speech becomes dysarthric and gradually deteriorates into muteness. The frequency of Huntington's chorea is about 5 cases per 100,000 in the United States, and it affects men and women in equal proportions.

Patients exhibit nonspecific atrophy primarily in the caudate nucleus and prefrontal and parietal lobes. The involvement of the caudate nucleus in Huntington's chorea leads to degeneration of intrinsic striatal cholinergic and striatonigral GABA-ergic neurons. Enzymes that biosynthesize acetylcholine and GABA are also decreased, contributing to further loss of GABA inhibition. Subsequent to the loss of striatonigral inhibition is disinhibition of dopaminergic cells in the substantia nigra. The nigrostriatal projections primarily inhibit pallidal output to the thalamus, resulting in the choreic movements of Huntington's disease. If a patient with Huntington's disease is given L-dopa, the choreic movements get worse. Furthermore, patients with Parkinson's disease who are given too much L-dopa develop choreic, athetotic, and dystonic movements, as previously discussed. Involuntary movements are caused by an imbalance from lesions anywhere along the dopaminergic–cholinergic–GABA-ergic loop.

WILSON'S DISEASE: HEPATOLENTICULAR DEGENERATION

Wilson's disease is a progressive disease of early life, with the onset of clinical manifestations between 10 and 25 years of age. It results from a disorder of copper metabolism leading to the degeneration of internal brain regions, particularly the basal ganglia, and to cirrhosis (damage to and degeneration of hepatic cells) of the liver. First investigated in the 1880s, it is clinically characterized by **increased muscular rigidity**, **tremor**, **dysarthric speech**, and **progressive dementia**. Corneal pigmentation (Kayser-Fleischer ring) is perhaps the most important diagnostic attribute of Wilson's disease. It has been related to autosomal recessive inheritance.

Basal Ganglia and Psychiatric Disorders

The movement disorders related to neuropathologies in basal ganglia are also known to have psychiatric concomitants. For example, there is a high incidence of depression in patients with Parkinson's disease; similarly, patients with Huntington's chorea exhibit a high suicide rate along with personality and mood disorders. Research has revealed important analogies between the neurotransmitter dysfunctions in movement disorders and in psychiatric illnesses such as schizophrenia and depression. Furthermore, a wide range of motor disorders, including rigidity, dystonias, and tardive dyskinesia, are known to result from the use of neuroleptic medications. These medications used for treating psychiatric conditions cause dysfunction of the striatal dopaminergic system, by either blocking or changing the sensitivity of dopaminergic receptors, which results in dyskinesias.

The discovery of the Huntington's gene, which is localized to chromosome 4, has revealed how molecular genetics is involved with the mind–body relationship. This gene encodes the protein huntingtin, which gradually accumulates and damages dopaminergic receptors with its accumulation. Identification of the gene has contributed to the development of the genetic test to diagnose Huntington's disease prenatally or before symptoms appear.

Summary of Basal Ganglia

The basal ganglia include a series of interconnected anatomical loops that are functionally contiguous with the thalamus and neocortex. The interconnected loops are the sites of reverberating circuits of electrical currents sustaining and modulating motor activity. The subthalamic nuclei and rostral brainstem also tie into the circuit, contributing to its stability. Lesions in one or more components of the system result in dyskinesias of varying types. Ballism is the only dyskinesia known to be produced by a single lesion in the subthalamic nucleus. The rest of the dyskinesias seem to be associated with diffuse lesions in different parts of the system. The neurotransmitter dopamine is deficient in parkinsonism owing to the degeneration of the substantia nigra dopaminergic cells that project to the striatum. Dopamine replacement therapy and surgical intervention have been helpful in relieving parkinsonian tremors, but neither is a cure. In recent years, chronic electrical stimulation in the thalamus was also found to control some forms of dyskinesia, such as Parkinson's disease. Many basal ganglia disorders cause significant cognitive deficits.

Case Studies

Patient One

A 60-year-old woman had sudden partial paralysis (weakness or paresis) in her left leg while sewing. Within 24 hours the paralysis was replaced by involuntary movements in her leg and arm. She was admitted to a hospital. On testing, she exhibited the following signs:

- Wild flinging movements of the left arm and leg that gradually became more intense
- Flaccid muscle tone

Magnetic resonance imaging revealed an infarct in the right subthalamic nucleus. The flinging movements gradually became more intense. Several weeks of conservative therapy did not decrease the movements, so an electrolytic lesion was stereotactically placed in the right subthalamic nucleus, relieving the dyskinesia. She could then walk and eventually feed herself, and there were no complications.

Question: Can you explain how the infarct of the subthalamic nucleus affects the basal ganglia mechanism?

Discussion: The subthalamic nucleus renders inhibitory influence on the globus pallidus. The irritative infarct impaired the smooth flow of electrical impulses from the basal ganglia, resulting in hemiballism in the limbs contralateral to the lesion site.

Patient Two

A 64-year-old salesperson saw his physician after he began having muscle rigidity and mild involuntary movements in his hands. This tired him and affected his ability to work. Examination revealed the following:

- Expressionless, tense face
- Impaired ability to initiate a movement
- Pill-rolling tremor in the hands

- Shuffling gait
- Dysarthric speech (his words were uttered quickly)
- Somewhat stooped posture

Question: Based on these characteristics, the physician suspected Parkinson's disease. Can you identify the brain site associated with this condition?

Discussion: Parkinson's disease, the most commonly studied basal ganglia disease, results from a bilateral degeneration of the substantia nigra. Its clinical symptoms include tremor at rest, cogwheel muscular rigidity, bradykinesia (slowed execution of body movements), akinesia (slow beginning or inability to initiate a movement), shuffling gate, expressionless face, flexed posture, and dysarthria. The muscle rigidity in Parkinson's disease is commonly treated with L-dopa, a dopamine replacement drug.

Patient Three

A 37-year-old schoolteacher began to have limb weakness and uncontrollable clumsiness in his movements. He also exhibited dysarthric speech, some confusion, and mild cognitive impairments. This changed his personality, and he gradually became a recluse. His wife took him to the family doctor, who made the following observations:

- Postural imbalance
- Mild weakness of the upper and lower limbs
- Hypotonia and hyporeflexia
- Choreic movements involving the shoulders, head, and tongue
- Dysarthria
- Father and grandmother who died young with similar symptoms, including dementia

Based on these characteristics, the patient's age, and the family history, the physician suspected Huntington's chorea.

Question: What characteristics helped the physician make this diagnosis?

Discussion: Huntington's chorea, an autosomal dominant disease, has four clinical characteristics: heredity, onset in early adult age, chorea, and cognitive deficits (dementia). Personality changes and mood disorders, including severe depression, are also present. This neurological condition is associated with degenerative changes in the corpus striatum (putamen and caudate nucleus) followed by changes in other cortical areas.

SUMMARY

Both the reticular formation and basal ganglia play important roles in motor activity. The reticular formation uses integrated sensory and motor input to regulate spinal motor activity and influence muscle tone. The basal ganglia, consisting of a series of interconnected anatomical loops, is the site of reverberating circuits of electrical currents that sustain and modulate motor activity. Further, the abnormalties of neurotransmitters in the basal ganglia also produce specific dyskinetic conditions, such as Parkinson's disease and Huntington's chorea.

Technical Terms

acetylcholine
akinesia
athetosis

autosomal dominance
ballism
basal ganglia

bradykinesia
chorea
cogwheel rigidity
decerebrate rigidity
dopamine

GABA-ergic neurons
reticular formation
tardive dyskinesia
tremor
vasomotor center

Review Questions

1. Define the following terms:

   acetylcholine
   akinesia
   athetosis
   autosomal dominance
   ballism
   basal ganglia
   bradykinesia
   chorea

   cogwheel rigidity
   decerebrate rigidity
   dopamine
   GABA-ergic neurons
   reticular formation
   tardive dyskinesia
   tremor

2. Describe the mechanism of reticular control of muscle tone and explain how its disorder can cause muscle rigidity.
3. Describe the anatomy of the basal ganglia with a labeled diagram.
4. Discuss the role of the basal ganglia in motor functions.
5. Illustrate the major basal ganglia feedback loops with a labeled diagram. Specifically, describe afferent and efferent projections of the caudate nucleus, globus pallidus, substantia nigra, subthalamic nucleus, and thalamus.
6. Where in the subcortical region is the cerebellar output to the cortex integrated with basal ganglia projections to brain?
7. Describe the suggested pathophysiologies of athetosis, ballism, chorea, dyskinesia, and tremor.
8. Describe the functions of basal ganglia neurotransmitters and discuss how an imbalance of these neurotransmitters results in the genesis of Parkinson's and Huntington's diseases.
9. Differentiate between and describe the symptoms of Huntington's disease and Parkinson's disease.
10. A 50-year-old man saw his doctor because of involuntary movements in his left arm. On examination, the involuntary movements were diagnosed to be violent and flinging. The muscles were hypotonic between the movements. A lesion in which of the basal ganglia structures might account for the left ballism?
11. What hereditary disease with onset in adult life is characterized by progressive choreoathetosis and mental deterioration?
12. Provide four signs of dysfunctioning in the basal ganglia, and identify the associated structures.
13. Describe the functions and characteristics of the substantia nigra.
14. Projections to the corpus striatum come from which structures?
15. Match the following numbered definitions to the associated lettered term.

    i. wild, flinging movements that usually involve one side of the body
    ii. rhythmic pill-rolling movements of fingers at rest accompanied by akinesia and rigidity
    iii. rhythmic, quick, involuntary movements of muscles in distal extremities
    iv. accessory movements associated with a desired motor act
    v. slow twisting movements in muscles of upper extremities

    a. athetosis
    b. chorea
    c. ballism
    d. dyskinesia
    e. tremor

14

Motor System 4: Motor Cortex

Learning Objectives

After studying this chapter, students should be able to do the following:

- Discuss the roles in motor movements of the primary motor cortex and surrounding cortical area
- Describe the functions of corticospinal and corticobulbar pathways
- Discuss the bilateral cortical innervation of speech-related cranial nerve nuclei
- Describe the location of upper motor neurons
- Explain the pathophysiology and signs of upper motor neuron syndrome
- Differentiate between upper motor neuron and lower motor neuron syndromes
- Explain the pathophysiology of spastic hemiplegia
- Discuss the pathophysiology of pseudobulbar palsy and describe its effects on speech muscles
- Discuss the pathophysiology of alternating hemiplegia and describe its clinical symptoms

Up to this point, motor functions have been discussed in relation to the **spinal cord, cerebellum, brainstem reticular formation**, and **basal ganglia**. These structures represent various motor organizational levels that do not initiate volitional motor movements on their own but instead act on efferent information that originates in the cerebral cortex and/or sensory information derived from various parts of the body and the environment.

The efferent impulses from the primary motor cortex activate spinal motor neurons and induce contraction of specific muscles; cortical motor projections manipulate discrete and skilled motor movements, such as finger tapping, dancing, running, and speaking. In addition to the activation of lower motor neurons (LMN) in the brainstem and spinal cord, the **motor cortex**, in conjunction with the **premotor, prefrontal, sensory**, and

associational cortices, participates in the planning of motor activity. This planning includes integration of sensory information regarding what and where the object is, calculation of the extent of muscle movements, determination of body parts that must be recruited, and generation of efferent signals for regulating specific muscles. The cerebral motor cortex executes movements with constant and updated feedback to and from the adjacent cortical and subcortical areas.

ANATOMY OF MOTOR CORTEX

The primary motor cortex is in the precentral gyrus of the frontal lobe (Figs. 2-5 and 14-1), which is rostral to the **central sulcus**. The primary motor cortex (Brodmann area 4) contains large **Betz cells**, which are unique to this area and are important in voluntary motor movement. A very low intensity of electric stimulation can evoke motor acts from this cortical area. The motor representation (**motor homunculus**) of the body is organized in the primary motor cortex. The face, speech muscles, and head are represented in the lower third of the motor cortex near the **sylvian fissure**; the arms and trunk relate to the upper motor cortical region (Fig. 14-1A); and the legs are in the midsagittal surface of the motor cortex (Fig. 14-1B). In comparison, the face and mouth occupy a large cortical area caudal to the premotor area. This dominant representation of the face and mouth in the human corresponds to the unique elaborate apparatus required for speech, an important point for professionals in communicative disorders.

The motor neural impulses that travel in the **pyramidal tract** originate from the three cortical regions (Fig. 14-2): **primary motor cortex, premotor cortex**, and **primary sensory cortex**. In the human, only about 25 to 30% of the pyramidal tract fibers are known to arise from the primary motor cortex (Brodmann area 4). Of those, only

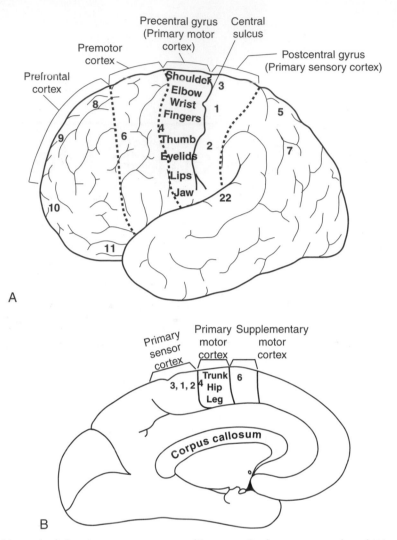

Figure 14-1.   Human body in primary motor cortex and important Brodmann areas on lateral (**A**) and medial (**B**) brain surfaces.

2% come from the large Betz cells. The Betz cells are pyramidal cells whose long axons extend to the lower limbs and thus require large cell bodies for metabolic support. There are relatively few large motor cells because the human has a much greater need of the shorter cortical projections to the cranial nerve nuclei (corticobulbar projections) and upper limb levels in the cord (corticospinal projections). Therefore, the small neurons in the motor cortex give rise to the remaining pyramidal fibers. Approximately 30% of the remaining descending pyramidal fibers arise from the premotor cortex (Brodmann area 6), which is rostral to the motor cortex and extends midsagittally as the supplementary motor area (Fig. 14-1B). The remaining 40% of the motor fibers arise from the primary sensory cortex (Brodmann areas 3, 1, and 2) in the parietal lobe (Figs. 14-1 and 14-2), and the adjacent somatosensory association cortex (Brodmann areas 5 and 7).

The motor cortex is organized into columns of neurons arranged vertically from the surface into the depth of the cortex. Each single column provides circuitry responsible for directing a group of muscles. Thus, the simultaneous and sequential organization of fine movement patterns, but not the individual muscles, are considered to be organized in the motor cortex. Direct control from the cortex allows higher primates, including humans, to control individual and grouped proximal and distal muscles to perform specific movements, such as finger movement.

This cortical motor system is maintained and enhanced by a thalamocortical excitatory loop, which itself is modulated by the intrinsic inhibitory basal ganglia functions (see Chapter 13) and excitatory afferents from the cerebellum (see Chapter 12). To maintain the precision, accuracy, smoothness, and sequential nature of the motor activity, the motor cortex depends on constant feedback from the adjacent cortical and subcortical regions. The cortical input includes afferents from the premotor cortex (Brodmann area 6), which with input from the prefrontal cortex (Brodmann areas 8, 9, and 10) is

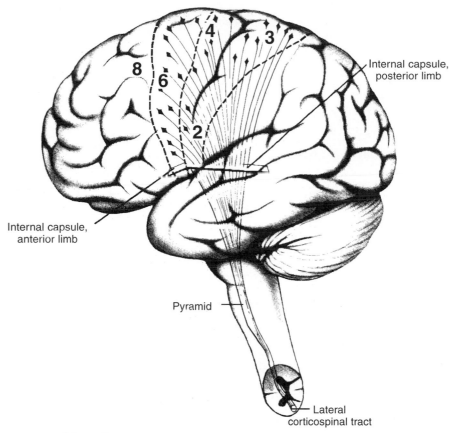

Figure 14-2. Pyramidal tract fibers originating from sensorimotor cortex, including premotor, motor, and sensory cortical areas. Numbers refer to Brodmann areas.

concerned with setting up a motor plan of a skilled movement pattern involving specific limbs. The prefrontal cortex, the site of reasoning, thinking, and planning, receives inputs from the occipital, parietal, and temporal lobes. The supplementary motor cortex (Brodmann area 6) is known to regulate planning and bilateral aspects of motor pattern control. Projections from the somesthetic cortex (Brodmann areas 3,1, and 2) modulate sensory feedback, whereas fibers from the association somesthetic cortex (Brodmann areas 5 and 7) regulate higher-order spatial aspects of the sensorimotor plan.

Much of a highly skilled movement is learned through a background of species-specific built-in capabilities. The sensory feedback aspects of the sensorimotor cortex and corticospinal projections to the spinal cord contribute to the process of motor learning. Once a skilled movement pattern is well learned, these feedback systems are usually not required unless a deterrent to the movement is encountered.

Lesions of the motor cortex and its descending fibers (upper motor neuron, or UMN) result in paralysis and slowed movement that interrupt voluntary and precise motor control, especially of distal limb muscles used in fine manipulative skills and muscles involved in vo-

cal and facial expression in the acute stage. However, there can be a gradual return of gross function.

INNERVATION PATTERN

The motor cortex is organized **contralateral** to output and input. The short (corticobulbar) and long (corticospinal) efferent projections from the motor cortex cross the midline to innervate **contralateral** cranial nerve and spinal output nuclei. Consequently, a lesion of the motor fibers above the pyramidal decussation produces clinical signs **contralateral** to the locus of damage. In the case of a lesion below the pyramidal decussation in the caudal medulla, spinal UMN and LMN clinical signs are **ipsilateral** to the side of the damage.

DESCENDING PATHWAYS

Impulses from the motor cortex to the LMNs travel on one of two direct pathways (Fig. 14-3): the **corticospinal tract** or the **corticobulbar tract**. The corticospinal tract, which contains approximately 30% of the motor fibers, mediates voluntary movements of the skeletal muscles through the spinal α-motor neurons. The corticobulbar tract, which contains about 70% of motor fibers, controls the facial and associated muscles through

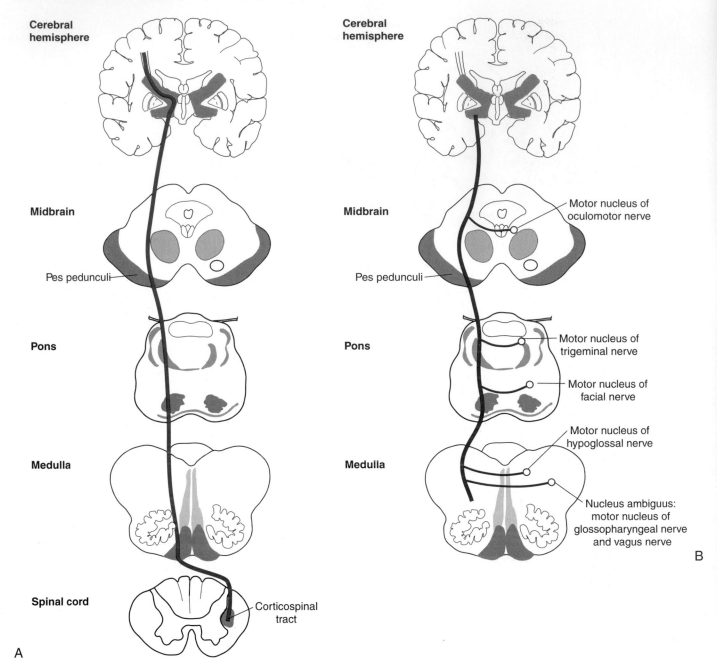

Figure 14-3. Origin and course of pyramidal fibers. **A.** Corticospinal fibers projecting to spinal motor nuclei. **B.** Corticobulbar fibers projecting to motor nuclei of cranial nerves. Most motor nuclei of cranial nerves receive motor commands from contralateral motor cortex; motor nucleus for upper face and tongue is known to receive bilateral projections.

activation of cranial nerve nuclei in the brainstem. Virtually all efferent fibers in both tracts cross the midline before synapsing upon their respective motor neurons.

Corticospinal Tract

The corticospinal fibers arise from the upper two-thirds of the primary motor cortex (precentral gyrus), premotor cortex, and sensory cortex. These fibers travel through the **corona radiata**, then descend through the posterior limb of the **internal capsule** of the forebrain. Later they run through the midbrain **pes pedunculi**. These descending fibers separate into diffuse fascicles in the pons, mingling with the pontine nuclei. Some fibers terminate in the pontine nuclei, while the rest continue to the medulla to form the **pyramids** (source of the term pyramidal tract) before crossing at the caudal end of the medulla. After crossing, the motor fibers descend into the **lateral corticospinal tract** (Figs. 14-2, 14-3A), named after the location of these fibers in the lateral funiculus of the spinal cord. Through the fibers of the lateral corticospinal tract, the motor cortex participates in digital control of the skeletal muscles of the distal limbs (fingers and toes) required for fine manipulative skills.

An uncrossed smaller fasciculus of motor fibers (**anterior corticospinal tract**) descends in the ventral funiculus of the spinal cord, which eventually crosses the midline before synapsing on the α-motor neurons (Fig. 11-7). The anterior corticospinal tract fibers are known to control the proximal axial and girdle muscles, which provide the postural platform required for digital skilled movements.

The UMN fibers of the lateral corticospinal tract terminate on the interneurons and α-motor neurons (LMNs) in the spinal anterior gray horns to initiate movements. Some of the fibers also terminate on γ-motor neurons, providing a means for the motor cortex to modulate the stretch reflex. This ensures an appropriate level of tone in the muscles in which the α-LMNs are influenced to provide the motor control. Some fibers also synapse on the sensory cells in the dorsal gray horns through which the cortex modulates somesthetic feedback data, which is largely in the form of error messages of deviations from what the premotor cortex planned and the motor cortex actuated. On its way to the spinal motor neurons, the corticospinal tract also emits multiple collaterals to the basal ganglia, thalamus, brainstem reticular formation, and pontine nuclei. The axonal processes of the LMNs exit at all levels of the spinal cord, terminating in the skeletal muscles.

Corticobulbar Tract

The corticobulbar fibers are similar to the fibers of the corticospinal tract in terms of their function of fine motor control. However, they exclusively control the muscles of the head and face through cranial nerves. The corticobulbar fibers arise from the lower third of the motor cortex and adjacent area, travel through the internal capsule and pes pedunculi, and cross the midline in the brainstem before synapsing on the cranial LMNs (Fig. 14-3B). The corticobulbar regulation of some cranial nerve LMNs is bilateral (see Chapter 15). The corticobulbar fibers from the left motor cortex innervate both the left and right motor nuclei of some of the cranial nerves. Similarly, projections from the right motor cortex control the functioning of some cranial nerve nuclei on both sides, which include the nuclei of the **trigeminal, facial, vagus**, and **glossopharyngeal nerves**.

An important clinical point is that because muscles of the jaw, larynx, and upper face receive projections from the bilateral motor cortices, a unilateral cortical lesion does not profoundly impair the function of some cranial nerves (facial, trigeminal, and vagal) and spares mastication, phonation, and speech. The functions of such cranial nerves are severely affected only in the case of a bilateral cortical pathology or after a LMN lesion.

CLINICAL CONSIDERATIONS
Spastic Hemiplegia

Interruptions of the corticospinal fibers result in spastic hemiplegia. Lesions of the corticospinal tract at various neuraxial locations usually produce different symptoms concomitant to the hemiplegia. As a result, involvement of the corticobulbar fibers additionally results in the paralysis of facial, lingual, palatal, and laryngeal muscles. Since corticospinal fibers cross the midline at the medulla, any lesion involving the pyramidal system in the brainstem above pyramidal decussation produces clinical symptoms **contralateral** to the locus of damage. However, in the case of a lesion below the decussation point, the spinal UMN and LMN clinical signs occur **ipsilateral** to the side of the damage.

Common causes of spastic motor dysfunctions are cerebrovascular accidents, tumors, and degenerative diseases of the nervous system. None of these causes respect the anatomical boundaries; therefore, most clinical pictures evolving from these are mixed, and they may also implicate extrapyramidal structures.

Typical spastic hemiplegia consists of a flexed upper arm, thumb, and fingers and the neck bent toward the affected side (Fig. 14-4A). While walking, the patient circumvents the affected leg. The clinical symptoms appearing immediately after an acute pyramidal tract lesion include profound weakness, especially in contralateral distal muscles; loss of delicate and manipulative skills; loss of abdominal and cremasteric reflexes; positive Babinski reflex; and flaccid tone in affected muscles. Within about 1 to 4 weeks, the muscle tone not only returns but increases and becomes spastic. The spasticity is most evident in passive manipulation of the affected limb, as there is a resistance to limb extension. If the pressure is persistently applied, the muscle resistance may suddenly disappear. This is called clasp-knife spasticity. Extreme levels of hypertonia and clasp-knife characteristics of the limbs are rarely seen in lesions restricted to the corticobulbar system. Furthermore, corticobulbar damage does not usually produce the same level of spasticity as that which develops in distal limbs after a corticospinal tract lesion.

The gradual emergence of spasticity is related to the outgrowth of local stretch afferents, which fill the depopulated synapses on the α-LMNs after a cortical lesion. This axonal outgrowth takes considerable time, explaining the span of several weeks that it takes for spasticity to appear.

Pseudobulbar Palsy

Bilateral spastic paralysis of the speech musculature is called pseudobulbar (supranuclear) palsy. This indicates that the lesion is not in the medulla but rather

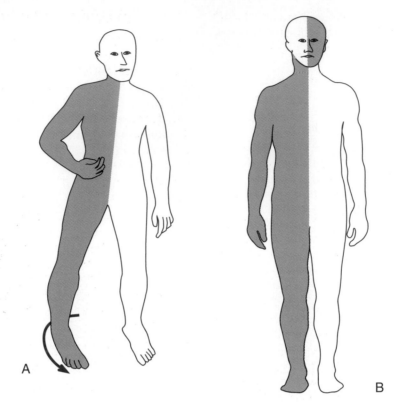

Figure 14-4. **A.** Right spastic hemiplegia. **B.** Left alternating hemiplegia, which is characterized by left facial palsy and right-sided hemiplegia and hemianesthesia.

in the motor pathways to the pons and medulla. It results from bilateral involvement of the corticobulbar pathways, which causes a supranuclear paralysis of the bulbar nerves. The patient has difficulty controlling facial muscles for delicate and discrete motor control such as in speech; however, there is little spasticity in facial and neck muscles.

Furthermore, the facial emotional response pattern remains intact. Consequently, when the patient attempts to move the facial muscles, they respond poorly. However, the patient's facial muscles respond strongly to an emotional stimulus, which is not considered under direct control by the cerebral cortex. The pathways that are activated during a true emotional response are not as fully understood as are the direct pathways that control voluntary actions. The emotional response may involve some limbic afferents. When the cranial nerve motor nuclei are activated through the so called intact emotional pathways, the facial response is actually exaggerated; when asked to show the teeth or perform a voluntary smile, the patient may assume the appearance of a Greek mask of tragedy, with forceful contraction of the same muscles that otherwise appear to be weak. Often these exaggerated emotional responses are accompanied by excessive laughter, sobbing, or choking, and they may pose a hazard to the patient who is eating.

Alternating Hemiplegia

Lesions at the brainstem level commonly produce **alternating hemiplegia**, which can result from the obstruction of small brainstem arteries. A lesion on one side of the brainstem affects the cranial nerve motor nuclei and/or nerves (motor units) extending to the innervated muscles. The LMN signs are **unilateral** to the side of the lesion. The lesion also interrupts the unilateral corticospinal fibers, which descend to cross the midline in the caudal medulla. A brainstem lesion results in an alternating pattern of symptoms: **ipsilateral** pharyngeal, facial, and/or ocular palsy symptoms and **contralateral** hemiplegia (Fig. 14-4B).

The unilateral damage to the motor nucleus of vagus nerve (LMN) produces flaccid paralysis of the pharyngeal and/or laryngeal muscles resulting in a weak and hoarse voice and swallowing difficulty; unilateral involvement of the motor nucleus of the facial nerve (LMN) causes facial asymmetry and affects eating and articulation; unilateral damage to the motor nucleus of the hypoglossal nerve (LMN) produces flaccid paralysis of the intrinsic and extrinsic lingual muscles, resulting in eating and speaking disturbance. If the lesion is large and extends to the lateral brainstem, it also produces contralateral hemianesthesia because of an interruption of the ascending somesthetic fibers. A lesion impairing the LMNs alone (Figs. 11-15 and 14-5, area B) produces the symptoms of the flaccid paralysis, absent reflexes, muscular fibrillation, and eventual atrophy of the involved muscle.

Upper Motor Neuron Syndrome

Interruption of the descending motor (corticospinal and corticobulbar) tracts have two clinically important components: the UMN (central nuclei and fibers) and the LMN (spinal and cranial nuclei and peripheral fibers). The UMNs relate to the cell bodies in the motor cortex and descending axonal processes before they synapse on the cranial or spinal motor neurons. The LMNs are the cell bodies in the anterior gray column in the spinal cord or cranial motor nuclei in the brainstem (see Chapters 11 and 15). The LMNs provide the output pathway to peripheral functions via their axons and innervate muscle fibers. The difference between the locations of the UMNs and LMNs has important clinical implications (Fig. 14-5, Table 14-1). Lesions of the corticospinal fibers (Fig. 14-5, area A) result in UMN syndrome, which is characterized by immediate flaccid muscle weakness; this is followed by increased muscle tone (spastic hemiplegia) after several weeks. Additional symptoms are a positive Babinski sign, hyperreflexia, and the loss of abdominal and cremasteric reflexes. With the loss of the pyramidal motor system, there is no cortical motor control on limb muscles and the patient loses precise and delicate motor control of the distal limb muscles used in fine manipulative skills, along with the head and neck muscles used for speech and facial expression. However, the paralyzed muscles do not atrophy (degenerate), because with intact LMNs their reflexive functions are preserved.

Flaccid in the beginning, the muscles gradually become spastic because of both pyramidal and extrapyramidal involvement. Spasticity, which includes hyperexcitability of reflex, takes 1 to 4 weeks to develop. This is largely due to collateral sprouting (scrambled wiring) of the type Ia (annulospiral) endings to spinal motor neurons, which fill depopulated or denuded corticospinal synapses. Contralateral spinal reflexes are hyperactive (Table 14-1). Abdominal and cremasteric reflexes are absent, with no muscle contraction in response to stroking the abdomen and inner thigh. The positive Babinski sign (Fig. 14-6B) is characterized by an extension of the toes in response to stroking the bottom of the foot with a pointed object.

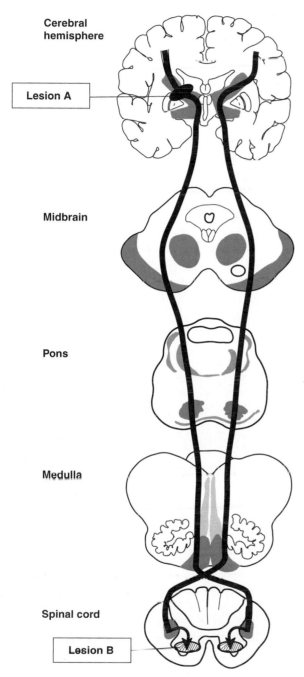

Figure 14-5. Lesion sites implicated with upper and lower motor neuron syndromes. Each site results in a different set of clinical symptoms. *Lesion A* (upper motor neuron lesion). Contralateral hemiplegia (flexed arm and extended leg), increased muscle tone (spastic), hyperactive reflexes, no muscle atrophy, Babinski's sign. *Lesion B* (lower spinal motor neuron lesion). Ipsilateral paralysis of specific muscles, absent muscle tone (flaccid), hypoactive or absent reflexes, muscular atrophy, muscle fasciculations.

Table 14-1. Characteristics of Upper Motor Neuron and Lower Motor Neuron Syndromes

UMN Syndrome	LMN Syndrome
Spastic paralysis or weakness	Flaccid paralysis or weakness
No signs of muscle denervation	Muscle denervation: fibrillations, fasciculations, and muscle atrophy
Increased muscle tone	Decreased muscle tone
Positive Babinski's	No Babinski's or cremasteric reflexes
Increased reflexes	Decreased reflexes
Involvement of multiple muscles or limbs (monoplegia, hemiplegia or quadriplegia)	Involvement of a single limb or selected muscles

Labels on figure: Cerebral hemisphere, Lesion A, Midbrain, Pons, Medulla, Spinal cord, Lesion B

A positive Babinski sign in a child is not an indication of disorder. Prior to maturation of the corticospinal system during the first 5 to 7 years of development, earlier reflexes, often called primitive, are pronounced; these include the protective flexor–withdrawal reflex. As the developing corticospinal system begins to dominate, Babinski and related primitive reflexes disappear. Corticospinal damage removes this domination, and the earlier reflexes including Babinski reappear.

There is always some recovery from spastic paralysis, and it may result in varying degrees of flexion in the upper extremity and hyperextension in the lower limbs (Fig. 14-6C). In general, gross motor movements recover, with proximal muscles displaying the greatest recovery.

No treatment is available to alleviate UMN symptoms other than to minimize the damage by reducing cerebral edema and by enhancing blood supply to the damaged tissue. Future treatment is concerned with finding a way to get UMN axons to grow past the damage and reinnervate former targets, an extremely challenging task. This nerve growth factor would have enormous implications for rehabilitation.

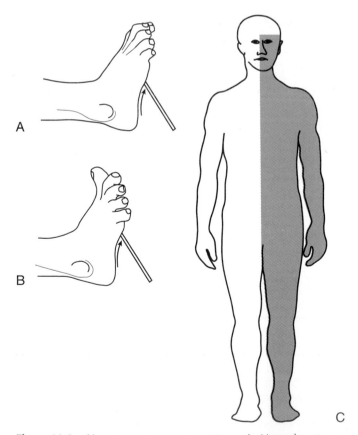

Figure 14-6. Upper motor neuron symptoms. **A.** Normal motor response. **B.** Babinski's sign in adults indicates dysfunctioning of corticospinal system. **C.** Left hemiplegia.

LESION LOCALIZATION

Rule 8: Upper or Lower Motor Neuron Lesion

PRESENTING SYMPTOMS

Increased reflexes in a symptomatic (sensorimotor) limb indicate an UMN lesion, while reduced reflexes in the same symptomatic limb would imply a peripheral or LMN lesion.

RATIONALE

The UMN influence on LMNs via the corticospinal and corticobulbar systems is excitatory. A lesion interrupting the excitatory projections from the upper motor levels first produces early signs of loss of precise motor control, especially of distal limb muscles; muscle weakness; flaccid tone; and hyporeflexia. However, in several weeks, the hyporeflexia and flaccid tone are replaced by increased reflexes and spasticity, which result from the increased power of the stretch reflexes because of the filling of the denuded corticospinal synapses to the LMNs.

The hyperactive antigravity stretch reflexes and spastic muscle tone take 1 to 4 weeks to have a clinical outcome. The LMN cell body provides the only output pathway to peripheral function via its axon, which traverses the ventral root and peripheral nerves to innervate a skeletal muscle, where it makes multiple axon branches to innervate and contract many muscle fibers. This entire single neuron–multiple muscle fiber functional unit is the motor unit. Damage to the LMN cell and/or its axon eliminates the entire function of a motor unit. This both weakens the muscles and reduces tendon reflexes. Additional LMN symptoms are flaccid muscle tone, muscle weakness, and muscle atrophy. These symptoms are seen in neurological conditions affecting motor units, diseases of the skeletal muscles (e.g., muscular dystrophy) and reduced nerve–muscle transmission (e.g., myasthenia gravis).

Rule 9: Brainstem Lesion

PRESENTING SYMPTOMS

An altered level of consciousness, cranial nerve impairments (facial paralysis, hearing impairment, nystagmus, dysarthria, dysphagia) on the same side (ipsilaterally), paralysis of the body on the opposite side (alternating or crossed hemiplegia), and hemianesthesia all imply a brainstem lesion.

RATIONALE

In alternating hemiplegia, the involved cranial nerves do not cross the midline, whereas the descending corticospinal fibers have not yet decussated. Thus, the brainstem involvement results in crossed or alternating symptoms, whereas hemiplegia involves the body contralateral to the lesion and the cranial nerve signs occur on the side of the brainstem lesion. Furthermore, dysarthria (laryngeal, pharyngeal, facial, or glossal dysfunctions) and dysphagia imply the involvement of cranial nerves and their nuclei, which are present in the brainstem. Disorders of consciousness can result from either the involvement of the reticular formation, which is essential for alertness and consciousness, or extensive bilateral cortical destruction or lesions.

Case Studies

Patient One: Hemiplegia

A 47-year-old woman had a stroke while sleeping. When she awoke, her left arm and leg would not move. She could talk, but her speech was dysarthric (imprecise articulation and weak voice). She was rushed to a hospital, and on testing, she exhibited the following:

- Weakness in the left upper and lower limbs
- Drooping lower left face
- Distorted smile with the mouth pulled to the normal (right) side
- Intact upper facial functions: frowning and eye closing
- Loss of proprioceptive, discriminative, and pain sensation on left side of the body
- Hyperactive deep tendon reflexes, including a positive Babinski's sign.

Magnetic resonance imaging revealed an infarct in the posterior region of the right internal capsule.

Question: Based on your understanding of the motor and sensory fibers, can you explain how this lesion caused these UMN symptoms?

Discussion: The internal capsule lesion affected the following structures:

- Damaged corticospinal fibers caused the left spastic hemiplegia.
- Damaged portions of the corticobulbar fibers supplied the motor nucleus of the facial nerve (loss of delicate motor control for left lower facial muscles), hypoglossal nerve (imprecise speech), and vagus nerve (weak voice). There was a differential effect of the lesion on the muscles of the larynx, lower face, and tongue. The effect was minimal on phonation because of the bilateral innervation of the nucleus ambiguus, and maximal on articulation because of the unilateral innervation of the facial and hypoglossal nuclei (see Chapter 15, which also discusses the distinction between UMN and LMN Bell's palsy).
- Interruption in the medial lemniscus projections resulted in loss of proprioceptive and discriminative touch on the left half of the body
- Damage to the thalamocortical projections accounted for the left-sided loss of pain and temperature sensation.

Patient Two: Alternating Hemiplegia

A 61-year-old man had a stroke while confined to a hospital for heart disease. He suddenly felt that he had no control of his left arm and leg and could not move his mouth. He was seen by a physician, who observed the following:

- Weakness in the right half of the face
- Inability to close his right eye and a widened palpebral fissure
- A weak bite on the right side
- No pain and touch sensation in the right half of his face
- Spastic paralysis of the left upper and lower limbs
- Positive left-sided Babinski's sign

Magnetic resonance imaging revealed a massive infarct in the right ventrolateral pons extending rostrally, and this was diagnosed as a case of alternating hemiplegia.

Question: Based on your knowledge of the pontine anatomy, can you account for the discrepancy in the clinical features observed? How is it that there was sensorimotor loss of the right face and right masticator muscles and yet left hemiplegia?

Discussion: The ventrolateral pontine infarct on the right side affected the following structures:

- Damaged facial nucleus and nerve (LMN syndrome) caused the paralysis of the right half of the patient's face.
- Damaged trigeminal motor nucleus (LMN symptom) caused the weakness of the right mastication muscles.
- Damaged chief sensory nucleus and spinal trigeminal nucleus affected pain and touch sensation from the right half of the face.
- Damaged uncrossed corticospinal fibers resulted in paralysis of the left side of the body. These fibers cross the midline at the caudal medulla. A positive Babinski's sign implicates an UMN lesion site.

SUMMARY

The several motor cortices control voluntary manipulative and delicate motor movements and initiate motor performance. Descending cortical projections to the motor neurons travel via two pathways, the corticobulbar tract and the corticospinal tract, collectively called the pyramidal tract. These tracts control cranial and spinal motor neurons (LMN), respectively. Activity at the motor cortex is influenced by extensive feedback channels from the cerebellum, brainstem, thalamus, and basal ganglia.

A lesion interrupting the excitatory projections from the motor cortex results in a specific loss of delicate motor control. It also results in signs of muscle weakness, flaccid tone, hyporeflexia, and loss of abdominal reflex. However, in several weeks, the hyporeflexia and flaccid tone are replaced by increased reflexes (hyperreflexia) and spastic tone in muscles.

Technical Terms

abdominal reflex	precentral gyrus
alternating hemiplegia	premotor cortex
Babinski reflex	pyramidal decussation
corticobulbar tract	pyramidal tract
corticospinal tract	spastic hemiplegia
cremasteric reflex	supplementary motor cortex
motor homunculus	upper motor neurons
postcentral gyrus	

Review Questions

1. Define the following terms:

abdominal reflex	precentral gyrus
alternating hemiplegia	premotor cortex
Babinski reflex	pyramidal decussation
corticobulbar tract	pyramidal tract
corticospinal tract	supplementary motor cortex
homunculus	spastic hemiplegia
postcentral gyrus	upper motor neurons

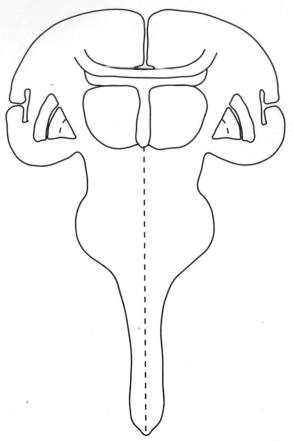

Figure 14-7. Exercise figure for illustrating motor pathway.

2. Describe the roles of the premotor, motor, and sensory cortices in the regulation of motor functions.
3. Outline the course of the pyramidal tract from the motor cortex to the spinal cord on Figure 14-7; also discuss the decussation points for the corticospinal and corticobulbar tracts.
4. What are the giant pyramidal cells (of Betz) and where in the cortex are they?
5. What cranial nerve nuclei are innervated by corticobulbar fibers?
6. Describe the pathophysiology of LMN and UMN syndromes.
7. Explain the reasons for spasticity, hyperreflexia, and hemiplegia after an UMN lesion.
8. Describe the clinical symptoms of alternating hemiplegia and explain how it is related to a brainstem lesion.
9. Why is examining the quality of a reflex important in the diagnosis of motor diseases?
10. Explain why muscles do not atrophy in the case of an UMN lesion.
11. Match the following conditions to the associated lettered lesion type.

   i. muscle atrophy   a. LMN lesion
   ii. loss of stretch reflex   b. UMN lesion
   iii. spasticity
   iv. fasciculation
   v. hypotonia
   vi. hypertonia
   vii. positive Babinski's sign

15

Cranial Nerves

Learning Objectives

After studying this chapter, students should be able to do the following:

- List the cranial nerves
- Relate the cranial nerves' numbers to their names
- Follow the rationale for the functional classification of cranial nerves
- Discuss the locations of the attachments of cranial nerves in the brainstem
- Identify the brainstem locations of cranial nerve nuclei
- Discuss the cranial nerve nuclei that receive bilateral or unilateral cortical projections
- Explain the clinical implications of the bilateral or unilateral innervation of motor nerve nuclei
- Discuss the branchial and somatic bases of muscles
- List the muscles derived from various branchial arches
- Identify functional components for each cranial nerve
- Relate cranial nerve nuclei and their projections to specific sensorimotor functions
- Explain idiosyncratic distributional patterns and innervational properties of cranial nerves
- Discuss clinical symptoms associated with disorders of cranial nerves and nuclei
- Describe function-based cranial nerve combinations
- Perform an oral–facial examination in accordance with the pertinent functional components of cranial nerves
- Relate patterns of facial paralysis to their respective lesion sites
- Differentiate between UMN and LMN symptoms of cranial nerves

The cranial nerves in the human are the result of an evolutionary modification of a basic vertebrate pattern of CNS organization, which was constructed of approximately 40 bilaterally symmetrical repeating segments, each with a dorsal horn and a ventral horn. Each CNS segment innervated the corresponding head or body region by means of the nerve roots on each side, the dorsal root and the ventral root. The peripheral process of the ganglion in the dorsal root innervates the tissue of the body segment as receptor endings, while its central axons travel to the dorsal horns of the corresponding CNS segment. The ventral root, containing efferent axons, innervates the somite-derived skeletal muscles of the body. Early in evolutionary development, there were additional (intermediate) roots of efferent fibers between the dorsal and ventral roots. These were present in only the rostral 15 segments of the CNS, extending from the head to cervical C-5 segments. The efferent axons leaving the intermediate roots innervated ancient muscles related to gill opening and closing and used to filter food from the water. In mammals these gill-related muscles have evolved into many of the skeletal muscles of the head and neck and have been modified for other purposes, such as **phonation** and **speech**, the area of most concern to students of human communication. This explains a differential evolutionary basis for the muscles now used for motor speech and is why the head and face muscles are treated as functionally different (see below the branchial origin of speech related muscles). The cranial nerves that innervate the head and neck muscles are the evolutionary remnants of the intermediate nerve roots.

The stable arrangement of afferent (sensory) neurons, transmitting their afferents to the CNS, and efferent (motor) neurons to innervate somatic muscles on each side of each spinal segment continues in the brainstem. The peripherally located afferent neurons of the cranial nerves are homologous to the spinal dorsal root ganglia and have names, such as spinal trigeminal nucleus and nucleus solitarius. The efferent neurons of the cranial nerves are homologous to the spinal α- and γ-LMN motor neurons in the spinal ventral horn; they lie within various nuclei, such as the nucleus ambiguus and facial nucleus.

Cranial nerves (CN) I and II are part of the forebrain; the other 10 are attached to the brainstem (Fig. 15-1). Some cranial nerves serve only sensory functions;

others serve only motor functions. However, many of the nerves are mixed, serving both sensory and motor functions.

FUNCTIONAL CLASSIFICATION OF CRANIAL NERVES[a]

Spinal nerves serve general motor and general sensory functions only, involving both somatic (that are derived from the somite) and visceral (internal organ) muscles, resulting in four functional components (Table 15-1). Besides serving the general motor and general sensory functions, however, cranial nerves use special receptors and neurons to serve additional functions that are classed as special. The general and special

___

[a] Consult Chapter 1 for definition of terms used in the functional classification.

functional components of cranial nerves can be further classified by whether the nerve innervates somatic muscles or visceral structures and whether it is involved with sensory (afferent) or motor (efferent) information (Table 15-1). The somatic component of cranial nerves with special functions contains only the afferent fibers, whereas the visceral component contains both afferent and efferent fibers (see Chapter 1 for a discussion of these embryological terms). This results in seven functional types of cranial nerves (Table 15-2). The cranial nerves have the following sensorimotor components.

Efferent

General somatic efferent (GSE): Innervates the skeletal muscles derived from somites. This functional component includes the innervation of ocular (oculomotor [III],

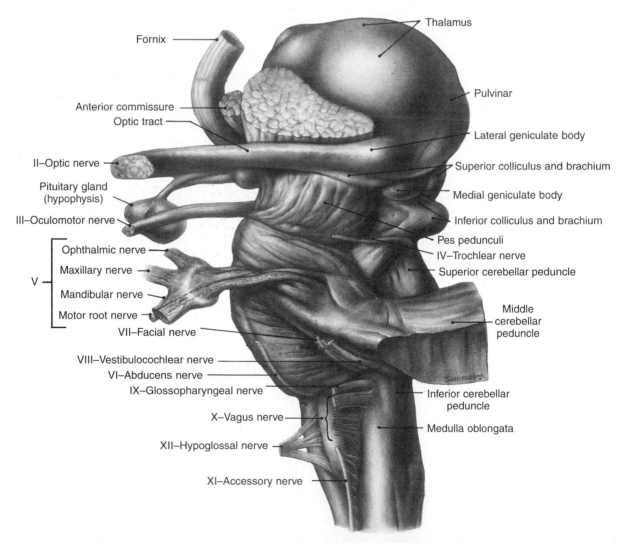

Figure 15-1. Cranial nerve roots and other structures on lateral surface of brainstem.

Table 15-1. Functional Components of Nervous System

	General		Special	
	Somatic Efferent	Visceral Afferent	Somatic Efferent[a]	Visceral Afferent
Efferent (motor)			**Efferent (motor)**[a]	
1. *GSE* controls muscles derived from somites that include skeletal, extraocular, glossal muscles.			5. *SVE/BE* controls gill-related muscles of face, pharynx, larynx, neck that evolve from branchial arches.	
2. GVE regulates autonomic innervation of smooth muscles, cardiac muscles, glands.				
Afferent (sensory)			**Afferent (sensory)**	
3. *GSA* mediates somesthetic input: pain, temperature, touch from somatic muscles, skin, ligaments, joints.			6. *SSA* mediates special sensations of vision from retina; audition, equilibrium from inner ear.	
4. *GVA* mediates sensations of pain and temperature from visceral organs.			7. *SVA* mediates sensations of taste from tongue and olfaction from nose.	

[a] Special somatic efferent does not exist.
GSE, general somatic efferent; GVE, general visceral efferent; SVE, special visceral efferent; BE, branchial efferent; GSA, general somatic afferent; SSA, special somatic afferent; GVA, general visceral afferent; SVA, special visceral afferent.

trochlear [IV], abducens [VI]) and tongue (hypoglossal [XII]) muscles.

General visceral efferent (GVE): Regulates the autonomic innervation of smooth muscles. This consists of the visceral nuclei including the Edinger-Westphal nucleus (oculomotor [III]), superior salivatory nucleus (facial [VII]), inferior salivary nucleus (glossopharyngeal [IX]), and dorsal motor nucleus (vagus [X]); these nerves are responsible for pupillary constriction, gland secretion, and regulation of the muscles of the heart, trachea, bronchi, esophagus, and lower viscera.

Special visceral efferent (SVE), or **branchial efferent (BE):** Controls the muscles of the face, pharynx, larynx, and neck, which evolve from branchial arches. This functional component consists of the motor nucleus of the trigeminal (V), motor nucleus of the facial (VII), nucleus ambiguus of the glossopharyngeal (IX), vagus (X), and accessory motor nuclei (in upper cervical C-1 to C-5 segments). They are related to the spinal accessory (XI) nerve and control the muscles of expression, mastication, phonation, deglutition, head turning, and shoulder elevation.

Afferent

General somatic afferent (GSA): Mediates somesthetic input, including pain, temperature, and touch sensations from the skin and somatic muscles in the head, neck, and face; this functional category primarily includes the trigeminal (V) sensory nuclei (chief sensory nucleus and spinal descending nucleus).

General visceral afferent (GVA): Component mediates general sensation, including pain and temperature, from the visceral structures of the pharynx, palate, larynx, aorta, and abdomen; this component consists of the glossopharyngeal (IX) and vagus (X) nerves.

Special somatic afferent (SSA): regulates special senses that include vision (optic [II]) and audition and equilibrium (vestibuloacoustic [VIII]). This functional component also includes proprioception.

Special visceral afferent (SVA): Mediates taste (gustation) and smell (olfaction). This functional component includes olfactory (I), facial (VII), glossopharyngeal (IX), and vagus (X) nerves.

BRANCHIAL ORIGIN OF SPEECH-RELATED MUSCLES

The classification of speech and the related muscles of phonation, mastication, deglutition, articulation, head turning, and shoulder elevation as special visceral efferent is often confusing for students of communicative disorders, because these muscles are under voluntary control, in addition to reflex control, and are structurally the same as other skeletal muscles derived from the somites and classified as somatic (Table 15-3). The reason for classifying these muscles related to motor speech processes as visceral or branchial is that they are derived from the branchial arches and gill-related structures of the embryo. Thus, to minimize the confusion caused by their visceral efferent classification, these muscles have also been identified as branchial efferent (BE) in this chapter.

Early in human embryonic development, six branchial arches emerge (Fig. 15-2). The first four arches

Table 15-2A. Functional Components of Cranial Nerves

	General				Special			
	Afferent		Efferent		Afferent		Efferent	
	GSA	GVA	GSE	GVE	SVA	SSA	SVE/BE	SSE[a]
I					+			
II						+		
III			+	+				
IV			+					
V	+						+	
VI			+					
VII				+	+		+	
VIII						+		
IX		+		+	+		+	
X		+		+	+		+	
XI							+	
XII			+					

[a] This category does not exist.
GSE, general somatic efferent; GVE, general visceral efferent; SVE, special visceral efferent; BE, branchial efferent; GSA, general somatic afferent; SSA, special somatic afferent; GVA, general visceral afferent; SVA, special visceral afferent.

Table 15-2B.   Summary of Cranial Nerve Functional Components

	Cranial Nerve	Classification	Cell Nuclei	Function
I	Olfactory	SVA	Neuroepithelial cells in nasal cavity	Smell
II	Optic	SSA	Ganglion cells in retina	Vision
III	Oculomotor	GSE	Oculomotor nucleus in upper midbrain tegmentum	Eye movement: controls all eye muscles except the lateral rectus (V) and superior oblique muscles (IV); also regulates levator palpebrae superioris
IV		GVE	Edinger-Westphal nucleus in midbrain tegmentum; preganglionic projections to ciliary ganglion	Reflexive constriction of pupil, accommodation of lens for near vision
V	Trochlear	GSE	Trochlear nucleus in tegmentum of midbrain	Eye movements: innervates contralateral, superior oblique muscle
	Trigeminal	GSA	First order: trigeminal (semilunar) ganglion Second order: primary sensory (pons), descending spinal nucleus (pons, medulla, upper cervical levels), mesencephalic nucleus (midbrain)	Receives cutaneous and proprioceptive sensations from skin and muscles in face, orbit, nose, mouth, forehead, teeth, meninges, anterior two-thirds of tongue
		BE/SVE	Trigeminal motor nucleus in pons	Innervates muscles of mastication (masseter internal and external pterygoid, temporal), mylohyoid, anterior belly of diagastric, tensor velum palatini, tensor tympani muscles
VI	Abducens	GSE	Abducens nucleus in tegmentum of pons	Eye movements: innervates ipsilateral lateral rectus muscle
VII	Facial	GVE	Superior salivatory nucleus: preganglionic to ganglia associated with oral, nasal glands	Regulates secretions from nasal, palatal, lacrimal, submaxillary, sublingual glands
		SVA	First-order cells: geniculate ganglion Second-order cells: nucleus solitarius	Mediates gustatory sensation from taste buds in anterior two-thirds of tongue
		BE/SVE	Facial motor complex in lateral pons	Innervates muscles of facial expression and platysma, extrinsic and intrinsic ear muscles, and stapedius muscle
VIII	Vestibuloacoustic	SSA	First-order cells: superior, inferior vestibular ganglia Second-order cells: vestibular nuclei in medulla, pons	Equilibrium and orientation of head in space
		SSA	First-order cells: spiral ganglion Second-order cells: cochlear nuclei in medulla	Hearing
IX	Glossopharyngeal	GVA	First-order cells: inferior ganglion Second-order cells: nucleus solitarius	Mediates general sensation from palate, posterior third of tongue, oral pharynx, carotid sinus
		GVE	Inferior salivatory nucleus: preganglionic to otic ganglion	Regulates secretion from parotid gland
		SVA	First-order cells: inferior ganglion Second-order cells: nucleus solitarius	Mediates taste sensation from posterior third of tongue and oral pharynx
		BE/SVE	Nucleus ambiguus	Contributes to swallowing by controlling stylopharyngeus muscle
X	Vagus	GVA	First-order cells: inferior ganglion Second-order cells: nucleus solitarius	Receives general sensation from pharynx, larynx, thorax, abdomen, carotid body, and aortic body; regulates nausea, oxygen intake, lung inflation
		GVE	Dorsal motor nucleus: preganglionic parasympathetic innervation	Innervates glands, muscles in heart, blood vessels, trachea, bronchi, esophagus, stomach, intestine
		SVA	First-order cells: inferior ganglion Second-order cells: nucleus solitarius	Mediates taste sensation from sensory buds in epiglottis, pharynx
		BE/SVE	Nucleus ambiguus	Controls muscles of larynx, pharynx, soft palate for phonation, deglutition, resonance
XI	Spinal accessory	BE/SVE	Spinal accessory nucleus in C-1–C-5 ventral horns	Controls head and shoulder by innervating trapezius, sternocleidomastoid muscles
XII				Controls tongue movement by regulating

GSE, general somatic efferent; GVE, general visceral efferent; SVE, special visceral efferent; BE, branchial efferent; GSA, general somatic afferent; SSA, special somatic afferent; GVA, general visceral afferent; SVA, special visceral afferent.

Table 15-3.   Branchial Arches, Associated Cranial Nerves, and Derived Muscles

Branchial Arch	Cranial Nerve	Muscles
First mandibular	Trigeminal (V)	Muscles of mastication: temporalis, masseter medial, lateral pterygoid Additional muscles: mylohyoid, anterior belly of digastric, tensor tympani, tensor veli palatini
Second	Facial (VII)	Muscles of facial expressions: buccinator, auricularis, frontalis, platysma, orbicularis oris, orbicularis oculi Additional muscles: stapedius, stylohyoid, posterior belly of digastric
Third	Glossopharyngeal (IX)	Stylopharyngeus
Fourth and sixth[a]	Superior laryngeal, recurrent laryngeal branches of vagus (X)	Pharyngeal and laryngeal muscles: cricothyroid, levator veli palatini, constrictors of pharynx, intrinsic muscles of larynx
Unnumbered gill structures	Spinal accessory nuclei in C-1–C-5	Sternocleidomastoid and trapezius muscle

[a] Fifth branchial arch is not developed in human embryo.

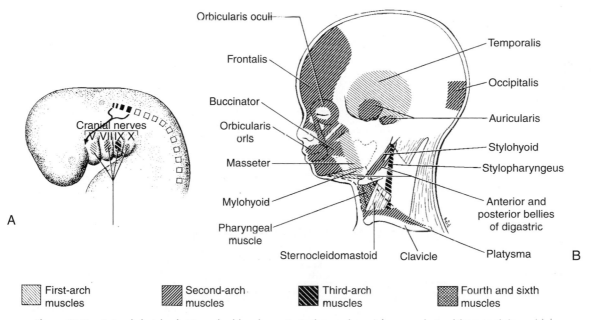

Figure 15-2.   Lateral sketch of a 4-week-old embryo. **A.** Arches and cranial nerves derived from each branchial arch. **B.** Major muscles derived from each arch.

are well marked; the fifth arch disappears during development; and the sixth arch, although present, is not obvious. Each branchial arch relates to specific groups of muscles (Table 15-3): the muscles of mastication (trigeminal nerve) relate to the first branchial arch; the muscles of facial expression (facial nerve) relate to the second branchial arch; and the stylopharyngeus muscles (glossopharyngeal nerve) relate to the third branchial arch. The remaining pharyngeal muscles (vagus nerve) are derived from the fourth branchial arch, and the laryngeal muscles (vagus nerve) are derived from the sixth branchial arch.

The spinal accessory nerve is also a branchial nerve, as it is related to a series of unnumbered gill structures that extended down to C-5 in mammals. The LMNs exiting the C-1 to C-5 form CN XI and innervate neck muscles.

CRANIAL NERVES AND THE AUTONOMIC NERVOUS SYSTEM

The cranial nerves also serve autonomic functions. The parasympathetic efferents of the autonomic nervous system (ANS) (see Chapters 2 and 16) exit the CNS from the craniosacral region (cranial segments and spinal segments S-2 to S-4). Therefore, autonomic components of the cranial nerves have only parasympathetic functions via the innervation of postganglionic neurons in the peripheral ganglia. These functions, classified as general visceral efferent, are carried out by the preganglionic LMNs in the brainstem of the Edinger-Westphal nucleus (CN III), superior salivatory (facial nerve complex), inferior salivatory nucleus (CN IX), and the dorsal vagal nucleus (CN X).

CRANIAL NERVE NUCLEI

Most of the cranial nerve nuclei are in the ventricular floor of the brainstem (Fig. 15-3). Depending on what functions they serve, some of the nuclei are connected to several related nerves. The intramedullary locations of the cranial nerve nuclei are shown in Figures 15-3, *A* and *B*.

Midbrain

There are three cranial nerve motor nuclei in the midbrain tegmentum: the **Edinger-Westphal nucleus** (CN III), the **oculomotor nucleus** (CN III), and the **trochlear nucleus** (CN IV). The Edinger-Westphal nucleus contains preganglionic parasympathetic efferents to innervate the ciliary muscle and the sphincter of the pupil. The oculomotor nucleus contains the LMNs that control most of the muscles of the eye. The trochlear nucleus contains the LMNs that innervate the superior oblique, one of the muscles of the eye.

Pons

Six major cranial nerve nuclei lie in the pontine tegmentum. There are the three sensory nuclei of the trigeminal nerve: the **primary sensory** nucleus, the **spinal trigeminal** nucleus, and the **mesencephalic** nucleus. The first two nuclei join to form the sensory branch of the trigeminal nerve. The mesencephalic nucleus contains afferents from muscle spindles and regulates jaw reflex. Adjacent to the sensory trigeminal com-

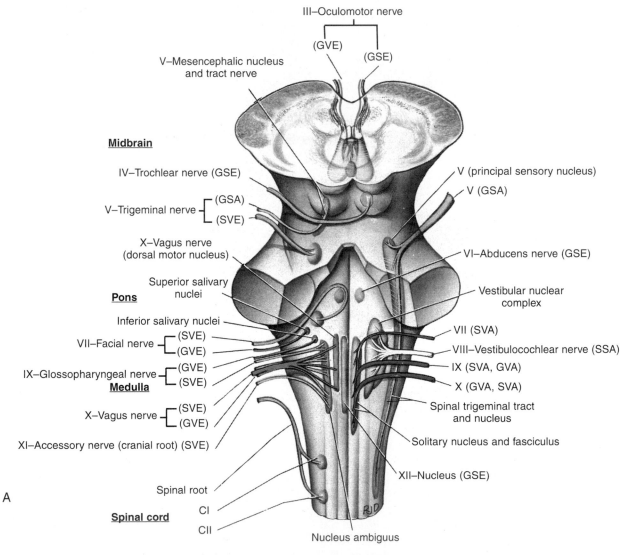

Figure 15-3. A. Intramedullary cranial nerves, their nuclei of origin, and their functional classifications.
(Figure continues)

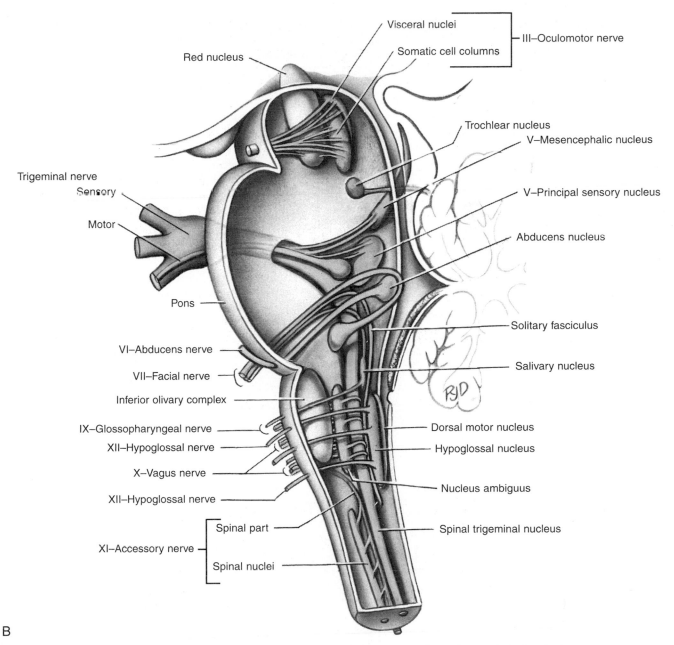

Figure 15-3. B. *(continued)* Intramedullary nuclei of cranial nerves on a midsagittal view of a hollow brainstem. All cranial nerves and associated nuclei except vestibulocochlear nerve are presented.

plex is the **trigeminal motor** nucleus, which contains LMNs to innervate the muscles of mastication and other associated muscles. Dorsal in the pontine tegmentum is the **abducens motor nucleus**, which contains LMNs to innervate the lateral rectus muscle of the eye. Ventrolateral to the abducens nucleus is the **facial motor nucleus**, which contains LMNs to innervate the muscles of facial expressions (Fig. 15-3*B*).

Medulla

There are nine major cranial nerve nuclei in the medulla. The **cochlear** and **vestibular nuclear com-**

plexes, which are not shown in Figure 15-3, are lateral at the junction of the pons and medulla (see Chapters 9 and 10). At the rostral medulla is the **salivary nucleus** (shared by facial, glossopharyngeal, and vagus nerves), a visceral motor nucleus responsible for controlling secretion from various glands. The **dorsal motor nucleus** of the vagus nerve controls autonomic motor activity of various visceral organs. Medial to the dorsal motor nucleus is the **hypoglossal nucleus**, whose LMNs innervate extrinsic and intrinsic muscles of the tongue. The nucleus solitarius, a visceral sensory nucleus responsible for taste, nausea, heart rate, respiration, and blood pressure, is shared by the facial and glossopharyngeal nerves. Lateral to the nucleus solitarius lies the **spinal trigeminal nucleus**. The **nucleus ambiguus**, which is between the inferior olivary nucleus and the spinal trigeminal nucleus, contains LMNs and controls the movements of laryngeal and pharyngeal muscles. This nucleus is also shared by the glossopharyngeal and vagus nerves.

The **spinal accessory nucleus**, the only cranial nerve nucleus outside the brainstem, is in the ventral horns of the upper cervical (C-1 to C-5) segments.

PATHWAYS

Motor, or Efferent, Pathways

The cranial nerve nuclei receive their motor projections from the corticobulbar fibers (Fig. 15-4). Corticobulbar fibers arise from the motor cells (UMN) in the lower part of the precentral cortex and descend through the internal capsule to synapse on the motor cranial nerve nuclei (LMN) in the brainstem. Before synapsing on the cranial nerve motor nuclei, most corticobulbar fibers cross the midline at different brainstem locations. However, a substantial bilateral cortical innervation of the cranial motor nuclei has been clinically reported for the muscles of the face, jaw, larynx, and pharynx.

Damage at the cortical level interrupts the corticobulbar projections, resulting in UMN symptoms of increased deep tendon reflexes and contralateral paralysis (see Chapter 14). The many aberrant corticobulbar fibers in the brainstem provide for safety from damage to cranial nerve motor functions, and therefore, pyramidal loss generally does not result in profound spasticity and weakness in cranial muscles. Lesions of the brainstem cranial motor nuclei and their axons (nerves) produce an LMN syndrome, which is characterized by flaccid mus-

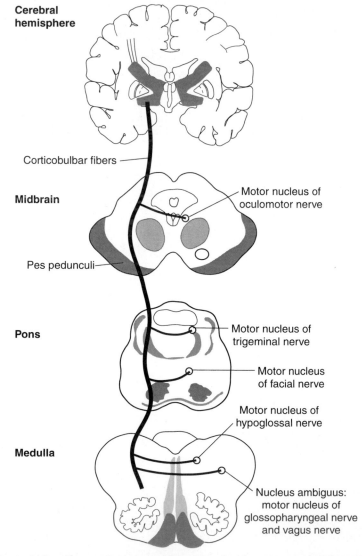

Figure 15-4. Corticobulbar fibers projecting to motor nuclei of oculomotor, trigeminal, vagal, and hypoglossal nerves in the brainstem.

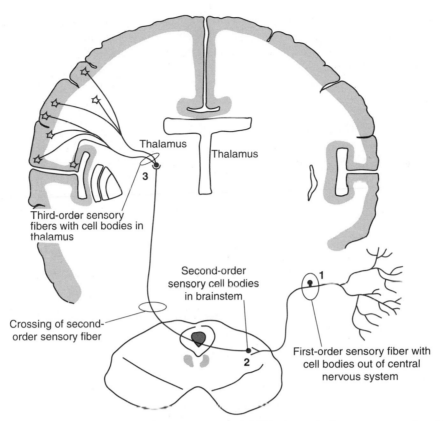

Figure 15-5. Sensory pathway for cranial nerves. First-order fibers, with cell bodies external to central nervous system, transmit information from periphery to second-order nuclei in the brainstem. Second-order fibers, with cell bodies in the brainstem, cross the midline and terminate in the thalamus. Third-order fibers, with cell bodies in the thalamus, project to lower parts of postcentral gyrus.

cle tone, absent reflexes, paralysis of the involved muscles, fibrillations (single denervated fiber), fasciculation (spontaneous firing of motor units), and atrophy of the muscles (see Chapters 11 and 14).

Sensory, or Afferent, Pathways

Most of the sensory pathways of the cranial nerves consist of three-order nuclei and their fibers (Fig. 15-5). The cell bodies of the **first-order fibers** are outside the CNS. The **second-order fibers**, with cell bodies in the gray matter of the brainstem, cross the midline and terminate in the thalamus. The **third-order fibers**, with cell bodies in the ventral posterior medial nucleus of the thalamus, project to the sensory cortex in the parietal lobe. Smell, audition, and vision are exceptions to the sensory organization of three-order cells and fibers.

PATTERN OF INNERVATION

The corticobulbar regulation of many branchial motor nuclei is bilateral (Fig. 15-6). The nuclei of such cranial nerves receive corticobulbar input from both sides of the cortex, though contralateral innervation is

somewhat stronger. The exception to this rule is control of the lower face muscles (CN VII), the sternocleidomastoid and trapezius muscles (CN XI), the tongue muscles (CN XII), and the ocular muscles (CN III, IV, and VI). This implies that a unilateral cortical lesion will not profoundly impair the function of the facial, trigeminal, vagal, and glossopharyngeal nerves, since their motor nuclei receive corticobulbar projections from both sides of the motor cortex. Such cranial nerve functions are severely affected only in the case of a bilateral cortical destruction or after an LMN lesion. The presence of many aberrant corticobulbar fibers further provides for safety from spasticity in cranial muscles in the case of pyramidal (UMN) lesions.

The pyramidal tract provides minor cortical regulation of eye movement (CN III, IV, and VI). For innervation of ocular muscles, a powerful corticobulbar projection to the midbrain conjugate gaze control center coordinates the movement of the eyes as a unit. For example, activation of the left frontal cortex leads to activation of the right pontine gaze center and subsequently to activation of the right abducens (lateral rectus) and left oculomotor nucleus (medial rectus). This results in contraction of the right lateral rectus and left medial rectus muscles and turns the eyes toward the right.

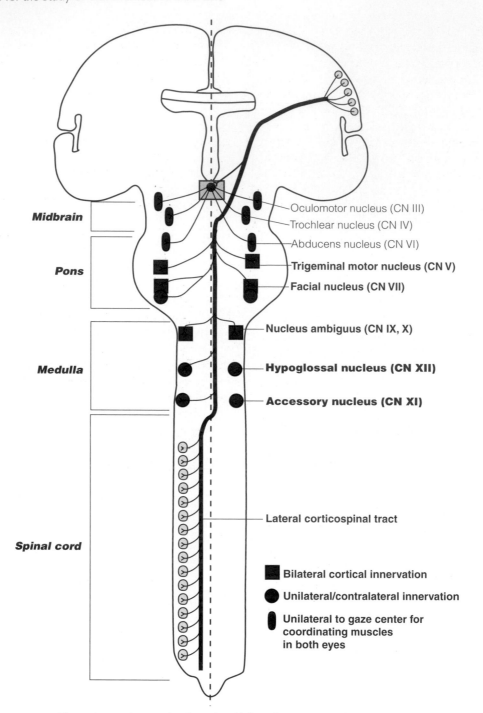

Figure 15-6.   Pattern of unilateral and bilateral innervation of cranial nerves.

CRANIAL NERVES AND THEIR SENSORIMOTOR FUNCTIONS

Olfactory Nerve

The olfactory system consists of the afferent neuron in the olfactory mucosal membrane, the olfactory bulb, the olfactory tract, part of the temporal cortex, and a limited region of the inferior fronto-orbital cortex. The cortical olfactory area develops on the basomedial surface of the cerebral hemisphere and includes the uncus, the periamygdaloid nucleus, the anterior hippocampal gyrus, and parts of the temporal lobe.

SPECIAL VISCERAL AFFERENT

The SVA begins with neurosensory cells that transduce odor molecules. These are embedded in the olfactory epithelium, a yellowish patch of cells in an area of the roof of the nasal cavity that is approximately 2 cm^2

(Table 15-4; Fig. 15-7). Also found in the epithelium are the sensory endings of the trigeminal nerve, which responds to noxious sensation, such as concentrated ammonia. The unmyelinated axons of the neurosensory (olfactory) neurons group together to form the olfactory nerve. The olfactory receptor cells are unique: they are the only mammalian neurons that are replaced with new cells in 30 to 60 days. The olfactory fibers that form the nerve pass through the foramina in the ethmoid cribriform plate, terminating on the mitral and other cells in the olfactory bulbs on the basal surface of the frontal lobe. The axonal projections from the mitral and associated cells in the olfactory bulb form the olfactory tract, which travels caudally to the olfactory trigone area and divides into subtracts (Fig. 15-8).

The olfactory tract divides into three major bundles (striae) of fibers: the **intermediate, medial,** and **lateral bundles.** The intermediate stria terminates in the trigone area and the anterior perforated substance anterior to the optic chiasm (Fig. 15-8). Some medial stria fibers terminate in the subcallosal area and are closely associated with the limbic lobe. Other medial stria fibers cross the midline through the anterior commissure and connect with the opposite olfactory bulb. Fibers of the lateral stria that form the central connections travel along the anterior perforated substance and terminate in the vicinity of the medial temporal lobe of the (primary) olfactory area, called the pyriform cortex because of its pear shape (Fig. 15-9). This includes the cortex of the uncus, the amygdaloid nucleus, and the anterior part of the parahippocampal gyrus. The primary cortical region mediates olfactory awareness. Various projections from the primary olfactory cortex to the neocortex and limbic region help integrate smell with the emotional brain and serve many vegetative functions. These extrinsic olfactory connections include the projections from the olfactory cortex to the orbitofrontal cortex and the insular cortex, which plays a role in odor discrimination. Direct olfactory projections to the hypothalamus play an important role in feeding behavior.

CLINICAL INFORMATION

At approximately 65 years of age, humans gradually begin to lose acuity of the sense of smell. This is largely caused by ongoing degeneration of olfactory sensory cells. The primary complaint in many such patients with chemosensory disturbance is the loss of taste, which is mostly related to impaired olfaction. A lesion that interrupts the olfactory fibers or the primary olfactory cells causes **anosmia,** a condition in which the ability to smell is partially or fully impaired. Two associated conditions are **hyposmia** and **hyperosmia.** In hyposmia there is decreased olfactory sensation, whereas in hyperosmia there is an abnormally acute sense of smell. Olfactory loss is also seen in patients with seizure activity involving uncinate fibers (uncinate fits) in addition to altered consciousness.

Olfactory loss may involve the neural mechanism of olfaction unilaterally or bilaterally. Bilateral lesions drastically restrict olfactory function. Olfactory nerve function is tested by asking the patient to identify various odors.

Optic Nerve

Many do not consider the optic nerve to be a nerve in the true sense because it, like the olfactory nerve, is merged with the brain and functions like a CNS tract. However, it has been included in the book as a cranial nerve.

Table 15-4. Functional Description of Olfactory Nerve

Classification	Nuclei	Function
S (special) V (visceral) A (afferent)	Neuroepithelial cells in nasal cavity	Smell

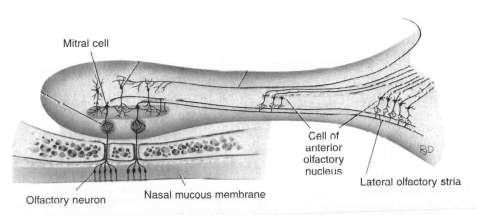

Figure 15-7. Olfactory neurons in the nasal mucosa, bulb, and centrally projecting fibers.

Labels: Mitral cell; Cell of anterior olfactory nucleus; Lateral olfactory stria; Olfactory neuron; Nasal mucous membrane

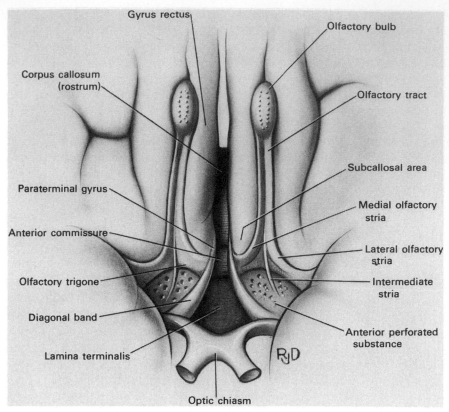

Figure 15-8. Olfactory structures on ventral surface of frontal lobe.

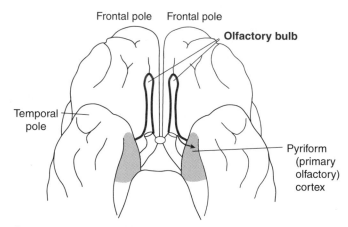

Figure 15-9. Primary olfactory (pyriform) cortex and associated structures on ventral surface of frontal and temporal lobes.

SPECIAL SOMATIC AFFERENT

As discussed in Chapter 8, outlined in Table 15-5, and illustrated in Figure 8-9, light rays entering the eye are bent (refracted) by the curvature of the cornea and lens and converge on rods and cones in the retina. The rod cells populate the peripheral regions of the retina and are sensitive to white light and to movement. Rods are capable of considerable adaptation to low-intensity stimulation, such as that needed for night vision. The cone cells populate mostly the central retinal region (fovea), where visual acuity is highest. Cones mediate color vision, which results from the differential sensitivity of three classes of cones: red, green, and blue. The retina also contains interneurons, which modulate and transform visual input including bipolar cells and retinal ganglion cells.

The photoreceptor cells transduce light energy into nerve potentials that travel through their axons. These axons form the optic nerve, optic chiasm, and optic tract. At the optic chiasm, fibers from the eyes cross the midline. The optic tract fibers, which are formed by the postchiasmatic fibers, travel posteriorly around the pes pedunculi and terminate in the lateral geniculate body, the thalamic relay center for vision. The geniculocalcarine projections, also called optic radiations, travel to the visual cortex in the occipital lobe. The visual cortex, in the upper and lower banks of the calcarine fissure, re-

Table 15-5.   Functional Description of Optic Nerve

Classification	Nuclei	Function
S (special) S (somatic) A (afferent)	Retinal ganglion cells	Vision

ceives projections from both eyes. In addition to the primary visual cortex in the pole and medial surface of the occipital lobe, other specialized visual cortical areas in the lateral cortex analyze visual information in terms of color, motion, location, and depth.

CLINICAL INFORMATION

Injury to any part of the visual pathway results in selected visual field loss. The area and type of visual field loss depend on the site and extent of the lesion. A lesion of the entire optic nerve leads to complete blindness in one eye. Cerebrovascular accidents and neuritis, an inflammation of the optic nerve, are common causes of optic nerve disorders. Common visual field defects are **bitemporal hemianopsia**, **homonymous hemianopsia**, **homonymous superior quadrantanopia**, and **homonymous inferior quadrantanopsia** (Fig. 8-14).

Visual field loss can be informally tested by having a patient close one eye and fix the other eye on a point straight ahead of him or her. The clinician then moves his or her index finger from the periphery to the midline from all directions (left, right, up, and down) and the patient is asked to report the point at which the finger is seen.

Oculomotor Nerve

All ocular movements are controlled by six extrinsic muscles: medial rectus, lateral rectus, superior rectus, inferior rectus, superior oblique, and inferior oblique. These muscles are controlled by three cranial nerves, the oculomotor, trochlear, and abducens, which are interconnected through the medial longitudinal fasciculus, a longitudinal fiber bundle in the brainstem (see Chapters 3 and 10). The combined function of these cranial nerves is to track moving objects and maintain visual fixation.

Functional components of the oculomotor nerve consist of the somatic and visceral motor nuclei (Table 15-6). The somatic motor nucleus innervates the extrinsic ocular muscles. The visceral motor (Edinger-Westphal) nucleus provides parasympathetic projections to the constrictor (circular) fibers of the iris and ciliary muscle, regulating pupillary constriction in response to light and enabling the lens to accommodate for near vision (see Chapter 8). The oculomotor nuclear complex is in the upper tegmentum (periaqueductal gray) of the midbrain at the level of the superior colliculus under the cerebral aqueduct. The oculomotor fibers travel ventrally through the midbrain tegmentum, the red nucleus, and basis pedunculi, exiting from the ventral surface of the brainstem at the junction of the pons and the midbrain (Figs. 15-10 and 15-11).

GENERAL SOMATIC EFFERENT

The oculomotor nerve splits in the orbital cavity to supply the following ocular muscles: superior rectus, medial rectus, inferior rectus, and inferior oblique (Fig. 15-11). In addition, the oculomotor fibers innervate the levator palpebrae superioris, the muscle responsible for raising the eyelid and implicated with ptosis (upper eyelid paralysis). Each muscle makes an individual contribution to the total eye movement: the superior rectus moves the eyeball upward and inward; the medial rectus adducts the eyeball medially; and the inferior rectus moves the eyeball downward and inward. The inferior oblique, along with the superior rectus, contributes to upward gazing and rotating the eye upward and outward (Table 15-10). These ocular muscles never work alone; they require synergistic participation from all of the muscles of the eye. For example, looking to the left entails contraction of the lateral rectus of the left eye and the medial rectus of the right eye with simultaneous relaxation of their opposite muscles.

GENERAL VISCERAL EFFERENT

The Edinger-Westphal nucleus, the visceral oculomotor nucleus (Fig. 15-10), is responsible for the parasympathetic innervation of the intrinsic eye muscles, such as the iris and ciliary muscles. It supplies the circular (constrictor) fibers of the iris muscle, causing pupillary constriction in response to light. The light reflex does not involve the visual cortex. The parasympathetic projections of the Edinger-Westphal nucleus to the ciliary muscles regulate the refractive power of the lens by changing its shape during the accommodation reflex for near vision, which requires the participation of the visual cortex, as one has to see something to focus on it. This neuronal circuitry difference between light and accommodation reflexes is used to evaluate the extent of CNS damage.

The neural mechanism of the pupillary light reflex is displayed in Figure 15-12, and the associated physiological events are listed in Table 15-7. As light shines into an eye, the pupils in both eyes promptly react by constricting. The pupillary light reflex in both eyes is mediated through the Edinger-Westphal nucleus of

Table 15-6.   Functional Description of Oculomotor Nerve

Classification	Nuclei	Function
G (general) S (somatic) E (efferent)	Oculomotor nucleus in midbrain	Responsible for eye movement; involves all eye muscles except superior oblique and lateral rectus; also regulates levator palpebrae superioris
G (general) V (visceral) E (efferent)	Edinger-Westphal nucleus in midbrain tegmentum preganglionic projections to ciliary ganglion	Responsible for reflexive constriction of pupil, accommodation of lens for near vision

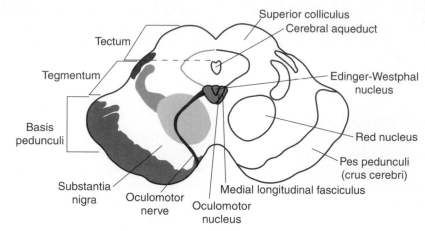

Figure 15-10. Section at superior colliculus level showing oculomotor nucleus and its fibers traveling through midbrain tegmentum.

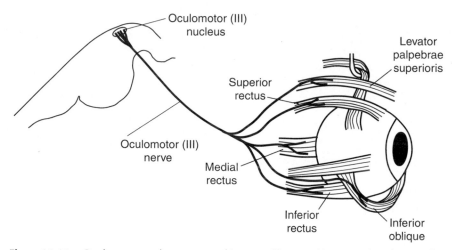

Figure 15-11. Oculomotor nucleus, course of its nerve fibers, and innervated ocular muscles.

both sides. Visual impulses from the retina travel via the optic tract, passing through the lateral geniculate body and the brachium of the superior colliculus to reach the pretectal area in the midbrain. The pretectal nucleus, anterior to the superior colliculus, projects to both Edinger-Westphal nuclei in the oculomotor complex. The Edinger-Westphal nuclei, which receive crossed and uncrossed projections, send the preganglionic parasympathetic projections along the oculomotor fibers to the ciliary ganglion lateral to the eyeball in the orbit. The postganglionic fibers from the ciliary ganglion supply the constrictor (circular) pupillary fibers of the iris (Fig. 15-12). The pupillary constriction in the illuminated eye is the direct light reflex and in the contralateral eye is the consensual reflex. In the dark, the activity of Edinger-Westphal nucleus is inhibited, and the dilation of the pupils is activated through the sympathetic projections to the dilator (radial) fibers of the iris muscle.

Accommodation–convergence reflex refers to adjustments in the shape of the lens to keep a nearing object in focus. It involves the visual cortex, because one has to see something to focus on it. This reflex consists of three components: ocular convergence, pupillary constriction, and lens thickening. This reflex is tested by asking a subject to focus on an object moving closer to the eyes. The ability to focus on the nearing object is achieved as the medial rectus muscle contracts for ocular convergence. The ciliary muscle contracts to regulate lens thickening. Its contraction narrows the optic globe, releasing the tension on the lens capsule and allowing the elastic lens to assume the natural rounded shape that is needed for near vision. The neural mechanism responsible for the accommodation reflex is slightly different from that of the light reflex, because it involves the visual cortex and superior colliculus. Impulses from the retina are relayed to the pretectal nucleus in the

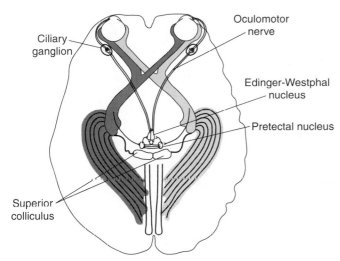

Figure 15-12. Pathway serving visual reflexes.

Table 15-7. Neuronal Events of Pupillary Light Reflex

1. Projection of light on photosensors in retina
2. Transmission of visual impulses on optic nerve and tract
3. Activation of pretectal nucleus in midbrain
4. Bilateral efferent projections to Edinger-Westphal (parasympathetic oculomotor) nucleus
5. Efferent projections through oculomotor nerve fibers to the ciliary ganglion
6. Activation of sphincter (circular) fibers of iris through the ciliary ganglion
7. Parasympathetic pupillary constriction

midbrain via the visual cortex and the superior colliculus. The crossed and uncrossed parasympathetic fibers from the pretectal nucleus reach the ciliary muscle through the Edinger-Westphal nucleus and ciliary ganglion (Fig. 15-12). The lens is connected to the ciliary processes through the suspensory ligaments. In accommodation, the reflexive contraction of the ciliary muscles pulls the ciliary processes forward, reducing the tension in the suspensory ligaments (zonules of Zinn). Reducing the tension in the suspensory ligaments releases the tension on the lens capsule and allows the elastic lens to assume its natural rounded shape. Consequently, the lens acquires the greater refractive power needed for viewing near objects. The opposite happens during relaxation of the ciliary muscles. As the ciliary muscles relax, they put tension on the suspensory ligaments and lens capsule, causing the lens to flatten and lose its refractive power.

CLINICAL INFORMATION

Oculomotor nerve pathology results in **external** and **internal ophthalmoplegia**. In external ophthalmoplegia, the extrinsic ocular muscles are paralyzed. This results in deviation of the ipsilateral eye to the lateral side (lateral strabismus) and ptosis in which the eyelid droops because of the paralysis of the levator palpebrae superioris.

In a normal physiological state, the simultaneous activation of all ocular muscles maintains the eyes slightly deviated to the midline in the horizontal axis. Oculomotor impairment may result in paralysis of the four extraocular muscles that are supplied by the third cranial nerve. This causes lateral inferior deviation of the involved eye because of the unopposed action of the intact superior oblique (trochlear nerve) and lateral rectus muscles (abducens nerve). A patient with oculomotor paralysis is likely to have difficulty looking up, down, and medially with the affected eye. Failure to direct both eyes toward an object (strabismus) in the direction opposite to the paralyzed side results in double vision (diplopia). As illustrated in Figure 15-13, a patient with left oculomotor nerve palsy is likely to have double vision when looking either straight or to the right. A patient with ptosis may compensate for the eyelid paralysis by using the frontalis muscle (facial cranial nerve) to raise the eyelid.

Internal ophthalmoplegia results from an interruption of parasympathetic fibers to the iris and causes permanent dilation of the pupil (mydriasis). This occurs because the fibers of the sphincter muscle become paralyzed and the sympathetic action on the dilator pupillary muscle fibers is unopposed.

Trochlear Nerve

GENERAL SOMATIC EFFERENT

The trochlear nerve, the second nerve contributing to ocular movement, is the only cranial nerve to exit dorsally from the brainstem (Fig. 15-3). The motor nucleus of the trochlear nerve is in the periaqueductal gray matter at the level of the inferior colliculus (Figs. 15-3B and 15-14A). The trochlear nerve fibers cross the midline in the anterior medullary velum and exit dorsally from the brainstem below the inferior colliculus (Fig. 15-3A). The nerve fibers enter the orbit with the oculomotor nerve and innervate the superior oblique muscle (Table 15-8). Contraction of this muscle causes the eye to move downward and laterally (Fig. 15-14B).

CLINICAL INFORMATION

Damage to the trochlear nerve results in paralysis of the superior oblique muscle, causing difficulty in looking downward and outward. The eye is fixed with an upward medial gaze because the actions of the inferior oblique, superior, and medial recti muscles (oculomotor nerve) are unopposed. An attempt to look down and outward results in diplopia because only one eye moves down and out, causing misalignment of the eyes.

Left oculomotor (III) nerve paralysis

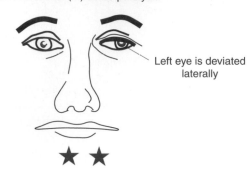

Left eye is deviated laterally

Diplopia on lateral movement to the right

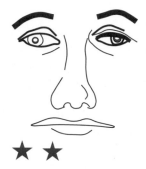

Diplopia disappears with lateral movement to the left

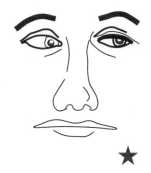

Figure 15-13.   Double vision caused by oculomotor nerve paralysis. In left oculomotor paralysis, eyelid droops (ptosis) and eye moves laterally, making the eyes disconjugate. As a result, when looking straight ahead (*center*), patient sees two images. Patient continues to see two images (*left*) when looking to the right because the left paralyzed eye cannot move beyond midline. However, a left movement of the right eye results in the eyes being conjugate (*right*). Hence, diplopia disappears.

Abducens Nerve[b]

GENERAL SOMATIC EFFERENT

The abducens is the third nerve contributing to ocular movements (Tables 15-9 and 15-10). The abducens motor nucleus is in the dorsal tegmentum of the pons within a loop formed by the facial nerve fibers (Fig. 15-3B). Fibers of the abducens nerve pass through the pontine tegmentum and pierce the corticospinal tract, exiting anteriorly from the pontomedullary junction (Figs. 15-3B and 15-15A). The abducens nerve enters the orbit and innervates the lateral rectus muscle, which moves the eye laterally (Fig. 15-15B).

CLINICAL INFORMATION

Because of its long intracranial course, the abducens nerve is highly susceptible to disruption. Its in-

juries cause the affected eye to turn in medially (medial strabismus), since the medial rectus muscle (oculomotor nerve) is functionally unopposed. With misalignment of the eyes, the patient has double vision (diplopia) when looking straight or to the affected side (Fig. 15-16). Isolated bilateral damage to the abducens nuclei and nerves results in medial deviation of both eyes because of unopposed activity of the medial rectus muscles.

The **medial longitudinal fasciculus** is an important brainstem tract with inputs from the vestibular complex and neck muscles. It projects to the motor nuclei of the ocular cranial nerves, the oculomotor, trochlear, and abducens (see Chapter 10). It coordinates the movements of the eye muscles for gaze control and

[b] To keep the discussion of the cranial nerves related to eye movements together, the abducens nerve is discussed out of order.

Table 15-8.   Functional Description of Trochlear Nerve

Classification	Nuclei	Function
G (general) S (somatic) E (efferent)	Trochlear nucleus in midbrain	Responsible for eye movement; innervates contralateral superior oblique muscle

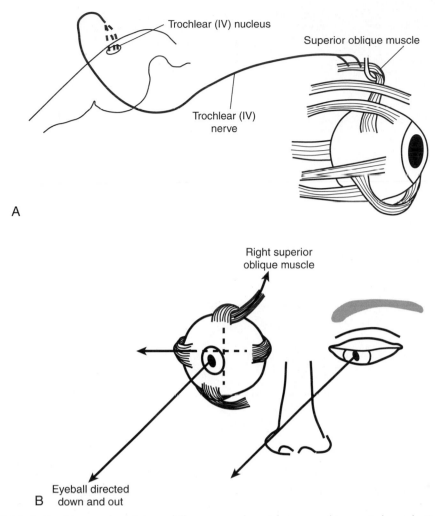

A

B   Eyeball directed down and out

Figure 15-14. A. Trochlear nucleus, intramedullary course of cranial nerve, and innervated muscle. **B.** Superior oblique muscle functioning.

Table 15-9.   Functional Description of Abducens Nerve

Classification	Nuclei	Function
G (general) S (somatic) E (efferent)	Abducens nucleus in tegmentum of pons	Responsible for lateral gaze; abducts eyeball via activation of the lateral rectus muscle

Table 15-10.   Cranial Nerves, Innervated Eye Muscles, and Their Functions

Cranial Nerve	Muscle	Functions
Oculomotor (III)	Inferior oblique	Elevates eyeball upward and outward
	Inferior rectus	Depresses eyeball downward and inward
	Medial rectus	Adducts eyeball medially and inward
	Superior rectus	Elevates eyeball upward and inward
Trochlear (IV)	Superior oblique (contralateral)	Rotates eyeball downward and outward
Abducens (VI)	Lateral rectus	Abducts eyeball laterally and outward

coordinates head position with eye movements. Lesions involving the medial longitudinal fasciculus severely affect gaze control.

Trigeminal Nerve

The trigeminal nerve is a functionally mixed nerve. As the principal sensory nerve for the head, face, orbit, and oral cavity, it mediates the sensations of pain, temperature, and discriminative touch (see Chapter 7). It has a small motor component that supplies the mastication (chewing) muscles along with other muscles (Table 15-11). The sensory and motor components together form the reflex arc for the jaw jerk reflex. It also mediates special somatic afferent (kinesthetic and proprioceptive awareness) information, which is responsible for stretch receptor feedback for the masticators.

GENERAL SOMATIC AFFERENT

The trigeminal nerve is responsible for cutaneous (touch, pain, and temperature) and proprioceptive

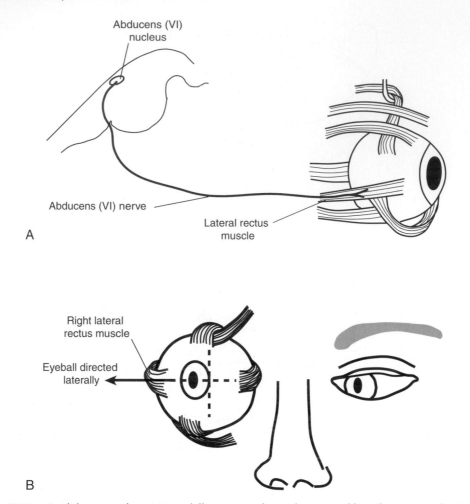

Figure 15-15. **A.** Abducens nucleus, intramedullary course of cranial nerve, and lateral rectus muscle. **B.** Lateral eye movement regulated by lateral rectus muscle.

(awareness of posture and muscle movement) sensations from the face, head, oral and nasal cavities, sinuses, teeth, anterior two-thirds of the tongue, anterior half of the pinna, external auditory meatus, and external surface of the tympanic membrane.

The sensory function of the trigeminal nerve is organized along three neurons (Fig. 7-9): the semilunar, or trigeminal, ganglion (first-order nerve cell), the trigeminal complex (second-order nerve cell), and the ventral posteromedial thalamic nucleus (third-order nerve cell). The trigeminal ganglion is external to the pons. The trigeminal nuclear complex, consisting of the chief sensory nucleus, descending spinal nucleus, and mesencephalic nucleus, is in the lateral tegmentum of the pons. Each of these sensory nuclei mediates different modalities of sensation. The chief sensory nucleus mediates discriminative sensation from the head and face. The descending spinal nucleus is primarily involved with pain and temperature and secondarily with diffuse touch. The descending spinal nucleus and its tract also receive GSA projections from the facial, glossopharyngeal, and vagus nerves. The mesencephalic nucleus mediates proprioceptive sensation from the jaw muscles.

The trigeminal nerve has three sensory branches: the ophthalmic, maxillary, and mandibular nerves (Fig. 15-17). These nerves project sensory information from the entire face and part of the head to the semilunar ganglion, the first-order trigeminal sensory nucleus. The ophthalmic nerve mediates the sensations of touch, pain, temperature, and proprioception from the skin of the forehead, anterior scalp, vertex, eyeball, upper eyelid, cornea, conjunctivum, anterior and lateral surfaces of the nose, frontal and nasal sinuses, and tentorium cerebelli. The maxillary nerve mediates sensation from the skin of the temples, posterior portion of the nose, upper cheeks, lower eyelids, and upper lips. Additional innervated oral structures include the upper gum, teeth (molar and premolar), mucosal membrane, and soft and hard palates. The maxillary nerve also receives sensations from the nasal cavity, the maxillary sinus, and the dura mater in the medial cranial fossa. The mandibular nerve, the largest of the trigeminal branches, mediates sensations from the skin on the sides of the scalp, the mucosal membrane of the lower gum, the mouth, and the meninges of the anterior and middle cranial fossae. Additional structures innervated by the trigeminal

Left abducens (VI) nerve paralysis

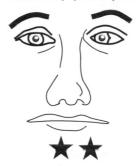

Left eye is deviated medially because of unopposed action of medial rectus

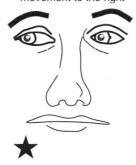

Diplopia disappears on eye movement to the right

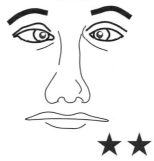

Diplopia on lateral movement to the left

Figure 15-16. Double vision caused by left abducens nerve paralysis. With paralysis of left lateral rectus muscle, the left eye moves medially because of unopposed action of the medial rectus muscle; this results in the eyes being disconjugate. Patient sees two images (diplopia) when looking straight ahead (*center*). Patient has double vision even when looking to the left (*right*) because the in-turned left eye remains disconjugate with the right eye. However, rightward movement of the right eye (*left*) results in conjugation of the eyes, causing diplopia to disappear.

Table 15-11.   Functional Description of Trigeminal Nerve

Classification	Nuclei	Function
G (general) S (somatic) A (afferent)	First-order: trigeminal ganglion Second-order: descending spinal nucleus Primary sensory nucleus	Responsible for cutaneous, proprioceptive sensation from face, head, oral cavity
B (branchial) E (efferent) or S (special) V (visceral) E (efferent)	Motor nucleus in pons	Responsible for innervation of muscles of mastication, tensor veli palatini, tensor tympani, anterior belly of digastric muscle

nerve include the anterior half of the pinna, external auditory meatus, external surface of the tympanic membrane, and anterior two-thirds of the tongue.

BRANCHIAL EFFERENT, OR SPECIAL VISCERAL EFFERENT

The motor nucleus of the trigeminal nerve lies in the mid pons, and its fibers exit with the mandibular branch of the nerve (Figs. 15-3B,15-18). The corticobulbar fibers from both motor cortices, although predominantly from the contralateral motor cortex, supply the trigemi-

nal motor nucleus. The trigeminal motor nucleus controls the muscles of mastication, which include the internal and external pterygoid, the temporalis, and the masseter; these are derived from the first branchial arch (Table 15-12). Other muscles supplied by the trigeminal motor nucleus include the mylohyoid, the anterior belly of the digastric, the tensor veli palatini (soft palate), and the tensor tympani (middle ear). The muscles of mastication (masseter, internal and external pterygoid, and temporalis), working jointly with other muscles, regulate the rotary and lateral motions of the jaw needed for chewing and the up and down motions required for speech. The tensor veli palatini, on contraction, brings the soft palate to one side. This palatal action prevents food from entering the nasal pharynx. The contraction of the tensor tympanic muscle has a pulling effect on the malleus in the middle ear; on exposure to very intense sound, the trigeminal nerve reflexively contracts the tensor tympani. Believed to be protective, this reflex restricts the movement of the tympanic membrane to prevent damage to the inner ear hair cells from very loud sounds.

CLINICAL INFORMATION

Sensory

The distribution of the trigeminal branches on the head, face, and oral cavity is well differentiated. Dam-

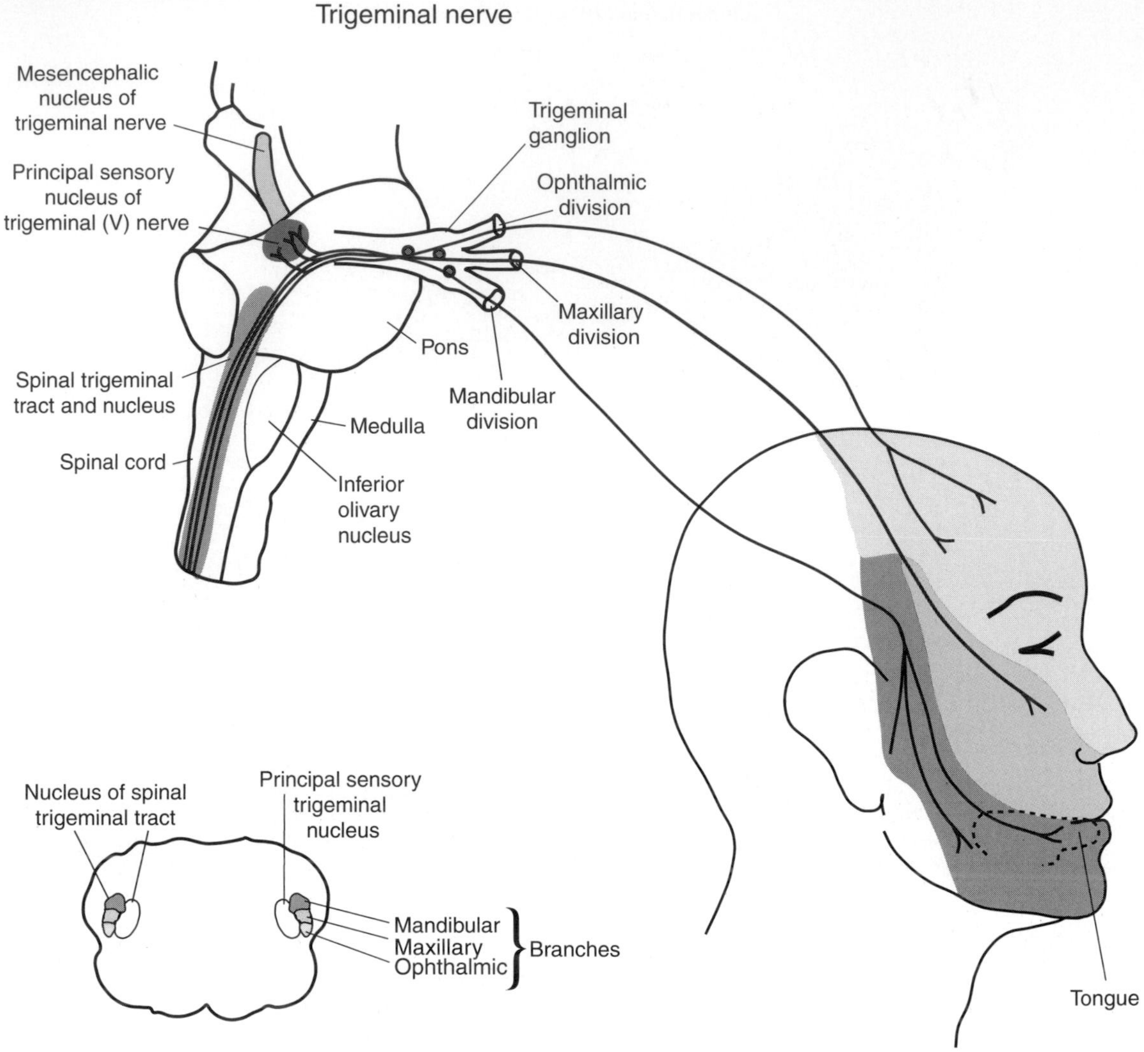

Trigeminal nerve

Figure 15-17. Trigeminal nuclear complex in the brainstem and divisions of trigeminal nerve.

age to any peripheral branch or branches results in an ipsilateral loss of sensation in the area of distribution for the nerve, which includes the face, rostral tongue, teeth and gingiva, and the cavities of the nose, orbit, and mouth. Sneezing and blinking reflexes are also lost because of the interrupted innervation of the nasal mucosa and the exterior surface of the eye. The affected branch of the nerve and the related modality (touch, pain, temperature) of sensation can be determined by clinical testing with various sensory stimuli (cotton and pinprick) and by assessing the sneeze and corneal reflexes. The most common trigeminal pathology is trigeminal neuralgia (pain), or tic douloureux. It is marked by an excruciating chronic pain of unknown cause, usually in the territory of the ophthalmic or mandibular branch. This pain, often described as burning or stabbing, can be elicited by the slightest tactile stimulus in the trigger zones of the trigeminal distribution. The recurrent stabbing pain of trigeminal neuralgia has often been surgi-

cally treated by transecting the involved nerve branch or by sectioning the sensory nerve root.

Motor

An injury in the trigeminal motor nucleus or its fibers produces a LMN syndrome characterized by a flaccid paresis or paralysis of the ipsilateral muscles of mastication. The jaw slightly deviates toward the side of the injury; this deviation is exaggerated on jaw protrusion. Along with this, the muscles twitch and gradually atrophy, and the jaw jerk reflex is absent. Since the muscles of mastication receive corticobulbar projections from the bilateral motor cortices (Fig. 15-6), any unilateral cortical or corticobulbar (UMN) injury is likely to have only a mild effect on the strength of the masticator muscles. Bilateral cortical (UMN) lesions, however, produce marked paralysis of the masticators bilaterally. With weakened elevator muscles, as in the case of a bilateral cortical lesion (UMN syndrome), the mandible

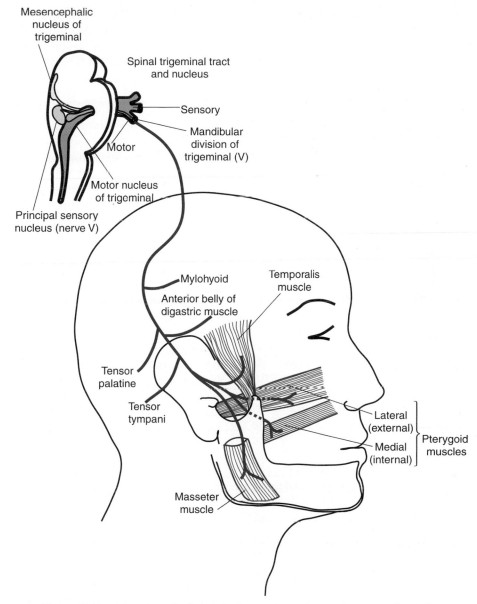

Figure 15-18.   Motor branch of trigeminal nerve, its nucleus, and innervated muscles.

Table 15-12.   Muscles of Mastication and Their Functions

Muscle	Function
Lateral and external pterygoid	Depresses and protrudes mandible toward opposite side; regulates movement side to side
Masseter	Elevates, closes, slightly protrudes mandible
Medial and internal pterygoid	Elevates, assists in mandible protrusion
Temporalis	Elevates, retracts mandible

hangs low, causing structural difficulty in the production of vowels and labial and lingual consonant sounds. The motor strength in patients with masticator palsy is assessed by asking them to bite down on a tongue depressor, move the jaw laterally against resistance, or open the jaw against resistance.

Facial Nerve

The facial nerve is functionally mixed. It is primarily a motor nerve for facial muscles and the stapedius muscle, but it also contains a small sensory component (Table 15-13). The facial nerve complex supplies the muscles of the face and scalp (facial expression), which are derived from the second branchial arch. It also contains secretory parasympathetic efferents to the lacrimal, sublingual, and submandibular glands and to the secretory glands in the mouth and nasal cavities. The sensory function of the facial nerve involves the mediation of taste sensation from the anterior two-thirds of the tongue and the nasopharynx.

The facial nuclear complex, which is in the laterocaudal pons at the level of the abducens nucleus, consists of three nuclei: the facial motor nucleus, the superior salivatory nucleus, and the nucleus solitarius (Figs. 15-3 and 15-19). The facial nerve fibers pass upward lateral to the abducens nerve nucleus, loop over the top of the nucleus at the floor of the fourth ventricle, and descend to exit laterally in the caudal pons (the junction of the pons and medulla). After exiting, the nerve fibers enter the internal acoustic meatus along with the vestibulocochlear nerve. At the end of the meatus is the geniculate ganglion (Fig. 15-19), where the facial nerve fibers separate from the vestibulocochlear nerve, enter the facial canal, and finally emerge from the stylomastoid foramen. After exiting, the nerve diverges to supply the muscles of facial expression and the stapedius muscle in the middle ear.

GENERAL VISCERAL EFFERENT

The GVE fibers of the facial nerve arise from the superior salivatory nucleus in the brainstem and supply the lacrimal, submandibular, and sublingual glands with visceral efferent impulses. The GVE fibers leave the facial nerve at the geniculate ganglion and carry the preganglionic parasympathetic fibers to the pterygopalatine ganglion and lacrimal nucleus. Postganglionic projections from the lacrimal nucleus and pterygopalatine ganglion are parasympathetic to the lacrimal glands in the eye and the glands in the nose and palate. The lacrimal gland produces tears, and the glands in the palate secrete saliva (Fig. 15-19*B*).

Some of the GVE fibers continue in the facial nerve and join the chorda tympani nerve, a sensory branch of the facial nerve that merges with the lingual branch of the trigeminal nerve. These GVE fibers transmit impulses to the submaxillary ganglion. The submaxillary ganglion provides the secretory parasympathetic fibers to the sublingual and submandibular glands, which regulate the secretions from the mucous membrane in the mouth and pharynx (Fig. 15-19*B*).

SPECIAL VISCERAL AFFERENT

The sensory root of the facial nerve carries gustatory sensation from the taste buds in the anterior two-thirds of the tongue. These taste-carrying afferent fibers travel along the lingual nerve of the mandibular branch of the trigeminal nerve and join the chorda tympani nerve. The fibers of the chorda tympani merge with the facial motor fibers toward the end of the facial canal in the middle ear. The sensory fibers with the first-order nerve cells in the geniculate ganglion enter the brainstem and terminate in the tractus and nucleus solitarius (Fig. 15-19), which sends this taste sensation to the sensory cortex through the ventral posterior medial nucleus of the thalamus.

BRANCHIAL EFFERENT, OR SPECIAL VISCERAL EFFERENT

The BE/SVE functional component of the facial nerve innervates all the muscles of facial expression. Fibers from the facial nucleus move toward the floor of the fourth ventricle in the pontine tegmentum and make a U-turn over the abducens nucleus (Fig. 15-3). The facial nerve fibers travel downward and exit from the lateral portion of the caudal pons (Fig. 15-19). After exiting, the nerve divides into the temporal, zygomatic, buccal, mandibular, and cervical branches to innervate the muscles of facial expression (depressor anguli oris, depressor labii inferioris, levator anguli oris, mentalis, orbicularis oculi, orbicularis oris, platysma, risorius, buccinator, and zygomaticus), which are jointly responsible for kissing, blowing, speaking, smiling, frowning, grimacing, raising the eyebrows, and exhibiting emotional expressions such as happiness, apathy, and sorrow (Table 15-14). The buccinator muscle in particular contributes to swallowing by compressing the cheeks to prevent food accumulation in the buccal (facial) sulci. The fibers of these facial branches also innervate the extrinsic muscles of the ear, the stapedius muscle of the middle ear, the stylohyoid muscle, and the posterior belly of the digastric muscle.

CLINICAL INFORMATION

The facial nerve fibers are responsible for different sensorimotor functions and thus take different routes to their destinations. The site of a given lesion determines which clinical signs emerge in the facial muscles. For example, an injury near the pons and surrounding area is likely to affect all three functions of the facial nerve, resulting in paralysis of the ipsilateral facial muscles, excessive secretion from the glands, and loss of taste from the anterior two-thirds of the tongue (Fig. 15-19). An injury in the facial nerve fibers at or beyond the stylomastoid foramen, where its fibers separate, is likely to result in paralysis of the ipsilateral half of the facial muscles, sparing glandular secretion and taste sensation. Similarly, an injury to the chorda tympanic fibers before they

Table 15-13.   Functional Description of Facial Nerve

Classification	Nuclei	Function
G (general) V (visceral) E (efferent)	Superior salivatory nucleus preganglionic to ganglia associated with glands	Secretions from lacrimal, sublingual, submaxillary glands
S (special) V (visceral) A (afferent)	First-order cells: geniculate ganglion Second-order cells: nucleus solitarius	Mediates taste sensations from anterior two-thirds of tongue and nasopharynx
B(branchial) E(efferent) or S (special) V (visceral) E (efferent)	Motor nucleus in lateral pons	Innervates muscles of facial expression, stapedius muscle

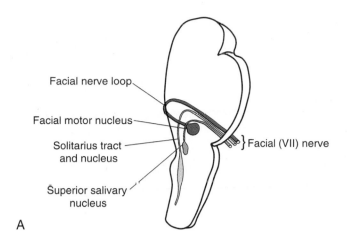

A

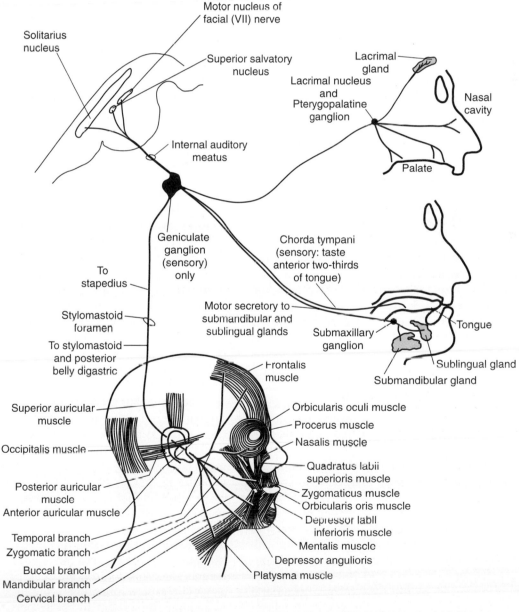

B

Figure 15-19.   Facial nuclear complex in the brainstem, sensorimotor branches, and innervated structures.

Table 15-14. Muscles of Facial Expression

Muscle	Function
Buccinator	Presses cheeks against teeth, forms stable lateral wall to oral cavity; prevents accumulation of food
Corrugator	Draws eyebrows together during expression of suffering
Depressor anguli oris	Draws mouth down and to the side in grimace and smile
Depressor labii inferioris	Draws corners of lips downward
Frontalis	Raises eyebrows and contributes to wrinkling of forehead
Levator anguli oris	Draws corner of lips and raises angle of mouth
Levator labii superioris	Lifts angle of upper lip and turns it outward
Mentalis	Raises, protrudes and wrinkles lower lip
Orbicularis oculi	Surrounds orbit; contributes to eye closing
Orbicularis oris	Contributes to closing lips, pressing lips against teeth, shaping lips for speech
Platysma	Pulls lower lip and corner of mouth downward; draws neck skin up; contributes to smiling
Risorius	Retracts corners of mouth
Superioris alaeque nasi	Elevates and protrudes upper lip
Zygomaticus major	Functions as a sling with depressor anguli oris; draws angle of mouth up and to the side
Zygomaticus minor	Raises upper lip, contributing to a broad smile

merge with the facial motor root affects only taste sensation from the anterior two-thirds of the tongue and secretion from sublingual and submandibular glands. Involvement of the GVE fibers to the pterygopalatine ganglion causes secretory dysfunctions of the glands in the eye and palate. Interruption of the efferents to the middle ear causes paralysis of the stapedius muscle (working jointly with the tensor tympani); impaired control of stapedius results in **hyperacusia**, a condition in which normal sounds seem very loud. The stapedius muscle, when functioning properly, reflexively dampens the ear drum and constricts ossicular movements.

The corticobulbar fibers differentially innervate the upper and lower face muscles (Figs. 15-6 and 15-20). The motor nucleus that controls the lower half of the face receives projections from the **contralateral** motor cortex alone. However, the facial nucleus innervating the upper facial muscles (frontalis and orbicularis) receives corticobulbar projections from both motor cortices (**bilateral innervation**). This scheme of motor innervation has significant clinical implications for UMN (supranuclear) and LMN (internuclear) syndromes. A dysfunction in the unilateral motor cortex (UMN) affects the muscles in the contralateral lower half of the face (Fig. 15-20A). The upper facial muscles are spared in the case of a contralateral cortical lesion. The patient is able to wrinkle the forehead and close the eye, because these muscles continue to re-

ceive partial projections from the **ipsilateral motor cortex**. Complete destruction of either the facial nucleus (LMN), which involves the nuclear regions for both the upper and lower face, or a bilateral cortical lesion is necessary to cause paralysis of all the upper and lower muscles in the face (Fig. 15-20B); it produces disastrous effects on the articulation of labial and labiodental sounds. Bilateral corticobulbar (UMN) lesions, also known as pseudobulbar palsy, produces bilateral facial palsy and results in profound impairments of motor speech. Patients lose delicate and discrete motor control, and muscles become paralyzed. In bilateral facial paralysis, the lips may be parted at rest and remain so during a smile and/or speech attempts.

A condition commonly associated with facial nerve dysfunctioning is Bell's palsy, an LMN syndrome. It is characterized by a sudden onset of paralysis of all ipsilateral upper and lower facial muscles (Fig. 15-20B). The muscles of the lower face sag, the fold around the lip and nose (nasolabial fold) flattens, and the palpebral fissure widens. On the side of the lesion, the patient is unable to wrinkle the forehead, close the eye, show the teeth, or purse the lips. With no motor control of the facial muscles, the corner of the mouth droops and food and saliva accumulate in the affected side of the mouth. The paralyzed side of the face is pulled toward the unaffected side. While the person is smiling, the lower portion of the face is pulled toward the unaffected side, resulting in a transverse shape of the lips. Furthermore, the corneal reflex is absent on the side of the lesion, but corneal sensation remains intact. Additional symptoms include impairments of sublingual and submandibular salivary secretion, hyperacusis, and loss of taste from the anterior two-thirds of the tongue.

Bell's palsy may result from a degenerative inflammatory injury or from an infection of the facial nerve after its exit from the brainstem. Depending on the site of the lesion, sensory and parasympathetic (gland secretions) functions may also be impaired in Bell's palsy. For example, all of the motor, secretory, and taste functions of the nerves are lost if the lesion is proximal to the geniculate ganglion (Fig. 15-19).

An interesting clinical observation in the case of facial paralysis from a supranuclear lesion in the motor cortex (UMN) is the preservation of emotional expression while the facial muscles are paralyzed for voluntary control. The paralyzed facial muscles continue to respond involuntarily to genuine emotional stimuli and states. One explanation is that pathways mediating preserved emotional expression differ from the ones originating in the motor cortex. Emotional pathways consist of extrapyramidal integrated prefrontal, limbic, basal ganglia, and hypothalamic projections to the brainstem premotor reticular generator that controls the muscles of facial expression.

The motor functions of the facial nerve are tested by asking the patient to smile, part the lips, show the teeth, puff out the cheeks, pucker the lips, and express

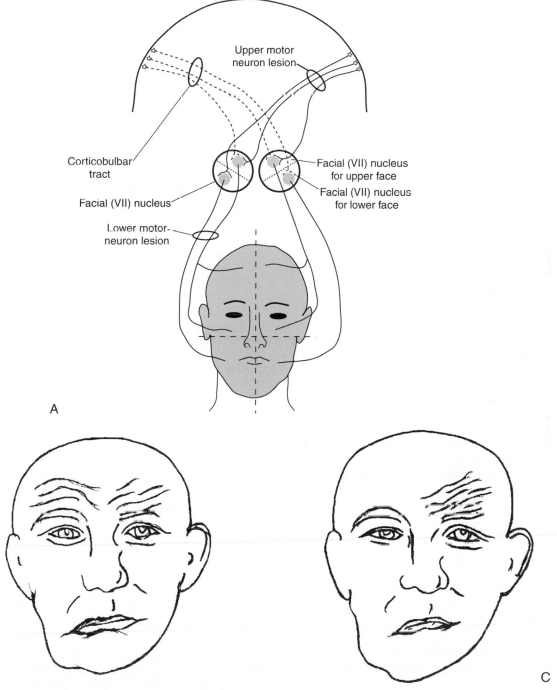

Figure 15-20. **A.** Distribution of facial nerve fibers carrying unilateral and bilateral projections from the cortex. Upper portion of face receives bilateral cortical projections, and lower half of face receives efferent commands from the contralateral motor cortex only. This differential neuronal organization for facial muscles accounts for different patterns of facial paralysis after UMN and LMN lesions. **B.** In UMN (left) syndrome, patient exhibits only lower facial palsy (loss of nasolabial fold and sagging of lower mouth) with preserved strength in frontalis and ocular muscles. **C.** In LMN (Bell's palsy) syndrome (right), one entire side of face is paralyzed.

emotions, while the examiner looks for signs of facial asymmetry. Sugar and salt are used to assess taste from the tongue.

Vestibuloacoustic Nerve

The vestibuloacoustic nerve has vestibular (see Chapter 10) and acoustic (see Chapter 9) branches (Table 15-15). Both branches are laterally attached to the brainstem at the junction of the medulla and pons (Fig. 15-1). The vestibular division mediates head position (equilibrium) in space, whereas the acoustic branch serves hearing.

SPECIAL SOMATIC AFFERENT

Vestibular Nerve

The vestibular system is a reflexive sensorimotor system that controls equilibrium, including regulation of neck position. In addition, the vestibular apparatus helps humans coordinate head and body movements and retain a stable visual fixation point in space during body and head movements. The vestibular branch of the vestibuloacoustic nerve originates from the vestibular (superior and inferior) ganglion equivalent of the dorsal root ganglia (DRG) neurons in the internal auditory meatus. The distal fibers of the vestibular ganglion innervate the hair cells in the cristae of the semicircular canals, saccule, and utricle. Their proximal axons make up the vestibular nerve and project impulses from the hair cells to the vestibular complex in the floor of the medulla's fourth ventricle (Fig. 10-4). The vestibular nuclei send ascending projections to the flocculonodular lobe of the cerebellum, reticular formation, medial longitudinal fasciculus, and motor nuclei of other cranial and spinal nerves (see Chapter 10). The descending projections from the vestibular nuclei to the spinal cord coordinate the limbs for standing balance. The importance of the vestibular system becomes evident in patients whose body equilibrium is impaired by vestibular dysfunctioning, as in Ménière's disease or because of a vestibuloacoustic schwannoma.

Auditory Nerve

The acoustic fibers of the CN VIII, which serve hearing, originate in the spiral ganglia (equivalent to DRG neuron); the peripheral processes of the cells in the spiral ganglia innervate the hair cells in the organ of Corti in the inner ear. The proximal axons of the spiral ganglion, the primary cell bodies of the auditory nerve, mediate auditory impulses to the cochlear nuclei in the rostrolateral medulla (Fig. 9-6). Some of the auditory fibers from the cochlear nuclei ascend ipsilaterally, while several others cross the midline through the trapezoid bodies. Most of the crossed auditory fibers terminate in the superior olivary nucleus, while some bypass it and ascend to the midbrain. The projections from the superior olivary nucleus form the lateral lemniscus, which ascends to the inferior colliculus of the midbrain. The fibers from the inferior colliculus travel through the brachium of the inferior colliculus to the medial geniculate body of the thalamus. The auditory fibers from the thalamus pass posterior to the internal capsule, then project to the primary auditory cortex in the temporal lobe. The auditory nerve has two important characteristics: (*a*) Its crossed and uncrossed fibers result in bilateral projections to the cortex. (*b*) Throughout its projections to the brain, a spatial tonotopic representation in tract fibers of various frequencies is discretely maintained .

CLINICAL INFORMATION

Injuries to the vestibuloacoustic nerve are associated with disturbances of equilibrium and audition. Symptoms of vestibular nerve dysfunctioning are impaired equilibrium, vertigo or dizziness (the sensation of moving around in space), and nystagmus (rhythmic movement of the eye in which the eye moves slowly away from the center and then returns rapidly).

There are two types of hearing impairment: conductive and sensorineural. The exact nature of the hearing impairment depends on the site of the lesion. Damage to the peripheral mechanism involving the tympanic membrane and/or middle ear ossicles results in conductive hearing loss, which may not be very disabling. Damage to the labyrinthine systems (organ of Corti, spiral ganglia, cochlear nerve, cochlear nuclei, and/or central auditory pathways) results in sensorineural impairment, which can be disabling. For example, if the cochlear nerve is damaged, hearing impairment in the affected ear may be permanent and profound. However, in the case of a brainstem lesion impairment is only partial because of the bilaterality of auditory projections to the cortex. An important symptom of sensorineural hearing loss is tinnitus, a sensation of ringing, buzzing, or other noises (see Chapters 9 and 10).

Glossopharyngeal Nerve

The glossopharyngeal and vagus nerves share similar anatomy and functions, although they follow different peripheral pathways. The glossopharyngeal nerve serves both sensory and motor functions (Table 15-16). The sensorimotor nucleus complex of the nerve consists

Table 15-15. Functional Description of Vestibuloacoustic Nerve

Classification	Nuclei	Function
S (special) S (somatic) A (afferent)	First-order cells: vestibular ganglia Second-order cells: vestibular nuclei in caudal pons;	Equilibrium and orientation in space
S (special) S (somatic) A (afferent)	First-order cells: spiral ganglia; Second-order cells: cochlear nuclei in caudal pons	Hearing

of the inferior salivatory nucleus, nucleus ambiguus, and nucleus solitarius (Figs. 15-21 and 15-22); the latter two nuclei are shared with the vagus nerve. After exiting laterally from the medulla posterior to the inferior olivary nucleus (Figs. 2-49 and 2-50), the nerve fibers leave the skull through the jugular foramen. At the opening of the foramen is the inferior ganglion, which contains the first-order cell bodies for cutaneous and taste sensation.

GENERAL VISCERAL AFFERENT

GVA fibers, which are primarily concerned with the initiation of reflexes, mediate the cutaneous touch,

pain, tension, and temperature sensations from intraoral visceral structures including the upper pharynx, tonsils, eustachian tube, soft palate, and posterior third of the tongue. With the primary sensory cell bodies in the inferior ganglion near the jugular foramina, the central processes from the inferior ganglion project to the nucleus solitarius in the medulla (Fig. 15-22). This sensory information later travels to the ventral posterior medial nucleus of the thalamus via the ventral secondary ascending trigeminal tract and subsequently to the sensory cortex in the rostral parietal lobe (see Chapter 7).

The GVA fibers also receive inputs from the chemoreceptors of the carotid body, the baroreceptors in the wall of the carotid sinus, and the middle ear. The carotid body chemoreceptors respond to changes in the carbon dioxide and oxygen content of the circulating blood and reflexively control the rate of respiration through modulation of the reticular respiratory center (see Chapter 16). The carotid sinus baroreceptors respond to increased blood pressure and reflexively control the flow of blood by dilating peripheral blood vessels. GVA afferents also mediate pain from the middle ear, which is often seen in the case of infection.

GENERAL VISCERAL EFFERENT

The GVE system is concerned with the autonomic control of visceral body organs including glands and cardiac muscles. The inferior salivatory nucleus mediates parasympathetic projections to the parotid gland. The preganglionic parasympathetic fibers from the inferior salivary nucleus supply the otic ganglion, which regulates secretion from the parotid gland in the oral cavity (Fig. 15-22).

Table 15-16.   Functional Description of Glossopharyngeal Nerve

Classification	Nuclei	Function
G (general) V (visceral) A (afferent)	First-order cells: inferior ganglion Second-order cells: nucleus solitarius	Mediates general visceral sensation from soft palate, palatal arch, posterior third of tongue, carotid sinus
G (general) V (visceral) E (efferent)	Inferior salivatory nucleus	Regulates secretion from parotid gland
S (special) V (visceral) A (afferent)	First-order cells: inferior ganglion Second-order cells: nucleus solitarius	Transmits taste sensation from posterior third of tongue and nasopharynx
B (branchial) E (efferent), or S (special) V (visceral) E (efferent)	Nucleus ambiguus	Contributes to swallowing by activating stylopharyngeus and upper pharyngeal constrictor fibers

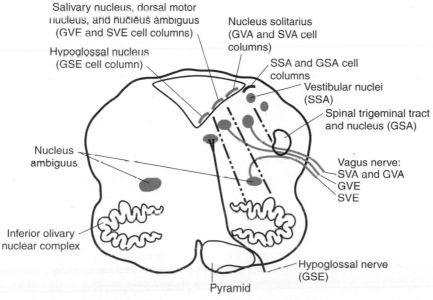

Figure 15-21.   A cross section of the medulla showing locations of nuclei: hypoglossal nucleus (GSE), salivary nucleus and dorsal motor nucleus (GVE), nucleus ambiguus (BE/SVE), nucleus solitarius (GVA and SVA), and vestibular and trigeminal nuclei (SSA and GSA). Many of these nuclei are shared by glossopharyngeal and vagus nerves.

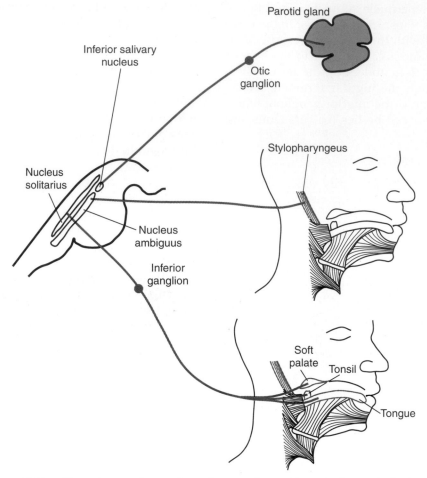

Figure 15-22.   Glossopharyngeal nerve, its nuclear complex, and its projections to the brainstem.

SPECIAL VISCERAL AFFERENT

The SVA fibers mediate taste information from taste buds in the posterior third of the tongue and scattered throughout the oral pharynx. The sensory processes, with their primary cell bodies in the inferior ganglion, send projections to the medulla, where they travel in the tractus solitarius, later terminating in the rostral nucleus solitarius (Fig. 15-22). Fibers from the nucleus solitarius proceed in the medial lemniscus to the ventral posterior nucleus of the thalamus and then to the tongue area in the primary sensory cortex.

BRANCHIAL EFFERENT, OR SPECIAL VISCERAL EFFERENT

The BE/SVE projections of the glossopharyngeal nerve contribute to swallowing by innervating the stylopharyngeus, a branchial or special visceral muscle derived from the third branchial arch (Fig. 15-2). The BE fibers of the glossopharyngeal nerve originate in the rostral region of the nucleus ambiguus, a column of motor nuclei also shared by the vagus cranial nerve. The nucleus ambiguus, dorsolateral to the inferior olivary nucleus (Fig. 15-21), receives UMN input from both sides of the motor cortex (corticobulbar tracts), with contralateral input being somewhat stronger. The fibers from the nucleus ambiguus exit the lateral medulla, supplying the ipsilateral stylopharyngeus muscle (Fig. 15-22).

CLINICAL INFORMATION

Because of the overlapping of nuclei and their proximity to other cranial nerves and nuclei, a lesion selectively affecting the glossopharyngeal nerve or its nuclei is rare. Nevertheless, a discrete lesion results in partial paresis of the unilateral stylopharyngeal muscle, impairing ipsilateral pharyngeal elevation in deglutition. An additional symptom is loss of general and taste sensation from the ipsilateral posterior third of the tongue. Impaired cutaneous sensation from the posterior tongue causes loss of the gag reflex. Furthermore, poor control of the parotid gland leads to excessive oral secretion. The symptoms are particularly pronounced following bilateral damage of the nerve. Dysfunctions of the glossopharyngeal nerve are usually assessed with the functions of the vagus nerve.

Vagus Nerve

The vagus, with more extensive distribution than any other cranial nerve, is 90% sensory and 10% motor (Table 15-17). From perspectives of students and professionals in communicative disorders, by far the most important function of the vagus nerve is its control of the muscles used for phonation and swallowing (deglutition). The vagus nerve innervates the cardiac muscles and smooth muscles of the esophagus, stomach, and intestine, and the branchial muscles of the pharynx and larynx. This nerve also mediates the cutaneous sensations from the muscles of the pharynx and larynx and visceral muscles of the epiglottis, thorax, and abdomen and the taste sensation from the pharynx and epiglottis. The vagus nerve also mediates general somesthetic input (GSA) and special somatic afferent (SSA with stretch feedback from pharyngeal muscles).

The vagal nuclear complex is in the ventricular floor of the medulla oblongata. It consists of the dorsal motor nucleus, the nucleus ambiguus, and the nucleus solitarius (Fig. 15-21). The nucleus ambiguus receives UMN input from both sides of the cortex, but the contralateral projection is somewhat stronger. The vagus nerve exits the brainstem from the lateral medulla between the inferior olivary nucleus and the inferior cerebellar peduncle (Fig. 15-1) and distributes its sensorimotor branches peripherally.

GENERAL VISCERAL AFFERENT

The cutaneous sensation is involved with the regulation of cardiovascular, respiratory, and gastrointestinal functions. The GVA component mediates general sensation, including touch, pain, tension, and temperature, from receptors in the walls of the viscera that include the pharynx, larynx, thorax, abdomen, heart, bronchi, and esophagus (Fig. 15-23). The primary cell bodies of these sensory fibers are in the inferior ganglion (equivalent of DRG), which is in the jugular foramen. The inferior ganglion projects to the tractus and nucleus solitarius. The afferent fibers from the nucleus solitarius travel in the medial lemniscus to a special part of the ventral posterior medial nucleus of the thalamus, then to the parietal superior opercular part of the sensory cortex in the sylvian sulcus.

GENERAL VISCERAL EFFERENT

As part of the ANS, the GVE fibers parasympathetically innervate the viscera, including the cardiac muscles and the smooth muscles of the trachea, bronchi, esophagus, stomach, and intestines. The dorsal motor nucleus, which is laterally in the ventricular floor, receives afferents from the hypothalamus and solitary tract. The long fibers leaving the dorsal motor nucleus send preganglionic projections to distal ganglia in the walls of the alimentary canal and digestive organs, including the trachea, bronchi, heart, esophagus, stomach, and intestines. The short postganglionic fibers regulate the functions of these structures (Fig. 15-24). The parasympathetic autonomic innervation of the rectum, bladder, and genitals is supplied from S-2 to S-4 spinal segments (see Chapter 16).

SPECIAL VISCERAL AFFERENT

The SVA fibers mediate taste sensation from the pharyngeal area. The sensory fibers from the base of the tongue, epiglottis, larynx, and pharynx have their cell bodies in the inferior ganglion (equivalent to DRG); they project to the tractus and nucleus solitarius in the medulla oblongata (Fig. 15-25). The fibers from the nucleus solitarius ascend in the medial lemniscus to the ventral posterior medial nucleus of the thalamus, from which fibers project to the sensory cortex in the parietal lobe. The primary (inferior ganglia) and secondary (solitarius) nuclei are shared by the glossopharyngeal nerve while serving the same SVA and GVA functions.

BRANCHIAL EFFERENT, OR SPECIAL VISCERAL EFFERENT

BE/SVE projections of the vagus nerve innervate muscles that are important to students of communicative disorders: those of the larynx, pharynx, and the upper part of the esophagus (Fig. 15-26). These motor fibers of the vagus nerve originate from the posterior two-thirds of the nucleus ambiguus (one-third of the nucleus is related to the glossopharyngeal nerve), which is known to receive corticobulbar projections from both sides of the cortex. The efferent fibers supply the branchial muscles of the pharynx, the muscles of the soft palate (except for the tensor palatini, which is served by

Table 15-17. Functional Description of Vagus Nerve

Classification	Nuclei	Function
G (general) V (visceral) A (afferent)	First-order cells: inferior ganglion Second-order cells: nucleus solitarius	Receives general sensation from muscles of pharynx, larynx, thorax, carotid body, abdomen; regulates nausea, oxygen intake, lung inflation
G (general) V (visceral) E (efferent)	Dorsal motor nucleus with preganglionic projections to visceral plexuses	Innervates glands, cardiac muscles, muscles of heart, trachea, bronchi, esophagus, stomach, intestine
S (special) V (visceral) A (afferent)	First-order cells: inferior ganglion Second-order cells: nucleus solitarius	Mediates taste sensation from posterior pharynx and epiglottis
B (branchial) E (efferent) or S (special) V (visceral) E (efferent)	Nucleus ambiguus	Controls muscles of larynx, pharynx, soft palate for phonation, swallowing, resonance

Vagus: general visceral afferent

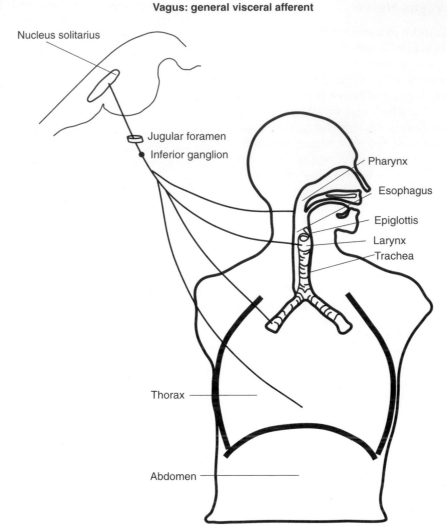

Figure 15-23. Nucleus solitarius with its GVA fibers, which mediate general sensation from muscles of pharynx, larynx, thorax, and abdomen.

the trigeminal nerve), the intrinsic muscles of the larynx, and the upper area of the esophagus.

The pharyngeal branch of the nerve supplies the three constrictor muscles (superior, middle, and inferior) of the pharynx and all soft palate muscles (palatoglossus and levator palati) except for the tensor palatini (trigeminal nerve). The superior laryngeal branch of the vagus divides into internal and external laryngeal branches. The external branch of the superior laryngeal nerve controls the cricothyroid muscle, an internal laryngeal muscle. The internal branch is sensory to mucous membrane as far down as vocal cord and the adjacent area. The recurrent laryngeal branch of the vagus takes different routes on the two sides. It curves around the subclavian artery before emerging on the right side but curves around the aortic arch on the left side. The recurrent laryngeal nerve fibers innervate the intrinsic muscles of the larynx and epiglottis and therefore play an important role in phonation (Fig. 15-26). While these branches provide motor control to the larynx, some of its

fibers are responsible for sensory innervation of the mucous membrane inferior to the vocal cords.

The nucleus ambiguus also receives afferent projections from the tractus solitarius, which contains stretch afferent feedback from the muscles innervated by the glossopharyngeal and vagus nerves (stretch reflexes). These afferent and efferent projections form the reticular neuronal circuitry that enables reflexes such as gagging, coughing, vomiting, and swallowing.

CLINICAL INFORMATION

The medulla oblongata, the site of many reticular networks, vital reflex centers, and several cranial nuclei, is a vitally important anatomical structure. Reflexes required for survival, such as swallowing, gagging, coughing, sneezing, vomiting, breathing, and cardiac rate require normal functioning of output nuclei, including nucleus ambiguus, dorsal vagus nucleus, and the hypoglossal nuclei and input association nuclei, especially the nucleus solitarius. Vagus nerve fibers par-

Vagus: general visceral efferent

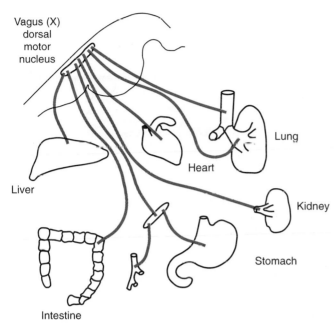

Figure 15-24. Dorsal motor nucleus of vagus nerve in medulla and its GVE projections to smooth muscle fibers of heart, trachea, bronchi, esophagus, stomach, and intestine.

ticipate in almost all of these functions. Most of the networks that organize and control these vital reflexes involve many regions of the reticular formation in the medulla, with hierarchical control from the higher CNS. Consequently, medullary lesions, especially large ones that damage both sides of the medullary reticular area, can damage aspects of these networks and their input and/or output nuclei, often with lethal consequences (see Chapter 16). For students of communicative disorders, the functions of the nucleus ambiguus are very important. A unilateral lesion of the nerve fibers and/or nucleus ambiguus is likely to result in ipsilateral paresis or paralysis of the soft palate, pharynx, and larynx. Injuries specifically to the pharyngeal branch of the vagus nerve cause paralysis of the pharynx and the soft palate, leading to swallowing difficulty. With unilateral paralysis of the levator muscle of the soft palate, the soft palate lowers on the affected side, and the uvula is pulled to the unaffected side (Fig. 15-27). With bilateral soft palate paralysis, despite symmetry, the soft palate hangs lower than its normal curvature (Fig. 15-27). Recurrent laryngeal nerve disorders lead to paralysis of the vocal folds. Unilateral LMN paralysis of the vocal folds causes breathy voice, diplophonia, and hoarseness but affects the ability to phonate only minimally. Vocal cord paral-

Vagus: special visceral afferent

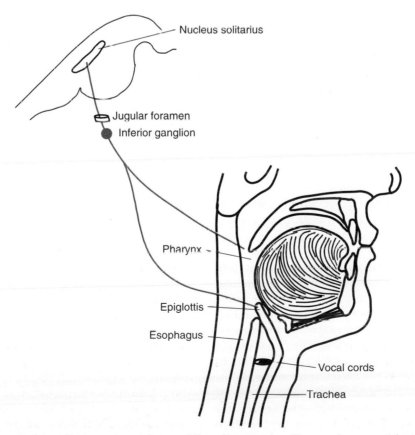

Figure 15-25. Nucleus solitarius and special visceral fibers from muscles of larynx, pharynx, epiglottis, and palate.

Vagus: special visceral efferent

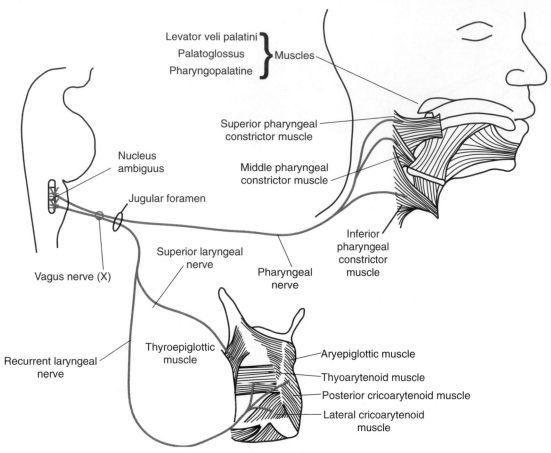

Figure 15-26. Vagus nucleus ambiguus with its BE/SVE projections to branchial muscles of larynx and pharynx.

ysis may also cause choking and pulmonary aspiration. Bilateral injury to the recurrent laryngeal nerve, however, produces inspiratory stridor and aphonia. It can also be life threatening if the paralyzed vocal cords impair air flow. Unilateral central (UMN) lesions in the brainstem involving the corticobulbar fibers cause harsh voice quality. However, such lesions do not produce severe phonatory and swallowing symptoms, since the nucleus ambiguus receives UMN input from both sides of the cortex (Fig. 15-6).

With vagus nerve injuries, many autonomic functions and visceral reflexes, such as coronary circulation, heart rate, and relaxation and contraction of tracheal and bronchial muscles, are impaired. Altered autonomic reflexes include vomiting, coughing, sneezing, sucking, hiccuping, and yawning. Damage to the sensory nuclear complex of the vagus leads to anesthesia of the larynx, pharynx, and associated structures and to loss of taste sensation from the pharyngeal and epiglottic areas. Because the glossopharyngeal, vagus, and spinal accessory nerves all pass through the jugular foramen, peripheral lesions involving the vagus nerve

alone are uncommon. Loss of vagus nerve functions are tested by visual examination of the soft palate and pharyngeal cavity and assessment of quality in phonatory and swallowing tasks.

Spinal Accessory Nerve

BRANCHIAL EFFERENT, OR SPECIAL VISCERAL EFFERENT

The spinal accessory is a branchiomeric motor nerve (Table 15-18) that receives projections primarily from the contralateral motor cortex. The corticospinal projections transmit nerve impulses through the spinal roots of the nerve. The remnants of gill-related muscles continue to C-1 through C-5. These fibers are classified as a cranial nerve, even though they originate from the spinal cord. The efferents from the LMNs in the ventral horns in C-1 through C-5 fuse longitudinally to enter the cranial cavity through the foramen magnus and leave the cranium via the jugular foramen (Figs. 15-1 and 15-3). They follow the vagus nerve, and the efferent fibers innervate two neck muscles, the trapezius and the stern-

Normal soft palate

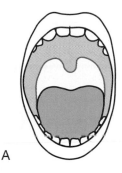

A

Left unilateral soft
palate paralysis

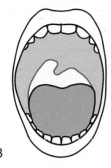

B

Bilateral soft
palate paralysis

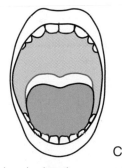

C

Figure 15-27. A. Normal soft palate. **B.** Paralysis of left soft palate and pharyngeal wall from a LMN lesion. Sagging of left pharyngeal wall and palatal arch moves uvula to the right, away from the side of the lesion. Muscles involved in this paralysis include levator veli palatini, palatoglossal, and palatopharyngeus. **C.** In bilateral soft palate paralysis, palatal arch remains symmetrical, although its curvature hangs lower than normal. Complete vagus nerve interruption causes many additional problems involving muscles of pharynx, palate, and larynx.

Table 15-18.   Functional Description of Spinal Accessory Nerve

Classification	Nuclei	Function
B(branchial) E(efferent) or S (special) V (visceral) E (efferent)	Spinal accessory nucleus in C-1–C-5 ventral horns of spinal cord	Controls head position by controlling trapezius, sternocleidomastoid muscles

ocleidomastoid (Fig. 15-28). The trapezius muscle tilts the head back and to the side and contributes to shrugging, and the sternocleidomastoid tilts the head forward and rotates it to the side opposite the muscle.

CLINICAL INFORMATION

The trapezius and sternocleidomastoid, combined with other adjacent neck muscles, contribute to tilt, forward and backward extension, and lateral rotation of the head. Accessory nerve dysfunctions affect the ability to control head movements. Accessory nerve function is tested by asking patients to turn their head and raise their shoulder against an opposing force provided by a clinician (Fig. 15-29). An interruption of the nerve sup-

ply to the trapezius muscle results in a dropped shoulder that cannot be raised. Damage to the sternocleidomastoid restricts head turning to the side away from the lesion. Paralysis of these muscles may also indirectly affect speech resonance.

Hypoglossal Nerve

GENERAL SOMATIC EFFERENT

The hypoglossal is a motor nerve (Table 15-19). The nerve fibers originate from the hypoglossal nucleus in the ventricular floor of the fourth ventricle close to the midline in the medulla (Figs. 15-1 and 15-3). The hypoglossal nucleus receives its direct corticobulbar input from the contralateral motor cortex (Fig. 15-6). The efferent fibers from the hypoglossal nucleus travel anteriorly, pass through the medullary substance medial to the inferior olivary nucleus, and exit lateral to the pyramidal tract (Fig. 15-21).

The hypoglossal nerve, which controls tongue movement, innervates all ipsilateral intrinsic and most extrinsic (genioglossal, styloglossus, and hyoglossus) tongue muscles except the palatoglossal, which is controlled by the vagus nerve (Fig. 15-30; Table 15-20). The afferent projections from the nucleus solitarius and

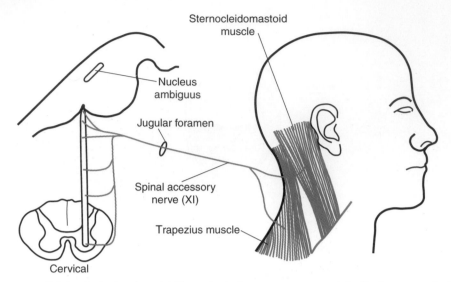

Figure 15-28.   Origin of spinal and cranial fibers of spinal accessory nerve and distribution to muscles in neck.

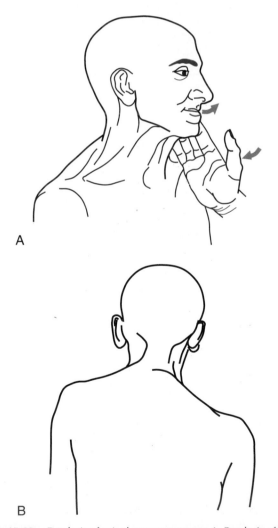

Figure 15-29.   Paralysis of spinal accessory nerve. **A.** Paralysis of sternocleidomastoid muscle restricts movement of face and neck opposite the side of damage. **B.** With paralysis of trapezius muscle, ipsilateral shoulder sags because of loss of normal contour between neck and shoulder.

trigeminal sensory nuclei are functionally linked with efferent hypoglossal fibers. This forms the neuronal circuitry for eating, sucking, and chewing reflexes.

CLINICAL INFORMATION

Unilateral damage to the hypoglossal nucleus or interruption of nerve projections in the distributions of the nerve results in LMN symptoms. Consequently, when the ipsilateral half of the tongue is paralyzed, it becomes flaccid and wrinkled. With voluntary control and reflexes absent over time, the paralyzed half of the tongue atrophies, which is characterized by loss of contour and corrugation of the edge. This weakness and muscle atrophy contribute to dysarthria and chewing difficulty, in which the patient has problems with formation and control of the bolus. On palpation, the affected side of the tongue appears soft and wrinkled. On protrusion, the tongue deviates to the side of the lesion (Fig. 15-31A). Bilateral LMN damage to the nucleus or nerve (Fig. 15-31B) is likely to cause severe difficulty in swallowing, eating, and speaking. After a unilateral supranuclear lesion, the loss of UMN influence on the contralateral hypoglossal nucleus (XII) results in significant loss of skill in using the contralateral half of the tongue during articulation and eating. However, the presence of some aberrant corticobulbar fibers may somewhat limit the impact of the loss. The affected and

Table 15-19.   Functional Description of Hypoglossal Nerve

Classification	Nuclei	Function
G (general) S (somatic) E (efferent)	Hypoglossal nucleus in medulla	Controls motor movements of tongue by regulating intrinsic, extrinsic glossal muscles

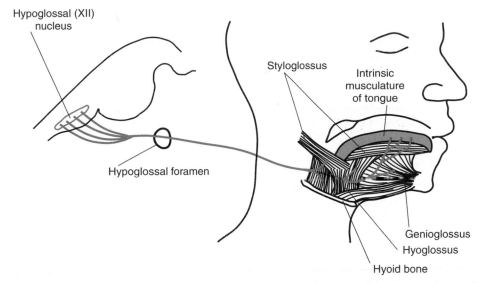

Figure 15-30. Hypoglossal nucleus in medulla, intramedullary course of nerve, and distribution of nerve fibers to glossal muscles.

Table 15-20. Muscles of Tongue

Muscle	Function
Extrinsic muscles	
Genioglossus (XII)	Raises hyoid bone, protrudes and retracts tongue
Hyoglossus (XII)	Retracts tongue and lowers its side
Palatoglossus (X)	Narrows fauces and elevates back of tongue
Styloglossus (XII)	Retracts and elevates tongue
Intrinsic muscles	
Superior longitudinal	Shortens and curls tip of tongue upward
Inferior longitudinal	Shortens and curls tip of tongue downward
Transverse	Elongates, narrows and raises sides of tongue
Verticalis	Flattens and broadens tongue

weakened tongue in such a case moves away from the side of the supranuclear (UMN) lesion.

The hypoglossal nerve is tested by asking the patient to protrude, retract, raise, and move the tongue laterally.

FUNCTION-BASED CRANIAL NERVE COMBINATIONS

There are two important aspects of cranial nerve functions. The first is multiple innervation, in which two or more cranial nerves innervate the same anatomical structure. For example, several cranial nerves combine to serve eye movement, sensory innervation of the tongue, and soft palatal and pharyngeal movements. The second is that some cranial motor (branchial) nuclei nerves receive corticobulbar projections from both motor cortices, although the contralateral projection is somewhat stronger. This has significant clinical implications.

Motor Control of Eye Muscles

The ocular movements of each eye are controlled by six muscles that are regulated by three different cranial nerves: the oculomotor, trochlear, and abducens (Fig. 15-32A). The oculomotor nerve innervates four ocu-

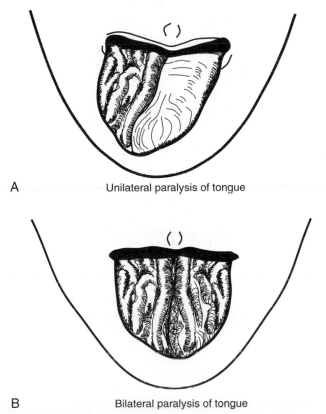

A   Unilateral paralysis of tongue

B   Bilateral paralysis of tongue

Figure 15-31. Paralysis of right half of tongue. **A.** Loss of bulk is evident, and on protrusion the tongue deviates to side of weakness. **B.** Bilateral palsy of tongue, characterized by general atrophy.

lar muscles: the medial rectus, inferior rectus, superior rectus, and inferior oblique. The trochlear nerve controls the superior oblique muscle, and the abducens nerve regulates the lateral rectus muscle. Each of these muscles, combined with others, makes specific contributions to eye movements (Fig. 15-32B). All of the ocular muscles work together and are coordinated by the gaze centers in the midbrain and pons, which receive coordinated corticobulbar signals from the motor cortex. The motor nuclei of these three cranial nerves are interconnected by the fibers of the medial longitudinal fasciculus (see Chapter 10). This brainstem tract ensures that the activity of muscles in the two eyes is coordinated and that the eyes move in the same direction concurrently with head movement.

The midbrain conjugate gaze control center coordinates the movement of both eyes together. For example, activation of the left frontal cortex (premotor area) leads to activation of the right pontine gaze center and thence to activation of the right abducens (lateral rectus) and left oculomotor nucleus (medial rectus). This results in contraction of the right lateral rectus and left medial rectus muscles to ensure a smooth turn of both eyes toward the right.

Sensory Nerve Supply to Tongue

The tongue displays a distinctive pattern in which three cranial nerves innervate general (cutaneous) and special (taste) sensations from its anterior and posterior regions (Fig. 15-33). The general sensations of pain, touch, and proprioception from the anterior two-thirds of the tongue are carried in the lingual branch of the trigeminal nerve (V). General sensations from the posterior third of the tongue are relayed by glossopharyngeal nerve (IX) branches (Table 15-21).

Two cranial nerves also participate in the mediation of the special sensation of taste from the tongue. Special sensation of taste from the anterior two-thirds of the tongue is carried by the chorda tympani, a branch of the facial (VII) nerve complex. Taste sensation from the posterior third of the tongue is carried by the fibers of the glossopharyngeal (IX) nerve.

Motor Nerve Supply to Soft Palate and Pharynx

The soft palate and the tube-shaped pharyngeal cavity are important in swallowing and speech resonance. The soft palate seals the nasopharynx to prevent the entrance of food during swallowing. It also regulates speech nasality. The circular constrictor (superior, middle, and inferior) muscles of the pharynx perform squeezing actions on the bolus, and vertical muscles (stylopharyngeus, palatopharyngeus, and salpingopharyngeus) elevate the larynx during swallowing. The motor innervation of the muscles of the soft palate and pharyngeal cavity is

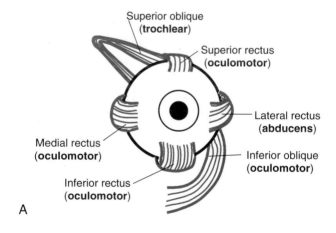

A

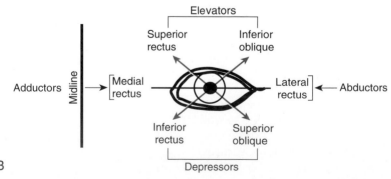

B

Figure 15-32. **A.** Muscles of left eye and cranial nerves responsible for their innervation. **B.** Group actions of ocular muscles of left eye.

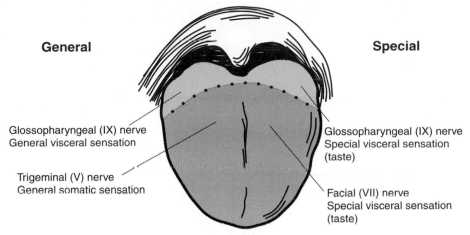

Figure 15-33. General and special sensory innervation of tongue.

Table 15-21. Sensory Innervation of Tongue

Cranial Nerve	General Sensation	Taste Sensation	Tongue Region
Lingual branch of trigeminal nerve	+		Anterior two-thirds of tongue
Glossopharyngeal nerve	+		Posterior third of tongue
Chorda tympani of facial nerve		+	Anterior two-thirds of tongue
Glossopharyngeal nerve		+	Posterior third of tongue

supplied by the pharyngeal branches of the vagus (X) nerve, except for the tensor veli palatini and stylopharyngeus. The tensor veli palatini is controlled by the trigeminal (V) nerve, and the stylopharyngeus muscle is controlled by the glossopharyngeal nerve (IX) (Fig. 15-34).

Sensory Innervation of Soft Palate and Pharynx

The glossopharyngeal and vagus nerves are responsible for general sensation from the pharynx, a visceral structure. The vagus alone carries the general sensation from the larynx, another visceral structure. However, the trigeminal nerve mediates the general sensation from the nasopharynx and soft palate.

UPPER AND LOWER MOTOR NEURON SYNDROMES

Lesions involving the UMNs and LMNs affect the function of buccofacial muscles differently. Interruption in corticobulbar projections from the motor cortex to the cranial nerve motor nuclei on the opposite side results in UMN syndrome, which is characterized by a loss of discrete and delicate motor control, muscle weakness, and brisk reflexes. The substantial number of aberrant corti-

cobulbar fibers probably provides safety from damage in the brainstem for cranial nerve functions. This explains why damage to the pyramidal fibers after they have separated from the major pyramidal tract does not result in any more than a minimal spasticity in cranial muscles. Furthermore, most buccofacial muscles that receive corticobulbar projections from both sides of the cortex may not be severely impaired by a unilateral UMN lesion. Bilateral involvement of UMN (pseudobulbar palsy), which profoundly affects cranial muscle function and motor speech, is characterized by hypotonia and loss of discrete motor control, again with little or no spasticity in cranial muscles. LMN lesions affect the motor cranial nuclei (final common pathways) or their projections and produce the LMN symptoms, which include flaccid paralysis, absent or reduced reflexes, muscular fibrillations and twitching, and muscle atrophy. The muscular twitching results from spontaneous firing of an α-LMN cell body or its axons, resulting in an entire motor unit firing at the same time. It is caused by irritation, infection, or hyperexcitability of the LMN cell body. If the LMN cell body dies, the innervating terminals (neuromuscular junctions) degenerate, and fasciculation ceases. When deprived of efferent impulses (reflexive or voluntary) from the LMN cell body, the muscle fibers eventually atrophy and degenerate. LMN lesions greatly affect the functioning of the buccofacial, glossal, laryngeal, and neck muscles.

UMN signs are **contralateral** to the locus of damage, while LMN signs are **ipsilateral** to the damage of the cell body or axon in the brainstem.

Case Studies

Patient One

A 60-year-old man had several lacunar strokes (deep cortical infarcts) bilaterally in the region of the internal capsule and basal ganglia, as

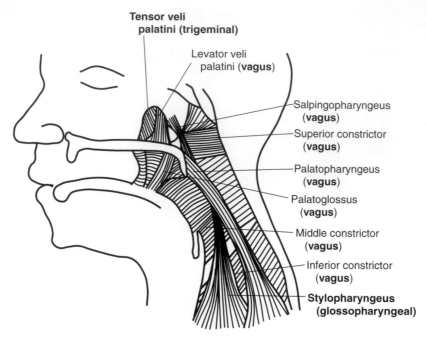

Figure 15-34.   Nerve supply to muscles of soft palate and pharynx.

demonstrated on magnetic resonance imaging. The bilateral UMN lesions to the corticobulbar fibers affected multiple cranial nerves along with sensorimotor dysfunctions in the extremity. Neurological examination revealed the following abnormalities:

- Mild cognitive decline (short-term memory was impaired)
- Stiff gait with slow, short steps
- Hyperactive muscle stretch reflexes and bilateral Babinski signs
- Impaired control of facial muscles, with inability to show his teeth, pucker his lips, or wrinkle his forehead
- Exaggerated facial movement when he laughed
- Difficulty controlling excessive laughter and sobbing
- Difficulty protruding tongue
- Difficulty chewing and swallowing; food accumulating in his mouth
- Failure of the soft palate to rise on phonation

Question: What cranial nerves control the muscles of facial expression, mastication, and deglutition? Can you account for this clinical picture based on lesions affecting those nerves?

Discussion: The functions of facial movement are mediated by the facial (VII) nerve; mastication is mediated by the trigeminal (V) nerve; deglutition involves the pharyngeal plexus of the glossopharyngeal (IX) and vagus (X) nerves, and tongue is controlled by the hypoglossal (XII) nerve. In this case, the lacunar lesions impaired voluntary control of the connected muscles by injuring the corticobulbar pathways from the cortex to the nuclei of those nerves. This is known as an UMN lesion. This clinical picture is often called pseudobulbar palsy, which is associated with bilateral cortical lesions. The name indicates that the problem is not really *in* the medulla and does not affect the LMNs; rather, it involves the motor pathways *to* the brainstem. Another term used to refer it is supranuclear paralysis (injury above or rostral to the cranial nerve nuclei of the brainstem) due to bilateral involvement of corticobulbar, or corticonuclear, pathways.

When the patient attempts to move his facial muscles, the muscles respond poorly; but they respond strongly to an emotional stimulus, which is not under direct control by the cerebral cortex through the corticobulbar pathways that have been damaged. The pathways that are functional during a true emotional response are not as well understood as are the direct pathways controlling voluntary actions. The pathways involved

with emotions are known to escape injury from lacunar strokes or cortical lesions in typical locations. When the cranial nerve nuclei are activated through the indirect and spared pathway known to mediate emotions, the facial response is actually exaggerated; the patient's face may assume an expressive mask, with forceful contraction of the muscles that appeared to be weak when he was asked to show his teeth or perform a voluntary smile. An emotional smile, in contrast, results in an exaggerated emotional expression accompanied by sobbing. It is important to avoid emotional stimulation when the patient is eating to minimize the risk of aspirating food or saliva.

Slow gait with hyperactive muscle stretch reflexes (also known as deep tendon reflexes) and extensor plantar responses (also known as Babinski signs) imply UMN symptoms. This means that the nerves of LMNs directly supplying the muscles have not been damaged, but the descending corticospinal motor pathways from the brain have been damaged, and the resulting syndrome of spastic weakness with impaired voluntary control but uninhibited reflex activity (the hyperactive knee jerks and ankle reflexes, for example) is UMN syndrome (see Chapter 14).

The reason the reflex activities of laughing and crying are not just intact but actually overactive or exaggerated in pseudobulbar palsy is similar to the reason for hyperactive knee reflexes at the spinal level: the reflexes are normally modulated, or somewhat inhibited, by activity in the intact corticonuclear or corticospinal pathways (corticonuclear [corticobulbar] for the display of emotion in the face; corticospinal for the stretch reflexes in the limbs). When that inhibition is removed as the result of the lesions, the responses are uncontrolled, or hyperactive.

The signs of cognitive impairment in this patient resulted from multiple cortical infarcts.

Patient Two

A 63-year-old man had a stroke and woke up in confusion and panic. In the emergency room the examining physician noticed the following:

- Complete left-sided facial paralysis
- Inability to move his left eye laterally (the eye was adducted medially)
- Hearing loss in the left ear
- Absence of pain and touch sensation on the left side of the face
- Some weakness in jaw movement

Magnetic resonance imaging revealed a small stroke in the superior tegmentum of the pons on the left that affected the LMN nuclei of the facial, abducens, and trigeminal nerves. The lesion also extended laterally, affecting the cochlear nuclei within the substance of the brainstem.

Question: Can you account for these cranial nerve–related sensorimotor symptoms on the left side and no paralysis in the muscles of the extremities?

Discussion: The pontine tegmental lesion affected the four cranial nerves (abducens, trigeminal, facial, and acoustic), which caused adduction of the left eye (impaired abducens nerve function), analgesia and anesthesia on the left face (trigeminal nerve interruption), paresis in the jaw (trigeminal motor nerve involvement), left facial paralysis (facial nerve), and hearing loss (acoustic nerve). The typical location of the lesion did not affect the descending corticospinal fibers, so limb motor functions were spared.

Patient Three

A 60-year-old man developed gradually worsening ringing in his left ear; he also noticed decreased hearing in that ear. He began to hold the telephone to his right ear instead of the left. Shortly before consulting his physician, he began to walk with a stiffly extended right leg, tending to scrape the toe of the right foot. He was also somewhat clumsy with his right hand.

Examination by a physician revealed the following abnormal signs:
- Mild right-sided weakness of the hand and lower limb
- Increased muscle stretch reflexes (deep tendon reflexes) and Babinski sign on the right
- Tendency to stagger and fall to the left while walking (a sign of cerebellar or vestibular injury)
- Decreased sensitivity to temperature and pinprick on the left side of the face
- Normal light touch sensation
- Absence of left corneal reflex
- Mild left-sided weakness when wrinkling his forehead, forcibly closing his eye, and retracting the corner of his mouth
- Loss of hearing in left ear, with lateralization of the tuning fork to the right ear on the Weber test and severely diminished air and bone conduction on the left

Magnetic resonance imaging revealed an egg-shaped mass in the left cerebellopontine angle that was expanding the internal auditory meatus of the temporal bone, compressing the left cerebellar hemisphere from below, and indenting the pons and upper medulla on the left side.

Questions: Can you account for these cranial nerve symptoms based on the tumor mass at the cerebellopontine angle? Can the location of the mass account for the spastic (UMN) weakness of the right side of the body (the side opposite the lesion) and the tendency to fall to the left side ipsilateral to the lesion? How does cranial nerve injury explain the sensory findings on the face and facial weakness? Does the hearing loss indicate disease of the middle ear or of the statoacoustic nerve? If it is nerve injury, would you expect any other abnormality of function of the statoacoustic nerve?

Discussion: UMN signs produced by a lesion anywhere above the decussation of the pyramids in the caudal medulla manifest on the opposite side of the body. Therefore, a mass at the level of the pons and rostral medulla on the left can account for right-sided hemiparesis. Cerebellar signs of unsteadiness appear on the same side as the lesion, and injury to the left cerebellar hemisphere accounts for falling to the left, the side of the lesion. Therefore, a single site of lesion can account for both of these clinical abnormalities. The decreased sensation on the face can be explained by partial injury to the trigeminal (V) cranial nerve on the left, with pain perception more affected than perception of touch. It may also be explained by injury to the sensory pathway for pain and temperature sensation inside the brainstem on the left, because fibers mediating pain and temperature sensation (known as the descending or spinal tract

of the trigeminal nerve) enter the brainstem at mid pons as part of the trigeminal nerve, then descend through the caudal pons and medulla as far as the high cervical spinal cord before synapsing and sending second-order sensory neurons across the midline to ascend to the thalamus on the right. The fibers mediating touch do not follow this descending course. They synapse, and the second-order axons cross at the level of entry in mid pons.

Absence of the corneal reflex can be explained by the loss of pain sensation on the cornea. The weakness of eye closure is also relevant to loss of the reflex, but without the sensory loss, some response of eye closure to touching the cornea with a wisp of cotton is likely, and the patient would feel the irritation of the stimulus.

The weakness of the face affects all components. When there is UMN facial weakness, the functions of forehead muscles are usually intact, because they are controlled by both ipsilateral and contralateral descending motor pathways. Therefore, in this case, the weakness appears to be of the LMN variety (involvement of the nerve itself). This is consistent with the mass on the left at the level of the lateral recess of the medulla, where the CN VII and VIII enter the brainstem. The loss of hearing is the sensorineural type, affecting both air and bone conduction. Therefore, it is likely to originate in the nerve and is not consistent with middle ear disease, in which bone conduction is preserved.

The slow development of symptoms is consistent with benign tumor. Usually a tumor in the cerebellopontine angle develops on the vestibular division of the CN VIII, from nerve sheath cells. The tumor is often called an acoustic neuroma, but better names for it are schwannoma (or Schwann cell tumor) and neurolemma. It is necessary to remove a schwannoma surgically to prevent further compression of vital structures of the medulla. Because the tumor tends to surround the facial nerve but not destroy it, facial weakness, if present, is usually mild prior to surgery. It may not be possible to preserve the nerve during the operation, however, because it is engulfed in tumor, and the face may be paralyzed postoperatively. Similarly, hearing is usually not restored, and because the tumor most often develops on the vestibular division of the nerve, caloric testing (irrigating the ear canal with warm or cold water) gives no response; that is, there is no vertigo or nystagmus when the test is performed on the damaged side. This is true before the operation as well, if the test is performed during the diagnostic workup.

Patient Four

A 60-year-old priest was taken to an emergency room for sensorimotor problems that developed abruptly while speaking to the members of his church during a Sunday mass. The attending physician noted the following:
- Unintelligible speech because of dysarthria
- Hypernasality with lowered left palate
- Dysphagia
- Sensation loss on the left side of the face
- Difficulty balancing, with falling to the left
- Left-sided facial paralysis
- Weakness in the right leg and arm

Magnetic resonance imaging revealed an infarct in the left caudal lateral ventral pons and medulla.

Question: Can you account for these symptoms of the left face and the paralysis of the right half of the body?

Discussion: A left pontine and medullary lesion had affected the following:
- The effects on the facial and trigeminal nerve fibers, along with the rootlets of the vagus, were facial motor disturbance, loss of sensation from the face, palatal paralysis, and swallowing difficulty.
- Involvement of the vestibular nuclei resulted in the equilibrium problem.
- Interruption of the long descending pyramidal (corticospinal) fibers above the point of decussation produced paralysis in the right arm and leg.

SUMMARY

The human cranial nerves are the result of evolutionary modifications to a basic vertebrate pattern of CNS organization, constructed of approximately 40 bilaterally symmetrical repeating segments. In the development, the first 2 nerves (olfactory and optic) became elaborated as the forebrain and involve the thalamus before reaching the cortex. The remaining 10 cranial nerves originate from the brainstem and innervate the muscles of the head, neck, face, larynx, tongue, and pharynx. These muscles serve speech, resonance, swallowing, facial expression, chewing, and phonation. Besides serving special senses such as vision, audition, smell, and taste, the cranial nerves regulate autonomic secretive functions of glands in the oral, nasal, and orbital cavities.

Some cranial nerves mediate only sensation, whereas others exclusively serve motor functions. However, most nerves have both sensory and motor functions. Some cranial nerves serve only a single functional component, whereas others contain fibers to serve two or more functional components. Several motor cranial nuclei receive corticobulbar projections from both sides of the motor cortex. This bilaterality of projection has important clinical implications for the motor speech processes.

Technical Terms

accommodation	lower motor neuron
atrophy	neuralgia
Bell's palsy	ophthalmoplegia
branchial arch	paralysis
ciliary muscle	postganglionic neuron
cranial nerves	preganglionic neuron
cutaneous	somatic
flaccid	strabismus
hypotonia	upper motor neuron
iris	visceral muscles
light reflex	

Review Questions

1. Define the following terms:

anosmia	light reflex
Bell's palsy	neuralgia
branchial arch	ophthalmoplegia
conductive hearing loss	pseudobulbar palsy
conjugate gaze	postganglionic neuron
ciliary muscle	preganglionic neuron
diplopia	sensorineural hearing loss
fasciculation	strabismus

2. List the four general and three special functional components of cranial nerves, giving examples of their sensorimotor functions.
3. Match the following numbered classifications to the associated lettered function.

i. GSA	a. pain, tension, and temperature
ii. GSE	b. vision and audition
iii. SSA	c. eye movements
iv. SVA	d. speech, phonation and swallowing
v. BE/SVE	e. taste and smell

4. List the branchial arches and associated cranial nerves.
5. Where do most corticobulbar fibers cross the midline?
6. Describe the syndrome of bulbar palsy.
7. Explain the causes of anosmia.
8. Describe the functional classifications, locations of nuclei, and functions of the oculomotor, trochlear, and abducens nerves.
9. Describe the neuronal events of the pupillary light reflex and lens accommodation–convergence reflex.
10. Describe the idiosyncratic decussation for the fibers of the trochlear nerve.
11. In the case of right oculomotor nerve injury, in what gaze direction is diplopia likely to occur?
12. A 45-year-old woman has decreased hearing in the right ear; the entire right side of her face is paralyzed; and she has no reflex to touch in the cornea of the right eye. What cranial nerves are suspected of being damaged?
13. A 25-year-old man received a head injury in an auto collision. Subsequently he claimed that food had no flavor. What cranial nerve or nerves may have been damaged, and how may the damage have contributed to the loss of taste?
14. Some clinical signs demonstrated by a stroke patient included left ptosis, pupil unresponsiveness to light, dilated left pupil, and deviation of the eye to the left. Discuss what cranial nerve is involved.
15. When a certain stroke patient looks to the right, the right eye does not fully abduct. What cranial nerve is likely to be involved?
16. Describe the functional classifications, locations of nuclei, and sensory and motor functions of the trigeminal nerve.
17. Discuss trigeminal neuralgia (tic douloureux) and the motor functions of the trigeminal nerve.
18. Discuss the sensory distribution of the trigeminal nerve.
19. Describe the functional classifications, locations of nuclei, course of fibers, and functions of the facial nerve.
20. Discuss the clinical picture of Bell's palsy.
21. Discuss the differential innervation for the upper and lower face and its clinical implications for UMN and LMN syndromes.
22. Describe the functional classifications, locations of nuclei, courses of fibers, and functions of the glossopharyngeal and vagus nerves.
23. Describe the functional classification and functions of the hypoglossal nerve.
24. What symptoms would result from an injury to the hypoglossal nerve within the medulla?
25. Review clinical findings associated with unilateral and bilateral lesions of the speech-related cranial (facial, trigeminal, vagus, and hypoglossal) nerves.
26. Describe which nerves and fiber tracts are involved when a patient suddenly develops left hemiplegia, paralysis of the right upper and lower face, and failure to abduct the right eye.
27. Which cranial nerve participates in cardiovascular reflexes?
28. Explain the lesion site that can account for sensory loss on the left side of the face and right side of the body.
29. Discuss the lesion site that may account for loss of motor control on the right side of the face and left side of the body.
30. What are the clinical signs of a lesion of the right or left recurrent laryngeal fibers of the vagus nerve?
31. Describe cranial nerves that are responsible for general and special (taste) sensation from the entire tongue.

32. Discuss the motor function of all extrinsic eye muscles.
33. Describe the motor nerve supply to the soft palate and pharynx.
34. Describe the innervation of the tensor and levator palatini muscles.
35. Which cranial nerve motor nuclei receive bilateral projections from the corticobulbar system?
36. Damage involving what cranial nerve may enhance hearing?
37. Explain why the right frontalis muscle (wrinkling the forehead) is less affected than the right orbicularis oris muscle (moving the mouth) after a lesion in the left motor cortex.
38. Describe the effects of the pseudobulbar palsy on motor speech processes.

Autonomic Nervous System, Limbic System, Hypothalamus, and Reticular Formation

Learning Objectives

After studying this chapter, students should be able to do the following:

• Describe the structural organization of the autonomic nervous system
• Discuss the functions of the sympathetic and parasympathetic systems
• Explain the central neural mechanism that controls the autonomic nervous system
• Describe the anatomical organization of the limbic system
• Discuss the functions of the cingulate gyrus, amygdala, and hippocampus
• Describe the anatomical organization and functions of the hypothalamus
• Describe the functions of common hormones
• Describe the anatomical organization of the reticular formation
• Discuss the important functions of the reticular formation including swallowing and respiration

The autonomic nervous system (ANS), limbic lobe, hypothalamus, and reticular formation are functionally and anatomically integrated and are identified as the limbic–axial brain. As early-developing parts of the brain, these structures control basic physiological functions and behaviors at the unconscious level. Together, the four components of the limbic–axial brain control all visceral and somatic activities vital to sustaining body functions. The ANS regulates functions of the heart, lungs, and blood vessels and organs of the digestive, reproductive, and urogenital systems. As a transitional structure, the limbic lobe (central unit of the limbic system) connects the thinking (neocortical) brain to the nonthinking and older (subcortical) axial brain and regulates drives, moods, motivation, and visceral activities that relate to the emotional aspects of sensorimotor behaviors. The hypothalamus, a visceral–somatic and metabolic control system, is func-

tionally related to the limbic system, controls activity of the ANS, and influences behaviors including copulation, defecation, urination, alimentation, and aggression. In addition, the hypothalamus contains centers that control respiration, blood pressure, pulse rate, temperature, electrolyte balance, fluid balance, food intake, metabolism, diurnal rhythms, and endocrine production. Furthermore, it contributes to our internal emotional state of well-being and pleasure. The brainstem reticular formation influences brain activity by regulating the alerting mechanism. In addition, as the integrator of the sensory and motor mechanisms, the reticular formation participates in generation of well-coordinated motor functions such as speech, eye–body coordinated movements, swallowing, respiration, and vomiting. It also regulates blood pressure, pulse rate, respiration, and sleep and awake states.

All four components of the limbic–axial brain are connected by a system of complex fibers whose exact functions are not completely known. Only the basic anatomy of these related systems and their important functions are discussed in this chapter.

AUTONOMIC NERVOUS SYSTEM

The ANS involuntarily regulates visceral body functions by controlling the cardiac muscles, smooth muscles, and glands. This brings together all vital body functions, including the cardiovascular, pulmonary, digestive, urinary, and reproductive systems, maintaining body homeostasis. The ANS is tightly integrated with automatic and volitional sensorimotor behaviors.

The ANS is composed of the sympathetic and parasympathetic systems (Table 2-1). The sympathetic system mobilizes the vital organs for discharging energy, as in cases of danger, whereas the parasympathetic system is responsible for the restitution of metabolic energy and thus promotes relaxation and growth. Most of the smooth muscles, glands, and cardiac muscles are under the influence of both divisions. This dual innervation is largely reciprocal. Each system renders its influence, which is often antagonistic to the effects of the other system. Exceptions are the piloerector muscles and sweat glands, which are regulated solely by the sympathetic system.

The responsibilities of the sympathetic and parasympathetic systems can best be understood by examining a common experience and analyzing the respective bodily changes associated with each division. Suppose you are driving during rush hour on an icy road in freezing rain with poor visibility. You must be home soon because your child's school bus arrives within 20 minutes. Another driver suddenly slides into your lane, and you just escape a head-on collision. The possibility of a nearly fatal accident may trigger an anxiety attack and bodily responses. Your heart beats rapidly, pupils dilate, skin becomes pale because of decreased blood circulation, and visceral organs transiently slow down. You begin perspiring profusely, and your body is cold. You are no longer conscious of the acute need to empty your bladder. In this time of distress, these visceral responses that represent body energy expenditures have been regulated by the sympathetic division of the ANS.

Later, after you are safely home, your internal system is no longer agitated. The anxiety-causing environmental stimuli are no longer present, and you feel relaxed. Consequently, your heartbeat and body temperature return to normal levels, pupils constrict to normal size, and blood circulation to the skin and visceral organs is restored. This visceral reaction is regulated by the parasympathetic division of the ANS.

Anatomical Organization

Unlike somatic motor system impulses, efferent projections of the ANS do not directly innervate the visceral organs. Instead, these efferents travel indirectly via secondary neurons in the peripheral nervous system (PNS). Efferents of the ANS are made of two neurons in tandem (Fig. 16-1). The cell body of the first neuron for each system is within the central neuraxis (brainstem and spinal cord) and is called the preganglionic autonomic neuron. Preganglionic fibers traveling from the cell body project to a second neuron outside the CNS, the postganglionic autonomic neuron. Postganglionic fibers terminate on specific visceral organs. The postganglionic neuron of the sympathetic system is bilateral along the spinal cord, while that of the parasympathetic system is near the target organ. Postganglionic fibers influence the activity of the viscera and glands on which they terminate.

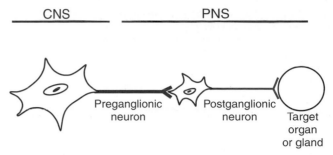

Figure 16-1. Two-neuron organization of peripheral nervous system (PNS): preganglionic and postganglionic. CNS, central nervous system.

Table 16-1. Sympathetic and Parasympathetic Systems

Structure	Sympathetic	Parasympathetic
General function	Expenditure of metabolic energy	Restoration of metabolic energy
Preganglion cells	Thoracic and lumbar cord	Brainstem and sacral segments of cord
Postganglionic cells	Sympathetic chain near vertebral column	Near target organs
Distribution	Scattered throughout body, projections render widespread influence on multiple visceral organs	Localized projections activate specific effectors

Visceral Efferent System

The ANS is largely motor, although it also has a sensory component in which afferent fibers carry sensory information from the visceral structures to the CNS. Its motor fibers project neural impulses to the visceral organs via the sympathetic and parasympathetic subdivisions of the ANS (Table 16-1). These two systems must work together to maintain optimal functioning of the visceral structures, such as the smooth muscles, glands (lacrimal, salivary, and sweat), cardiac muscles, blood vessels, and gastrointestinal system (Table 16-2). The locations of the postganglionic cell differ for the two systems; in the sympathetic system, the postganglionic cells lie closer to the spinal cord, whereas in the parasympathetic system, the postganglionic cells are farther from the neuraxis and closer to the target organs.

SYMPATHETIC SYSTEM

The sympathetic nervous system is also called the thoracolumbar system because the preganglionic cell bodies are in the intermediolateral gray matter between the sensory and motor columns in the thoracic and upper lumbar segments of the spinal cord (Fig. 16-2). These cell bodies give rise to preganglionic efferent fibers. Efferent fibers of preganglionic cells leave through the ventral spinal roots of the thoracic and lumbar segments and travel through the white communicating ramus of

Table 16-2. Differential Effects of Sympathetic and Parasympathetic Systems on Glands and Muscles

Structure	Sympathetic System	Parasympathetic System
Glands		
Nasal	Decreased secretion	Increased secretion
Lacrimal	Decreased secretion	Increased secretion
Intestinal	Decreased secretion	Increased secretion
Gastric	Decreased secretion	Increased secretion
Sweat	Decreased secretion	Increased secretion
Smooth muscles		
Iris	Pupil dilation	Pupil constriction
Ciliary	No effect	Contraction
Urinary bladder	Relaxation	Contraction
Anal sphincter	Constriction	Dilation
Digestive tract	Reduced activity	Increased activity
Bronchi	Dilation	Constriction
Lungs	Vasodilation	Vasoconstriction
Skin	Sweating, piloerection	None
Cardiac muscles	Increased activity	Decreased activity
Blood vessels	Vasoconstriction in viscera and skin; vasodilation in skeletal muscle and heart	None
Genitals	Vasoconstriction	Vasodilation

each spinal nerve (Fig. 16-3). They are white because most of the fibers are myelinated. These fibers terminate on the postganglionic neurons in the sympathetic chain or on other postganglionic sympathetic neurons in the abdomen around the aorta. The postganglionic neurons in the sympathetic chain are also known as the paravertebral ganglia, whereas the postganglionic sympathetic neurons close to the large abdominal arteries are called prevertebral ganglia. The prevertebral ganglia surround the visceral branches of the aorta and include the coeliac, superior mesenteric, and inferior mesenteric ganglia. The sympathetic ganglionic chain extends from the base of the skull to the coccyx along the anterolateral area of the vertebral column. The cervical portion of the sympathetic trunk contains three ganglia formed by a fusion of the original eight segmental ganglia: the superior, middle, and inferior cervical ganglia (Fig. 16-2). The cervical sympathetic ganglia innervate the smooth muscles and glands in the head and upper limbs. Postganglionic fibers from the 11 thoracic ganglia innervate the heart, lungs, and thoracic and abdominal viscera. Postganglionic fibers from the lumbar ganglia are distributed via the spinal nerves and innervate the upper abdominal viscera, intestines, bladder, and genitals. Some of the unmyelinated sympathetic postganglionic fibers rejoin the spinal nerves via the gray communicating ramus (Fig. 16-3). They travel with the spinal nerves and separate from them before innervating blood vessels, smooth muscles, and sweat glands.

The sympathetic system mobilizes metabolic energy for expenditure. This is common in stressful situations and emergencies, in which the heart rate accelerates, arterial pressure rises, blood sugar level increases, and blood flow is diverted from visceral structures to the skeletal muscles.

PARASYMPATHETIC SYSTEM

The parasympathetic system preserves or restores metabolic energy. This system is also known as the craniosacral system because the cell bodies giving rise to preganglionic fibers are in the brainstem and sacral region of the spinal cord. The parasympathetic efferent fibers innervate the visceral structures in the head, neck, thorax, much of the abdominal cavity, and pelvic organs (Fig. 16-4). The cranial section of the parasympathetic system includes the oculomotor, facial, glossopharyngeal, and vagus cranial nerves. The Edinger-Westphal nucleus, the visceral component of the oculomotor complex in the midbrain (see Chapter 15), sends preganglionic fibers to the postganglionic neurons in the ciliary ganglion. The postganglionic fibers from the ciliary ganglion innervate the sphincter of the iris and smooth muscle of the ciliary body. The facial preganglionic parasympathetic fibers supply the pterygopalatine and submandibular ganglia; the postganglionic fibers innervate the lacrimal glands and their blood vessels and mucous membrane glands. Postganglionic fibers of the facial cranial nerve also innervate the submandibular and sublingual salivary glands and the mucous membranes in the floor of the mouth. Postganglionic fibers from the otic ganglion of the glossopharyngeal cranial nerve activate the parotid gland. The largest source of preganglionic parasympathetic fibers is from the vagus nerve, which supplies practically all thoracic and abdominal viscera except for the pelvis. It supplies the parasympathetic ganglia in the heart, bronchial musculature, stomach, large and small intestines, liver, pancreas, and kidneys. In the intestinal system, short postganglionic fibers terminate in the smooth muscle and glands and serve motor and secretory functions. The sacral parasympathetic postganglionic fibers supply the urinary bladder, colon, rectum, accessory reproductive organs, and intestinal viscera not innervated by the vagus.

The parasympathetic system dominates during periods of relaxation because it reduces the activity of various organs and conserves metabolic energy. Common parasympathetic activities include decreasing heart rate, lowering blood pressure, constricting pupils, and increasing digestion.

Visceral Afferent System

Sensory fibers from the thoracic, abdominal, and pelvic viscera travel through sympathetic nerves, ultimately reaching the sympathetic chain. They enter the T-1 to L-2 regions of the cord via the white communicat-

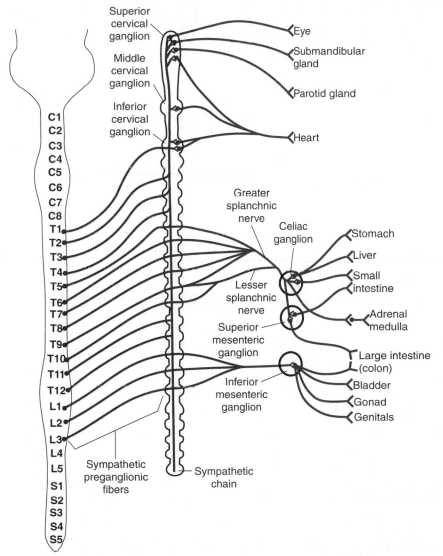

Figure 16-2.   Sympathetic autonomic nervous system.

ing rami. From there they ascend into the dorsal lemniscus and anterolateral systems. The visceral afferent fibers of the vagus nerve, whose cell bodies are in the inferior (nodose) ganglion, are distributed peripherally in the heart, lungs, and other viscera. Fibers from the bladder, rectum, and accessory genital organs travel through the splanchnic nerves and enter the spinal cord through the S-2 to S-4 nerves. Afferent visceral fibers are important for visceral and viscerosomatic reflexes that are mediated through the spinal cord, brainstem, and hypothalamus. For example, sacral visceral afferents from stretch receptors of the urinary bladder control the bladder reflex and sensations that occur with bladder distension. The nucleus of the solitary tract in the medulla receives stimuli from the walls of the digestive tract, respiratory tract, and heart and its vascular trunks. These projections mediate respiratory and cardiovascular reflexes that are regulated by the medulla and hypothalamus.

Most autonomic sensory reactions remain subconscious but cause visceral pain, distress, nausea, hunger, and other less well localized visceral sensations. A constant stream of visceral impulses allows for the general feeling of either internal well-being or malaise. Almost all visceral abdominal pain is projected in the sympathetic system. Intense visceral pain from internal organs is often felt on a skin area supplied by the somatic fibers arising from the same cord segment (referred pain) (see Chapter 7).

Neurotransmitters

Acetylcholine is the main neurotransmitter for the preganglionic and postganglionic fibers of the parasympathetic system and for the preganglionic fibers of the sympathetic system. The postganglionic sympathetic nerves secrete norepinephrine as a transmitter (Table 16-3).

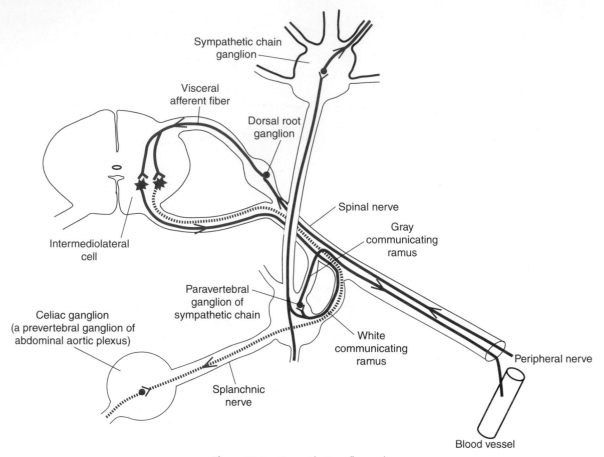

Figure 16-3. Sympathetic reflex arch.

Table 16-3. Sympathetic and Parasympathetic Neurotransmitters

Structure	Sympathetic	Parasympathetic
Preganglionic cells	Acetylcholine	Acetylcholine
Postganglionic cells	Norepinephrine	Acetylcholine

Central Autonomic Pathways

The hypothalamus centrally controls the ANS. The hypothalamic regulation of the ANS is mediated in part by a series of synaptic relays from the neocortex, limbic system, diencephalon, brainstem, and spinal cord. Activation of the anterior hypothalamus stimulates the parasympathetic system, whereas activation of the posterior lateral hypothalamus stimulates the sympathetic system. Hypothalamic impulses are transmitted to the midbrain via a descending component of the medial forebrain bundle, the mamillotegmental tract, and through other descending projections. Continuing from the midbrain, the hypothalamic impulses are relayed caudally through synaptic relays in the brainstem reticular formation, which in turn conveys the impulses to visceral motor nuclei of the brainstem and spinal cord.

Clinical Information

Interruptions of the autonomic regulation of visceral functions are characterized by impaired control of blood pressure, respiration, cardiovascular activity, gland secretion, sexual activity, bladder incontinence, and urinary retention. In the case of disturbance in the sympathetic system, unopposed parasympathetic control of visceral structures results in symptoms indicating the restoration of metabolic energy in activities such as decreased heart rate, lowered blood pressure, constriction of the pupils, and increased digestion. The reverse is true in cases of parasympathetic disturbance, in which unopposed activity of the sympathetic system results in expenditure of metabolic energy, for example acceleration of heart rate, elevation of arterial pressure, and increased blood flow to the skeletal muscles.

Summary of Autonomic Nervous System

The ANS regulates visceral functions and maintains homeostasis by regulating vital body systems including the cardiovascular, pulmonary, digestive, urinary, and reproductive systems. The ANS uses its sympathetic and parasympathetic systems, two functionally antagonistic components, to render opposite effects on

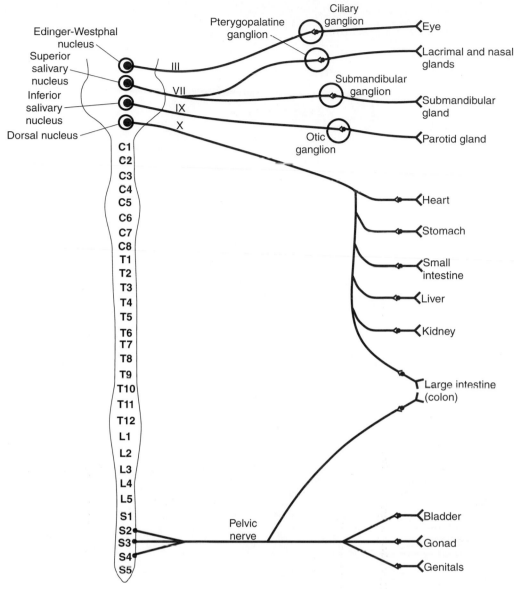

Figure 16-4. Parasympathetic autonomic nervous system.

organ activities. For instance, sympathetic neurons expand metabolic energy by dilating the pupils, accelerating the heartbeat, inhibiting intestinal movements, and contracting the rectal sphincters. Conversely, the parasympathetic neurons constrict the pupils, slow the heart, increase peristaltic movement, and relax the sphincters. The parasympathetic system is concerned with anabolic activities, such as the restoration and conservation of energy. The sacral parasympathetics activate the excretion of intestinal and urinary wastes.

LIMBIC SYSTEM

The limbic system (visceral brain) refers to closely related functional structures of the limbic lobe, diencephalon, septum, and midbrain. The limbic lobe in-

cludes the subcallosal gyrus, cingulate gyrus, isthmus, parahippocampal gyrus, hippocampus, olfactory cortex, uncus, and amygdala (Figs. 16-5 and 16-6). The septum, located at the rostral diencephalon, forms the septohypothalamomidbrain continuum. It is essential for completing the limbic system's bidirectional circuitry, connecting the limbic lobe to the hypothalamus, thalamus, and midbrain. The fornix, a large C-shaped bundle of bidirectional fibers, serves as the main circuitry that connects the limbic lobe to the diencephalon and visceral centers of the hypothalamus.

The limbic system regulates emotional and motivational aspects of behavior. Limbic projections to the forebrain contribute to emotions and provide motivation for behaviors fundamental to survival (feeding, mating, aggression, and flight). The limbic structures

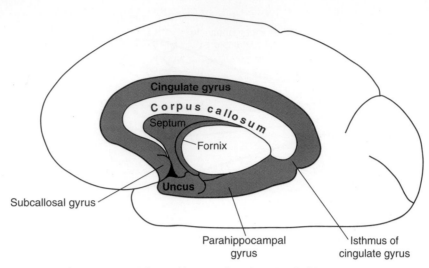

Figure 16-5. Midsagittal brain surface depicting limbic structures.

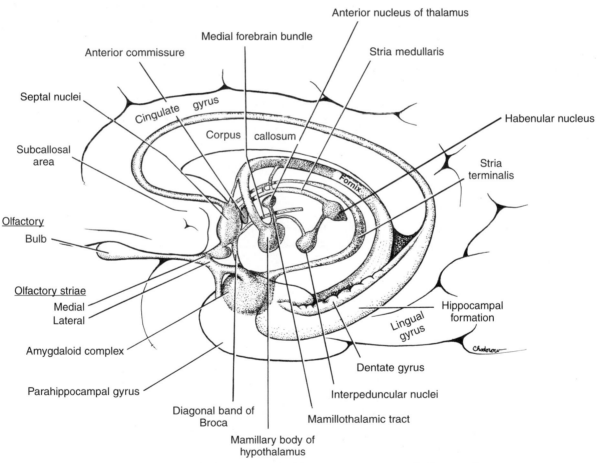

Figure 16-6. Major limbic structures and their connections on medial brain surface.

also participate in memory and learning. Most understanding of limbic behaviors and pathologies, such as Klüver-Bucy syndrome, is primarily based on animal experiments. Humans with dementias, carbon monoxide poisoning, and temporal lobe seizures may exhibit the behaviors found in animals with impaired limbic systems.

Anatomical Structures

The key limbic structures are connected by an extensive network of afferent and efferent fibers. These interconnecting fibers account for the limbic influence on virtually all cortical, brainstem, and visceral functions and the regulation of emotions. Not all limbic connections are completely understood. Major inputs to the limbic lobe are from the neocortex, olfactory bulb, thalamus, septum, and reticular formation. The limbic output goes to the neocortex, hypothalamus, thalamus, and reticular formation. Projections to the prefrontal lobe in the neocortex regulate affective aspects of emotion, such as moods and feelings. Projections to the hypothalamus and reticular formation regulate ANS activities and motor aspects of emotions, such as fear, flight, and sex. Major ascending and descending tracts of the limbic system (Fig. 16-7) include the medial forebrain bundle, stria medullaris, stria terminalis, mamillothalamic tract, mamillotegmental tract, and medial longitudinal fasciculus.

The septum is connected with the amygdala through the stria terminalis (Fig. 16-6) and with the hypothalamic mamillary bodies through the fornix and ascending and descending fibers of the medial forebrain bundle. The stria medullaris forms the limbic–thalamic pathway that reciprocally connects the septum with the thalamus. The mamillothalamic tract mediates limbic outputs to the neocortex via the anterior nucleus of the thalamus. The limbic descending projections travel to the brainstem reticular formation via the mamillotegmental tract and medial forebrain bundle.

In addition to the structures already mentioned, the fornix and cingulum are two major pathways that interconnect the major limbic structures. The cingulum, a massive fiber bundle, circulates limbic information from the cingulate gyrus to the parahippocampal gyrus and then to the hippocampus. The fornix is the major link between the forebrain and midbrain. It connects the hypothalamus with both the hippocampus and the olfactory cortex. Despite this structural complexity, basic limbic functions are served by four structures: **amygdala, hippocampal formation, cingulate gyrus,** and **septum.**

AMYGDALA

The amygdala is beneath the uncus in the medial anterior cortex of the temporal lobe (Figs. 2-16 and 3-30). Posteriorly, it borders the hippocampus and the tail of the caudate nucleus. The amygdala is reciprocally connected to the hypothalamus, reticular formation, olfactory system, orbital region, hippocampal formation, and neocortex. It also projects to the medial dorsal nucleus of the thalamus, septum, cingulate gyrus, and prefrontal region (Fig. 16-6). Along with bidirectional projections to the prefrontal orbital cortex and hypothalamus, the amygdala directly controls drive and motivation associated with visceral brain activities and the accompanying internal feelings.

The stimulation-based investigations of the amygdaloid function in animals suggest that its activation with high-threshold stimulation can produce all of the behaviors that are elicited from the hypothalamus. These functions include defecation, micturition, pupillary dilation, hair erection, pituitary hormone secretion, blood pressure and heart rate changes, and gastrointestinal motility and secretion. Other behaviors include

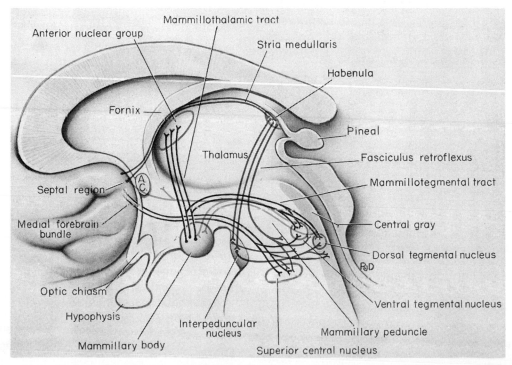

Figure 16-7. Major limbic pathways: medial forebrain bundle, mamillothalamic tract, mamillotegmental tract, and stria medullaris.

sexual activities such as erection, copulatory movements, ejaculation, ovulation, uterine activity, and premature labor. Rage, escape, punishment, and fear are also associated with the amygdala. Stimulation of the amygdala has resulted in motor activities that include head movements, circling, dystonic movements, licking, chewing, swallowing, and vomiting. Combined stimulation of the amygdala and hypothalamus facilitates rage reactions. Amygdala stimulation may increase or decrease hypothalamic induced rage. Bilateral ablation of the amygdala and surrounding temporal tissues is associated with Klüver-Bucy syndrome, which is characterized by indiscriminate eating, oral exploration, fearlessness, loss of aggression, psychic blindness, and inappropriate hypersexuality. Complex partial seizures (see Chapter 20), which emanate from the amygdala and surrounding temporal lobe structures, are characterized by automatic aggressive behaviors, memory impairment, and automatisms (impaired ability to monitor behavior and face the consequences).

HIPPOCAMPUS

The hippocampus is in the ventromedial temporal lobe beneath the hippocampal gyrus. It forms the ventromedial wall of the lateral ventricle temporal (inferior) horn (Fig. 3-30). The principal sources of afferents to the hippocampus are the polysensory association cortical areas. Impulses to the hippocampus travel via the parahippocampal and occipitotemporal gyri (Fig. 16-6). The hippocampus also receives projections from the septum, hypothalamus, and midbrain via the medial forebrain and fornix fiber bundles. Primary efferents from the hippocampus are to the amygdala, septum, and hypothalamus. Hippocampal stimulation and ablation implicate endocrine and autonomic functions generated in the hypothalamus. However, the hippocampus is best known for its involvement with memory and learning.

In the early 1950s, drastic anterograde memory deficits were noted to have occurred after radical bilateral ablations of the hippocampal formation that extended posteriorly in the region of the caudal parahippocampal and fusiform (occipitotemporal) gyri. Patients could not remember their experiences from one moment to the next. A hippocampal lesion was associated with severe anterograde amnesia with preserved retrograde memories. In other words, patients lost newly acquired data but retained memory of events that preceded the lesion. Clinical and experimental findings suggest that the anterograde memory deficit may have been due to the interruption of reverberating cortical circuits that connect the polysensory association cortices with the parahippocampal and fusiform gyri.

CINGULATE GYRUS

Lying above the corpus callosum (Figs. 2-10, 16-5, and 16-6), the cingulate gyrus receives projections from the hypothalamic mamillary bodies by way of the mamillothalamic tract and the anterior thalamic nucleus. The cingulate gyrus projects to the hypothalamic mamillary bodies via the fornix fibers that arise in the entorhinal cortex. This limbic circuit has been clinically associated with anxiety and obsessive-compulsive behaviors.

SEPTUM

The septum consists of two parts. Dorsally, it consists of a midline fibrous sheet attached to the corpus callosum (Figs. 2-11, 16-5, and 16-6). Ventrally, it consists of a collection of nuclei. In conjunction with the diencephalon and brainstem, the septum is a major component of the axial brain, forming the septohypothalamomidbrain continuum. It provides a vital portal entry connecting the limbic lobe with the diencephalon and brainstem. It is also actively involved in processing autonomic, visceral, endocrine, sensorimotor, reproductive, neurotransmitter, emotional, and motivational functions.

Clinical Information

Clinical symptoms that appear after limbic system lesions involve emotions and motivation. They are characterized by uninhibited instinctual behavior, altered sexual behavior, excessive fear, aggression and disturbances in circadian rhythm.

Summary of Limbic System

Anatomically, limbic structures form the inner brain neural circuitry that connects the cortex to the diencephalon and midbrain structures. Functionally, they regulate all visceral, endocrine, and sensorimotor functions. With rich interconnections, the limbic system forms the neural mechanism responsible for motivational drive and emotions.

HYPOTHALAMUS

Consisting of only 4 g of gray matter and occupying a small area in the anterior region of the diencephalon beneath the thalamus, the hypothalamus has importance that greatly exceeds its size. Interconnected with the forebrain, brainstem, and spinal cord, the hypothalamus is the central structure for controlling autonomic and visceral behaviors, such as vasodilation, body homeostasis (internal body environment), anger, reproduction, hunger, and thirst. With its projections to the limbic lobe, it provides the substrates for regulating motivation and emotions. The neurosecretory cells of the hypothalamus regulate the production and circulation of hormones by the pituitary gland.

Anatomical Structures

The hypothalamus is fully exposed on the medial surface of the brain and lies symmetrical along the lateral walls of the third ventricle (Figs. 2-11 and 2-12). Dorsally delineated by the hypothalamic sulcus, the hypothalamus extends from the optic chiasm to the posterior border of the mamillary bodies. The anterior commissure identifies its rostral limit, whereas caudally it extends to the central gray matter in the midbrain tegmentum. The internal capsule marks the lateral limit of the hypothalamus.

On the midsagittal surface, the hypothalamus is divided into the **anterior, tuberal,** and **posterior regions** (Fig. 16-8). The anterior hypothalamus is the region above the optic chiasm. The tuberal region is enclosed by the optic chiasm, optic tract, and mamillary bodies. The posterior hypothalamic region includes the mamillary bodies and the nuclei above them. Coronally, the hypothalamus is divided into three areas: **periventricular, medial,** and **lateral.** The principal hypothalamic nuclei are preoptic, supraoptic, ventromedial, dorsomedial, paraventricular, anterior, posterior, and mamillary body (Fig. 16-8).

The infundibulum is the stalk of the pituitary gland, and it comes from the floor of the third ventricle. As the transitional structure between the CNS and the peripheral endocrine system, the infundibulum is the interface between the brain and pituitary gland. The median eminence (tuber cinereum) lies just caudal to the infundibulum. Above this tuberal level are the ventromedial and dorsomedial hypothalamic nuclei.

The hypothalamus is connected to the cerebral cortex, thalamus, and midbrain with extensive afferent and efferent fiber tracts. Afferents to the hypothalamus come primarily from the limbic region of the forebrain, brainstem, and spinal cord. The bidirectional connections of

the hypothalamus to the brainstem and spinal cord regulate visceral and autonomic functions. However, its interconnections to the limbic lobe account for motivational drive and emotions (Fig. 16-7). The major fiber bundles that interconnect the hypothalamus with other neuraxial structures include the medial forebrain bundle, stria terminalis, fornix, and mamillothalamic, mamillotegmental, and dorsal longitudinal fasciculi (Figs. 16-7 and 16-9).

AFFERENTS

The medial forebrain bundle mediates the forebrain input to the hypothalamus and is the major bidirectional tract formed by the cells in the olfactory region, septum, and amygdala. This pathway mediates information basic to the emotional drives. Other important input for emotional drives comes from the amygdala, which is connected to the hypothalamus via the stria terminalis (Fig. 16-6). The fornix, a large bidirectional pathway, curves around the thalamus and connects to the hypothalamic mamillary bodies via the septum. The bidirectional fibers of the mamillothalamic tract connect the mamillary bodies to the anterior nucleus of the thalamus, which projects to the cingulate gyrus of the limbic lobe (Fig. 16-7). The brainstem and reticular input to the hypothalamus enter by way of the mamillary bodies, dorsal longitudinal fasciculus (Fig. 16-9), and in part the medial forebrain bundle (Fig. 16-7).

EFFERENTS

Efferents of the hypothalamus project to the forebrain limbic structures (septum, hippocampal formation, and

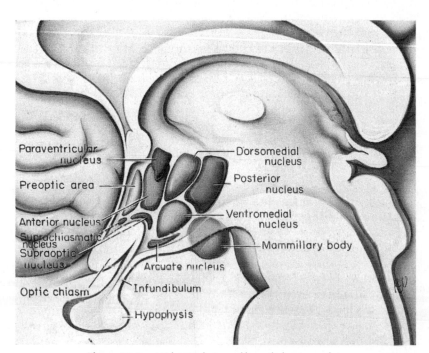

Figure 16-8. Midsagittal view of hypothalamic nuclei.

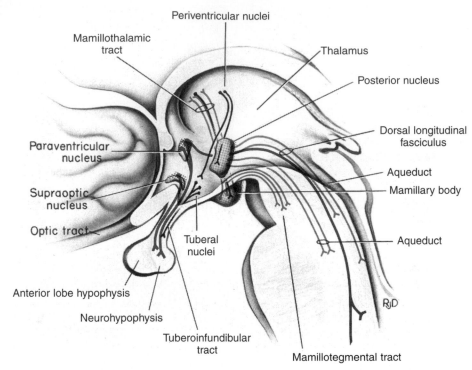

Figure 16-9. Major hypothalamic primarily efferent pathways.

amygdala). Projections also reach the brainstem reticular region, which includes the periaqueductal gray matter, by way of bidirectional fibers in the tracts just described under afferents. The efferent hypothalamic projections to the limbic lobe travel via the septum to the hippocampus and via the mamillothalamic tract to the cingulate gyrus (Fig. 16-9). The mamillothalamic fibers connect the hypothalamus to the anterior thalamic nucleus (see Chapter 6), which in turn connects to the cingulate gyrus, another limbic structure. Hypothalamic projections to the amygdaloid nucleus travel primarily via the stria terminalis and hypothalamoamygdaloid fibers. The multisynaptic outputs travel through the fibers of the dorsal longitudinal tract to the sympathetic and parasympathetic preganglionic cranial and spinal cells. Because of this, the hypothalamus controls the autonomic system and regulates eating and drinking. Additional projections to the lower brainstem and spinal preganglionic autonomic nuclei come from the reticular formation, which in turn receives hypothalamic input via fibers of the mamillotegmental tract (Fig. 16-9). Other important neural projections of the hypothalamus travel to the posterior pituitary gland. Hypothalamic neuronal influence on the anterior pituitary gland controls the secretion of gonadotropic, adrenocorticotropic, and thyrotropic hormones.

Hypothalamic Functions

Most understanding of hypothalamic functions is based on the electrical stimulation of the hypothalamus and/or observations of impaired functions after lesions induced in the hypothalamus of animals. In addition to regulating autonomic (sympathetic and parasympathetic) functions, the hypothalamus has specific centers for controlling eating, drinking, reproduction, aggression, and biological body rhythms. The hypothalamus also contributes to blood electrolyte balance and temperature control. Most important, it controls endocrine-monitored behaviors through the secretion of hormones. Only a few hypothalamic functions are discussed here.

AUTONOMIC INNERVATION

The posterior hypothalamic region controls activity of the sympathetic nervous system. Electrical stimulation of this region activates thoracolumbar outflow, which increases metabolic and somatic activities typical of emotional stress and aggression. The activities include pupil dilation, piloerection, somatic hyperactivity, inhibition of the gut and bladder, increased heart rate, blood pressure, and respiration.

The control center for the parasympathetic system is in the anterior and medial hypothalamic regions, which on activation increase vagal and sacral autonomic responses. Such responses include reduced heart rate, peripheral vasodilation, and increased tone and motility of the alimentary and bladder walls.

BODY TEMPERATURE REGULATION

Body temperature regulation involves the balanced coordination of the sympathetic and parasympathetic nervous systems. Neurons in the anterior hypothalamus are sensitive to increases in blood temperature. They react to an increase in temperature by dissipating excess heat through sweating (a sympathetic activity) and by inhibiting the sympathetic system, causing cutaneous blood vessels to dilate. The posterior hypothalamus, however, preserves heat by inhibiting the sympathetic system in constricting cutaneous vessels and stopping sweat secretion. This is accompanied by shivering (a somatic activity) and decreased visceral activity. An anterior hypothalamic lesion impairs the heat dissipation mechanism and results in **hyperthermia,** whereas a posterior hypothalamic lesion impairs the pathways responsible for both heat conservation and dissipation, resulting in a **poikilothermic state** in which body temperature is governed by environmental temperature.

WATER INTAKE REGULATION

Adequate water input and output, essential for normal body activity, is regulated by vasopressin, an antidiuretic hormone. Synthesized in the supraoptic nucleus of the anterior hypothalamus, vasopressin is released into the bloodstream per physiological circumstances by way of the posterior pituitary gland. Vasopressin production is controlled by blood osmotic pressure and hydration. A rise in blood osmotic pressure or a reduction in circulating vascular volume increases vasopressin production, causing fluid retention. A dehydrated state activates the supraoptic hypothalamic vasopressin system. Vasopressin is resynthesized and stored in the posterior pituitary gland after water balance is reestablished.

Activation of the anterior hypothalamus causes increased water intake. In fact, the anterior hypothalamus regulates both food and water intake. Small lesions in the lateral hypothalamus cause adipsia (a lack of desire to drink), and large lesions cause both adipsia and aphagia (inability to eat). A lesion in the supraoptic nucleus results in increased water intake (polydipsia) and increased urine output (polyuria), a condition clinically known as diabetes insipidus.

FEEDING

The feeding (phagic) center is in the lateral hypothalamus. A lesion in this area causes anorexia, a decreased desire to eat. The ventromedial nucleus of the hypothalamus is the site of a satiety center. Lesions of the ventromedial nucleus of the hypothalamus cause hyperphagia, obesity, and aggressive behavior.

PUNISHMENT

Feelings such as fear, terror, and the desire to flee, engendered by challenging situations, arise from stimulation of the periventricular hypothalamus. These structures extend posteriorly to the central gray surrounding the cerebral aqueduct or aqueduct of Sylvius in the midbrain. Prolonged stimulation in these areas may cause death. By varying the electrical parameters, stimulation of the ventromedial hypothalamus may elicit fear, rage, and aggression. Stimulation of the more rostral midline preoptic area elicits the fear and anxiety associated with escape. In generating these behaviors, the cerebral cortex, in conjunction with various environmental inputs, must recruit somatic and hypothalamic visceral systems. Together they control the expression of pleasure or displeasure associated with the behavior.

HYPOTHALAMIC REGULATION OF PITUITARY GLAND (HYPOPHYSIS)

Nicknamed the master gland, the pituitary gland forms the central endocrine system and works with the nervous system to maintain body homeostasis. The pituitary gland controls the functioning of other glands and tissues in the body by secreting hormones and chemical messengers. The pituitary gland consists of a large anterior lobe (adenohypophysis) and a small posterior lobe (neurohypophysis) (Fig. 16-10).

Release of hormones produced in the neurosecretory hypothalamic cells stimulates the adenohypophysis to secrete the following hormones: growth hormone, thyrotropin, adrenocorticotropin, gonadotropin, and prolactin. The releasing hormones are transported into the anterior lobe of the pituitary gland through the hypothalamic hypophyseal portal (blood) circulation (Fig. 16-10 and Table 16-4).

Thyrotropic hormones stimulate and regulate thyroid gland hormone secretion. Adrenocorticotropin regulates steroid secretion by the adrenal cortex. Gonadotropin (follicle-stimulating hormone) stimulates production of ova and sperm. Prolactin (lactogenic hormone), in conjunction with other hormones, stimulates and maintains milk secretion by the mamillary glands. Growth hormones stimulate and maintain the growth of bones and muscles. Hyposecretion and hypersecretion of growth hormones are directly related to dwarfism and gigantism. These growth hormones also regulate the rate of protein synthesis, fat burning, and conversion of glycogen into blood glucose.

Two peptide hormones, vasopressin and oxytocin, are released from the posterior pituitary gland (Table 16-5). Vasopressin is predominantly synthesized in the supraoptic nucleus, whereas oxytocin is synthesized in the paraventricular nucleus of the hypothalamus. They are both transported axonally to the posterior hypophysis, where they are stored and then released into the bloodstream. Vasopressin is an antidiuretic hormone that increases water reabsorption in the kidney and is also used to raise blood pressure in states of hypotension. Lesions of the posterior lobe cause diabetes insipidus, which is marked by the excretion of 10 to 15 L of urine per day. Oxytocin-induced contraction of the

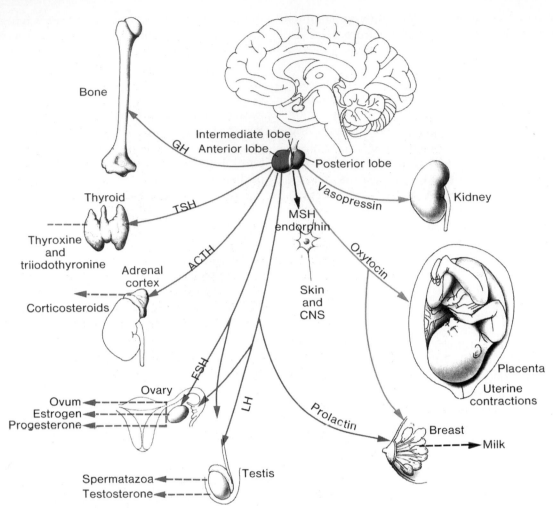

Figure 16-10. Commonly secreted pituitary hormones in adenohypophysis and neurohypophysis. Hormones of anterior pituitary gland or adenohypophysis include growth hormones (*GH*), thyrotropin, adrenocorticotropic hormone (*ACTH*), gonadotropin, and prolactin. Posterior pituitary lobe or neurohypophysis contains vasopressin and oxytocin.

Secreted by cells in supraoptic and paraventricular hypothalamic nuclei, they regulate kidney function (*vasopressin*) and glands of the breasts (*oxytocin*). *CNS*, central nervous system; *FSH*, follicle-stimulating hormone; *LH*, luteinizing hormone; *MSH*, melanocyte-stimulating hormone; *TSH*, thyroid-stimulating hormone.

Table 16-4. Anterior Pituitary Gland Hormones and Their Functions

Hormones	Primary Functions
Growth hormones	Control general body growth
Thyroid-stimulating hormones (thyrotropic)	Control thyroid hormone secretions
Adrenocorticotropic hormones	Control secretion of adrenal cortex hormones
Gonadotropic hormones	Initiate sperm production in males; promote development of ova in females
Prolactin	Promotes milk secretion by mammillary glands

Table 16-5. Posterior Pituitary Gland Hormones and Their Functions

Hormone	Primary Function
Oxytocin	Stimulates uterine contraction and mamillary gland alveoli, causing milk secretion
Vasopressin	Decreases urine volume and raises blood pressure by constricting arterial lumen, particularly during hemorrhage

smooth muscle cells of the uterus assists in the delivery of a baby. It also assists in milk ejection by contracting the cells of the mammary gland.

An imbalance in the secretion of hormones results in endocrine disturbance, which is marked either by decreased hormone secretion (hyposecretion) or increased hormone secretion (hypersecretion). Hypersecretion and hyposecretion of various hormones are associated with specific clinical symptoms (Table 16-6).

Neurotransmitters and Behaviors

Neurotransmitters play an important role in the regulation of behaviors mediated by the hypothalamus. The interaction of vasopressin with noradrenergic synapses is known to influence memory consolidation.

Table 16-6. Disorders Associated with Hormone Disturbances

Growth hormones	
Hyposecretion	Dwarfism
Hypersecretion	Gigantism
Thyrotropic hormones	
Hyposecretion	In infancy results in low metabolism, low body development, mental retardation; in adults causes lethargy, excessive sleeping, slow mental activity
Hypersecretion	Increased metabolic rate; makes person hungry, increasing food intake
Adrenocorticotropic hormones	
Hyposecretion	Impaired synthesis of glucose and loss of sodium in urine
Hypersecretion	Decreased immune response and excessive fat deposits
Gonadotropic hormones	Impaired sexual functions
Vasopressin	Water imbalance

Norepinephrine released in the hypothalamus may block visceral drives such as eating, drinking, and sexual behavior. This suggests that while norepinephrine activates the neocortex, it inhibits the competing visceral drives. Excessive production of norepinephrine causes manic psychosis, whereas insufficient production of it causes depression. Stimulation of the dopamine projections to the hypothalamic area enhances eating and fighting drives. A bilateral hypothalamic lesion that impairs the dopaminergic systems reduces these drives.

Clinical Information

Clinical symptoms that commonly result from hypothalamic dysfunction are characterized by disturbances of food intake, water balance, libido, menstruation, and temperature control. Also, pituitary hormone changes can affect body growth, the ability to reproduce, and milk secretion.

Summary of Hypothalamus

The hypothalamus is the central structure for controlling autonomic and visceral behaviors. It is the central generator of motivational and emotional–motor behaviors, and it controls visceral functions including vasodilation, body homeostasis (internal body environment), reproduction, hunger, and water and food intake. Its neurosecretory cells regulate pituitary gland hormone production and release.

RETICULAR FORMATION

The reticular formation consists of a group of neurons that are interconnected by parallel and serial running neuronal circuits. Composing most of the brainstem (medulla, pons, and midbrain), it is also functionally wired to nuclei in the thalamus and spinal cord (Fig. 2-23). With their central location, the neuronal circuits of the reticular formation inhibit, facilitate, modify, and regulate all cortical functions and further integrate all sensorimotor stimuli with internally generated thoughts, emotions, and cognition. It is also responsible for maintaining the homeostatic state of the brain, which is essential for regulating visceral, sensorimotor and neuroendocrine activities, including arousal, consciousness, sleep, blood pressure, posture, and movement. It also regulates emotions, mood, and cognition. Furthermore, it energizes the reticular activating system (RAS) that controls arousal and consciousness. A single lesion of the RAS can produce complex illnesses and altered states of arousal or permanent unconsciousness, such as coma, insomnia, headaches, depression, tremors, aggression, and forgetfulness. Descending reticular fibers regulate the quality of motor movement and muscle tone. They also inhibit sensory inputs at the spinal level. Finally, two important functions of the reticular formation for students of communicative disorders are its regulation of respiration and swallowing.

Anatomical Structures

The reticular circuitry is characterized by multiple parallel and serial running circuits. These neuronal circuits inhibit, facilitate, modify, and regulate brain and spinal cord functions. They also contribute to reticular sensorimotor integration and behavior generation. Because of its organization, one reticular nerve cell has the potential to influence more than 25,000 to 30,000 neurons in the brainstem. This architectural property enables the reticular cells first to amplify a weak impulse and second to disseminate the amplified signal to thousands of other nuclei. The reticular formation can concentrate impulses from thousands of neurons to a single neuronal circuit. It can also channel and screen information and respond to the amount of information rather than to the details.

The reticular cells are longitudinally arranged in transverse modules and project to overlapping dendrites, which generally lack dendritic shafts. The dendritic processes look like radiating spokes of a wheel. Each dendrite shaft receives input from different combinations of axons throughout the neuraxis. The axons, the efferent component of the reticular cells, are long (Golgi type I) and tend to bifurcate and project in opposite directions to distant structures. Projections run caudally to the spinal cord and rostrally throughout the brainstem, diencephalon, limbic structures, basal ganglia, and cortex.

The brainstem reticular cells are arranged in three broad longitudinal columns: median, medial, and lateral (Fig. 13-1). The median reticular cell column contains the midline nucleus raphe, which forms a continuous cellular column in the brainstem and consists of regions that provide projections to the brain and spinal cord. The medial cell column consists of a central group of reticular nuclei, including the gigantocellular reticular nucleus, whereas the lateral cell column contains small to intermediate-sized nuclei.

AFFERENTS

Overlapping afferents, of which some are inhibitory and others facilitatory, converge on a given reticular neuron. Reticular afferents consist of collaterals from the ascending and descending spinal tracts (pain, proprioception, tactile, temperature, vibration), cranial nerve nuclei, cerebellum, midbrain, thalamus, subthalamus, hypothalamus, striatum, limbic lobe, and various cortical areas.

EFFERENTS

Through its direct and indirect projections, the reticular formation influences all nervous system functions. It sends projections to somatic and autonomic nuclei in general, to autonomic and somatic motor nuclei of cranial nerves in the brainstem, and to interneuronal pools in the spinal cord. Direct and indirect reticular projections also travel to the cerebellum, red nucleus, substantia nigra, midbrain tectum, subthalamic nuclei, thalamus, hypothalamus, and limbic lobe (septum, hippocampus, amygdala, and cingulate gyrus).

Functional Considerations

Within the diffuse reticular core of nuclei in the brainstem, specific nuclear cell aggregates form closed-loop circuits and serve as the reticular centers for regulating various sensorimotor, visceral, and cortical activating functions. Reticular centers may combine to form reticular networks that help regulate complex sensorimotor and visceral behaviors, such as eating, swallowing, vomiting, coughing, sneezing, copulation, and fighting.

Examining all of the unifying functions of the reticular formation is beyond the scope of this chapter. However, to provide a simpler way to describe functions, the reticular functions have been divided into three types: cortical arousal, sensorimotor elaboration, and visceral integrated activity.

REGULATION OF CORTICAL AROUSAL

The activation and regulation of cortical arousal are perhaps the best known functions of the reticular formation. The serotonergic, cholinergic, and catecholaminergic cells of the ascending reticular activating system and their projections from the brainstem to the neocortex and limbic structures collectively contribute to cortical arousal. The reticular activating system is indiscriminate to variations between sensory input and its modality; rather, it responds best to stimulus intensity and novelty.

Clinically, cortical electrical activity is the best indicator of cortical arousal and brain functions. Various patterns of the brain's electrical activity are known to relate to different mental states of arousal. For example, if a person is relaxed with eyes closed, the usual electrical activity observed is the α-rhythm (see Chapter 20). Opening the eyes or exposing the subject to other sensory stimuli causes the α-rhythm to change to a high-frequency, low-amplitude (electroencephalographic [EEG] activation) wave pattern. This electrical activity reflects changes in the arousal or alertness of the cerebral cortex and is related to functions of the reticular system.

Sleep is related to the state of arousal and consciousness and is directly involved with the functioning of the reticular activating system. In general, there are two sleeping states: deep sleep, or non–rapid eye movement (NREM) and paradoxical, or rapid eye movement (REM) sleep. NREM sleep has several substages, representing progressively deeper states of unconsciousness characterized by slower and higher-amplitude EEG patterns. EEG recordings of deep sleep are characterized by slow-frequency waves of large amplitude from which one can recover with full restoration of awareness and cognitive functions.

Deep sleep is periodically interrupted by REM sleep, in which the individual is as physically relaxed as in deep sleep but displays the EEG pattern characteristic of being awake. This is associated with the dream state. REM sleep is also characterized by variations in heart rate, blood pressure, and respiration. Being awake is accompanied by a low-voltage and fast-frequency desynchronized wave form. Electrical stimulation of the reticular formation can change EEG patterns of deep sleep to the pattern of wakefulness, indicating that the reticular activating system may regulate levels of cortical arousal and wakefulness.

The median raphe nucleus (serotonergic) and locus ceruleus (noradrenergic) are two important reticular neurotransmitter nuclei (Fig. 13-1B) concerned with sleep; their alternating actions trigger NREM and REM stages of sleep. The median raphe nucleus generates the high-voltage, slow waves of deep sleep. A lesion of the raphe nucleus causes constant wakefulness or insomnia. Conversely, the nucleus locus ceruleus generates REM sleep. If the locus ceruleus is damaged, REM does not occur.

Most coma-causing lesions are at the midbrain, hypothalamic, and thalamic junctions. The lesion can result from traumatic injury, vascular occlusion, tumors, or encephalitis. Impairment of the brainstem reticular formation may be a major causative factor, especially at the midbrain level.

REGULATION OF SENSORY FUNCTIONS

The reticulospinal projections also modulate the quantity and quality of sensory information and employ the gating mechanism that screens information at both spinal and thalamic levels. The brainstem collateral terminals of primary sensory fibers are under direct reticular influence. The reticular formation affects sensory impulse transmission in presynaptic and postsynaptic terminals.

Reticular nuclei also send input to brain structures such as the cochlear and vestibular nuclei, tectal and pretectal structures, geniculate nuclei, and thalamic nuclei that process specialized and general sensory input. The direct reticular projections influence information processing by either accentuating or attenuating the sensory (audition, vision, olfaction, pain, temperature, and tactile) stimuli. There is a reticular pain monitoring and control system at the midbrain level and posterior diencephalic reticular formation, especially in the tegmental and periaqueductal regions.

INTEGRATED MOTOR FUNCTIONS

Integrated motor functions include unconscious activities that are vital to survival and are controlled by the brainstem reticular nuclei. The reticular formation uses convergent multimodal input and diffuse divergent output to control the vital centers of the brainstem that regulate cardiac activity, respiration, and swallowing. The reticular modulation of the lower motor neurons and resultant altered muscle tone are discussed in Chapter 13.

Cardiovascular Activity

The reticular nuclei regulating vasomotor functions of the heart extend from the rostral medulla to the mid pons. These nuclei receive extensive projections from peripheral receptors and are in part controlled by the hypothalamus. They project information via fibers of the vagus nerve. Stimulation of the lateral reticular pressor center increases heart rate and causes vasoconstriction. However, stimulation of the depressor center in the lower medulla decreases heart rate and causes vasodilation. Most spinal nerves and some cranial nerves, when stimulated, raise arterial pressure by exciting the pressor region and inhibiting the depressor region. Lesions of the medullary center for cardiovascular control can cause cardiac irregularities and blood pressure changes, both of which are life-threatening.

Respiration

Respiration is the basic process underlying speech, though its primary purpose is to maintain a proper level of oxygen and carbon dioxide in the body tissue through the regulated cycles of inhalation and exhalation. Changes in the concentration of any of these constituents renders an immediate effect on the respiratory activity. For example, the concentration of carbon dioxide, which is detected by chemoreceptors located in the carotid and aortic bodies, can directly stimulate the respiratory center through inspiratory and expiratory signals to the respiratory muscles. The primary muscles of respiration are the diaphragm, internal and external intercostals, and abdominal muscles. The contraction of the diaphragm and external intercostal muscles increases the intrathoracic volume and decreases the pleural cavity pressure, thus prompting the inspirational phase, where air is forced into the pleural cavity according to Boyle's law. Expiration is a passive process controlled by the elasticity of the lungs and the walls of the abdomen and chest. However, forced expiration, as during coughing and defecating, requires muscle contraction from the abdominals and internal intercostals.

The control of respiration is not as clear as generally depicted. The regulation of breathing involves two controls, voluntary and automatic. The nuclei forming the voluntary respiratory control center are in the motor cortex. The automatic brainstem respiratory center consists of several groups of scattered neurons in the reticular formation; it can be divided into two distinct centers: pontine pneumotaxic center and medullary respiratory center. The medullary respiratory center is further divided into the dorsal respiratory group and the ventral respiratory group of neurons (Fig. 16-11). A lesion in the pontomedullary respiratory center causes asphyxia and eventually death if artificial respiration is not administered.

Voluntary Respiration Control. Temporary increases and decreases in the rate and depth of breathing due to different motor activities are regulated by the voluntary respiratory center. This center is in the motor cortex. Projections from the motor cortex descend through the internal capsule (diencephalon), pes peduncle (midbrain), and pyramidal fibers (medulla) before innervating the spinal motor neurons in the cervical, thoracic, and lumbar regions of the spinal cord. The neuronal projections from the cervical and thoracic regions of the cord control the activity of muscles of respiration, such as the diaphragm, intercostals, and abdominal muscles.

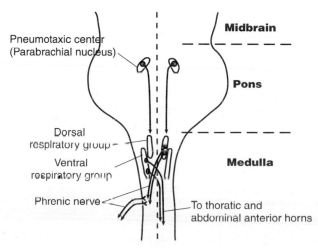

Figure 16-11. Autonomic (pontine and medullary) respiratory centers.

Automatic Respiration Control.   The automatic center of the brainstem includes the pneumotaxic center of the pons and dorsal and ventral respiratory nuclei of the medulla (Fig. 16-11). The function of the pontine pneumotaxic center is to limit the duration of the inspiration phase in the lungs. Based on physical activity and bodily needs, the strong signals from the pneumotaxic center temporarily shorten the filling phase of the lungs. However, weaker signals from this center lengthen the inspirational phase, resulting in excessive filling of the lungs. By limiting the duration of inspiration, this pneumotaxic center also regulates the duration of expiration, and it controls respiratory depth and its rate by constant inhibition of the medullary respiratory centers. In normal physiological conditions, the activity of the pontine pneumotaxic center, in conjunction with vagal afferents from the branchial stretch receptors, inhibits the strong inspiratory activity.

The dorsal medullary respiratory center contains reticular nuclei, including the nucleus of the tractus solitarius, which is responsive to afferents from the carotid and aortic chemoreceptors through the vagus and glossopharyngeal nerves. These signals, along with the sensory information from the lungs, help control respiratory activity. The fibers descending from the dorsal medullary respiratory neurons cross to activate the anterior horn cells of the cervical region of the cord. Efferent projections from C-3 to C-5 (predominantly from C-4) form the phrenic nerve, which causes contraction of the diaphragm, the main muscle of respiration. Contraction of the diaphragm increases the intrathoracic volume, beginning the cycle of inspiration. The dorsal respiratory area is known to regulate respiratory rhythm.

Next to the dorsal respiratory group of nuclei is the ventral group of respiratory nuclei, which is inactive during the normal respiratory cycle. It is known to become active when high levels of pulmonary ventilation are required. Projections from the ventral medullary respiratory nuclei cross the midline to activate the contralateral thoracic motor nuclei; their projections regulate the activity of the spinal intercostal and abdominal muscles. Both the dorsal and ventral respiratory nuclei of the medulla contain the mechanism responsible for controlling the rhythmic activity of the respiratory muscles.

The most important motor function of the spinal cord for motor speech is its control of the muscles that regulate respiration (Table 16-7), a patterned cycle of inhalation and exhalation that not only is vital for survival, but also contributes to the loudness of speech. Respiration involves about 15 muscles, the four major groups of which are the diaphragm, abdominals, and external and internal intercostals. Sternocleidomastoid and scalenus are also important accessory muscles. The motor nuclei from the anterior horns of the C-3-C-5 (with predominance from C-4 through phrenic nerve)

Table 16-7. Motor Innervation of the Muscles of Respiration

Spinal Roots	Muscles	Functions
C-3 to C-5, mainly C-4	Diaphragm	Increasing intrathoracic volume for inspiration
T-1 to T-12	External intercostals	Increasing intrathoracic volume by raising ribs for inspiration
T-1 to T-12	Internal intercostals	Decreasing intrathoracic volume by depressing ribs for expiration
T-6 to T-12	Abdominal muscles	Increasing intrathoracic pressure for expiration

innervate the diaphragm. The efferents to the internal and external intercostals exit from T-1 to T-12. The abdominal muscles receive efferents from the motor nuclei of T-6 to T-12. The diaphragm and external intercostals are the primary muscles of inspiration, whereas the abdominal and internal intercostals participate in forced expiration.

During the inspiratory phase, contraction of the diaphragm and external intercostals increases the intrathoracic volume, which lowers the pressure within the lungs and thoracic cavity. The reduced intrathoracic pressure forces air into the lungs through the trachea. Exhalation is initiated by an increase in intra-abdominal pressure and a decrease in intrathoracic volume caused by the abdominal and internal intercostal muscles. In quiet inspiration, the diaphragm and external intercostals actively participate, whereas quiet exhalation does not require active muscular activity because the elastic recoil of the lungs restores intrathoracic volume to the resting level. However, forced inspiration (during exercise) and expiration (during blowing out a candle or coughing) requires active muscle contraction. These facts are clinically important, since spinal lesions involving motor nuclei at different levels differentially affect respiration. For example, a patient with a complete spinal lesion above C-3 has complete paralysis of all respiratory muscles and is likely to lose the ability to breathe spontaneously. Such a patient requires artificial respiration/tracheostomy for survival. Patients with a spinal injury below C-4 and above T-12 have varying degrees of paralysis of all primary respiratory muscles except the diaphragm. With basic control over the diaphragm, such a patient may continue to inhale and quietly exhale because of the elastic recoil of lungs. With full control of diaphragm, inspiration is not a problem for such a person. However, with reduced or impaired control over the abdominal and internal intercostal muscles, such a patient would not be able to undertake the forced exhalation needed for coughing, bowel movements, and blowing. In the case of any lesion below T-12, the patient's control of respiratory muscles is likely to remain intact.

Swallowing

The physiology of deglutition, or swallowing, has recently become an important clinical issue in communicative disorders, as many clinicians are diagnosing and managing disorders of swallowing. As with respiration, the reticular nuclei regulate the act of swallowing by integrating the functions of the trigeminal, facial, glossopharyngeal, vagus, and hypoglossal nerves. Swallowing is a reflexive action instigated by the sensory and motor components of these cranial nerves along with reticular participation.

Swallowing has two stages: **voluntary** and **involuntary.** The voluntary stage consists of masticating a bolus and moving it into the pharyngeal cavity. The involuntary stage is the passage of the bolus through the pharynx and esophagus. The voluntary stage covers the act of chewing and the movement of the bolus in the oral cavity. It ends as the upward and backward motion of the tongue forces the bolus against the palate. As the bolus presses against the palate to enter the pharynx, the involuntary stage begins through sensory projections from the posterior palate to the reticular swallowing center in the lower pons and upper medulla. The reticular swallowing center directs projections to the adjacent respiratory center and to the nuclei of trigeminal, facial, glossopharyngeal, vagus, and hypoglossal nerves, which initiate a series of reflexive motor actions that ensure proper breathing management while the bolus passes through the pharynx. Major reflexive actions include the upward movement of the palate to close the nasopharynx, backward and downward movement of the epiglottis to seal off the glottis, raising of the larynx to close the airway, and enlarging the esophageal opening to allow entrance of the bolus. As the bolus passes the pharyngeal phase, the reticular respiratory center regulates the reopening of the respiratory passageway. Brainstem lesions interrupting the afferent and efferent projections of the reticular formation can alter the integrity of the swallowing reflex and cause aspiration. Common disturbances of swallowing seen in neurogenic patients are poor mastication, delayed swallowing reflex, reduced peristalsis of the bolus through the pharynx, and aspiration.

Vomiting

The reticular nuclei that regulate vomiting are in the medulla. They receive inputs from the oropharynx and gastrointestinal tract. Noxious impulses mediating irritations of the intestinal tract and oropharynx initiate reflexive vomiting. Projections from the vomiting center in the medulla descend through the fibers of cranial nerves X and IX and coordinate the contraction of the abdominal, diaphragmatic, and intercostal muscles. The oropharyngeal musculature, which facilitates vomiting, works with all of these muscles.

Coughing

Afferents mediating irritation from laryngeal and tracheal lining tissues initiate the coughing reflex via cranial nerve X and the solitary tract nuclei. As with the vomiting reflex, the diaphragm, abdominal, and intercostal muscles are involved; however, they contract alternately, not simultaneously.

Autonomic Functions

The reticular formation contributes to the autonomic system through its reticulobulbar and reticulospinal fiber projections. Input to the reticular autonomic regulatory system comes from limbic and diencephalic structures of the forebrain, which include the orbitofrontal cortex, cingulate gyrus, amygdala, hippocampus, hypothalamus, and the medial, anterior, and dorsal groups of the thalamic nuclei. Reticular projections regulate hypothalamic centers specializing in endocrine production and release, temperature, food and fluid intake, sexual activity, diurnal body rhythms, blood electrolyte balance, visceral and autonomic functions, emotional states, and learning.

Biological Rhythms

A self-regulated internal clock, a characteristic of all living systems, determines the turnover rates of macromolecules, annual seasonal variations, and daily environmental changes in the body. Biological rhythms govern reproductive cycles, development, cell division, and cell death. Many rhythms depend on an intact hypothalamus with its multiple connections, including those from the reticular formation. The reticular formation is also indirectly involved in neural control of the pineal gland, a structure that participates in regulating circadian rhythms (repetitive cycles, or biorhythm).

Self-Awareness

Deep cellular layers of the superior colliculus receive multimodal inputs that outline the space around the body. This input stems from overlapping visual, auditory, and somatic stimuli, representing various temporal and spatial reference points surrounding the body. These stimuli form a three-dimensional body image in the midbrain reticular formation. The reticular formation projects this image to nonspecific and specific thalamic nuclei and thus enables humans to have conscious self-awareness. The thalamus in turn relays the information to the neocortex for further in-depth analysis.

Head and Eye Movement

The reticular formation regulates the rotation of the head and eyes. Through fibers of the medial longitudinal fasciculus, the reticular formation mediates impulses connecting various participating cranial and cervical muscles that control head and eye movements.

Their integrated activity is responsible for head and body movements, such as circling in one direction.

RETICULAR NEUROTRANSMITTERS

The reticular formation uses various neurotransmitters to communicate with the brain, spinal cord, and neighboring reticular regions. These neurotransmitters are synthesized by a specialized population of cells (see Chapter 5). A monoamine imbalance can generate somatic and psychic symptoms of excitement, agitation, anxiety, and insomnia, among others. For example, an overabundance of norepinephrine can lead to the somatic symptoms of speech dysfluency, rapid heart rate, increased blood pressure, dry mouth, and cessation of intestinal peristalsis.

Serotonin

Electrical discharge firing rates of serotonin and noradrenergic neurons fluctuate with sleep and wakefulness. Therefore, they participate in the general activity level of the CNS. Serotonin is thought to be concerned with overall levels of arousal and slow-wave sleep as well as severe depression. In the treatment of depression, antidepressant drugs appear to enhance the concentration of serotonin at the synapse by reducing its uptake. Serotonin is also an important contributor to the descending pain control system.

Norepinephrine

The locus ceruleus is the major noradrenergic reticular nucleus. Noradrenergic projections have a profound influence on brain function and are known to regulate brain tone by inhibiting background activity, enhancing the signal-to-noise ratio in the brain. Behaviorally, the locus ceruleus contributes to the generation of REM sleep. Along with other noradrenergic neurons, the locus ceruleus is also thought to mediate attention and vigilance. Depression can be treated with drugs that enhance the transmission of norepinephrine at the synapse.

Dopamine

Degeneration of dopamine-producing cells has been associated with parkinsonism, a motor disorder consisting of a shaking palsy, akinesia, a masked face, drooling, and a shuffling gait (see Chapter 13). Dopamine projections to the cortex and limbic structures seem to influence cognitive functions and motivation. Cocaine and amphetamine, drugs that enhance the action of dopamine, induce syndromes resembling paranoid schizophrenia. Drugs of substance abuse cause dopamine release in the nucleus accumbens, suggesting that this mesolimbic projection may be associated with a sense of pleasure. Thorazine and related drugs used in the treatment of schizophrenia block dopamine receptors, which suggests that the mesolimbic and mesocortical dopaminergic systems may be involved in this psychotic disorder.

Enkephalins

Enkephalins in the reticular formation contribute to pain suppression. As a subgroup of endorphin opiates, they are primarily present in the PNS. They form local neuronal circuits that are found in the gastrointestinal system, which responds to opiates by reducing gastrointestinal motility. Abdominal pain (colic) often responds best to opiates.

Substance P

The substance P neurotransmitter has a slow and long-lasting inhibitory effect on neuronal firing. It attenuates pain and is present in the reticular formation and spinal dorsal root ganglia. Fibers of the opiatelike enkephalin cells form axoaxonic synapses with substance P fibers. This connectivity is thought to control the pain that may occur with movement disorders such as Parkinson's disease.

γ-Aminobutyric Acid

γ-Aminobutyric acid (GABA), the most prevalent inhibitory transmitter, dominates in local circuit neurons. It is produced from the decarboxylation of glutamate. GABA serves as the inhibitory neurotransmitter from the Purkinje cells to the deep cerebellar nuclei, from the striatum to the globus pallidus and substantia nigra, and from the globus pallidus and substantia nigra to the thalamus.

Tranquilizers such as diazepam (Valium) bind to GABA receptors and increase the effects of the transmitter released at GABA synapses. Abnormal movements, as seen in Huntington's chorea, are due to the loss of GABA neurons in the caudate and putamen. This elevates the ratio of dopamine to acetylcholine, producing abnormal movements. However, a reduced ratio of dopamine to acetylcholine causes the abnormal motor movements of parkinsonism.

Clinical Information

Clinical symptoms that may occur after lesions of the reticular formation are irregularities in sleep, blood pressure, pulse rate, respiration, vigilance, and states of consciousness. Motor dysfunctions may include tremors and altered muscle tone, ranging from hypertonic rigidity to flaccidity. Speech and swallowing disorders may occur after lesions in the caudal brainstem reticular formation.

Summary of Reticular Formation

A diffuse core of nuclei in the brainstem, the reticular formation serves as a fine-tuner of cortical functions. With extensive dendrites and axons, it regulates sensorimotor, visceral, and cognitive functions. An important function of the reticular formation is to regulate cortical arousal, which is measured by various patterns of brain electrical activity. It also regulates functions such as sleep and awake states.

Case Studies

Patient One: Autonomic System Dysfunction

A 55-year-old schoolteacher consulted his physician for what he thought was a strange feeling of nervousness. This was marked by bladder incontinence that caused him embarrassment. Other sensorimotor functions were normal. Magnetic resonance imaging (MRI) revealed a tumor in the sacral region of the spinal cord.

Question: Based on your understanding of the sympathetic and parasympathetic ANS, can you explain how the sacral lesion caused bladder incontinence?

Discussion: With the tumor compressing the sacral cord, all afferent and efferent impulses of the spinal reflex to the bladder were interrupted. Bladder control was lost and the bladder became flaccid. Once the bladder was full, the urine dripped out gradually.

Patient Two: Autonomic Nervous System

A 45-year-old schoolteacher consulted his physician about asymmetrical pupil sizes. On examination, he exhibited right pupil constriction (meiosis). Additional signs included ptosis of the right upper eyelid and inability to perspire on the forehead. The attending physician suspected Horner's syndrome, an autonomic nervous system impairment, and MRI confirmed an infarct in the right cervical sympathetic chain.

Question: Based on your understanding of the ANS, can you explain how a cervical sympathetic chain lesion caused these symptoms?

Discussion: (a) Horner's syndrome results from a lesion of the sympathetic pathways to the eye and forehead. Clinical characteristics are miotic (constricted) pupil, ptosis of the upper eyelid, and inability to sweat on the forehead. (b) Pupil constriction (meiosis) is regulated by parasympathetic impulses, whereas pupil dilation (mydriasis) is controlled by sympathetic impulses. Sympathetic impulses originate in the ipsilateral hypothalamus and descend to the motor neurons in the T-1 to T-2 segments. Preganglionic neuron projections travel to the superior sympathetic cervical ganglion, which projects to the smooth dilator muscle of the iris.

Damage to the superior cervical ganglia affected the sympathetic projections, resulting in unopposed actions of the parasympathetic system. This caused the pupil constriction and contributed to the inability to sweat.

Patient Three: Hypothalmus

A 25-year-old schoolteacher was very slim and had a history of poor appetite, weight loss, and episodes of high fever. She had lost interest in sex, and her menses were irregular. She drank large quantities of water but considered her behavior to be normal. Her physician suspected hypothalamic involvement and anorexia.

Question: How can hypothalamic damage cause these symptoms?

Discussion: Hypothalamic damage usually causes an imbalance in food and water intake and temperature control and a decrease in sexual drive. Weight loss is commonly seen in patients with anorexia. A vasopressin (antidiuretic hormone) deficiency causes excessive thirst and accompanying urinary output. Alterations in gonadotropic hormones lead to changes in the cycle of menses. Furthermore, hypothalamic damage causes a disturbance in temperature control.

Patient Four: Limbic System

A 35-year-old man had a history of temporal lobe seizures. During his seizure attacks, he would become very violent, throwing objects at people. He frequently harmed his wife and abused his children. Strangely, he retained no memory of his actions.

Question: How did seizure activity in the temporal (limbic) lobe affect memory?

Discussion: Abnormal electric discharges of the temporal lobe stimulated the hippocampus and amygdala, resulting in automatic behaviors for which there was loss of conscious control. The involvement of association cortices during his seizures impaired his memory.

Patient Five: Reticular Formation

A 25-year-old automobile salesperson was in a head-on car collision in which his forehead slammed against the dashboard. He was unconscious for a week. When he recovered, he had no memory of the accident and the events preceding it. According to his wife, he became a very different person after regaining consciousness. He lost energy and had no ambition. Physically, his actions were slow. With faulty reasoning, he could not think abstractly or make decisions. He also lost interest in grooming and hygiene.

Question: Can you explain the loss of consciousness, memory loss, and personality changes in this patient?

Discussion: The laceration and concussion of the prefrontal lobe account for his personality changes and cognitive deficits. The temporarily impaired functioning of the brainstem reticular formation was related to his loss of consciousness.

SUMMARY

The ANS, limbic lobe, hypothalamus, and reticular formation are four functionally integrated structures with nebulous anatomical borders. Working together, they influence the vital automatic and unconscious bodily functions that are indispensable for reproduction and survival. The system's interwoven cellular networks modulate visceral, somatic, autonomic, endocrine, alimentary, vascular, respiratory, and sexual behaviors. Each of these systems is represented by specialized overlapping cellular networks that extend throughout the septum, hypothalamus, and brainstem reticular formation. By using sympathetic and parasympathetic projections, the autonomic nervous system controls visceral functions, regulating body homeostasis and the functioning of the cardiovascular, pulmonary, digestive, urinary, and reproductive systems.

The integrated activity of the limbic system regulates the emotional and motivational aspects of behavior fundamental to survival, such as feeding, mating, aggression, and flight.

The hypothalamus, as the central regulator of the ANS and endocrine functions, controls visceral functions including vasodilation, body homeostasis, reproduction, hunger, and the intake of water and food. The neurosecretory cells of the hypothalamus regulate pituitary gland hormone production and endocrine body functions.

By integrating stimuli with internally generated thoughts, feelings, and emotions, the reticular formation regulates the homeostatic state of the brain essential for controlling sleep and vigilance. It also controls metabolic, respiratory, visceral, sensorimotor, neuroendocrine, emotional, and cognitive activities. A single lesion of the reticular system may generate complex illnesses characterized by various symptoms including insomnia, headaches, depression, tremors, aggression, and forgetfulness.

Technical Terms

acetylcholine	parasympathetic system
adenohypophysis	peristalsis
adipsia	polydipsia
akinesia	polyuria
α-rhythm	portal system
amnesia	postganglionic
amygdala	preganglion
anabolism	preoptic
aphagia	pterygopalatine ganglion
asphyxia	raphe nucleus
autonomic ganglia	serotonergic
catecholaminergic	subcallosal gyrus
cholinergic	supraoptic
cingulate gyrus	sympathetic
colic	tegmentum
diurnal	tremors
Edinger-Westphal nucleus	uncus
gonadotropic	vasodilation
hippocampus	vasopressin
insomnia	visceral
Klüver-Bucy syndrome	viscerosomatic
noradrenergic synapses	

Review Questions

1. Define the following terms:

adenohypophysis	amygdala
adipsia	anabolism
akinesia	aphagia
α-rhythm	asphyxia
amnesia	autonomic ganglia
catecholaminergic	postganglionic
cholinergic	preganglion
cingulate gyrus	preoptic
colic	pterygopalatine ganglion
diurnal	Purkinje cells
gonadotropic	raphe nucleus
hippocampus	serotonergic
infundibular portal circulation	subcallosal gyrus
insomnia	supraoptic
Klüver-Bucy syndrome	sympathetic
locus ceruleus	tegmentum
osmotic pressure	thyrotropin
parasympathetic system	uncus
peristalsis	vasodilation
polydipsia	vasopressin
polyuria	visceral
portal system	viscerosomatic

2. What are the two divisions of the ANS, and what functions do they serve?
3. Describe the role played by the preganglionic and postganglionic neurons in the autonomic innervation.
4. Describe how the sympathetic and parasympathetic systems differ in terms of the locations of their preganglionic nuclei.
5. Describe the antagonistic effects of the sympathetic and parasympathetic systems on the following structures:

Glands	Intestinal
Muscles	Gastric and sweat
Nasal	Smooth muscles of iris ciliary,
Lacrimal	bladder, lungs; cardiac muscles

6. Describe functions of the limbic system and name its major structures.
7. Describe how limbic projections to the cortex and brainstem participate in emotions.
8. What do we know about functions of the limbic structures, such as amygdala, hippocampus, and cingulate gyrus?
9. Describe the anatomy and functions of the hypothalamus.
10. Describe major afferents and efferents of the hypothalamus.
11. Discuss the hypothalamic mechanisms for regulating water intake, food intake, and body temperature.
12. Name the major hypothalamic hormones; discuss the functions of these hormones and describe the disorders associated with hormone disturbances.
13. Discuss the functions of the anterior (adenohypophysis) and posterior (neurohypophysis) pituitary gland.
14. Describe the major afferents and efferents of the reticular formation and discuss primary functions of the reticular formation.
15. Describe the reticular mechanism for regulating cortical arousal, cardiovascular activity, respiration, swallowing, vomiting, coughing, and biological rhythms.

Vascular System[a]

Learning Objectives

After studying this chapter, students should be able to do the following:

- Discuss the importance of blood circulation to the brain
- List the major arteries that transport blood to the cerebrum
- Describe the cortical region supplied by each major artery
- Discuss the blood supply for the brainstem, cerebellum, and spinal cord
- Explain common symptoms associated with involvement of major arteries
- List common points of anastomoses in the vascular system
- Explain the significance of potential collateral circulation
- Describe the venous–sinus system
- Discuss common types of cerebrovascular accidents
- Explain the physiology of cerebrovascular accidents
- Describe the mechanism regulating blood flow to the brain
- Discuss the nature of medical treatment for stroke
- Discuss the concept and clinical significance of the blood-brain barrier

Blood supplies brain cells with needed nutrition, such as glucose and oxygen. It also removes carbon dioxide from nerve cells. Nerve cells, which depend on an uninterrupted supply of oxygenated blood, cannot use any other source of energy, such as fat, nor have they the mechanism for storing glucose and oxygen. The brain's metabolic needs are disproportionate to its size. Although its mass comprises only 2% of body weight, it consumes approximately 20% of the total cardiac output and uses more than 20% of oxygen and metabolized glucose. Blood flow to the brain is approximately 50 mL/100 g tissue per minute; an average of 750 mL blood is pumped to the brain per minute. After

perfusion in the brain, the circulated blood is drained through the veins and sinuses back to the heart and pumped through the lungs for the reoxygenation of hemoglobins.

Without adequate blood supply, the brain can function for only a short time before irreversible damage to its cell bodies. The conventional understanding is that approximately 5 to 8 seconds of circulatory interruption to the brain may result in unconsciousness, and circulatory deprivation sustained for 20 to 25 seconds can eliminate the electrical activities in the affected brain cells. Vascular interruption for 4 to 6 minutes results in irreversible brain damage. This rule applies only to the cells in the center of the infarct, not to the ones that are at the periphery and are partially impaired. Knowledge of brain cell tolerance of oxygen deprivation emphasizes the importance of timing in providing cardiopulmonary resuscitation. Furthermore, the cells in the cerebral cortex are highly susceptible to oxygen deprivation, whereas cells in the brainstem and spinal cord can sustain oxygen deprivation for a longer period. This has important implications for the disorders of higher mental functions and sensorimotor systems.

VASCULAR NETWORK

Blood circulation to the brain depends on an elaborate network of arteries and veins. Arteries carry oxygenated blood away from the heart to the brain, and veins return the deoxygenated and circulated blood back to the heart.

Large arteries divide into arterioles, arteries smaller in diameter that deliver blood to capillaries, the terminal extensions of the arterial network. Unlike large arteries, capillaries do not permit rapid flow of blood. The primary function of the slow circulation of blood at

[a] Technical detail that appears in small type is necessary for completeness of information.

the capillary level is to exchange nutritive substances and waste products between the blood and brain cells. Capillaries also connect the arterioles with venules, the smaller extensions of the venous system.

Veins form the part of the vascular network responsible for draining circulated blood from brain tissues and transporting it back to the heart. Venules, the smallest extensions of the venous system, are deep in the cortical substance. They receive blood from the capillaries and transport it to larger veins on the cortical surface that in turn empty blood into the sinuses.

Veins are composed of essentially the same three coats, or tunics, of walls as arteries: the tunica interna, tunica media, and tunica externa. However, the walls of the veins are less thick than those of arteries. This difference is related to the thinner coat of tunica media and relative lack of smooth muscles in veins. Consequently, the average blood pressure in veins is considerably lower than arteries. This may also explain why more strokes involve arteries than veins.

Cerebrovascular Supply

The brain receives its blood supply from two arterial systems, the carotid and the vertebral basilar. These arterial systems (Fig. 17-1A) join at the circle of Willis

(Figs. 17-1B and 17-2) at the base of the brain. Cortical and subcortical (central) penetrating arteries that originate from the circle of Willis supply blood to the internal and external structures of the forebrain.

CAROTID SYSTEM

The carotid system begins with the common carotid artery, which ascends on each side of the neck. Posterior to the jaw, the common carotid artery divides into the external carotid and internal carotid (Fig. 17-1A). The external carotid artery and its branches supply blood to the facial muscles, forehead, and oral, nasal, and orbital cavities. The internal carotid artery, a major source of blood to the brain, enters the cranium through the carotid foramen in the petrous bone and curves forward and medially to enter the cavernous sinus. At that level, the anterior choroidal and ophthalmic branches arise from the internal carotid artery. The ophthalmic artery supplies blood to the eyeball and ocular muscles. Its branches connect with branches of the external cerebral artery and form the basis for a potential collateral circulation. The internal carotid artery emerges from the cavernous sinus, joins the circle of Willis, and divides to form two cortical arteries, the anterior cerebral (ACA) and the middle cerebral (MCA).

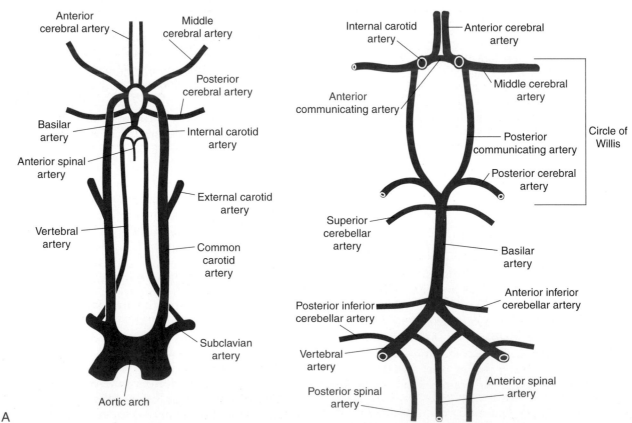

Figure 17-1. Vascular network to brain and arterial circle at base of brain. **A.** Carotid and vertebral basilar systems. **B.** Circle of Willis.

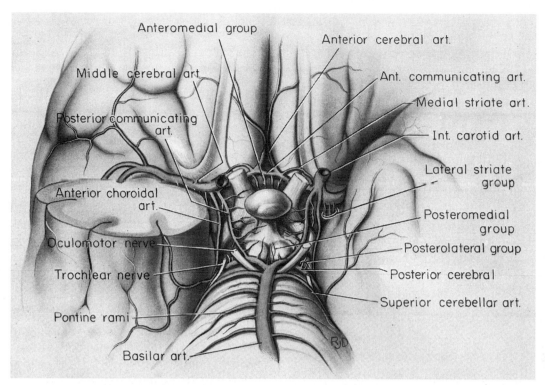

Figure 17-2. Cerebral arterial structure at base of brain depicting large and small arteries.

Table 17-1. Arteries of Brainstem, Cerebellum, and Spinal Cord

Structures	Arteries
Midbrain	Posterior cerebral artery
Pons	Basilar artery
	Anterior inferior cerebellar artery
Medulla	Posterior spinal artery
	Anterior spinal artery
	Basilar artery
Cerebellum	Posterior inferior cerebellar artery
	Anterior inferior cerebellar artery
	Superior cerebellar artery
Spinal cord	Posterior spinal artery (posterior third of cord)
	Anterior spinal artery (anterior two-thirds of cord)

Table 17-2. Signs of Vertebral Basilar Involvement

Area Supplied	Signs of Involvement
Vertebral Arteries	
Medulla (pyramid, medial lemniscus, cranial nerves IX–XII), cerebellum (posterior inferior cerebellar arteries), choroid plexus of 4th ventricle	Contralateral hemiplegia and discriminative touch loss, impaired pain and temperature sensation from ipsilateral face (trigeminal tract and nucleus) and from contralateral trunk and limb (lateral spinothalamic tract), ipsilateral ataxia (cerebellum), vertigo, nystagmus, vomiting (vestibular nucleus), dysphagia and dysarthria (paralysis of pharynx, palate and vocal folds and tongue; CN IX, X, and XII)
Basilar Artery	
Lateral pons, cerebellum (anterior inferior cerebellar and superior cerebellar artery), cranial nerves (V, VII, VIII)	Cranial nerve symptoms: deafness, vomiting, nystagmus, vertigo (CN VIII, nucleus), facial paralysis (CN VII, nucleus), loss of facial sensation (CN V, nucleus), hemiplegia (pyramidal tract), ataxia (cerebellum)

VERTEBRAL BASILAR SYSTEM

Two vertebral arteries arise from the subclavian arteries and ascend through the bony foramen of the upper cervical vertebrae. They enter the posterior cranial fossa of the skull through the foramen magnum and continue along the ventrolateral surface of the medulla oblongata. At the level of the caudal pons, both vertebral arteries merge to form a single basilar artery that courses upward along the pontine midline, eventually joining the circle of Willis (Figs. 17-1 and 17-2).

Before terminating in the circle of Willis, the vertebral basilar arteries give rise to numerous small branches that supply blood to the spinal cord, medulla, pons, midbrain, and cerebellum (Tables 17-1 and 17-2). Each vertebral artery gives rise to three major arteries: the posterior spinal, anterior spinal, and posterior inferior cerebellar (Figs. 17-1 and 17-2). Some of the branches of the descending posterior spinal artery also supply the dorsal medulla, while the remaining travel caudally to supply the dorsal third of the spinal cord. The dorsal medullary column, relay nuclei (nucleus gracilis and nucleus cuneatus), and dorsal spinal column fibers receive projections from the spinal dorsal lemniscal system. Consequently, circulatory disorders in the posterior spinal artery cause medullary symptoms and a loss of epicritic sensation in half of the body.

The anterior spinal artery from each vertebral artery merges and descends along the midline. Some of its branches supply the lower median medulla, which contains the pyramidal fibers, pyramidal decussation, and medial lemniscus fibers. The remaining branches supply the ventral two-thirds of the spinal cord. Interruption of the vascular flow of the anterior spinal artery affects sensory and motor fibers and causes hemiplegia and epicritic and protopathic hemisensory loss. Occlusion of the anterior spinal artery branches that supply the medulla results in alternating hemiplegia, which is associated with ipsilateral paralysis of the face and tongue and contralateral paralysis of the extremities. In alternating hemiplegia the lesion is above the pyramidal decussation in the medulla. This syndrome is discussed in detail in Chapter 14.

Each posteroinferior cerebellar artery supplies the ipsilateral posteroinferior cerebellum, which plays a significant role in the coordination of rapid movements. Immediately after its formation, the basilar artery gives rise to anteroinferior cerebellar arteries, which proceed downward and laterally to serve the anterior and lateral surfaces of the cerebellum. At the pontine level, the basilar artery gives rise to many rami bilaterally that supply the pontine structures (Fig. 17-2). One of the most important basilar branches is the internal auditory artery. This branch delivers blood to the cochlea and the vestibular apparatus in the inner ear. Immediately before the basilar artery joins the circle of Willis and forms the posterior cerebral artery (PCA), it gives rise to the superior cerebellar arteries at the level of the midbrain. These arteries supply the anterior and dorsal surfaces of the cerebellum, and their branches anastomose (open one structure into another by connecting blood vessels) with the other cerebellar arteries. Pathology implicating the cerebellar arteries may result in motor incoordination, impaired balance, and dysarthric speech.

Circle of Willis

The wreath-shaped circle of Willis is at the ventral surface of the brain, and it connects the carotid arterial system with the vertebrobasilar system (Figs. 17-1B and 17-2). The circle of Willis consists of the anterior and posterior communicating arteries and the proximal portions of the anterior, middle, and posterior cerebral arteries. The ACAs are rostrally interconnected via the anterior communicating artery. The posterior communicating arteries connect the internal carotid arteries with the basilar artery. The circle of Willis is an important anastomotic point that serves to equalize the vascular blood

Table 17-3. Vascular Supply to Brain Surface and Lobes

Brain Area	Artery
Frontal lobe	
Lateral surface	Middle cerebral artery
Medial surface	Anterior cerebral artery
Inferior surface	Middle and anterior cerebral arteries
Parietal lobe	
Lateral surface	Middle cerebral artery
Medial surface	Anterior cerebral artery
Occipital lobe	
Lateral and medial surfaces	Posterior cerebral artery
Temporal lobe	
Lateral surface	Middle cerebral artery
Medial surface	Jointly by middle cerebral, posterior cerebral, posterior communicating, and anterior choroidal arteries
Inferior surface	Posterior cerebral artery

supply to both sides of the brain. However, because of usual pressure equalization in both arterial systems, very little blood normally flows through the communicating arteries to the left and right sides of the circle.

Two types of arteries, cortical and central, arise from the circle of Willis. The cortical (circumferential) branches are large arteries that primarily supply the external brain structures (Table 17-3) and give rise to branches to anastomose with other cortical arteries. The central (penetrating) branches are small arteries that penetrate the ventral surface of the brain to supply internal brain structures.

CORTICAL ARTERIES

Anterior Cerebral Artery

After arising from the bifurcation of the internal cerebral artery at the circle of Willis, the ACA travels rostrally in the interhemispheric fissure along the midsagittal surface of the brain. It follows the genu of the corpus callosum and continues posteriorly along the dorsal surface of the corpus callosum (Fig. 17-3). Its branches are the orbital, frontopolar, callosomarginal, and pericallosal arteries, which supply the orbital and medial cortical surfaces of the frontal and parietal lobes. In the posterior medial cortical area, the branches of the ACA anastomose with branches of the PCA. Many terminal branches of the ACA cross over to the lateral cortical surface and develop anastomosing continuity with the branches of the MCA in the watershed region, where the distribution of major cerebral arteries overlaps.

The interruption of blood circulation in the ACA usually results in paralysis of the legs and feet because of decreased blood supply to the midsagittal extension of the motor cortex (Figs. 2-6 and 14-1; Table 17-4). The vascular impairments of this artery may also lead to many prefrontal lobe symptoms, which include disor-

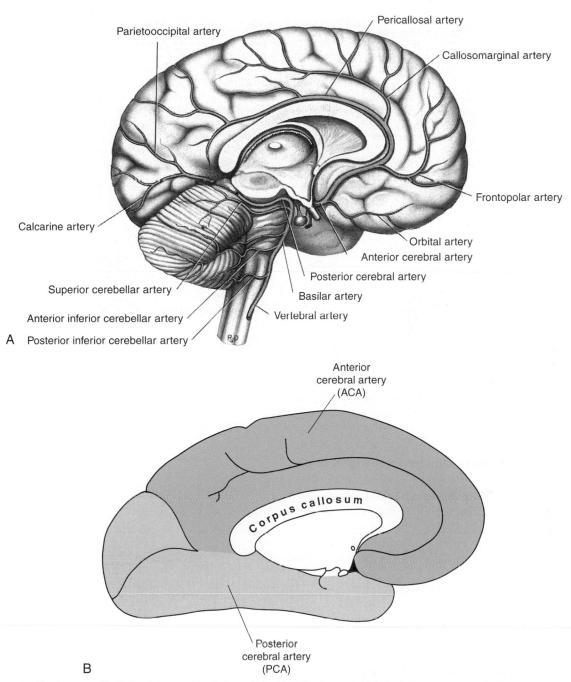

Figure 17-3. **A.** Anterior and posterior cerebral arteries together with cerebellar and brainstem arteries on midsagittal brain surface. **B.** Diagram of the midsagittal territory covered by the anterior cerebral and posterior cerebral arteries.

ders of thinking, reasoning, abstracting, self-monitoring, and planning. Additional impairments include decreased spontancity, motor inaction, impaired judgment, and limited concentration.

Middle Cerebral Artery

The MCA, the largest of the cortical arteries, is the direct continuation of the internal carotid artery. After leaving the circle of Willis, it runs laterally and emerges through the sylvian fissure on the lateral brain surface.

On the lateral surface, it divides into the temporal (anterior and posterior), frontal (rolandic and prerolandic), and parietal (anterior, posterior, and angular) artery branches (Fig. 17-4, *A* and *B*). The MCA branches supply blood to the entire lateral surface of the brain, including the site of speech, language, and a large part of sensorimotor areas. The important areas are the somatosensory cortex in the postcentral gyrus, motor cortex in the precentral gyrus, Broca's area in the premotor region, frontal cortex, primary auditory cortex in the transverse

Table 17-4. Signs of Involvement of Cortical Arteries

Area Supplied	Signs of Involvement
Anterior Cerebral Artery	
Medial aspect of frontal lobe and anterior 80% of corpus callosum; partial supply to basal ganglia (caudate head and putamen)	Paralysis of opposite leg and foot, sensory loss of foot and leg, mental impairments (lack of spontaneity, easy distraction, reduced abstraction, indecisiveness)
Middle Cerebral Artery	
Entire lateral surface of cerebral hemisphere (including sensorimotor area, premotor area, language cortex, and associational cortex), inferior frontal lobe, basal ganglia (body and head of caudate, lateral globus pallidus, putamen), internal capsule	Contralateral hemiplegia with spared leg, foot (precentral gyrus), contralateral hemianesthesia (postcentral gyrus), homonymous hemianopsia (visual radiations fibers in parietal and temporal lobes), aphasia (dominant hemisphere), constructional apraxia (nondominant hemisphere), cognitive impairments (prefrontal lobe). Hemiplegia, hemianesthesia without aphasia from involvement of lateral striate arteries (internal capsule).
Posterior Cerebral Artery	
Medial surface of occipital lobe; inferior surface of occipital, temporal lobes	Contralateral homonymous hemianopsia (calcarine branch), low pain threshold (thalamic syndrome), upper midbrain symptoms (coma), hemiballism (involvement of the subthalamus)

Heschl's gyrus on the superior surface of the first temporal gyrus, Wernicke's area in the superior posterior temporal lobe, and angular and supramarginal gyri in the inferior parietal lobe (Fig. 17-4).

While passing through the lateral sulcus, the MCA emits lateral and medial lenticulostriate branches that supply the basal ganglia and diencephalon (Fig. 17-5). The medial lenticulostriate artery supplies blood to the globus pallidus, the posterior internal capsule, and the medial ventral area of thalamus. The lateral lenticulostriate artery supplies the entire pulvinar and caudate nucleus except for its anterior portion, which is served by the ACA.

Impaired vascular circulation of the MCA results in contralateral hemiplegia (motor disorder) and impaired sensory functions that include discriminative and diffuse touch, position sense, and pain and temperature (Table 17-4). Other symptoms are aphasia, constructional apraxia, temporospatial deficits, homonymous hemianopia, and reading and writing deficits. Lenticulostriate artery damage results in involuntary motor movements and sensorimotor symptoms.

Posterior Cerebral Artery

The basilar artery bifurcates to form two posterior cerebral arteries. Each of these arteries receives a potential anastomotic flow from the posterior communicating artery, and each curves laterally and caudally along the inferior brain surface, where it supplies blood to the anterior and inferior temporal lobe, the uncus, the inferior temporal gyri, and the inferior and medial occipital lobe, including the primary visual cortex in the calcarine region. The end branches of the artery also cross over to the lateral surface and anastomose in the watershed region with the terminal branches of the MCA.

Occlusion of the PCA results in homonymous hemianopsia. Occlusion of the basilar artery, which provides blood to both posterior cerebral arteries, can result in total blindness and numerous pontine and cerebellar symptoms (Table 17-4).

CENTRAL ARTERIES

The central arteries are the branches that arise either from the proximal portions of the cortical arteries or from the circle of Willis and penetrate the inferior surface of the brain (Fig. 17-2). These supply blood to the subcortical structures: the thalamus, hypothalamus, caudate nucleus, putamen, globus pallidus, basal ganglia, internal capsule, choroid plexus, and others (Table 17-5). One important aspect of the circulation by central arteries is the marked overlapping of blood supply as the branches distribute to the subcortical areas. The overlapping blood supply facilitates the development of anastomotic channels in response to occlusive or ischemic vascular problems. Important central arteries are the anteromedial, medial striate, anterior choroidal, posterior choroidal, posteromedial, and posterolateral (Fig. 17-2).

The anteromedial arteries arise from the anterior communicating and anterior cerebral arteries and penetrate the anterior perforated area to supply the hypothalamus and suprachiasmatic regions of the brain. Involvement of these arterial twigs results in disorders of the autonomic nervous system (ANS) and hypothalamus. The medial striate arteries arise from the ACA and supply blood to parts of the caudate nucleus, putamen, and anterior limb of the internal capsule. The lenticulostriate branches of the MCA supply the remaining parts of the caudate nucleus and putamen. Circulatory disturbances in these arteries result in motor movement disorders.

The anterior choroidal artery supplies blood to the choroid plexus, hippocampus, portions of the globus pallidus, posterior internal capsule, putamen, tail of the caudate nucleus, and lateral geniculate body. Signs of its occlusion consist of contralateral hemiplegia, hemianesthesia, involuntary movements, and memory disturbances. Circulatory involvement of the hippocampus results in memory impairment.

The posterior choroidal artery (not shown) originates from the PCA and supplies blood to the choroid plexus of the third ventricle, tectum, and pineal gland. The posteromedial arteries supply blood to parts of the thalamus, red nucleus, substantia nigra, medial portion

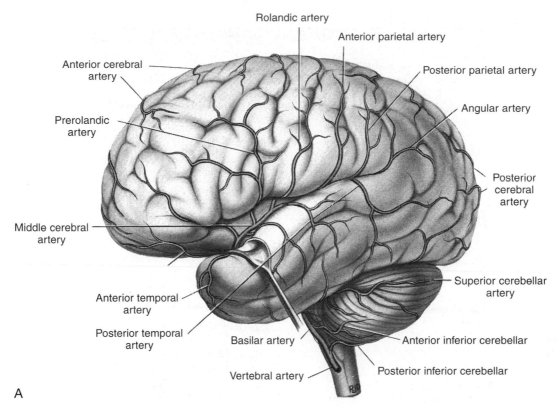

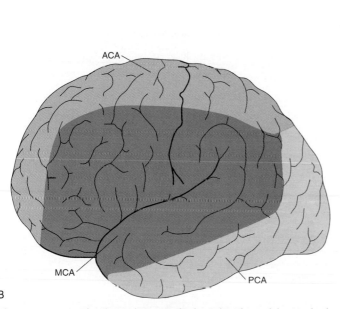

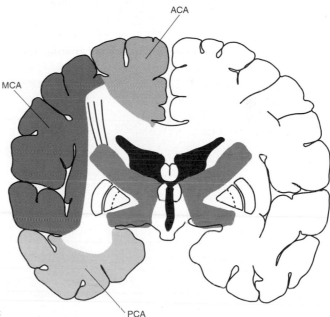

Figure 17-4. **A.** Blood circulation to the lateral surface of the cerebral hemisphere and cerebellum. **B.** Diagram of the lateral cortical surface marking the territories of three cortical arteries. **C.** Coronal illustration of the territories of three cortical arteries. ACA, anterior cerebral artery; MCA, middle cerebral artery; PCA, posterior cerebral artery.

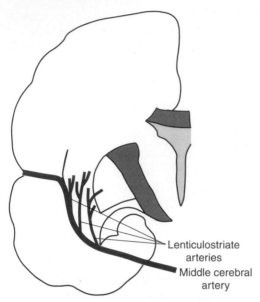

Figure 17-5. Lenticulostriate arteries.

Table 17-5. Vascular Supply to Subcortical Structures

Structure	Artery
Thalamus	Posteromedial, posterolateral, choroidal
Hypothalamus	Anteromedial and posteromedial
Caudate nucleus	Anterolateral, medial striate, and lenticulostriate
Putamen	Lenticulostriate, medial striate, anterior choroidal
Globus pallidus	Anterior choroidal
Subthalamus	Posteromedial
Red nucleus and substantia nigra	Posteromedial

of the cerebral peduncle, subthalamic nucleus, midbrain reticular formation, and superior cerebellar peduncle. Occlusion of these arteries results in multiple problems. Damage to the red nucleus leads to contralateral ataxia; damage to the substantial nigra leads to involuntary movements; damage to the subthalamic nucleus leads to hemiballism, and most important, damage to the midbrain reticular formation results in a coma.

The posterolateral arteries penetrate the inferior surface of the brain to supply blood to the parts of the lateral thalamus and the posterior pulvinar. Occlusion of this artery results in somatosensory disturbances in the opposite half of the body. Threshold to various sensory stimuli is lowered, resulting in intense pain from stimuli that would usually not be painful.

Blood Supply to Spinal Cord

Blood is supplied to the spinal cord by two major longitudinal arteries, the anterior and posterior spinal arteries, both of which originate from the vertebral arteries (Figs. 7-1 and 17-6). The anterior spinal artery from each vertebral artery joins to form a single descending artery along the midline, giving rise to branches on the left and right to serve the anterior two-thirds of the spinal cord, which contain sensorimotor fibers and motor neurons. Interruption in the vascular flow of the anterior spinal artery affects sensory and motor fibers and causes hemiplegia and protopathic hemisensory loss.

The posterior spinal arteries descend on the dorsal surface of the cord and supply the dorsal spinal area (Fig. 17-6), which contains the dorsal lemniscal fibers and dorsal gray column. Circulatory disorders in the posterior spinal artery result in a loss of epicritic sensation.

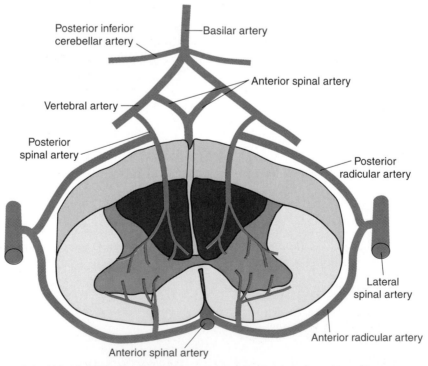

Figure 17-6. Spinal blood distribution through posterior and anterior spinal arteries and its augmentation by the radiculospinal arteries.

The vascular supply to the spinal cord is further augmented by the segmental radicular arteries; these arteries descend from the aorta and enter the spinal column through the intervertebral foramina along with the spinal nerves. Each of the radicular of spinal arteries supplies blood to about six spinal segments, except the great radicular artery of Adamkiewicz. At the lower thoracic and upper lumbar level, one of the radicular arteries enlarges to form the artery of Adamkiewicz; this supplies most of the caudal third of the cord. A clinical implication of the enlarged vessel is that this artery should not be compromised because of its importance.

Collateral Circulation

Collateral circulation refers to the alternative supply to a given structure after it has lost its primary arterial blood supply. Collateral circulation is important in the natural recovery process of damaged brain structures. There are many potential channels for alternative blood circulation; however, not all are effective. The variability in arterial anatomy and the degree of vascular pathology are two factors that contribute to the development of collateral circulation. In general, better collateral circulation develops if an artery is blocked near the main arterial trunk or major branches. Obstruction of the terminal arteries or capillaries after they have penetrated deep into the brain reduces the capabilities of developing collateral circulation. The arterial system from one hemisphere can never adequately perfuse the other hemisphere. A gradually developing arterial insufficiency facilitates the maximum development of compensatory circulation. A sudden arterial occlusion, as in stroke, usually does not lead to the development of a substantial source of alternate circulation.

There are four common points of collateral circulation within one hemisphere or across both. First, the anterior communicating artery connects the two anterior cerebral arteries. Second, the vertebral basilar system feeds through the posterior communicating artery if the internal carotid artery blood flow is insufficient. Similarly, the posterior communicating arteries may feed into the posterior cerebral arteries if the vertebral basilar arterial system is occluded. Third, although infrequent, thromboembolic involvement of the internal carotid artery can trigger retrograde blood flow from the external carotid artery through the ophthalmic artery branches in the eye. Fourth, the terminal branches of all three cortical (anterior, middle, and posterior cerebral) arteries may anastomose in the watershed zone on the lateral brain surface, which is highly probable in the case of reduced blood volume through any one of the three cortical arteries. The watershed area constitutes the terminal distribution of blood supply to a given area in relation to its source.

Vascular Pathology

Vascular diseases of the brain are the most frequent causes of neurological deficits and in the United States are ranked as the third most common cause of death after cancer and heart disease. Vascular interruption deprives the brain tissues of life-sustaining oxygen. Without oxygen, the brain cells die (infarction).

Strokes, or cerebrovascular accidents, are characterized by sudden development of focal neurological deficits, which fall into three common types: occlusive vascular pathology (thrombosis or embolism), hemorrhage (bleeding from ruptured vessels), and arteriovenous malformations (Table 17-6).

OCCLUSIVE VASCULAR PATHOLOGY

Atherosclerosis, which consists of hardened arterial walls, is the primary cause of local arterial occlusion. Atherosclerosis is a slow process in which various lipids, blood platelets, calcium deposits, fatty particles, and other undissolved substances in the blood gradually accumulate along the inner walls of blood vessels and cause narrowing of the arterial lumen. An atheroma takes years to form. The adherence of lipids and platelets usually occurs at an ulcerated or injured site, commonly a point of bifurcation. Increased blood coagulability can contribute to an occlusive disease. Since a narrowed or blocked arterial lumen (channel) decreases or stops blood flow, the brain

Table 17-6. Principal Types of Stroke

Type	Location	Time of Occurrence	Warning Signs
Thrombosis	Occlusion at atherosclerotic lesion	During sleep, periods of low physical activity	TIAs, headaches, seizures
Embolism	Occlusion of smaller artery by displaced clot moving peripherally	When awake and active	None; possible headaches, seizures
Hemorrhage	Rupture of arterial wall or aneurysm	Anytime, usually during awake hours	None
Arteriovenous malformations	Twisted arteriovenous malformation	Anytime, usually during awake hours	Recurrent headaches

suffers from ischemia (insufficient blood supply). A transient ischemic attack (TIA) is a temporary interruption of blood circulation to the brain. This is caused by various mechanisms that interfere with blood supply to the brain, such as occlusive carotid disease, emboli from heart, and infrequently spasms of arterial muscles. The exact symptoms depend on the brain area affected. A patient with TIA may have several of the following symptoms: focal weakness, double vision, headache, paresthesia, hemianesthesia, dysarthria, and dizziness. These may last from a few minutes to several hours. A TIA rarely lasts more than 24 hours, though it may cause brain damage. The transient symptoms of a TIA are clinically significant, since their presence indicates that a larger stroke may be in progress. Administration of blood-thinning medication at this stage may prevent a major cerebrovascular accident. In arteriosclerosis, the heart initially compensates for the reduced blood flow by pumping blood with greater force. However, this compensation may lead to high blood pressure (hypertension). Once the atherosclerotic process has begun (Fig. 17-7A), it interrupts the blood supply by forming either an embolism (Fig. 17-7B) or a thrombosis (Fig. 17-7C).

Embolism is blockage in a distal artery with a narrow lumen. An embolus is a clot that breaks free from a thrombosis and enters the bloodstream, eventually blocking a small end artery. Cerebral emboli produce rapid development of neurological signs that usually do not progress. Embolic strokes usually occur during a period of activity and often affect young people.

Thrombosis is a local buildup of fatty substances and blood platelets in a cerebral vessel that is caused by an atherosclerotic plaque; the buildup mostly occurs at sites of arterial bifurcation or at sites subjected to injury and inflammation. The presence of plaque causes the degeneration of the vessel wall, and damage to the endothelial layer attracts fibrin and blood platelets to the site. The thrombosis grows slowly; it can take several years before the arterial lumen closes. Thrombosis becomes symptomatic only in the mid and late years (Fig. 17-7). By then, the arterial lumen is mostly blocked. Most thrombotic strokes occur during sleep or a period of inactivity. Patients, unaware of their deficits, awaken to find themselves paralyzed. The reason a thrombotic stroke tends to occur during sleep is that the lower blood pressure during inactivity allows vessels to narrow or close. The warning signs of a thrombotic stroke include TIA (occurring in 40–60% of patients).

HEMORRHAGE

Hemorrhagic strokes are associated with sudden onset of neurological symptoms and may cause coma and stupor that may progress with time. Hemorrhagic strokes result from bleeding of ruptured blood vessels. They occur when a weakened arterial wall ruptures un-

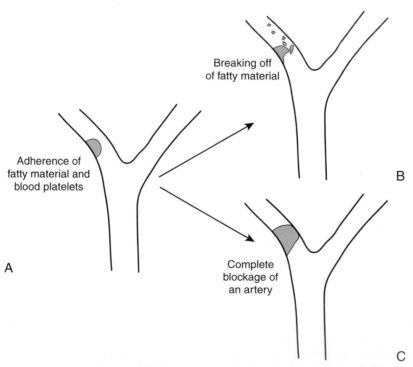

Figure 17-7. Thromboembolism. **A.** Thromboembolism forms in vascular system. **B.** Embolus is a detached part of thrombosis, which occludes a smaller vessel at a distance from the original site. **C.** Thrombosis completely blocks a blood vessel by local accumulation of undissolved substances, including globules of fat, clumps of bacteria, and blood platelets.

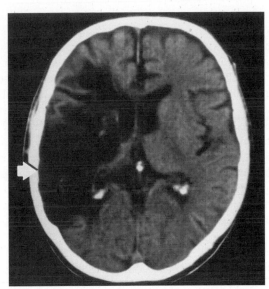

Figure 17-8. Large right middle cerebral artery infarct (*arrow*) on an axial CT image.

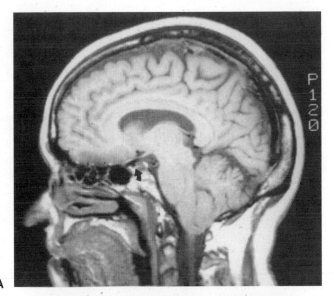

A

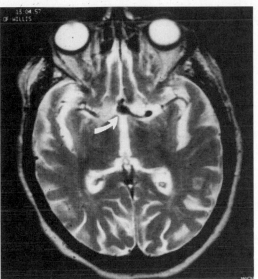

B

Figure 17-9. **A.** Sagittal T1-weighted MRI of aneurysm (*curved arrow*) of the internal carotid artery. **B.** T2-weighted axial MRI of an anterior communicating artery aneurysm (*curved arrow*).

der the pressure of constant blood flow. Hemorrhages can occur anywhere in the arterial system; however, the lenticulostriate arteries that supply the thalamus and basal ganglia are the most common sites. The major types of hemorrhagic strokes are lacunar strokes, intracerebral hemorrhage, subdural hematoma, and subarachnoid hemorrhage.

Lacunar strokes involve small arteries of the basal ganglia and thalamus. They occur abruptly or in spurts over days. They are commonly found in individuals with idiopathic hypertension. Intracerebral hemorrhages are space-occupying lesions involving the rupturing of an intracranial artery. Blood released from the ruptured artery, if not surgically drained, accumulates to form a hematoma, which encroaches on vital cortical centers. Intracerebral hemorrhages usually occur during an active or awake state. The full extent of deficit is seldom present at the outset but develops over several hours.

In subdural hematoma, which can result from a traumatic injury, a blood vessel ruptures in the arachnoid tissue beneath the dura mater. The accumulated blood, if not surgically drained, will expand and compress the soft underlying brain tissues, causing irreversible brain damage. Another potential site for hemorrhage is the subarachnoid space, which usually develops after physical exertion. It is often accompanied by a headache and stiff neck. Subarachnoid hemorrhage is commonly seen with bleeding of an arteriovenous malformation (AVM) or aneurysm.

Aneurysm, a vascular condition associated with hemorrhage, is a local balloonlike dilation of an artery (Fig. 17-9). It usually occurs at points of bifurcation of major cerebral arteries. The outpouchings of an aneurysm are due to either weakness in the vessel wall or congenital arterial defect. An aneurysm causes neu-

rological symptoms in two ways: (*a*) the mass effect of arterial dilation can compress the surrounding structures; (*b*) the aneurysm can no longer withstand the blood flow pressure, and it ruptures, releasing blood into the brain or onto its surface.

ARTERIOVENOUS MALFORMATIONS

Arteriovenous malformations are congenital conditions in which tangled dilated arteries and veins become connected in a local area (Fig. 17-10). With age, they may become large and are susceptible to hemorrhage because of their thin walls. These malformations often cause seizures and recurrent headaches (mimicking migraines). Depending on the location of the malformations, they can also cause language impairments,

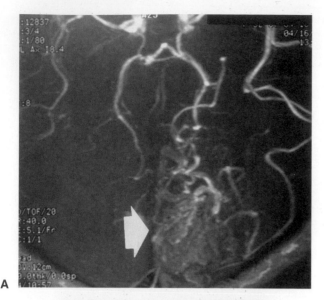

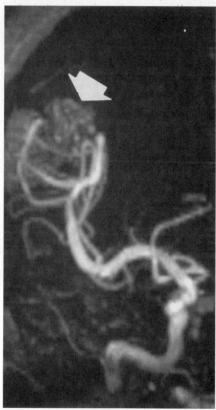

Figure 17-10. **A.** Axial MRI of a left occipital AVM (*arrow*) in the branches of the left PCA. **B.** Reconstructed MRI of the right cerebral artery AVM.

motor speech problems, visual disorders, sensory loss, and hemiplegia.

SELECTIVE VULNERABILITY TO ANOXIA

Since the brain receives its energy supply entirely from the oxidative metabolism of glucose supplied by the blood, a reduction in the vascular supply in stroke results in sudden onset of neurological symptoms because of anoxia in the brain cells. However, the nerve cells in various regions of the brain are differentially vulnerable to anoxia. The general rule seems to be that the brain cells that are inherently active at all times because of constant sensory input are the most susceptible to anoxia. This perhaps accounts for the high vulnerability of the cerebral cortex, cerebellum (Purkinje cells), and the cells of the hippocampus. The constant state of inherent sensorimotor activity also makes the parietal, frontal, and occipital lobes, along with the anterior and dorsomedial thalamus, highly susceptible to anoxia.

RISK FACTORS

Hypertension, heart disease, diabetes mellitus, high cholesterol, and smoking are the most common risk factors for a stroke. Untreated hypertension can damage the arterial walls so that they become sites of atherosclerotic plaques. High blood pressure is the single most common risk factor for strokes, and controlling hypertension contributes to a significant decline in the incidence of stroke.

Heart disease is another frequent cause of the embolic stroke, as clots leaving the heart can block brain arteries. People with coronary heart disease (heart attack and chest pain) are at twice as much risk of having a stroke as the general population. Diabetic mellitus, another cause of stroke, is known to accelerate the development of atherosclerosis. Also, high cholesterol levels cause buildups on arterial walls, narrowing their passageways and leading to heart attack and stroke. Smokers are also known to be highly susceptible to coronary artery disease.

VENOUS SINUS SYSTEM

Veins and sinuses collect deoxygenated blood and transport it back to the heart and lungs for reoxygenation. Drainage of the blood first begins at the capillary level, where the intraparenchymal capillaries unite to form small veins that are called venules. Venules collect the blood from capillaries and transfer it to the network of large veins. Veins drain the surface and deep brain structures and empty blood into the sinuses. The sinuses, which consist of large spaces between the periosteal and meningeal layers of dura mater, are in the cranium (Fig. 2-43).

Dural Sinuses

The dural sinuses form a network of cavities in and around the brain (Figs. 2-43 and 17-11). The superior sagittal sinus runs along the dorsomedial line on the vertex in the falx cerebri, receiving blood from the superior cerebral veins and cerebrospinal fluid drained through the arachnoid villi. The inferior sagittal sinus

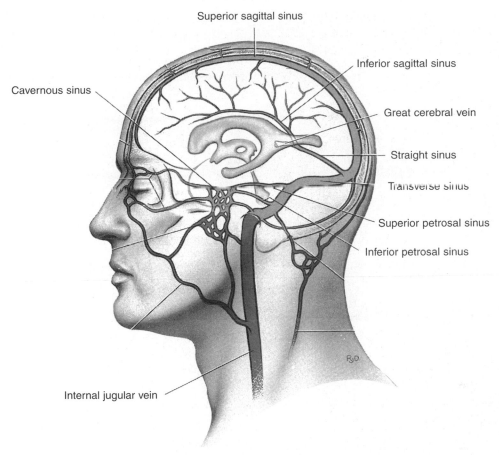

Superior sagittal sinus

Inferior sagittal sinus

Cavernous sinus

Great cerebral vein

Straight sinus

Transverse sinus

Superior petrosal sinus

Inferior petrosal sinus

Internal jugular vein

Figure 17-11.   Dural venous sinuses and their major connections.

runs in the inferior margin of the falx cerebri over the dorsal edge of the corpus callosum. Posteriorly, it joins the straight (rectus) sinus, which runs posteriorly and empties into the sinus confluence. The paired transverse sinuses arise from the confluence of sinuses, which course laterally, rostrally, then down and forward to form the internal jugular vein. The cavernous sinus, a large irregular network of smaller veins, lies around the pituitary gland. The cavernous sinus drains into the transverse sinuses through the petrosal sinuses. The sinuses siphon off all of the collected blood and shunt the cerebrovascular fluid to the internal jugular veins, through which it returns to the heart.

Cerebral Veins

Veins collect the circulating blood from the cortical and subcortical areas and empty it into the sinus network. There are two types of cerebral veins, superficial and deep. The superficial cerebral veins collect circulated blood from the neocortex and subcortical white matter and drain it into the superior sagittal sinus (Fig. 17-12). The large superficial veins include the superior, inferior, and superficial middle cerebral veins. The superior cerebral veins collect blood from the middle surface and the vertex and drain into the superior sagit-

tal sinus. The inferior cerebral veins drain the basal surface of the brain and empty blood into the cavernous, petrosal, and transverse sinuses. The superficial middle cerebral veins collect blood from the lateral brain surface and drain it into the cavernous sinus.

The deep cerebral veins include numerous smaller veins, such as the internal cerebral, basal, choroidal, and thalamostriate. They all drain blood from the subcortical structures, including the striatum, thalamus, choroid plexus, and hippocampus, and empty into the great cerebral vein of Galen. The great vein opens to the straight sinus.

Veins of the Spinal Cord

The venous drainage system of the spinal cord is similar to the arterial network. The anterior and posterior spinal veins are joined by the anterior radicular veins. The spinal venous system also communicates with internal and external venous plexuses adjacent to the spinal dural sac and the vertebral column.

REGULATION OF CEREBRAL BLOOD FLOW

The vascular circulatory system is a closed system in which the movement of blood requires constant pres-

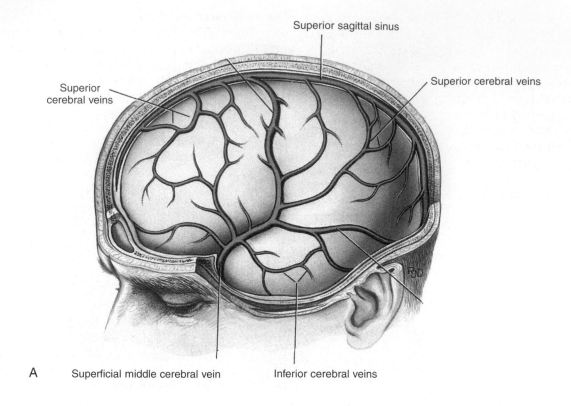

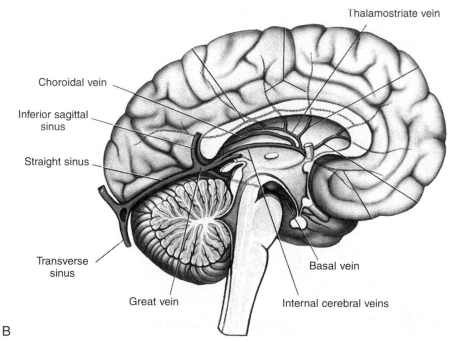

Figure 17-12. Superficial and deep veins. **A.** Large veins on the lateral surface include branches of superior cerebral and inferior cerebral veins and superficial middle cerebral veins. **B.** Midsagittal view of internal cerebral veins.

sure. To a large extent, arterial response and regulation of blood flow are automatically adjusted. The internal arterial response and the brain's metabolic needs are also important in the regulation of blood flow. Contraction and expansion of arterial walls, made possible by their elasticity, contributes to the maintenance of constant blood flow. With increasing age, however, the arteries lose this elasticity because of hardening of their walls (arteriosclerosis). When this happens, blood can flow though arteries only in spurts, causing an increase in internal blood pressure. The arteries also respond to metabolic states in brain tissues. Increased carbon dioxide content in the brain dilates arterial walls, allowing greater blood flow to the brain. On the other hand, increased oxygen constricts the arterial walls, decreasing the blood flow. The arteries respond to the volume of blood by altering their resistance to blood flow from the heart. They respond by dilating if the volume of blood pumped through the artery is reduced. When the volume increases, arteries constrict.

TREATMENT OF VASCULAR DISEASES

The goal of medical management of a stroke patient is to restore normal blood circulation and to contain the size of the infarction. Treatment may include medication and/or surgical intervention. The exact treatment depends on the location in the brain and whether the disease is occlusive or hemorrhagic. In thromboembolic processes, anticoagulant drugs, such as heparin or warfarin (Coumadin) are found to reduce stroke by preventing further embolization.

Platelet-inhibiting drugs, such as acetylsalicylic acid (aspirin), dipyridamole (Persantine), clopidogrel bisulfate (Plavix) and ticlopidine (Ticlid) have been successfully used to reduce the risk of recurrent TIAs. Cerebral vasodilating drugs, such as papaverine, when used on patients with thromboembolic strokes, have had limited success. The discovery of thrombolytic agents such as tissue plasminogen activating agents (TPA) are very effective in restoring blood flow by dissolving the clot. However, the TPA treatment is effective only if it is administered within 3 hours of the onset of a stroke. A common problem in the use of TPA drugs is that they are associated with an increased risk of cerebral hemorrhage. Another treatment of patients with atherosclerosis is surgical removal of the plaque (endarterectomy). This procedure is highly favorable for patients with 77 to 99% stenosis of one or both carotid arteries. In case of a hemorrhagic condition, medically optimal treatment is the reduction of elevated blood pressure.

Medical management of an aneurysm entails reducing blood pressure to prevent bleeding; clipping is surgically used to obliterate the neck of the aneurysm, thus disabling it. Aneurysms are also treated without opening the skull through coiling, which involves placing a platinum coil in the aneurysm. This coil causes a blood clot to form, sealing off the aneurysm.

BLOOD-BRAIN BARRIER

The blood-brain barrier (blood-cerebrospinal barrier) is an important clinical concept. It restricts movement of specific substances, such as infectious microorganisms, from the bloodstream to the brain tissue and extracellular fluid, which is similar to the cerebrospinal fluid. The blood-brain barrier applies only to the central nervous system (CNS) because in brain capillaries, unlike the muscle capillaries, endothelial cells form a continuous interior lining membrane. These cellular elements are tightly joined, and there are no adjacent intracellular pores or fenestrations. The endothelial cell membrane in the CNS is further surrounded by the end feet of astrocytes outside the capillary wall (Fig. 17-13). Both of these add to the selective membrane permeability, restricting the flow of certain substances in the blood to the extracellular space and restricting flow from the choroidal capillaries to the cerebrospinal fluid. Information regarding which substances cross the blood-brain barrier is important in the administration of medicine. Although it keeps harmful microorganisms out of the brain, the blood-brain barrier also keeps many helpful antibodies out, making it difficult to treat many cerebral infections.

Some disease states in the brain disrupt the blood-brain barrier by enabling some normally excluded substances to enter into the cerebrospinal and cellular interstitial fluids. Meningitis and brain tumors are two conditions that alter the blood-brain barrier and allow toxic substances to enter the brain. In brain tumors, new proliferating capillaries are known to have intracellular pores, which affect the capillary permeability. This has some diagnostic significance, because radioactive amino acid can exit through pores into the brain, allowing localization of the tumor.

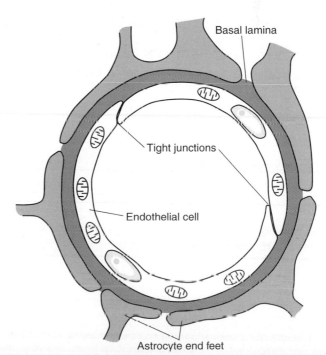

Figure 17-13. Structural properties that contribute to the blood-brain barrier.

LESION LOCALIZATION

Rule 10: Vascular System Disorder

PRESENTING SYMPTOMS (A)

Sudden development of contralateral hemiplegia of the lower face, arm, and upper extremity more than the leg with accompanying sensory loss results from occlusion of the MCA, which may be caused by either thrombosis or embolism. The symptoms discussed under rule 1 (see Chapter 2) may also appear. An abrupt onset of symptoms usually indicates vascular pathology, while gradual progression of symptoms indicates a mass lesion.

RATIONALE

The regions of the motor cortex involved with the representation of different body parts are served by two arteries, the MCA and ACA. The MCA supplies the area of motor control for the face, hand, and upper extremity, while the ACA serves the motor area for the leg (Figs. 14-1 and 17-4).

Involvement of the somatomotor cortex and corticospinal fibers accounts for the contralateral paralysis of the upper face, trunk, and upper extremity. Involvement of somatosensory cortex and thalamocortical fibers results in hemianesthesia for the trunk, face, and upper extremity.

PRESENTING SYMPTOMS (B)

Toe, foot, and leg paralysis, sensory loss, and mental impairments (distractibility, indecisiveness, and lack of spontaneity) are associated with ischemia due to embolism or thrombosis in the ACA distribution.

RATIONALE

The ACA supplies the medial frontal cortex, which serves higher mental functions and motor control for the leg (Figs. 14-1, 17-3, and 17-4).

PRESENTING SYMPTOMS (C)

Homonymous hemianopsia is associated with PCA involvement. Low pain threshold is also seen because of the thalamic involvement.

RATIONALE

The PCA supplies the visual cortex in the occipital lobe and the thalamus (Fig. 17-3).

Case Studies

Patient One

A 55-year-old woman was admitted to a hospital for high blood pressure. She had a stroke while sleeping. When she awoke, her right hand and leg would not move, and her head felt heavy. She could not find appropriate words to explain the loss of motor control. She was examined by a neurologist and at his recommendation, a speech pathologist. They observed the following:

- Right hemiplegia with intact sensation for touch, pain, and temperature
- Moderate difficulty finding words
- Limited verbal output
- Impaired verbal repetition
- Impaired reading and writing
- Near-normal auditory comprehension

Within a few days her speech improved, but it still was sparse and consisted of only a few words. She used many gestures and pointed with her left arm. Failure to communicate frustrated her, and she was depressed.

Magnetic resonance imaging (MRI) revealed a large infarct in the left frontal lobe anterior to the central sulcus that involved the anterior language cortex and a large part of the motor cortex.

Question: Based on your knowledge of vascular circulation, can you relate the manifestations of aphasia with the site of infarct?

Discussion: A stroke involving the anterior branches of the MCA affected the motor cortex and Broca's area (Brodmann area 44 and 45).

Patient Two

A 65-year-old right-handed businessman was admitted to a hospital after sudden development of confusion. Initially, the man did not speak much except some jargon and stereotyped expressions. After 3 weeks of care and recovery, he exhibited the following:

- Severe receptive aphasia
- Fluent and copious verbal output
- Severe anomia marked with many (related and unrelated) paraphasic errors and perseverations
- Excessive usage of general pronouns
- Semantically empty speech
- Limited repetition
- Severe difficulty in understanding others
- Moderate alexia
- Poor writing
- Intact somatosensory and motor functions
- Right visual field defect

MRI revealed an infarct in the posterior left superior temporal gyrus and parts of the inferior parietal lobe.

Question: Based on your knowledge of vascular circulation, can you relate the manifestations of receptive aphasia with the temporoparietal site of infarct?

Discussion: A stroke in the posterior branches of the MCA affected the temporal cortex, including the classical Wernicke's area (Brodmann area 22), which impaired comprehension and expression in this patient. The temporal lesion also affected the geniculocalcarine visual radiation fibers. Intact sensorimotor function was related to the spared ascending branches of the MCA.

Patient Three

A 59-year-old woman woke up blind in the right eye. She was taken to a hospital, where the attending physician noted the following:

- A history of elevated blood pressure
- No history of trauma
- No previous episode of TIA
- Right homonymous hemianopia

With selective visual symptoms, a vascular cause was suspected. However, computed tomography (CT) of the head produced normal findings. Since patient's visual difficulty persisted, a repeat CT of the head, undertaken after 3 days, showed an infarct in the left occipital lobe.

Question: Can you account for these symptoms on the basis of your understanding of the vascular supply and the functional organization in the brain?

Discussion: The stroke involving the left occipital lobe accounts for the focal symptom of the right homonymous hemianopsia.

- The sudden emergence of the symptom implies a vascular cause (gradual appearance of the symptoms indicates a tumor).
- The stroke affected the PCA, which supplies blood to the visual cortex in the occipital lobe (Figs.17-3 and 17-4).
- The infarct was visualized only on a repeat CT because it takes nearly 36 hours for infarcts to show on CT.

Patient Four

A 60-year-old priest was taken to an emergency room for sensorimotor problems that developed abruptly while he was getting ready to go to church to speak for a Sunday mass. The attending physician noted the following:

- Unintelligible speech because of dysarthria
- Hypernasality (with lowered left palate)
- Dysphagia
- Sensation loss on the left side of the face
- Difficulty balancing with falling to the left
- Left-sided complete facial paralysis
- Weakness in the right leg and arm

MRI revealed an infarct in the left caudal lateral–ventral pons extending to the medulla.

Questions: Can you account for these symptoms of the left face and the paralysis of the right half of the body? Can these symptoms be related to the involvement of the supply blood to the pontomedullary area?

Discussion: Small lateral arterial branches of the basilar artery supply the pons and part of medulla. The lateral medulla, which contains sensorimotor fibers, is supplied by the posterior inferior cerebellar artery, a branch of the vertebral artery.

- A pontomedullary stroke involving these arteries affected the trigeminal, facial, and acoustic nerves, and rootlets of the vagus nerve. Effects on the facial and trigeminal nerve fibers along with the rootlets of the vagus resulted in facial motor weakness, loss of sensation from the face, palatal paralysis, and swallowing difficulty.
- The involvement of vestibular nuclei resulted in impaired equilibrium with a tendency to fall to the left.
- The interruption of the descending pyramidal (corticospinal) fibers above the point of decussation produced right (contralateral) paralysis in the right arm and leg. The implicated cranial nerve fibers had already crossed, so there was left (ipsilateral) facial paralysis. This clinical picture is called alternating hemiplegia (see Chapter 14).

SUMMARY

The CNS depends on an adequate supply of blood, oxygen, and metabolized glucose. The heart pumps oxygenated blood to the CNS through two arterial systems, the vertebral basilar and the carotid. Both of these arterial systems ascend and join the arterial circle of Willis at the base of the brain. Three cortical branches and numerous penetrating subcortical branches arise from the circle of Willis and supply blood to the brain. After perfusion, the deoxygenated blood is collected by veins and drained into the sinus system responsible for transmitting the collected blood and cerebrospinal fluid back to the heart for reprocessing.

Technical Terms

anastomose
aneurysm
arteriosclerosis
arteriovenous malformations
atheroma
atherosclerosis
autoregulation
blood-brain barrier
carotid vascular system
cerebrovascular accident
circle of Willis
coagulation

collateral circulation
embolism
hemorrhage
ischemia
metabolism
paresthesia
sinus
thrombosis
vasoconstriction
vasodilation
watershed infarction

Review Questions

1. Define the following terms:
   anastomose
   aneurysm
   arteriosclerosis
   arteriovenous malformations
   atheroma
   atherosclerosis
   autoregulation
   blood-brain barrier
   carotid vascular system
   cerebrovascular accident
   circle of Willis
   coagulation
   collateral circulation
   embolism
   hemorrhage
   ischemia
   metabolism
   paresthesia
   sinus
   thrombosis
   watershed infarction
2. Describe the importance of the uninterrupted supply of oxygen to brain cells; also discuss the relative length of time that brain cells can sustain blood deprivation.
3. Discuss the mechanism that regulates blood flow to the brain.
4. Explain the difference between cortical (circumferential) and central (penetrating) arteries.
5. Outline the cortical area that the ACA distributes blood to and discuss important functional impairments that would follow its interruption.
6. Discuss the functional impairments that would follow vascular interruption to the MCA.
7. Describe the cortical area supplied by the PCA and discuss functional impairments that would follow its interruption.
8. Describe vascular circulation to the brainstem (midbrain, pons, medulla).
9. Describe the blood supply to the cerebellum.
10. Discuss vascular circulation to the spinal cord.
11. Discuss the importance of collateral circulation and list common sites of collateral circulation.
12. Explain the clinical significance of the circle of Willis.
13. Name the arteries included in the circle of Willis.
14. Describe common types of vascular pathology.
15. Describe the venous–sinus system.
16. Discuss the blood-brain barrier and its clinical advantages.
17. Outline the blood supply to the basal ganglia and thalamus.
18. A thrombosis of which artery is most likely to result in complete blindness?
19. Describe the process of cerebral embolic occlusion.
20. Name the arteries that supply the watershed area.
21. Discuss the basics of medical treatment in thrombotic and hemorrhagic vascular accidents.
22. A stroke involving which of the arteries is most likely to result in Wernicke's aphasia?
23. A stroke involving which of the cortical arteries is most likely to result in cognitive impairments with and without the paralysis of legs?
24. A stroke involving which of the subcortical arteries would result in thalamic syndrome?

Cerebrospinal Fluid

Learning Objectives

After studying this chapter, students should be able to do the following:

- Discuss the functions of cerebrospinal fluid
- Describe the mechanism of cerebrospinal fluid production
- Outline the circulation of cerebrospinal fluid
- Discuss the types of circulatory disorders
- Explain the diagnostic significance of cerebrospinal fluid
- Discuss the treatment of hydrocephalus

Cerebrospinal fluid (CSF) is a clear, colorless fluid. It is produced by the choroid plexus in the ventricular system and circulates from the ventricles to the subarachnoid space around the CNS. By forming a mechanical cushion around the CNS, CSF protects the brain and spinal cord from sudden and violent body movements. The buoyancy effect of the floating CSF in the subarachnoid space reduces the brain's weight by more than 95%. Thus, a brain weighing 1300 to 1400 g in the air weighs only 60 to 70 g when floating in CSF. This is an important aspect of the protective mechanism. As an active transport mechanism, CSF may also participate with the vascular system in the removal of harmful substances and waste resulting from cellular metabolic activities. CSF is also known to regulate extracellular environments.

CHOROID PLEXUS

Extending from the ventricular surface into the ventricular cavity, the choroid plexus is formed by an extensive network of infolded vascular capillaries, which are surrounded by the vascular pia mater (tela choroidea) and connective tissue. This also receives a layer of epithelium from the ependymal lining of the inner ventricular surface. The choroid plexus is a fenestrated structure with tight junctions around its apical regions and with a minutely folded surface. The pores or fenestration are formed by epithelial cells. The tight junctions between adjacent cells contribute to the barrier for the exchange of solutes between the blood and CSF. The choroid plexus is primarily located in the center of the lateral and fourth ventricles, with its largest formation around the collateral trigone region of the lateral ventricles. No choroid plexus is present in the small opening of the cerebral aqueduct of Sylvius nor the anterior and posterior horns.

CSF is mainly produced by the choroid plexus. The average total volume of CSF present in the human is approximately 100-140 mL. The human brain produces about 0.35 mL of CSF every minute, totaling 500 mL/day. CSF is normally replaced three times within 24 hours. Because it is secreted through the modified capillary–pia membranous network, in general CSF is a filtered form of blood. It resembles blood plasma but differs from blood in its molecular composition; for example, CSF contains less protein, fewer cells, and half the glucose found in blood. Diseases of the CNS change the constituent composition of CSF, an alteration that has diagnostic importance for identifying pathologic changes that occur in the brain and spinal cord.

CEREBROSPINAL FLUID CIRCULATION

CSF circulates in the ventricles and the subarachnoid space. There are four ventricles in the brain (Fig. 18-1): two lateral ventricles, one in each hemisphere; the third ventricle in the diencephalon; and the fourth ventricle in the brainstem. CSF flows from both lateral ventricles in the cerebral hemispheres to the third ventricle via the interventricular Monro's foramen. The third ventricle runs vertical between the two thalami, and its fluid

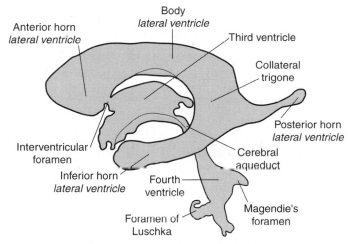

Figure 18-1. Lateral view of ventricles.

flows to the fourth ventricle through the cerebral aqueduct. From the fourth ventricle, CSF enters the subarachnoid space through three apertures, two lateral foramina of Luschka and one mediodorsal Magendie's foramen (Fig. 18-1). The subarachnoid space wraps around the entire CNS between the arachnoid membrane and the pia mater. The subarachnoid space varies from region to region: it is narrow over the gyri and wide over the fissures. The arachnoid, which rests on the dura mater, is separated from the dura by a potential subdural space, while the pia mater closely adheres to the cortical surface. Arachnoid trabeculae extend from the arachnoid to the pia mater and contribute to the maintenance of the subarachnoid space (Figs. 2-46A and 18-2). The subarachnoid space houses many large cisterns that form large pockets of CSF. The important cisterns are the cerebellomedullary, superior, interpeduncular, chiasmatic, pontine, and lumbar. The cerebellomedullary, the largest cistern, is between the medulla and the cerebellum, which receives fluid from the fourth ventricle. The interpeduncular cistern is the large pocket of fluid ventral to the midbrain. The chiasmatic cistern lies in front of the optic chiasm, while the pontine cistern is in front of the pons. The lumbar cistern extends from L-2 to S-2 and contains fibers of the cauda equina nerve roots and filum terminale (Figs. 2-48 and 18-2).

Once in the subarachnoid space, CSF flows up toward the convexity of the brain or down toward the spinal cord. Some CSF infiltrates the depths of the cerebral cortex along the blood vessels that penetrate the brain. This area around the penetrating blood vessels is the perivascular space, the site for possible diffusion of metabolic solutes from CSF into extracellular fluid. The diffusion of metabolites has important implications for medical treatment.

ABSORPTION OF THE CEREBROSPINAL FLUID

CSF is absorbed through the arachnoid granulations, which are one-way openings. These tufted structures lie dorsal along both sides of the superior sagittal sinus (Fig. 2-46B). The arachnoid granulations protrude into the dural sinus and empty CSF into the superior sagittal sinus, which also receives venous blood.

CLINICAL CONSIDERATIONS

The draining of CSF from the subarachnoid space is a pressure-sensitive process. Emptying CSF into the superior sagittal sinus requires a pressure differential between the subarachnoid space and the venous–sinus system. A pressure difference of at least 30 to 60 mm H_2O regulates normal CSF drainage through the arachnoid villi. If for any reason this pressure differential alters and the sinus pressure exceeds the ventricular pressure, the one-way openings of the arachnoid villi close, ending the draining and elevating intracranial pressure.

The rate of CSF production, however, is independent of its absorption and interventricular pressure. CSF continues to be produced even after an interruption in its drainage into the sinus system. A dissociation between production and absorption rates of CSF results in hydrocephalus, a condition to which three factors contribute: the increased production of CSF, the blocking of the draining passage through which CSF reaches the subarachnoid space, and the impaired absorption of CSF. Choroid tumors have also been implicated with hydrocephalus. Regardless of the underlying cause, in hydrocephalus, an excessive amount of CSF pressure increases pressure in the brain. Sustained pressure causes enlargement of the ventricles and damage to the surrounding vital cortical tissues (Fig. 18-3). If hydrocephalus begins in infancy, the increased CSF pressure also enlarges the cranial vault.

Circulatory Disorders

There are two types of hydrocephalus: communicating and noncommunicating. In communicating hydrocephalus, the problem is impairment of drainage into the sinus. CSF is not adequately drained into the sinus system even though it can reach the subarachnoid space through the foramina of Magendie and Luschka. Tumor or inflammation of the brain often causes communicating hydrocephalus. In noncommunicating hydrocephalus, the CSF flow from the ventricles to the subarachnoid space is blocked because of an obstruction within the ventricular cavity. The obstruction can occur either in the ventricular system itself or in Luschka's and Magendie's foramina in the fourth ventricle. The most common site of blockage is the narrow aperture of the cerebral aqueduct in the midbrain. Regardless of the

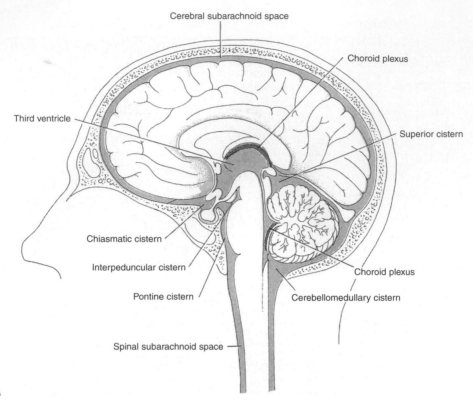

A

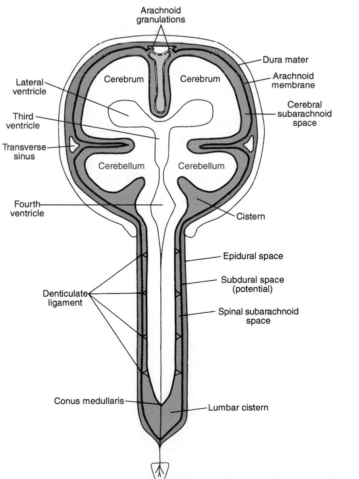

B

Figure 18-2. **A.** Subarachnoid space (*shaded*) and major subarachnoid cisterns. **B.** Brain and spinal cord showing locations of subarachnoid spaces.

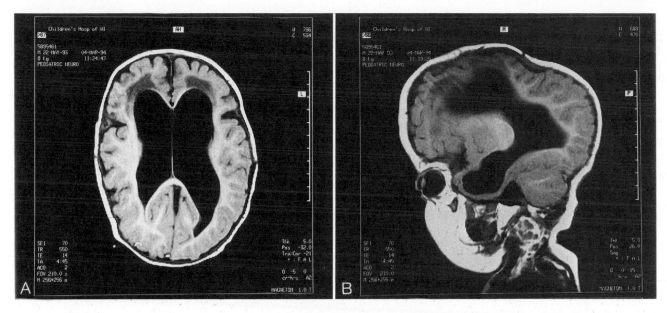

Figure 18-3.   Magnetic resonance image of enlarged lateral ventricles in a hydrocephalic child. **A.** Transaxial view. **B.** Sagittal view.

hydrocephalic type, the final result is the same: CSF pressure rises in the ventricles. It enlarges the ventricles and compresses the surrounding white and gray matters (Fig. 18-3), affecting vital cortical functions that include sensorimotor and higher mental functions. In hydrocephalic children, the head becomes pyramidal, with the face being disproportionately small and the eyes turned outward. In the most advanced cases of hydrocephalus, a coronal section of the brain reveals nothing but two large compartments of the lateral ventricles, whereas the cortical mantle is reduced to a thin layer between the ventricles and the skull.

Treatment

Hydrocephalus no longer has to be fatal. If diagnosed early, it can easily be treated surgically. Treatment involves diverting the blocked ventricular CSF to another body cavity for absorption. A thin rubbery tube is surgically inserted into the enlarged ventricular cavity and used to divert CSF flow to the peritoneal cavity in the abdomen, the pleural space, the ureter, or the right atrium of the heart. Usually the tube has a valve system to help regulate the pressure inside the skull, preventing complete collapse of the brain. This system is called a shunt. Draining into the peritoneal cavity is the most common procedure because it is easiest and safest. Other locations can also effectively absorb CSF, but they require more extensive surgery and/or have a higher failure rate.

Diagnostic Significance of Cerebrospinal Fluid

Changes in the pressure and composition of CSF have diagnostic significance. CSF pressure is measured by lumbar puncture. A needle is inserted into the lumbar subarachnoid space between the fourth and fifth lumbar vertebrae, because spinal penetration at this point does not injure any nerve fibers. Once CSF starts flowing, the needle hub is attached to a manometer or other pressure-sensitive device. Normal pressure in an adult is 80 to 150 mm H_2O. Increased intracranial pressure occurs in response to increased amounts of CSF, brain swelling, and brain tumors. A pressure level higher than normal suggests a pathological process. Ventricular pressure can also be measured by inserting a catheter into the lateral ventricles.

Spinal puncture is also used to administer anesthesia in the lower spinal region. A fluid anesthetic, such as lidocaine, is injected into the spinal subarachnoid space to suppress pain and other sensations from the lower body up to the level of the spinal injection. The anesthesia prevents nerve impulses from being conducted through the spinal nerves.

Brain pathology also alters the composition of CSF. Consequently, chemical analysis of it may provide important diagnostic information. For example, acute bacterial meningitis, viral infection, or cerebral infarction increases the number of white blood cells. Elevated protein content in CSF suggests a block in the subarachnoid space by a compressive lesion. Blood pigments in CSF may indicate an intracranial hemorrhage.

SUMMARY

CSF, which the choroid plexus produces in the ventricles, circulates from the ventricles to the subarachnoid space. Along with the meningeal membranes,

CSF protects the brain. Its other function is to regulate extracellular environments. It collects harmful substances and waste products that result from cellular metabolic activities. Inadequate drainage of the CSF results in excessive accumulation of CSF followed by increased intracranial pressure and hydrocephalus. Hydrocephalus can be treated by surgically implanting a shunt. However, if not adequately treated, the increased intracranial pressure that accompanies hydrocephalus enlarges the ventricular cavity and causes irreparable brain damage.

Technical Terms

arachnoid granulations	**ependymal cells**
cerebrospinal fluid	**hydrocephalus**
choroid plexus	**intracranial pressure**
lumbar puncture	**subarachnoid space**
meningitis	**venous sinus system**
peritoneal cavity	**ventricles**
spinal anesthesia	

Review Questions

1. Define the following terms:

arachnoid granulations	peritoneal cavity
choroid plexus	spinal anesthesia
ependymal cells	subarachnoid space
hydrocephalus	venous sinus system
intracranial pressure	ventricles
lumbar puncture	

2. Discuss the functions of CSF.
3. Discuss the production and circulation of CSF.
4. Discuss the common types of CSF circulatory disorders.
5. Describe the mechanism, clinical implications, and treatment of hydrocephalus.

Cerebral Cortex: Higher Mental Functions[a]

Learning Objectives

After studying this chapter, students should be able to do the following:

- Describe the functional importance of the primary and associational cortical areas
- Discuss major cortical functions
- Describe the relationship between cerebral dominance and handedness
- Describe the neurological diagnosis of behavioral deficits
- List the major types of aphasia and describe their neurolinguistic characteristics
- Discuss the neurology of apraxias
- Discuss the neurology of reading and writing
- Describe the neurology of motor speech
- Discuss the neurology of cognition in reference to dementia and traumatic brain injuries
- Provide a clinical discussion of dementia

Chapters 1 to 18 focus on the structural organization of the nervous system and the sensorimotor functions that are bilaterally organized in the brain. What testifies to the uniqueness of the human brain is its possession of higher mental functions, such as thought processes, language, and speech, and their asymmetrical organization. The asymmetrical cerebral specialization for higher mental functions, or cerebral dominance, relates to the unique cytoarchitectural organization of the brain.

The cerebral cortex is a massive, convoluted structure that is the site of higher mental functions. It has an area of about 2.5 square feet and contains as many as 14 billion neurons. The brain is divided into four primary lobes: frontal, parietal, temporal, and occipital. Each lobe

---

[a] This chapter was written by Howard S. Kirshner, MD, Department of Neurology, Vanderbilt University Medical Center, Nashville, Tennessee.

has a relatively constant cortical anatomy that is divided by sulci or fissures into discrete gyri (Figs. 2-4 and 2-5).

METHODS OF STUDY

Neurology is the study of diseases that affect the nervous system. Classically, neurology depended on evidence gathered during the medical examination of stroke patients and the correlation with brain lesions seen at autopsy.

In the modern era, brain imaging modalities permit the simultaneous visualization of brain structure and examination of associated behavior. **Computed tomography (CT)**, **magnetic resonance imaging (MRI)**, **positron emission tomography (PET)**, and **single photon emission computed tomography (SPECT)** are commonly used neuroimaging methods (see Chapter 20). Another area of advance in brain localization is electrical stimulation. The electroencephalogram is an electrical study of neuronal firing patterns in the brain. Computer-assisted techniques such as brain electrical activity mapping increase the anatomical accuracy of the electroencephalogram but are still less precise in anatomical localization than are CT and MRI. Electrical stimulation of the awake patient, used as a guide for excision of epileptic foci in the brain, has further delineated areas of the brain important for language and speech (Ojemann, 1989, Bhatnagar, et al., 2000).

FUNCTIONAL LOCALIZATION IN THE BRAIN

Clinical data obtained from patients with stroke, traumatic brain injury, brain tumors, and epilepsy; from surgery; and from emerging studies using PET and SPECT have helped reveal functional regional anatomy of the brain in terms of the four major lobes and their cortical gyri. These gyri, or parts of them, operate as modules dedicated to specific cognitive or behavioral functions. The modules act somewhat like the "brain centers" that 19th century physicians described, but they are organized not as individual centers but as parts of interacting networks that connect modules in different regions or lobes. The cortical modules also have connections with subcortical centers such as the basal ganglia and other deep brain structures. What follows, then, is a simplified description of the major functions of the four lobes of each hemisphere of the brain.

In general, the cortex of the brain is divided into primary motor areas, primary sensory areas (for vision, hearing, touch, smell, and possibly taste), and association areas. The association cortex is divided into a unimodal association cortex, such as the visual and auditory association cortices, and heteromodal association cortex. The heteromodal cortical areas include the parietal cortex, which is a sensory association area for interaction between the senses, and the frontal region, which is thought of as the "executive function" for the entire brain. These heteromodal association cortices represent the areas of largest expansion of the brain from apes to man, and they are likely to make possible the extraordinary cognitive and behavioral capabilities which our species, *Homo sapiens*, has demonstrated.

Frontal Lobe

The posterior limit of the frontal lobe, on the lateral surface of the brain, is the precentral gyrus, which contains motor cells of the primary motor cortex (Brodmann area 4). This cortical strip carries a map of the contralateral side of the body (homunculus), with cells programmed to produce contractions of specific muscles or specific movements (Fig. 2-6). The motor homunculus has its face and lips in the most inferior part of the gyrus, just above the sylvian fissure; the hand and arm lie above that; the leg and foot extend over the superior part of the gyrus and continue downward on the medial aspect of the hemisphere. Stimulation of cells in the motor cortex produces specific movements of contralateral parts of the body. The large size of the cortical representation of the thumb, fingers, and hand compared with the arm reflects the importance of fine finger movements. Similarly, the large space reserved for the mouth and lips indicates the importance of speech.

Anterior to the premotor area is the **premotor cortex**, which is involved in the initiation and planning of skilled motor movements. Just anterior to the face area of the motor strip is the cortical Broca's area (Brodmann area 44), thought to program patterned movements of the vocal apparatus to produce phonemes and words. Brodmann area 8, in the superior frontal lobe, is involved in movement of the eyes and head to the contralateral side. The supplementary motor cortex is on the medial side of the hemisphere anterior to the leg area of the primary motor cortex. Stimulation of this area produces complex postures or patterned movements. Lesions in this area also disrupt the initiation of speech.

Another function of the dorsolateral frontal lobe, one of the two heteromodal association cortices of the brain, is the executive function of deciding what elements of incoming stimuli should be attended to and which motor outputs should be activated (Goldman-Rakic, 1996). The dorsolateral frontal lobe is also important for working memory, or immediate attention span.

Functions of the **prefrontal cortex** anterior to the premotor area and the orbitofrontal cortex are quite complex and poorly understood. Lesions of the frontal cortex may produce disinhibition of speech and other behaviors, known as **frontal lobe syndrome**. Patients with lesions of the orbitofrontal cortex may have normal intelligence and memory, but they may have totally changed personality, with short temper, irritability, poor impulse control, sociopathic (anti-social) personality, and a general tendency to act out. Blumer and Benson (1975) referred to this behavior as **pseudopsychopathic**, in that it resembles the behavior of a sociopathic personality. Such syndromes are frequently seen after frontal head injuries. The lateral frontal convexities are also involved in the initiation of behavior. Bilateral lesions of this area tend to produce a reduction or cessation of behavior, often referred to as **akinetic mutism** or **abulia**. Patients may sit and stare passively, not speaking or responding only in a whisper. This type of frontal lobe syndrome is called pseudodepressed. In general, these frontal lobe syndromes resemble psychiatric disorders, because there are profound alterations of behavior and personality, yet the basic cognitive functions, such as memory, language, visuospatial functioning, and elementary motor and sensory functions, are intact.

On the medial surface of the frontal lobe lies the cingulum, or cingulate gyrus. This gyrus is a part of the **limbic system**, or **Papez's circuit**, of projections from the hippocampus via the septum and fornix to the mamillary bodies and then to the anterior thalamic nuclei. Projections then go to the cingulate gyrus and back to the hippocampus. This circuit is important to memory and to elementary limbic functions, such as motivation and drive (see Chapter 16).

Parietal Lobe

The parietal lobe contains Brodmann areas 1 to 3, which are devoted to sensory function. In the inferior parietal lobule are Brodmann areas 39 and 40, the angular and supramarginal gyri. The inferior parietal lobule in the left hemisphere is tied to language function, especially reading and naming, and to calculations and arithmetic. This region is the second part of the heteromodal association cortex, along with the dorsolateral frontal lobe. The parietal association cortex may be thought of as a center for the association of information from different sensory modalities, such as vision, hearing, and touch. Gerstmann (1930) associated four deficits with lesions of the left inferior parietal lobule: agraphia, acalculia, right–left confusion, and finger agnosia (loss of the ability to know which finger is which). The inferior parietal lobule in the right hemisphere is involved with the body schema. Right inferior parietal lobe lesions produce neglect of the left side of the body. The superior parts of the parietal cortex are devoted to visuospatial and constructional functions, higher-level "cortical" sensory functions, such as stereognosis (recognition of palpated shapes) and graphesthesia (ability to recognize letters or numbers drawn on the skin).

Lesions of the right parietal lobe produce important neurobehavioral deficits, including left-side neglect, denial of the presence of a motor deficit (anosognosia), and dressing apraxia (inability to place garments correctly in relation to body parts). Other spatial and topographical dysfunctions associated with right parietal lobe lesions include difficulty finding one's way around and an inability to draw or read a map. Constructional tasks, such as copying figures, drawing a clock or a house, or bisecting a line, may reveal difficulty with spatial relationships or neglect of the left side of space. Although speech and language are relatively well preserved in patients with right parietal lesions, the emotional intonation of speech may be lacking, as may the ability to comprehend emotional tone in the speech of others. These patients often fail to grasp sarcasm or humor. These paralinguistic disorders are disabling to patients in the social world. Emotional indifference often characterizes the mood of these patients; they may be undisturbed by this left-sided paralysis or by the impending loss of ability to work. All of these right-hemisphere deficits amount to a change in the personality of the patient, and changes in personality are often more difficult for families to accept than the loss of language ability seen with left-hemisphere lesions.

Temporal Lobe

The superior temporal gyrus of each hemisphere contains the primary auditory cortex (Brodmann areas 41 and 42), which lies buried within the sylvian fissure. Lesions of the primary auditory cortex cause cortical deafness. Bilateral superior temporal damage can cause pure word deafness (inability to understand spoken words) with preserved pure tone hearing and recognition of nonverbal sounds. Another bitemporal syndrome is auditory agnosia, or inability to recognize nonverbal sounds.

The left superior temporal gyrus contains Wernicke's area, which is critical to the comprehension of heard language. There may be a language comprehension area in the inferior temporal gyrus and adjacent fusiform gyrus, as identified by electrical stimulation (the basal temporal language area, or BTLA). Interestingly, no convincing evidence indicates a language deficit resulting from ablation of or damage to this area.

The BTLA may therefore be part of a network involved in understanding of language but not be necessary to functioning of the language comprehension system.

The right temporal lobe is a silent area of the brain, as surgical resection of this area produces only very subtle deficits. Appreciation of rhythm and musical qualities may be affected by right temporal lesions, as may be nonverbal memory. In general, the medial temporal areas, such as the hippocampus, together with their connections to the thalamus, septal area, and cingulate gyri of the medial frontal lobes, are most clearly related to memory. Bilateral lesions produce lasting loss of new learning and recent memory. Unilateral left medial temporal lesions produce disorders of verbal memory, whereas unilateral right temporal lesions produce nonverbal memory loss. Acute lesions of the right temporal lobe, as in strokes, may also cause confusion or delirium.

Occipital Lobe

The most posterior poles of the occipital lobes are the primary visual cortices (Brodmann area 17). Damage to this cortex on one side produces a contralateral hemianopic visual field defect for both eyes. Damage to both sides may produce cortical blindness. Some patients with cortical blindness are unaware of their blindness and confabulate descriptions of objects and scenes they claim to see. Adjacent occipital areas (Brodmann areas 18 and 19) are called the visual association cortex and are thought to contribute to complex visual analysis. Lesions of these areas on both sides produce complex visual syndromes called visual agnosia.

DISORDERS OF CORTICAL FUNCTIONS

Cerebral Dominance and Functional Specialization

Since Broca's observations in 1861, it has been known that in most humans the left hemisphere is at least relatively dominant for language. Virtually 99% of right-handed people and most left-handed people have left-hemisphere dominance for language. Handedness has some correlation to cerebral dominance, so left-handed people are more likely than right-handed people to have right-hemisphere language dominance. However, most left-handers still become aphasic if the left hemisphere is damaged, and only a few become aphasic if the right hemisphere is damaged. Some left-handed people appear to have mixed dominance, such as having speech expression in the left hemisphere and comprehension in the right hemisphere.

The right hemisphere, often called the minor hemisphere, serves many nonlanguage functions. As discussed with reference to the parietal lobes, right-hemisphere functions include visuospatial and constructional tasks, knowledge of maps and topography, dressing, emotional feeling and processing, production of emotional intonation of speech, and music appreciation.

Cerebral dominance may have structural correlates. Geschwind and Levitsky (1968) reported that right-handed people have a longer **planum temporale** in the left hemisphere than in the right (Fig. 9-10). Similar asymmetries have been described in newborn infants and in illiterate people, suggesting that these anatomical asymmetries are genetically programmed, not acquired through use. Cerebral asymmetries have recently been reaffirmed using CT and MRI. The relationship of such asymmetries to language dominance, as determined by the Wada test, is being investigated by many.

Speech and Language Disorders

Speech and language disorders have long held great interest for students of the nervous system. First, the ability to communicate verbally sets humans apart from other animal species. Second, language disorders were the first behavioral or cognitive impairments to be correlated with disease processes involving specific areas of the brain.

MOTOR SPEECH DISORDERS

Motor speech disorders consist of abnormal speech articulation in the absence of any language disorder. Abnormal motor speech control, or **dysarthria**, can involve abnormal strength or place of articulation, abnormal timing or speed of articulatory movement, or abnormal voicing. Dysarthric patients can comprehend both spoken and written language, and their speech output, if comprehensible, can be transcribed into normal language. Darley and colleagues (1975), in a comprehensive study of dysarthric speech at the Mayo Clinic, divided these neurogenic dysarthrias into the following six types: flaccid, spastic, ataxic, hypokinetic, hyperkinetic, and mixed.

Flaccid dysarthria results from lesions of the bulbar muscles, neuromuscular junction, cranial nerves, and anterior horn cells of the brainstem nuclei and is characterized by hypernasal breathy speech with imprecisely articulated consonants. **Spastic dysarthria** is seen in patients with bilateral lesions of the motor cortex or corticobulbar tracts. Speech characteristics involve harsh, strain-and-strangle speech, with a slow speaking rate, low pitch, and imprecisely articulated consonants. A variant of spastic dysarthria is unilateral upper motor neuron dysarthria, resulting from a unilateral lesion such as a stroke. The same characteristics pertain but are less severe. **Ataxic dysarthria**, seen in cerebellar disorders, involves irregular cadence or prosody of speech, with long pauses and sudden explosions of sound, abnormal and sometimes excessively equal stress on specific syllables, and imprecisely articulated consonants. This pattern is sometimes called scanning speech. **Hypokinetic dysarthria**, as classically seen in Parkinson's disease, is associated with decreased and monotonous

loudness and pitch, occasional rushes of syllables, occasional pauses, and some imprecisely articulated consonants. **Hyperkinetic dysarthria**, seen in chorea and related movement disorders, including Huntington's chorea, is characterized by variable rate, excessive variation in loudness and timing, and distorted vowels. In dystonia, this form of dysarthria can also involve harsh strain-and-strangle speech with imprecisely articulated consonants. **Mixed dysarthria** can involve combinations of any of the other five types. Common examples include **amyotrophic lateral sclerosis**, in which spastic and flaccid elements coexist, and **multiple sclerosis**, in which spastic and ataxic characteristics predominate. In practice, there is considerable overlap among the categories of dysarthria.

APRAXIA OF SPEECH

Apraxia of speech is difficult to separate from aphasia. Speech apraxia entails abnormal articulation of sequences of phonemes, usually with inconsistent error patterns from one attempt to the next, in contrast to the consistent misarticulations in dysarthrias. Apraxia of speech is inability to program sequences of sounds, especially consonants. Consonants are more often substituted than distorted. Apraxia of speech is most obvious with polysyllabic words. Difficulty with initial consonants is common, and speech takes on a hesitant, groping quality. A patient may attempt to say a word like *catastrophe* five times and produce five different errors or may achieve the correct pronunciation once or twice. Apraxia of speech is only rarely seen without aphasia. More commonly, apraxia of speech is part of an aphasic deficit, particularly Broca's aphasia.

APHASIA

Aphasia is an acquired disorder of language processing secondary to brain disease (Alexander and Benson, 1992). This definition excludes developmental or congenital language problems (dysphasia), motor speech or articulation disorders (dysarthria, dysphonia, and pure apraxia of speech), and impaired thought processes (dementia and schizophrenia).

Broca's Aphasia

French physician Paul Broca first described Broca's aphasia in 1861. It is characterized by nonfluent, often halting, dysarthric, and ungrammatical speech in which meaning is conveyed largely by meaning-carrying nouns and verbs, leaving out the minor structural words (Table 19-1). Naming is also deficient, but the patient can often pronounce the first letter or phoneme (tip-of-the-tongue phenomenon). Auditory comprehension often seems relatively normal, although deficits may occur in comprehension of multistep commands or in sentences with complex grammatical structure. Those with Broca's aphasia tend to have difficulty comprehending complex

Table 19-1. Language Features of Common Types of Aphasia

Feature	Broca's	Wernicke's	Global	Conduction	Anomia
Spontaneous speech	Nonfluent	Fluent, paraphasic	Nonfluent	Fluent	Fluent with pauses
Naming	Impaired	Paraphasic	Poor	Variable	Most impaired
Comprehension	Mildly impaired	Poor	Poor	Intact	Intact
Repetition	Impaired	Impaired	Impaired	Impaired	Intact
Reading	May be impaired	Impaired	Poor	May be intact	Intact
Writing	Impaired	Impaired	Poor	May be intact	Intact

syntax, just as they have difficulty producing such syntax. For example, a person with Broca's aphasia might have difficulty with a sentence such as "the book Bill gave to Betty was thick." The subject might understand that a book was given but could not specify who gave and who received the book. Deficits can virtually always be detected on standard language batteries. Repetition in Broca's aphasia is usually halting and reduced in fluency. Reading is often more strongly affected than auditory comprehension. Patients exhibit writing deficits, because most of them have right hemiparesis (paralysis of right arm and leg), forcing them to write with their nondominant left hand. Persons with Broca's aphasia not only have awkward handwriting but also spell poorly; many cannot write even single words or short phrases.

Lesions of Broca's aphasia involve the left frontal region. Broca identified the area as the posterior part of the inferior frontal gyrus, although both of his patients had much more extensive lesions. Mohr and colleagues (1978) found that patients with lesions in or near Broca's area exhibit an excellent recovery within weeks, whereas patients with lasting expressive deficits, such as Broca's original cases, have more extensive lesions involving most of the frontal and parietal lobes. Recent studies have also suggested that lasting nonfluent aphasia also includes damage to subcortical structures, particularly the subcallosal fasciculus and periventricular white matter (Naeser et al., 1989).

Aphemia, a variant of Broca's aphasia, is a rare syndrome of muteness or nonfluent speech with good language comprehension and preserved writing. Because there is very little true language disturbance, aphemia may not be true aphasia; it has been equated with the equally rare syndrome of pure apraxia of speech.

Wernicke's Aphasia

Carl Wernicke reported Wernicke's aphasia in 1874. In contrast to those with Broca's aphasia, patients with Wernicke's aphasia speak fluently and effortlessly, although their meaning is obscured by the paucity of meaningful nouns and verbs, the overabundance of stock phrases and idioms, and the presence of numerous verbal paraphasic errors (Table 19-1). Neologisms are usually present in severe cases, making the speech jargon. In milder cases, many paraphasic substitutions and

idioms take the sentences in directions not intended by the speaker. Naming in Wernicke's aphasia is paraphasic, often with bizarre substitutions. Auditory comprehension is usually so severely impaired that the patient cannot answer simple yes-or-no questions. Repetition is also paraphasic, and reading comprehension usually mirrors the poor language comprehension seen in auditory testing. In some cases, either auditory comprehension or reading may be less affected than the other (Kirshner et al., 1989), and this spared language modality can be used to communicate with the patient. Writing is also abnormal in Wernicke's aphasia. Unlike patients with Broca's, most of those with Wernicke's aphasia have no hemiparesis, and they can grip a pen and write without difficulty. The content of the writing, however, shows the same abnormality as the speech and is characterized by abnormal spelling patterns. Thus, writing samples may be a good way to detect mild Wernicke's aphasia, as in patients with slowly developing syndromes related to brain tumors.

Lesions associated with Wernicke's aphasia generally involve the posterior two-thirds of the left superior temporal gyrus, although in some cases they extend into other parts of the temporal lobe and into the inferior parietal lobule. Lesions that damage most of the traditional Wernicke's area are especially well correlated with lasting impairments of comprehension, whereas those involving primarily the inferior parietal lobule may be more associated with reading and writing disorders. As patients with Wernicke's aphasia recover, their deficits often evolve into the milder syndromes of conduction or anomic aphasia.

A variant of Wernicke's aphasia is *pure word deafness*, selective loss of auditory comprehension and repetition with preserved naming, reading, and writing. Many patients have mildly paraphasic speech. The syndrome classically results from bilateral temporal lobe lesions, which disconnect the auditory cortices from Wernicke's area. Cases resembling pure word deafness have been reported with unilateral temporal lobe lesions.

Global Aphasia

Global aphasia may be thought of as the sum of the deficits of Broca's and Wernicke's aphasias (Table 19-1).

Patients with global aphasia are nonfluent or mute, and they exhibit impaired comprehension. All elements of language—speech, naming, comprehension, repetition, reading, and writing—are severely impaired. Syndromes of less severe but equally generalized impairments of language are called **mixed aphasia**. Lesions associated with global aphasia involve much of the left middle cerebral artery territory of the frontal, temporal, and parietal lobes. Large lesions of the subcortical white matter and basal ganglia result in a similar syndrome. As the patient with global aphasia recovers, the deficit profile often evolves toward Broca's aphasia.

Conduction Aphasia

Although conduction aphasia occurs in fewer than 10% of aphasia cases, it teaches important lessons about language. In this syndrome, repetition is the most severely affected language modality (Table 19-1). Spontaneous speech is fluent, often with many literal paraphasic errors. The patient is aware of these errors and makes efforts at self-correction. Naming is variable, but auditory comprehension is usually normal. The patient understands well but cannot repeat what was said. Reading aloud may show similar deficits to repetition, as may writing to dictation. Wernicke originally postulated a lesion disconnecting the auditory word association area (Wernicke's area) in the left temporal lobe from Broca's area in the left frontal lobe. Modern studies have found two general locations of lesion in conduction aphasia: the left superior temporal region, with incomplete damage to Wernicke's area, and the inferior parietal lobule, especially the supramarginal gyrus. Benson and colleagues (1973) noted that patients with conduction aphasia secondary to parietal lobe lesions often have associated limb apraxia, whereas those with temporal lobe lesions do not. The supramarginal gyrus area may be important to the generation of phonemes in response to repetition or naming. An alternative explanation for conduction aphasia is a short-term memory deficit specific to auditory verbal material (Shallice and Warrington, 1977).

Anomic Aphasia

Also called amnesic or amnestic aphasia, anomic aphasia refers to syndromes in which naming is the most severe deficit. The patient speaks fluently, with some word-finding pauses and circumlocutions. Repetition, auditory comprehension, reading, and writing are intact. Many patients show no other abnormalities on neurological examination. The lesions producing anomic aphasia are more variable than those underlying the other aphasic syndromes discussed thus far. Some authors have emphasized lesions of the angular gyrus, although lesions there often produce other deficits, including alexia, constructional impairment, and the four elements of Gerstmann's syndrome. Anomic aphasia is also seen in conditions without clearly localized lesions,

such as in confusional states and dementing disorders like Alzheimer's disease. According to some sources, left frontal lobe lesions affect naming of actions (verbs), whereas left temporal lesions are more associated with misnaming of objects (nouns).

Transcortical Aphasias

The next three aphasic syndromes are transcortical aphasias; the responsible lesions affect not the primary language cortex or the circuit from Wernicke's to Broca's area but rather other areas of the brain that project to the language cortex. Specific lesions are quite variable, including cortical damage in the frontal, temporal, and parietal areas and subcortical white matter. Table 19-2 lists key features of the three transcortical aphasia syndromes.

The first transcortical aphasia is **transcortical motor aphasia**, in which the patient speaks little, much as in Broca's aphasia. In response to questions, the patient may either remain mute or may give a one- or two-word answer, often in a whisper or after a delay. As in Broca's aphasia, the patient utters the most important, meaningful words of a sentence, often communicating adequately. Unlike the patient with Broca's aphasia, however, a patient with transcortical motor aphasia can repeat normally. Auditory comprehension tends to be preserved, whereas naming, reading, and writing are more variable. Lesions associated with this syndrome usually lie in the left frontal lobe, anterior to, superior to, or beneath Broca's area. The most common location is the frontal cortex within the territory of the left anterior cerebral artery distribution.

The second transcortical syndrome, **transcortical sensory aphasia**, is a Wernickelike syndrome in which speech is fluent but paraphasic and auditory comprehension is severely impaired. Unlike the patient with Wernicke's aphasia, however, the patient with transcortical sensory aphasia can repeat phrases and sentences without difficulty. Naming is typically paraphasic, and reading comprehension and writing are impaired, similar to Wernicke's aphasia. Lesions of the left posterior temporo-occipital lobe have been described, and the syndrome also occurs in patients with Alzheimer's disease.

Table 19-2. Language Features of Transcortical Aphasias

Feature	Isolation	Transcortical	
		Motor	Sensory
Speech	Nonfluent, echolalic	Nonfluent	Fluent, echolalic
Naming	Impaired	Impaired	Impaired
Comprehension	Impaired	Intact	Impaired
Repetition	Intact	Intact	Intact
Reading	Impaired	May be spared	Impaired
Writing	Impaired	Impaired	Impaired

The final transcortical aphasic syndrome is **mixed transcortical aphasia** (syndrome of the isolation of the speech area). This syndrome is the transcortical equivalent of global aphasia. The patient cannot speak fluently, comprehend spoken language, follow commands, name objects, read, or write. Surprisingly, however, these patients can repeat fluently, and some are even echolalic. A patient reported by Geschwind and colleagues (1968) could even learn lyrics of new songs popular only after her illness, indicating that some memory storage of words was possible. **Isolation syndrome** is an extreme form of transcortical aphasia in which the perisylvian language cortex is intact but not connected to other cortical areas necessary for propositional speech or comprehension. It usually indicates extensive cortical damage to both cerebral hemispheres, sparing the perisylvian cortex, as in watershed infarctions seen in states of hypotension, hypoxia, carbon monoxide poisoning, or bilateral carotid artery occlusion.

Subcortical Aphasias

Subcortical aphasias are defined by lesion localization rather than by characteristics of the aphasia. Although aphasia usually reflects dysfunction of the language cortex, subcortical lesions can disrupt connections to the language cortex. The most common subcortical aphasia syndrome, often called the **anterior subcortical aphasia syndrome**, is seen in patients with lesions involving the head of the caudate nucleus, the anterior limb of the internal capsule, and the anterior putamen. Speech is usually dysarthric, with mild deficits of repetition and comprehension. Lesions of the dominant thalamus produce fluent aphasia with paraphasic errors but with relatively spared auditory comprehension. Subcortical lesions can also involve the temporal isthmus, cutting off connections to Wernicke's area and producing severe disturbance of comprehension. Delineation of the precise neuroanatomy of the subcortical aphasia syndromes is an active area of research.

ALEXIAS: NEUROLOGY OF READING

Disordered reading and writing are important aspects of most aphasia syndromes. In some syndromes, however, reading and writing are affected out of proportion to deficits in spoken language and auditory comprehension. French physician Joseph J. Déjérine delineated the two classical alexia syndromes, with and without agraphia, 100 years ago.

Alexia with Agraphia

Alexia with agraphia is acquired illiteracy: a patient becomes unable to read or write (Table 19-3). Although spoken language is relatively intact, most cases have a fluent paraphasic speech pattern. Auditory comprehension and naming are often impaired to some degree. The syndrome results from lesions in the left inferior parietal lobule, comprising the supramarginal and angular gyri. As such, the syndrome overlaps with Wernicke's aphasia, and some cases may evolve as a stage in the recovery of acute Wernicke's aphasia.

Alexia Without Agraphia

Pure alexia without agraphia can be thought of as a linguistic blindfold in which the inability to read is an isolated deficit (Table 19-3). These patients have normal spontaneous speech, repetition, and auditory comprehension; in fact, most patients can comprehend words spelled aloud, indicating that their spelling is not disturbed. There is often some naming difficulty, particularly for colors. Writing is intact, and one of the most intriguing aspects of the syndrome is that a patient may write a phrase or sentence but shortly afterward may be unable to read it. The inability to read is often complete at first, then improves such that the patient can spell out words letter by letter. Most of these patients have reduced short-term memory and right hemianopsia. The lesion is almost always a stroke in the territory of the left posterior cerebral artery, which supplies the medial occipital and medial temporal lobes and the splenium of the corpus callosum. Déjérine's explanation was that the left occipital lesion caused right hemianopsia and the lesion of the corpus callosum prevented visual information from being transmitted from the intact right occipital lobe to the left hemisphere language centers. Thus, the patient can see in the left visual field but cannot decode written language. This syndrome is a good example of a disconnection syndrome.

Aphasic Alexia

Aphasic alexia occurs in association with aphasic disturbances. Benson (1977) used the term **third alexia** to characterize the reading disorder of Broca's aphasia. In this classification, the first and second alexias are the classical syndromes of alexia with and without agraphia. Benson noted that most patients with Broca's aphasia have more difficulty with reading than with auditory comprehension.

Neurolinguists have developed a different classification of reading disorders based on mechanisms of the

Table 19-3. Language Features of Alexias

Feature	Alexia With Agraphia	Pure Alexia
Spontaneous speech	Mildly paraphasic	Intact
Naming	Often impaired	Normal except for colors
Comprehension	May be mildly impaired	Intact
Repetition	Intact	Intact
Reading	Poor	Poor; letter reading may be spared
Writing	Poor	Intact

disorder itself rather than on the pattern of associated language disorders or location of the responsible lesions. **Deep dyslexia** implies a defect in the basic reading process or the conversion of printed graphemes to spoken phonemes. The characteristics of the reading disorder in deep dyslexia include the inability to read nonwords, semantic and visual errors in reading words (*boat* for *schooner* or *perform* for *perfume*), and marked effects of word class and word "imageability" on reading performance. Nouns and verbs are generally read better than adjectives, adverbs, and prepositions, and concrete nouns, whose referents can be visualized, are more likely to be read correctly than abstract nouns. These patients appear to read more by direct recognition of familiar words or access of the semantic system directly from orthography (spelling) than by conversion of the grapheme into a phoneme and then into the semantic system. Most deep dyslexic patients have large left hemisphere lesions and significant aphasia of mixed or Broca's type.

A second alexia syndrome is **phonological dyslexia**, which is similar to deep dyslexia except that the reading of single-content words may be nearly normal, and semantic errors are rare. Reading of nonwords is difficult, as in deep dyslexia. In this syndrome, patients may be able to read aloud not only by recognition of the words' meaning but also by a process of conversion of words to phonemes (lexical–phonological route). However, conversion of individual graphemes to phonemes is still defective.

A third seemingly opposite type of dyslexia is **surface dyslexia**. This syndrome occurs in patients who can read phonetically by grapheme-to-phoneme conversion but cannot recognize words directly. In this syndrome, words of irregular spelling, such as *yacht* or *colonel*, are particularly difficult. This is a rare syndrome that has been reported in patients with anterior left hemisphere lesions.

A fourth neurolinguistic alexia syndrome, **letter-by-letter reading**, is synonymous with the syndrome of pure alexia without agraphia (see section on alexia without agraphia), in which patients have recovered enough reading ability to read letters and to spell words aloud letter by letter.

AGRAPHIA: NEUROLOGY OF WRITING

Writing, a basic element of language, is often disrupted in aphasic syndromes. The classical syndrome of **pure agraphia** affects patients with minimal or no aphasic deficits other than inability to write. The diagnosis of pure agraphia requires that the failure to write not be explainable by simple motor deficit (hemiparesis), apraxia (discussed later), or visuospatial difficulties. Lesions of pure agraphia are commonly found in the left superior frontal region, although left parietal lesions have been reported to cause pure agraphia as well.

Agraphia is divided into phonological and lexical types, corresponding to the process of writing by producing a whole word from the semantic meaning (lexical pathway) or by production of the phoneme and then derivation of the corresponding graphemes (phonological pathway). A patient with phonological agraphia can write common words from dictation but cannot write dictated nonword phonemes. The spontaneous writing of such a patient contains semantic errors or production of words of meaning that is similar but spelling that is dissimilar to the target word. There is also a preference for concrete over abstract nouns and both nouns and verbs over prepositions, adjectives, and adverbs. Phonological agraphia thus bears a close resemblance to the pattern of deep dyslexia, but the two deficits do not necessarily affect the same patient. In the other type of agraphia, **lexical agraphia**, the patient can write nonwords to dictation but cannot write irregularly spelled words and is confused by words of the same sound but different spelling (homophones). The clinical syndromes of phonological and lexical agraphia are still in an investigational stage in terms of correlation with lesion localizations, other aphasia phenomena, and practical use in rehabilitative therapy.

APRAXIAS: NEUROLOGY OF LEARNED MOVEMENT

Apraxia is a disorder of learned motor acts not caused by paralysis, incoordination, sensory deficit, or lack of understanding of the desired movement. In practical terms, apraxia is inability to carry out skilled motor acts to command when it can be demonstrated that the patient understands the command and can perform the same motor act in a different context (Geschwind, 1975; Kirshner, 1992). Liepmann, a 19th-century German physician, described three types of apraxia: **ideomotor apraxia**, **ideational apraxia**, and **limb kinetic apraxia**.

It is important to differentiate several diverse motor phenomena commonly confused with principal varieties of apraxia. These include constructional, dressing, oculomotor, and gait apraxia. **Constructional apraxia**, which is characterized by visuospatial difficulties, is associated with right hemispheric lesion. These patients may be unable to construct or copy a drawing of simple items (e.g., a clock or house). In most instances, this deficit is related to neglect of the left side of space or failure to appreciate the spatial relations of items, not to a motor planning deficit. In **dressing apraxia**, associated with right hemisphere lesions, the patients have difficulty with the spatial perception of the garment in relation to the body, and the difficulty is not a true motor apraxic deficit. **Oculomotor apraxia** refers to a difficulty with voluntary direction of the eyes in gaze and is associated with damage to the brainstem mechanism for control of eye movements. **Gait apraxia** refers to inability to walk that is not clearly explained by primary motor weakness, ataxia, or sensory loss. There is no easy way to demonstrate that the same sequential actions can be performed normally in a different context, and therefore it is unclear whether this gait disorder is a true apraxia. Perhaps even more problematic is speech apraxia, discussed in the section on apraxia of speech. Whether speech apraxia is a true apraxia is debated by aphasiologists.

Ideomotor Apraxia

Ideomotor apraxia refers to the failure to carry out a motor act in response to a verbal command when the patient understands the command and has the motor capacity to perform the same motor act under a different context. By Liepmann's model, the idea of the movement, decoded in Wernicke's area, is disconnected from its execution in the premotor cortex of the frontal lobe. Ideomotor apraxia often accompanies aphasia in patients with left hemisphere lesions (Geschwind, 1975). In published series, only a small percentage of patients with ideomotor apraxia have right-sided lesions. A high percentage of patients with aphasia and left-hemisphere lesions have ideomotor apraxia, whereas a much smaller percentage of nonaphasic patients with left-hemisphere lesions demonstrate such apraxia (DeRenzi et al., 1980). Patients typically fail to carry out the test act to verbal command, perform only slightly better in imitation of the examiner, but carry out the act almost normally if given the actual object.

According to the anatomical model of Liepmann, later modified by Geschwind, a lesion in the left temporal lobe, which also causes aphasia, prevents information regarding the desired act from reaching the left premotor area. Thus, ideomotor apraxia may be part of the deficit in Wernicke's aphasia, but the impairment of comprehension makes it questionable whether the patient has understood the command.

In conduction aphasia and Broca's aphasia, there may be associated ideomotor apraxia that interferes with the carrying out of commands with limbs on either side of the body. Finally, lesions of the corpus callosum can prevent motor information from reaching the right hemisphere motor area. This callosal apraxia affects movement of the left limbs. The existence of callosal apraxia implies that the left hemisphere is dominant not only for speech but also for learned motor acts, because the right hemisphere cannot program the movement independently.

This association of aphasia and apraxia may reflect the underlying symbolic nature of both speech and gestural expression, or it may simply reflect the anatomical contiguity of centers for speech–language function and those for learned motor acts. The association between apraxia and aphasia explains why most aphasia patients cannot learn complex linguistic gestural systems, such as American Sign Language.

Ideational Apraxia

Ideational apraxia is an even more complex phenomenon than ideomotor apraxia. There are two competing definitions of the term. First, some authors use it to mean apraxia for real objects. Ochipa and colleagues (1989) described a patient who could name objects but not demonstrate their use, as if he had lost the concept of what the object was for (apraxia for tool use). The second definition of ideational apraxia is loss of the ability to carry out a multistep activity, although each individual step may be performed appropriately. For example, a patient may not be able to fill, light, and smoke a pipe. This type of apraxia may reflect motor planning difficulty seen in frontal lobe lesions. It may also simply be a more sensitive test for apraxia than single motor commands.

Limb-Kinetic Apraxia

The third of Liepmann's types of apraxia is limb-kinetic apraxia, a deficit of fine motor acts involving only one limb. Patients with mild pyramidal tract lesions may not be weak in gross limb movements but may have difficulty with rapid or fine movements of the fingers. Such apraxia may be a sign of a partial corticospinal tract lesion with mild weakness.

AGNOSIAS: NEUROLOGY OF RECOGNITION

Agnosias are disorders of recognition. Most affect a single sensory system (visual, auditory, or tactile agnosia), while others involve selected classes of items within a modality (prosopagnosia, or agnosia for faces). In each case, the patient must be shown to have normal primary sensory perception, normal ability to name the item once it is recognized, and no general cognitive deterioration or dementia. For example, the patient with visual agnosia may fail to recognize a key ring by sight but identify and name it from the sound of the keys jingling or from the feel of the keys in his or her hand. Each sensory modality carries a somewhat arbitrary division between primary sensory cortical deficits and agnosia. Most agnosias require bilateral cortical lesions, cutting off input from the sensory modality to the left hemisphere language centers.

In the visual system, bilateral occipital lesions may cause cortical blindness. More partial lesions, however, may permit primary visual perception of the elements of an object or picture, such that the patient can even draw lines or angles representing the item but cannot identify the item. Shown a bicycle, the patient may report two circles and identify it as eyeglasses. Prosopagnosia, or failure to identify faces, is a subtype of visual agnosia in which patients cannot recognize family members or friends, though they can describe features such as hair color, a mustache or beard, or items such as hats or glasses. Frequently, the prosopagnostic patient identifies the person by voice or gait pattern. Oliver Sacks described prosopagnosia in "The Man who Mistook His Wife for a Hat."

Auditory agnosias also overlap with the syndrome of cortical deafness, resulting from bilateral lesions of the temporal cortex. Some patients with bilateral temporal lobe lesions have preserved pure tone hearing but cannot understand spoken language or repeat: pure word deafness. Geschwind postulated that pure word deafness results from a bilateral disconnection of the input from the primary auditory cortex (Heschl's gyrus) to Wernicke's area in the left hemisphere. More rarely, patients show preserved auditory comprehension but impaired nonverbal auditory recognition, for example identification of animal sounds or the characteristic sounds associated with objects such as bells and whistles. This deficit is called auditory nonverbal agnosia.

In the tactile modality, parietal lesions often disrupt the identification of objects by feel, a deficit called astereognosis. If the patient can describe the sensory characteristics of an object but not identify it, this can also qualify as tactile agnosia. Rare patients with bilateral parietal lesions have no ability to recognize objects by touch on either side.

DEMENTIAS: NEUROLOGY OF COGNITION

Dementia is defined as a gradual deterioration of previously intact cognitive functions secondary to diffuse rather than focal brain disease. The *Diagnostic and Statistical Manual of Mental Disorders*, fourth edition (DSM-IV), commonly used by psychiatrists, defines dementia in terms of memory loss and at least two additional cognitive functions, such as language, visuospatial functioning, or apraxia. Although the pattern of cognitive deterioration varies, memory loss is usually the first symptom, and other deficits follow. Tests of language function frequently show deficient naming, although fluency of spontaneous speech and repetition remains normal. In later stages, reading, writing, and auditory comprehension begin to deteriorate. Patients may evolve from an initial deficit of anomic aphasia to a pattern resembling Wernicke's or transcortical sensory aphasia. Other cortical deficits, such as apraxia and acalculia, are frequently present.

In contrast to this common pattern of language dissolution in dementing illness, which is typical of Alzheimer's disease, is a less common pattern in which focal deficits predominate early in the illness. For example, cases of primary progressive aphasia have apparently focal aphasic deficits that gradually progress over years. Some patients fail to show memory loss or other cognitive deficits for years post onset. Mesulam and colleagues first called this syndrome primary progressive aphasia, but more recent studies have placed this presentation within a broader category of frontotemporal dementia (discussed later in the chapter).

Dementia can be caused by any of a multitude of diseases. Three major groups of conditions cause dementia: systemic diseases, primarily involving organ systems outside the central nervous system; neurological diseases, marked by degeneration of other systems than the higher cortical functions; and diseases presenting primarily with loss of cognitive faculties.

Dementias Secondary to Systemic Diseases

Most of the dementia-causing systemic diseases are listed in Table 19-4. Because most of these conditions are treatable, identifying them is essential. Many metabolic disorders, which include disturbances of electrolytes such as hyponatremia, failure of the liver or kidneys, and calcium disturbances, present with an acute confusional state rather than chronic dementia. Toxic disorders include effects of chemical and heavy metal toxins, alcohol, and drugs. Chronic alcohol ingestion coupled with poor nutrition may cause symptoms of thiamine deficiency, Wernicke-Korsakoff syndrome. Technically, this syndrome is pure amnesia (loss of memory) rather than dementia, but there is evidence that chronic alcohol abusers may develop true dementia as well. Among toxins, prescribed drugs are among the most

Table 19-4. Systemic Diseases Associated with Dementia

Metabolic disorders
    Low sodium, low calcium; high calcium, aluminum
    Renal, hepatic, pulmonary failure
    Dialysis dementia
Nutritional
    Vitamin B_1, B_{12} deficiency, pellagra
Endocrine
    Hypothyroidism, hyperthyroidism, Cushing's, hyperparathyroidism
Toxic
    Heavy metals, organic compounds
    Drugs, polypharmacy, alcoholism
Infections
    Neurosyphilis
    Chronic meningitis: bacterial, fungal, tuberculous
    Parasitic diseases
    Sequelae of viral meningitis
    Subacute sclerosing panencephalitis
    Progressive multifocal leukoencephalopathy
    Creutzfeldt-Jakob disease
    AIDS dementia complex
Vascular diseases
    Multi-infarct dementia, Binswanger's disease
    Multiple cholesterol emboli
    Collagen vascular diseases, vasculitis
    Arteriovenous malformations
Neoplasms
    Brain tumor, increased intracranial pressure
    Multiple metastatic tumors
    Neoplastic meningitis
    Chemotherapy, radiation toxicity
    Limbic encephalitis

common treatable causes of dementia. Sedative effects of multiple medications may combine to cause chronic mental impairment. A few drugs cause confusional states when used alone; for example, anticholinergic effects of drugs such as tricyclic antidepressants, antihistamines, and neuroleptics may produce anticholinergic encephalopathy. A nutritional cause of dementia is vitamin B_{12} deficiency.

Infections are a relatively infrequent but important cause of dementia. The most treatable cause is infectious meningitis. Viral encephalitis is a more acute syndrome that may leave dementia in its wake. Dementia is also an aspect of AIDS. Although some patients have secondary infections and tumors affecting the nervous system, the HIV agent itself appears to cause chronic encephalitis resulting in dementia (AIDS dementia complex). Multiple strokes can also cause dementia.

Neurological Diseases Associated With Dementia

The second group of dementias involves neurological diseases that lead to cognitive deterioration. Normal-pressure hydrocephalus and basal ganglia diseases are the most common examples. Normal-pressure hydrocephalus is characterized by the gradual onset of mental slowing and then frank dementia, gait difficulty, and urinary incontinence. Brain imaging studies show dilation of the cerebral ventricles out of proportion to the degree of brain atrophy. Some cases respond dramatically to shunting procedures in which spinal fluid is rerouted from the cerebral ventricles into the abdomen, with return of mental function and improved gait and urinary continence.

Several diseases that affect the basal ganglia also produce a pattern of subcortical dementia. The most common is Parkinson's disease, which is characterized by bradykinesia (slowed movement), rigidity, resting tremor, masklike or impassive face, and dysarthric speech. Patients exhibit slowed mental processes.

Another neurological disease not considered primarily dementia is multiple sclerosis. Recent studies that have included neuropsychological test batteries have found that most patients with chronic multiple sclerosis have significant cognitive impairments. There is some suggestion from recent studies that multiple sclerosis plaques in the deep periventricular white matter, seen frequently on MRI in these patients, may correlate better with cognitive and mood disturbances than with physical disability. Dementia also occurs in some cases of Huntington's disease, progressive supranuclear palsy, and Wilson's disease.

Primary Degenerative Dementias

A few diseases primarily cause slowly progressive dementia. Alzheimer's disease is the most common, accounting for 50 to 60% of a random series of autopsied cases of dementia. The disease is defined by the presence of senile plaques in the neuropil of the cerebral cortex and neurofibrillary tangles (silver-staining strands) in the neurons of the cerebral cortex, hippocampus, and nucleus basalis of Meynert. The pathology of Alzheimer's disease is difficult to separate from that of normal aging of the brain, and recent studies have found that nearly 50% of people older than 80 years meet the clinical criteria for dementia (Evans et al., 1989). Careful examination and testing for treatable factors, as discussed earlier, are therefore essential for diagnosing Alzheimer's disease. Although many drug therapies are being tested in Alzheimer's disease, the ultimate cause of the neuronal degeneration and curative treatment remain to be discovered. Genetic defects have been found to underlie some early-onset cases of Alzheimer's disease, and a gene for the apolipoprotein E4 appears to increase the likelihood of development of the sporadic disease. Recently, drugs that block the acetylcholinesterase enzyme have been found to improve memory in patients with Alzheimer's disease. The drugs tacrine (Cognex), donepezil (Aricept), rivastigmine (Exelon), and galantamine (Reminyl) are the first agents to show clear benefit to patients with Alzheimer's disease. Other promising therapies include antioxidants such as Vitamin E, nonsteroidal anti-inflammatory drugs, and estrogen hormones, though recent trials of prednisone, nonsteroidal anti-inflammatory agents, and estrogen hormones have been disappointing.

Pick's disease is a similar but less frequent disease that has a predilection for the frontal and temporal lobes, often beginning unilaterally. The findings include silver-staining intraneuronal inclusions called Pick's bodies but few or no senile plaques and neurofibrillary tangles, which are seen in Alzheimer's disease. Pick's disease may be clinically indistinguishable from Alzheimer's disease, but many cases present with focal frontal lobe syndromes or isolated aphasia before progressing to general dementia.

Pick's disease is now considered to be part of a family of diseases called frontotemporal dementia, in which selective degeneration of the frontal and temporal lobes on one or both sides of the brain atrophy. Patients may present with progressive aphasia, usually of nonfluent type, or with behavioral disturbances similar to those already mentioned in the section on frontal lobe syndromes. A minority of patients also develop motor neuron disease. The syndrome of primary progressive aphasia, referred to earlier, is rarely secondary to Alzheimer's disease but can be considered a part of the spectrum of frontotemporal dementia. Disorders underlying this syndrome include Pick's disease, nonspecific neuronal loss and gliosis, and corticobasal degeneration. Some familial cases of frontotemporal dementia are associated with a gene defect on chromosome 17.

Another recent addition to the list of diseases causing dementia is diffuse Lewy body disease. It has been known for some years that some patients with Parkinson's disease become demented over the course of the disease, but some patients show cognitive deficits and hallucinations early in the course, when motor symptoms are mild. These patients tend to be older at onset than patients with idiopathic Parkinson's disease, and their progression is more rapid. At autopsy, the Lewy inclusion bodies found in the basal ganglia of patients with Parkinson's disease are widespread throughout the brain.

Creutzfeldt-Jakob disease is a rapidly progressive syndrome characterized by mood changes, dementia, seizures, myoclonus, and exaggerated startle responses. The course progresses from first symptoms to death in 6 to 12 months or less. The disease is rare; there is one case per million people per year worldwide. Creutzfeldt-Jakob disease is interesting because it was found to be transmitted by inoculation of tissues via contaminated surgical instruments, corneal transplants, and pituitary extracts. A variant of this disease is bovine spongiform encephalopathy (BSE), or mad cow disease, which has been transmitted by beef from infected British cattle.

TRAUMATIC BRAIN INJURY

Traumatic brain injury is a major cause of death and disability, particularly in young people. An acute blow to the head may cause instantaneous loss of consciousness and a brief period of retrograde amnesia, such that the patient does not remember the blow that caused the loss of consciousness. The term *cerebral concussion* implies a head injury with a brief loss of consciousness and brief retrograde amnesia but no other evidence of structural disruption of the brain. A great deal of research has concentrated on these minor head injuries and the resultant postconcussive syndrome. Such patients have normal brain imaging studies, including skull radiographs, CT, MRI, and electroencephalograms. Patients frequently complain of headaches, poor concentration and memory, insomnia, irritability, mood swings, and sometimes vertigo or dizziness.

More severe brain injuries may initially cause coma and evidence of contusion or bruising of the brain, shear hemorrhages into the brain tissue, or pooling of blood in the subdural or extradural space. Such patients are more severely impaired than patients with concussive injuries, and they frequently have motor deficits as well as impaired cognition. These patients commonly require prolonged rehabilitation, first in inpatient and later outpatient settings. Impaired memory and attention are common accompaniments, as are frontal lobe syndromes, such as impulsive or agitated behavior. In terms of language, high-level impairments are frequently found, especially in the organization of discourse.

SUMMARY

This chapter covers the functional organization of the human cerebral cortex and the principal syndromes of abnormal cortical functioning resulting from brain diseases. The emphasis throughout has been on speech and language disorders, including related disorders such as apraxia, agnosia, dementia, and traumatic brain injury. These topics constitute the part of neurology increasingly known as behavioral neurology or cognitive neuroscience.

Technical Terms

acalculia	dysarthria
agnosia	hemianopsias
agraphia	hemiparesis
alexia	hippocampus
Alzheimer's disease	hyperparathyroidism
amygdala	hyponatremia
anosognosia	metastasis
aphasia	myasthenia gravis
apraxia	neologisms
ataxia	neurofibrillary tangles
concussion	paraphasias
contusion	planum temporale
dementia	

Review Questions

1. Define the following terms:

acalculia	dementia
agraphia	dysarthria
alexia	hyponatremia
Alzheimer's disease	metastasis
amygdala	neologisms
apraxia	neurofibrillary tangles
ataxia	paraphasias

2. Name the higher mental functions for which left or right cerebral dominance has been established. Also describe the associated brain area.
3. Discuss the higher mental functions of each cerebral lobe.
4. Differentiate among dementia, aphasia, apraxia, and dysarthria.
5. Discuss common types of dysarthrias and list their clinical symptoms.
6. Differentiate between ideomotor and ideational types of apraxia.
7. Describe the clinical characteristics of the major types of aphasia.
8. Describe how word deafness differs from Wernicke's aphasia.
9. Describe the cognitive and linguistic features of dementia, and name common dementia-causing diseases.
10. Describe the major types of alexia and discuss their characteristics.

20

Orientation to Diagnostic Techniques and Neurological Concepts

Learning Objectives

After studying this chapter, students should be able to do the following:

- Explain common brain imaging techniques
- Describe the basics and significance of each brain imaging technique
- Explain the sodium Amytal infusion technique used for assessing cerebral dominance
- Explain the mechanism of electromyography and its clinical significance
- Discuss the mechanism of electroencephalography and its clinical value
- Describe the physiology of sleep and explain associated patterns of brain activity
- Discuss the concept of evoked potential technique
- Describe the functional aspect of the dichotic listening paradigm
- Explain common neurosurgical procedures and their treatment purposes
- Discuss the neurolinguistic significance of surgical procedures, such as corticography, subcortical implant, and stereotaxic surgery
- Discuss myopathic, neuropathic, and seizure disorders
- Explain common patterns of inheritance and genetic disorders

An array of diagnostic techniques and medical concepts apply to the management of neurologically impaired patients. Addressing or even listing all of them is beyond the scope of this chapter; only the most relevant clinical concepts, treatment procedures, and diagnostic techniques relating to the management of patients with neurological and neurolinguistic impairments are discussed.

BRAIN IMAGING

Brain imaging is the use of neuroradiological techniques to evaluate normal and abnormal brain struc-

tures. Since the beginning of the 20th century, imaging of the brain has progressed; however, the most major developments have taken place only within the past 2 decades. The earlier imaging techniques involved the use of ionizing radiation (x-rays) and consisted of applications such as **plain radiography, pneumoencephalography**, and **cerebral angiography**. Newer imaging techniques, not limited to x-rays, include **magnetic, radionuclide**, and **isotope technologies**. Each technique provides a different perspective of the live brain tissue and differs in terms of its tissue resolution.

Among the older techniques, pneumoencephalography, which is not included in the discussion here, was particularly invasive. It evaluated not only the ventricular cavity but also some characteristics of cerebral morphological distortion, mass effect, and the flow of cerebrospinal fluid (CSF). Cerebral angiography, another older invasive technique, is highly useful for providing morphological evaluation of the cerebral vasculature and establishing some understanding of cerebral blood flow dynamics.

Among the newer techniques, **computed tomography (CT)** has been in use since the late 1970s. It uses x-rays to display sectional brain anatomy with the aid of computer technology. More recently, development in **magnetic resonance technology** has spawned a number of exciting tools, such as **magnetic resonance imaging (MRI), functional magnetic resonance imaging (fMRI), magnetic resonance spectroscopy (MRS), magnetization transfer techniques**, and **perfusion- or diffusion-weighted imaging**. These newer methods of evaluation provide a clearer and more detailed view of the cerebral morphology and various aspects of brain function and internal physiological environment. **Regional cerebral blood flow (rCBF), single photon emission computed tomography (SPECT)**, and positron emission tomography (PET) employ the use of radioactive tracers or isotopes to evaluate some facet of brain function.

Cerebral Angiography

Among the earliest radiological techniques, cerebral angiography is still an excellent tool for evaluating the cerebral vascular structure. It is used to diagnose vascular disorders, such as atherosclerotic disease, aneurysms, and arteriovenous malformations. This procedure is invasive and is therefore associated with a significant risk factor, primarily stroke. When appropriately used, however, it can provide invaluable clinical information for planning medical and surgical treatment.

Cerebral angiography is frequently performed in a dedicated angiography suite designed solely for this procedure. Arterial access must first be established, commonly via a puncture of the common femoral artery. However, sometimes the carotid and axillary arteries or even the abdominal aorta is used, depending on the accessible route and the patient's condition. The selected artery, usually the femoral artery at the groin, is punctured. A catheter is inserted into the artery and guided by fluoroscopy to the arch of the aorta and then to the carotid or vertebral artery. Once the catheter is in place, a radiopaque contrast substance is injected into the catheterized artery. This is followed by a series of radiographs at various angles. The images taken early in the process depict the filling of the lumens of the injected arteries. The radiopaque material can outline the major (anterior, posterior, and middle) cerebral arteries; many smaller arteries may not be distinguishable, although some often appear (Fig. 20-1). Filming is continued to distinguish the opacifying capillary bed and the cerebral venous anatomy. Finally, the course of the contrast bolus is followed as it assumes the path of flowing blood, starting in the arterial phase and proceeding to the capillary and venous phases. The ability to visualize the pattern and extent of the opacified vasculature helps identify various arterial pathologies, such as thrombosis, hemorrhages, aneurysms (localized arterial dilation), and mass effect (irregularly displaced vessels). **Thrombosis** reveals little or no arterial filling beyond the blockage point, although this finding is not frequently demonstrable (Fig. 20-2). Other findings include poor capillary contrast staining

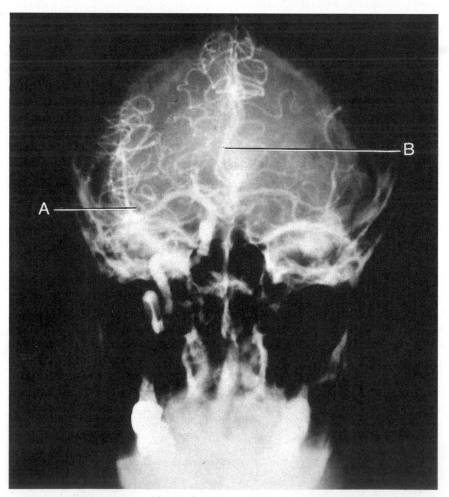

Figure 20-1. Normal carotid angiogram, anteroposterior view illustrating important arteries: middle cerebral artery branches (**A**) and anterior cerebral artery branches (**B**).

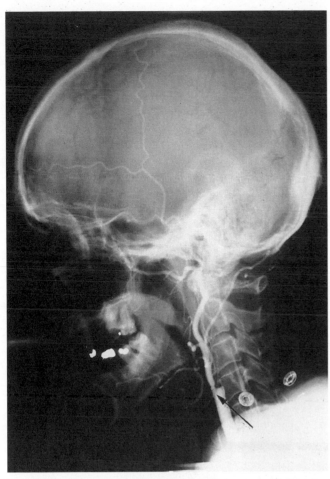

Figure 20-2. Angiogram, lateral view. Left internal carotid artery thrombosis (arrow), because there is no filling of internal carotid artery beyond its bifurcation from external carotid artery.

indicating early draining veins or retrograde arterial filling. Unfortunately, the paucity of angiographic findings does not exclude the diagnosis of thrombosis, and the presence of angiographic findings are not specific for this process. In the case of a **hemorrhage**, there is rarely an extravasation of injected dye with massive bleeding at the time of the study, although most cerebral hematomas are angiographically identified by their mass effect on the surrounding vessels and the relative paucity of the contrast staining. Local vascular dilation indicates **aneurysm**, whereas large feeding arteries, small clustered nidus, and dilated tortuous draining veins indicate arteriovenous malformations. Arterial displacement, which reflects mass effect, can also suggest brain tumor or a process outside the brain but inside the skull, such as a **subdural hematoma.**

Digital subtraction is a newer development in cerebral angiography. A computer is used to gather, digitize, and process the information from the radiograph, rather than simply allowing it to form a direct shadow on the film. This provides many advantages related to the ability to manipulate the accumulated data with computers. For instance, the contrast-filled lumen of the arteries can be rendered more conspicuous by subtracting the overlying bony structures, which would show up on routine plain radiographs. In digital subtraction, contrast medium is released into the artery through a catheter, after which a series of radiographs are taken and fed into a computer. The computer subtracts the images taken before the artery was outlined from the images taken after the introduction of contrast material. The acquisition speed and processing of the angiographic data present numerous advantages in the evaluation and display of the information, but the stunning advances are modulated by some disadvantages. For example, the improved contrast resolution of digital subtraction angiography is countered by the lower spatial resolution relative to conventional plain film angiography. Most modern-day angiography suites, however, are digital, and manufacturers continue to improve the spatial resolution. Digital substraction angiography requires a lesser amount of contrast than its conventional version. Further, it allows the evaluation of vessels in multiple projections.

Computed Tomography

Developed in the early 1970s, CT is considered to be a major breakthrough in brain imaging. For the first time, it allowed direct demonstration of brain structures without intracranial invasion. CT uses a narrow beam of x-rays to examine the head and brain in a series of thin slices. The newer generation of CT examines brain slices that are about 1 or 2 mm thick. The x-ray beam rotates around the head and passes through the brain. On the other side of the head, the transmitted radiation is recorded by a series of detectors that measure quality and quantity of the x-ray beams emerging from the head. Each image is displayed with varying shades of white, gray, and black to correlate with various areas of x-ray attenuation. The data of absorbed x-ray particles (photons) are processed by a computer, which creates a two-dimensional image of a particular slice the of brain based on a mathematical calculation of the x-ray data reaching the detectors. A number of strategies and techniques are used by various manufacturers to create this mathematical two-dimensional representation of the brain, but the theoretical cornerstone is the work of British senior research scientist G. N. Hounsfield, who was awarded the Nobel Prize in 1973.

CT diagnosis is based on detecting variations from the norms of x-ray particle absorption by brain structures (Fig. 20-3A). While it is common for a nonradiologist to relate the absorption of x-rays to the density of the material imaged, this is an oversimplified explanation of a complex phenomenon that is more accurately related to photon energy and the multiple types of interactions with electrons. For example, skull bones and blood are higher in density constructs and absorb more x-ray particles; thus, their computer-generated image appears mostly in the white range. White and gray matter and the fluid-filled ventricles are less dense and attenuate fewer x-ray

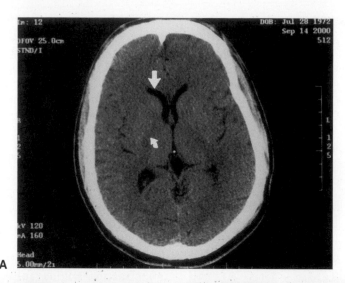

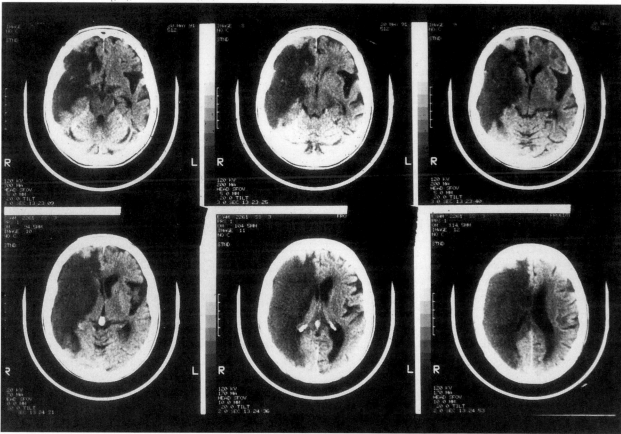

Figure 20-3. **A.** Axial CT of the normal brain. The lower density of the fluid-filled anterior horns of the lateral ventricle (*straight arrow*) can be clearly distinguished from the adjacent brain parenchyma. The basal ganglia (*curved arrow*) is also visible. **B.** An x-ray CT depicting a massive infarct in right hemisphere involving frontal, parietal, and occipital lobes.

particles, so their images are assigned a darker shade. Based on photon absorption coefficiencies, intracranial lesions are in general either **high-** or **low-density lesions**. High-density intracranial lesions especially significant to students in communicative disorders are acute hemorrhages and aneurysms. Important low-density lesions are cerebral chronic infarction, edema, and cystic lesions ((Fig. 20-3*B*). Tumors may be either high or low density. In the early days of CT, scientists hoped to characterize

cerebral pathology according to density measurements alone, but this was rapidly abandoned, as almost every disease entity proved to be a dynamic process that displayed a whole range of x-ray attenuation profiles, depending on the disease stage and other complicating factors. There is, however, an inaccurate but understandably persistent tendency to characterize lesions solely according to their density on CT.

Various radiopaque compounds are injected to

characterize pathological processes and to demonstrate certain vascular anatomy. The contrast-enhancing agents are injected into the intravascular space, which becomes more conspicuous because of the greater attenuation of x-rays by the contrast. However, some but not all pathological conditions show contrast staining as a result of a breakdown of the blood-brain barrier, allowing seepage of contrast from the intravascular compartment into the cerebral tissues. In addition, contrast enhancement in some pathological states only occurs during a certain stage of the disease.

CT has been used extensively in neurolinguistics for studying brain behavior relationships. In an excellent description of CT, Gado and colleagues (1979) provided a comprehensive framework for relating brain anatomy on CT with language regions and Brodmann areas. Thereafter, Naeser and Hayward (1987), Naeser and colleagues (1981, 1982), Damasio (1991) and many others used CT to demonstrate anatomical correlations for classical aphasias. Alexander and associates (1987) used CT to demonstrate the existence of subcortical aphasias.

Magnetic Resonance Imaging

MRI does not use any ionizing radiation or hazardous x-rays. Rather, it creates images by measuring the magnetic activities of the atomic nuclei of hydrogen, a strong resonator in brain tissue. Water is one of the main components of the body, and each water molecule contains two hydrogen nuclei. Body tissues differ in their water content. Without any external interference, the magnetic activity of hydrogen atoms is random, as one cell cancels the activity of another cell. Placement of the brain in a large external magnetic field (which is the foundation of the MRI procedure) causes the hydrogen atoms of brain tissues to align in a single plane. When arranged in such a manner, they conform to the external magnetic field, producing a strong magnet. The transmission of signals from an external radio frequency transmitter provides extra energy to these aligned hydrogen atoms, resonating and perturbing them to rearrange themselves in a different plane, depending on the tissue type. When the externally administered radio frequency signal ends, the hydrogen atoms return to the previous orientation. However, before returning to the magnetic field orientation, they discharge their electromagnetic signals. These radio frequency signals from the hydrogen atoms are collected by the computer and converted into shades of gray, black, and white. These shades represent different strengths of signals, creating images that correspond to differences in relaxation. Since bone contains limited water, it produces very few signals relative to the other cerebral structures (Fig. 20-4). The nuances of brain tissue characteristics are better demonstrated by MRI than by CT (Fig 20-5). Because gray matter contains more water than white matter, there is a remarkable difference between the images of

each. MRI has become the standard in the evaluation of many neurological disorders and so has also been used extensively in neurolinguistic investigations.

Advances in magnetic resonance techniques have allowed for the development of applications that evaluate brain function or physiology. Functional MRI, a new and promising technique, is capable of detecting changes in regional blood oxygen levels associated with cortical neuronal activity in time. This allows for precise mapping of a variety of brain functions by activating specific areas of the brain through appropriate stimuli and/or tasks. The creative application of carefully designed tasks or stimuli allows neuroradiologists to observe the differences in the activated brain regions from listening to Mozart to smelling roses. This tool not only is important to investigation of normal or basic brain function in vivo but also is a valuable source of information to guide

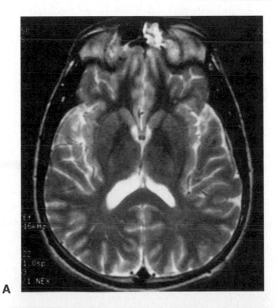

A

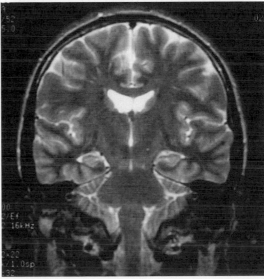

B

Figure 20-4. **A.** Normal T2 weighted (FSE) axial MRI of the brain; an incidental small amount of left frontal sinus disease is present. **B.** Normal T2-weighted (FSE) coronal MRI of the brain.

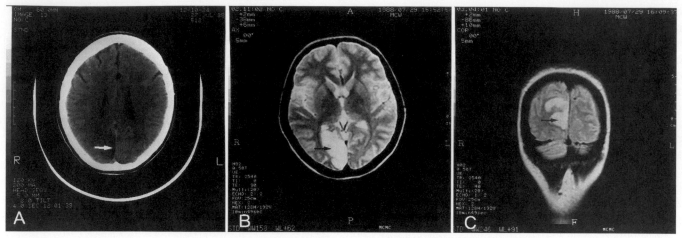

Figure 20-5. Three views of massive right occipital infarct in the same patient. **A.** X-ray CT. **B.** MRI, transverse view. **C.** MRI, coronal view.

treatment of pathological conditions. The localization of the sensorimotor cortex by fMRI has provided useful preoperative information to decrease the risk of paralysis from some cases of brain surgery.

MRI spectroscopy, another new application, uses the MRI scanner to evaluate the biochemical profile of a particular area of a sampled brain. In other words, the technique provides a biochemical fingerprint of the brain. MRI spectroscopy has been useful both in the study of basic brain biochemistry and clinically to evaluate diagnostically difficult cases in which brain morphology is normal but metabolism is abnormal. MRI spectroscopy is frequently used in conjunction with routine MRI imaging.

Magnetic resonance angiography is a new way of diagnosing vascular diseases by evaluating the vessels in different projections. It incorporates the principle of time of flight (TOF) where the signal is obtained from the blood moving within the vessels. The TOF imaging requires no contrast substance and is noninvasive. Contrast (gadolinium) bolus dynamic gradient echo magnetic resonance imaging is another way of evaluating the vessels. It uses intravenous contrast injection to enhance the signal to noise ratio and contributes to a better visualization of the vessels.

Regional Cerebral Blood Flow

rCBF measures the flow of blood to functionally active brain areas by monitoring a radioactive tracer. The principle underlying regional cerebral blood flow is that brain areas responsible for performing activities require increased blood flow. This increased blood flow is needed for the additional metabolic energy required by the tissue. rCBF was the first technique that revealed the dynamics of the functional brain. The technique for assessing cerebral blood flow entails the use of xenon-133, a radioactive isotope of the inert gas xenon. The isotope is dissolved in a sterile saline solution that is injected into an artery or inhaled. The presentation and washout

(radiation attenuation) of the isotope solute are monitored using a γ-ray camera, which consists of multiple scintillation detectors. The camera measures attenuated radiation around the head. The information obtained from the solute is fed into a computer, which delineates different levels of blood flow with various colors and hues. Because blood flow and local metabolic activity are directly related, the images provide insights regarding which brain areas participate in various activities. In a detailed study of specific brain function and blood flow by Lassen and colleagues (1978), observations of blood flow that were not uniform throughout the brain reaffirmed the conviction that there is functional localization in the brain, a belief held by classical neurologists. The study further demonstrated that there is greater blood flow to the prefrontal cortex, even during rest. Furthermore, the right nondominant hemisphere exhibited greater functional participation in speech than previously thought, and the supplementary motor area was also important, primarily in dynamic motor activity.

Positron Emission Tomography

The most recent advancement in neuroimaging, PET assesses physiological changes in brain cells. It entails the following three steps: (*a*) tagging radioactive substances (positron isotopes) with one natural body substance (water molecules or glucose), (*b*) injecting tagged radionuclide into the body, and (*c*) measuring spatial distribution of positron (radiation) emitting radioisotopes and their dissipated energy. PET measures glucose and metabolized oxygen distribution by looking at nerve cells and cerebral blood flow. The radionuclide fluorodeoxyglucose has been commonly used for determining the local cerebral metabolic rate of glucose by brain cells to study cognitive, language, and speech functions. The principle underlying PET is that the collision of the injected positron with an electron leads to their mutual annihilation and results in the emission of two γ-rays (photons). The two rays travel in opposite directions (180° from each other). Detectors circling the brain locate these photons and feed their path into a computer that generates the images (Fig. 20-6). Because oxygen metabolism by cells reflects physiological functioning, PET allows study of brain physiology that reflects mental and sensorimotor functions.

Changes in types of information processing, which depend on the underlying cognitive activity, produce differential neuronal activity patterns in local regions of the brain. PET has been used to examine the physiology of brains in normal subjects and brain-damaged patients to determine neuroanatomical correlates of functions (Fig. 20-7). Studies of cellular glucose metabolisms in aphasic patients have repudiated the belief that there is a strict localization of functions in the brain. Rather, they demonstrated that focal brain pathology also affected the functions of distant brain regions. These distant metabolic changes were common in the prefrontal cortex, basal ganglia, and thalamus. For a better understanding of PET applications to neuroanatomical pathologies in aphasic patients, consult a series of publications by Mazziotta and

colleagues (1981, 1982), Metter and Hanson (1985), Metter and colleagues (1986), and Metter (1987).

PET is also used for the detection of abnormal brain tissue causing seizures or psychiatric disorders in which the metabolism of glucose is different from the rest of the brain. This localization of abnormal brain tissue provides important diagnostic information prior to surgery. In addition to functional imaging, PET is also used for identifying the limit and spread of tumor in the body and the brain. Since the tumor cells in general are marked with increased metabolism, the tumor affected area shows increased cellular activity, which is measured using fluorine-18 tagged deoxyglucose. This increased cellular metabolism provides information on the tumor spread and helps in planning treatment and in determining disease outcome.

Single Photon Emission Computed Tomography

SPECT is functionally similar to PET in some ways, although it provides fewer details. Generally known for a refined blood flow measurement, SPECT is performed

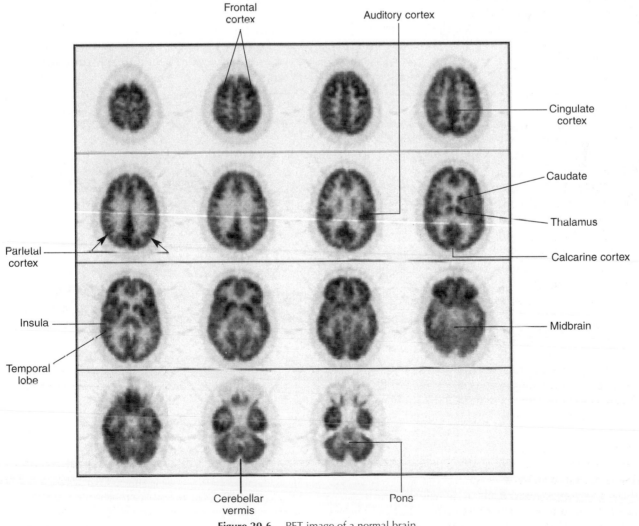

Figure 20-6.   PET image of a normal brain.

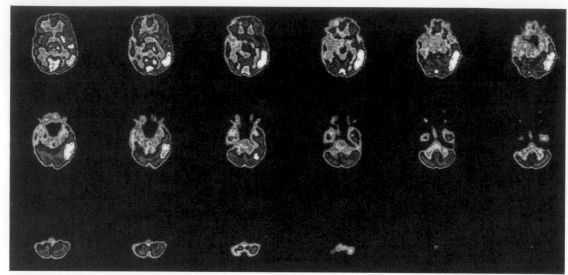

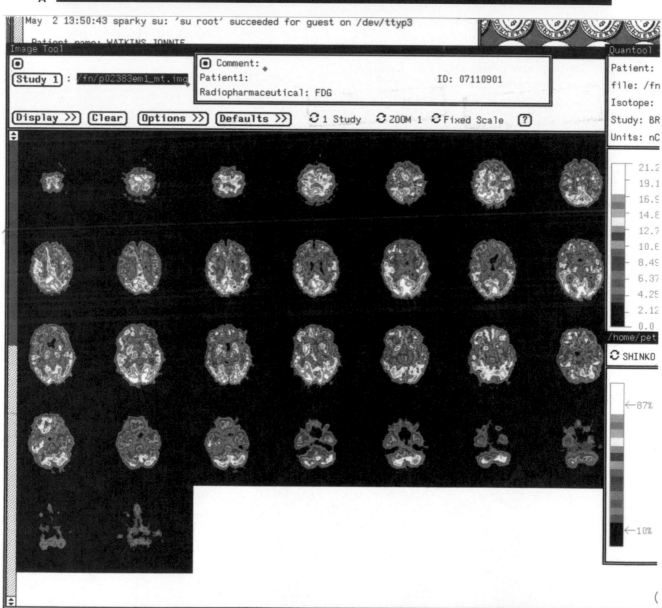

Figure 20-7. **A.** PET image exhibiting hypermetabolic activity in Wernicke's area and left inferior parietal lobule during a seizure. **B.** PET image indicating hypometabolism in bifrontal and bitemporal regions in a patient diagnosed with Pick's disease.

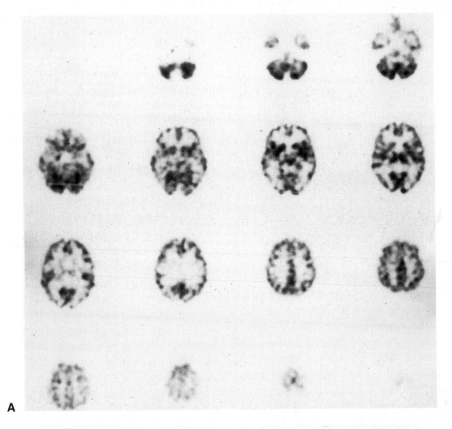

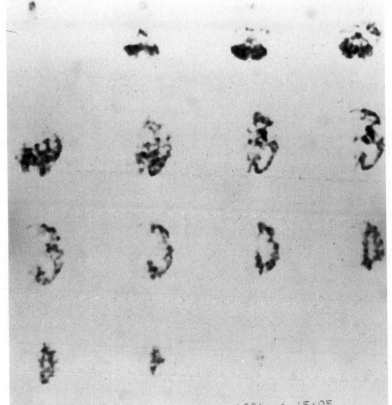

Figure 20-8.   **A.** Normal SPECT. **B.** SPECT of a stroke patient indicating decreased blood flow in right hemisphere.

after injection of a radiotracer substance tagged with a radiopharmaceutical. Tomographic techniques and a γ-detecting camera are used to measure the distribution of the radiopharmaceutical. Unlike PET, which involves dual photon emission, in SPECT the radiopharmaceutical substance emits a single γ-ray. By using the point of γ-emission and its trajectory, SPECT measures rCBF; it reconstructs data into three-dimensional images of blood flow in the brain (Fig. 20-8). Bhatnagar and colleagues (1989, 1990) and Tikofsky and Hellman (1991) have used SPECT to examine cognitive and language functions in neurosurgery and neurology patients.

SODIUM AMYTAL INFUSION FOR ASSESSING CEREBRAL DOMINANCE

Sodium Amytal infusion, also known as the Wada test, is a modified form of angiography used for determining cerebral dominance. The use of this technique began with the discovery of the surgical management of epilepsy and corticography undertaken at the Montreal Neurological Institute in 1940s and 1950s. Intracarotid injection of sodium amobarbital induces a functional loss in the injected hemisphere lasting 2 to 10 minutes. The underlying assumption of the test is that interruption of language functions after sodium Amytal infusion in either hemisphere should identify the hemisphere dominant for language. Sodium Amytal–based dominance assessment has been used in neurosurgical patients with intractable epilepsy. The drug is injected while the patient counts and maintains arms and fingers extended. As the drug anesthetizes one hemisphere, the contralateral arm becomes flaccid. Linguistic functions—ongoing counting and then confrontation naming—are also impaired if the injected hemisphere is dominant for language. This procedure has been extensively used for exploring the relationship between cerebral dominance and handedness. Do left-handed individuals have left cerebral dominance similar to right-handed individuals, or do they have a right-hemispheric or bilateral language and speech representation? When used to explore this relationship, the test confirmed that most right-handed persons have left-hemispheric dominance for speech (Table 20-1). However, so do most left-handed individuals. This test also revealed that a significant number of left-handed individuals also exhibit right-hemisphere language or their language is regulated by both left and right hemispheres (Wada and Rasmussen, 1960).

Table 20-1. Cerebral Dominance in Relation to Handedness Determined on Seizure Patients (Wada and Rasmussen, 1960)

Handedness	Total Cases	Left Hemisphere (%)	Right Hemisphere (%)	Bilateral (%)
Right	140	96	4	0
Left	122	70	15	15

ELECTROENCEPHALOGRAPHY

Brain cells normally generate electrical activity. The **electroencephalogram (EEG)** is a graphic representation of the potential differences between two separated points on the scalp surface that represent brain-transmitted electrical potentials or brain waves of the cortex below, specifically of the vertical pyramidal cells. The EEG has 8 to 16 channels for recording scalp-transmitted electrical activity. EEG brain wave recordings can be made simultaneously from the frontal, parietal, occipital, and temporal scalp areas. Comparisons can be made between corresponding areas of the two brain hemispheres and various areas within one hemisphere for evaluating symmetry in wave patterns, amplitudes, and durations.

Metal electrodes 5 to 10 mm in diameter are placed on the scalp for electrical recording. Eight basic points in the frontal, parietal, occipital, and temporal lobes are used in scalp recordings. In bipolar recordings, interconnecting electrodes are paired in the sagittal, transverse, and circular planes using the internationally standardized 10–20 system of electrode placement (Fig. 20-9). The earlobes and mastoid processes may be used as references for unipolar recordings.

Spontaneous cortical surface activity is generated from the fluctuating voltage differences between the apical and basal portion of cortical dendrites. The greatest voltages are found in areas containing masses of dendrites. EEG is an excellent diagnostic procedure for seizures. The dominant electrical brain activity appears to cluster within a few frequency ranges that are represented by Greek letters (Table 20-2). There is no specific frequency for specific brain regions, although the α-frequency tends to predominate in the occipital area.

The α-EEG frequency patterns represent normal cortical activity, predominantly in the posterior part of the brain. However, central and temporal regions may also have independent foci of α-rhythms. Eye opening and mental concentration usually suppress the α-activity. The fast frequencies of β-rhythms are present in the central and frontal areas. β-Activity has relatively low voltage, usually not more than 20 μV, while θ- and δ-activities are not frequent EEG patterns in normal subjects. The central brain areas may contain some θ-patterns, but they do not represent dominant EEG patterns. Brain potentials are measured in microvolts, and the waves may vary from 25 to 300 μV. A seizure may display 1000-μV discharge amplitudes. Frequencies are usually 0.5 to 35 cycles per second.

In normal conditions, the electrical patterns in homologous parasagittal areas are similar. In contrast, patterns in the two temporal areas are usually not synchronous. Abnormal brain wave patterns are usually irregular wave combination spikes of high voltage and varied frequencies. Focal discharge areas often display spike or sharp wave reversal patterns (see the section on

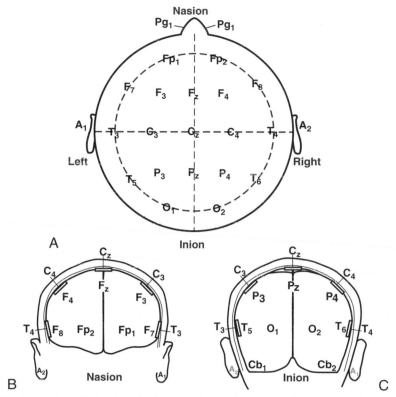

Figure 20-9. The international federation 10-20 electrode placement system for EEG recording. **A.** Dorsal view of head. **B.** Anterior view. **C.** Posterior view.

Table 20-2. Common Brain Wave Frequencies

Type	Range
Delta: generalized brain region	1–3
Theta: generalized brain region	4–7
Alpha: posterior cortex	8–13
Beta: anterior cortex	> 13

epilepsy). Similarly, asynchronized brain waves can be used to evaluate consciousness and reduced responsiveness of the brain (see the section on sleep).

The EEG is an excellent diagnostic tool to examine altered levels of consciousness, such as sleep, and to evaluate seizure disorders. However, in evaluation of seizures, problems arise in deciding when to perform the test. In some cases, such as grand mal seizures, it is impossible to run an EEG when the patient is having a seizure because of movement artifacts. Routine EEG tests undertaken between seizures may be positive for the diagnosis of seizures in only 70 to 80% of patients. Specific techniques are used to evoke transient seizures for diagnostic reasons. Specific seizure-evoking methods are **hyperventilation, photic stimulation, sleep induction,** and **drug administration**.

Hyperventilation is used to activate the epileptic brain, which may be in a state of relative low excitability (quiescence). It is most effective for evoking abnormal

discharges in patients with petit mal and psychomotor epilepsies. Photic stimulation, consisting of repeated flashes of light, can also elicit abnormal discharges in idiopathic epilepsy. An exaggerated response may occur in patients with a history of epilepsy. The response is most pronounced over the occipital and posterior parietal areas, especially in the α-frequencies. Sleep is effective for activating discharges in all forms of epilepsy and most productive in psychomotor epilepsy. In addition, sleep deprivation was found to elicit paroxysmal activity in epileptics.

ELECTROMYOGRAPHY

Electromyography is the visual record of muscular electrical activity during spontaneous and/or voluntary movements. During contraction, muscle fibers generate action potentials that represent the transmembrane current of muscle fibers. This electrical activity of muscles can be recorded by placing a small electrode on the skin surface over the muscle or by a needle inserted into the muscle.

Electromyography is used to diagnose diseases of the nerves or muscles (muscular atrophy, myoneural junction disorder, and denervation) when clinical evidence is absent or equivocal or must be confirmed. An examination of the quality, speed, and magnitude of electrical impulses in muscles can help detect nerve or mus-

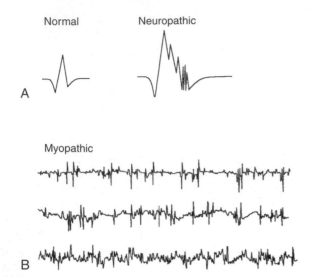

Figure 20-10. **A.** Normal motor action potentials have at least two phases. This phasic profile is altered in neuropathic lesions, which are characterized by high amplitude, long duration, and polyphasic motor unit action potentials. **B.** Myopathic lesions produce polyphasic motor action potentials with small amplitude and short duration.

cle damage (Fig. 20-10). It can also differentiate among muscle disease (myopathy), atrophy of spinal motor neurons (neuropathy), interruption of the nerve supply (denervation), and neuromuscular (myoneural) problems.

Muscle pathologies are determined by comparisons made with normal patterns of muscle electrical activities. For example, there is no electrical activity in a normally functioning muscle during rest. In addition, the electrical potentials that result from the nerve irritation consequent to electrode insertion do not last more than about a second in normal muscle tissues. However, in denervated (interrupted nerve) muscle fibers, there is spontaneous electrical activity, and the insertional potentials can last a long time. Furthermore, denervation produces high-frequency polyphasic discharges, fibrillations, and fasciculations. In paralyzed and atrophied muscle, there is no spontaneous electrical activity. In cases of muscle weakness due to myopathy (muscular disease) or neuropathy (motor neuron disease), low-amplitude, short-lasting motor unit potentials, fibrillation, and fasciculations are usually seen. Fibrillation is spontaneous action potentials of a single muscle fiber, whereas fasciculation is spontaneous discharge from an entire motor unit. Patients with neuromuscular junction disorders may exhibit one of the two following patterns: (*a*) progressively increasing motor unit action potentials with repetitive stimulation of the motor nerve, as in the case of presynaptic impairment or (*b*) gradually decreased response of muscle action potential with repetitive nerve stimulation, as in cases of postsynaptic myoneural junction disease.

Nerve conduction studies are used to identify disorders in the transmission of impulses to muscles. A peripheral nerve along its course is stimulated, and the resultant electrical activity from the muscle is recorded. The amplitude, speed, and direction of impulse conduction provide important clinical information. Measuring the amplitude of subsequent motor responses provides information about the number of muscle fibers activated, whereas recording nerve impulses at two points along the nerve helps determine the speed (velocity) of the nerve impulse and the time the impulse transmission takes. In denervating diseases, impulse transmission is slow.

EVOKED POTENTIALS

Evoked potentials are the normal electrical activities of the central nervous system (CNS) that occur in response to specific and controlled sensory stimulation. Whether the sensory stimulus is **visual**, **somatosensory**, or **auditory**, evoked brain responses are recorded using electrodes referred to the spinal cord, brainstem, and scalp. The amplitude of the evoked brain responses is quite small, ranging from 1 to 5 μV. The evoked activity can easily be obscured by the large magnitude of spontaneous electrical activity in the brain. To delineate the evoked potentials from spontaneous background activity, **signal averaging** is used: multiple responses to a single repeated stimulus are summated, averaged, and amplified by a computer. Through averaging, the time-locked evoked activity is incrementally measured from the background CNS activity, which as a random noise has a mean of zero and therefore cancels itself out in the averaging process. A careful analysis of the latency and amplitude of the evoked response peaks provides significant information about the physiology of neural pathways and the possible pathology sites in the CNS.

Visual Evoked Potential

Visual evoked potentials are used to evaluate electrical conduction along the optic nerve, optic tract, lateral geniculate, optic radiations, and visual cortex. The eye is stimulated with flashes of light, and electrical components of the visual response are recorded in the occipital area. Abnormalities of latencies, amplitudes, and wave patterns may occur in response to abnormalities at specific anatomical sites of electrical transmission.

Somatosensory Evoked Potential

Somatosensory evoked responses are elicited through the simulation of a contralateral peripheral nerve, such as the median nerve. Electric potentials that result from stimulation of the nerve are recorded from electrodes on the scalp. The intensity of the stimulation used is just below the parameters that elicit a thumb twitch. The latency of the wave gradually increases with distance from the primary sensory area. However, delayed latency or diminished amplitude of sensory evoked potentials indicates peripheral and CNS diseases. The lesion may be in the nerves, nerve roots, or spinal cord. Clinical conditions in which somatosensory evoked potentials have diagnostic value include multiple sclerosis, head injuries, brain death, posterior column spinal cord lesions, and lesions of the peripheral nerves.

Auditory Evoked Potential

Auditory evoked response audiometry is the electrophysiological assessment of auditory functions. It measures responses in the form of neural activity in the auditory system and pathway (eighth nerve, pons, and ascending pathway) in response to the controlled presentation of acoustic stimuli, primarily clicks but also tones and speech sounds. Evoked-response audiometry is used to assess the functioning of the auditory neural pathway to predict hearing thresholds in patients who are difficult to test and to help identify the site of dysfunction in the auditory system.

In evoked-response audiometry, the most commonly measured response is the **auditory brainstem response** (**brainstem auditory evoked response**). This is a test of synchronous neural firings from the brainstem auditory pathway that occurs within 10 to 12 msec of stimulus onset. Five positive wave patterns identified from the vertex represent the electrical activity produced in the auditory pathway (Fig. 20-11). Wave response classes appear to represent a specific anatomical point in the auditory pathway (Table 20-3). For example, wave I appears to arise from the peripheral and distal fibers of cranial nerve (CN) VIII; wave II, from the proximal or brainstem portion of the CN VIII; wave III, from the first brainstem synapse, including the cochlear complex and trapezoid body; and waves IV and V, from the auditory pathway to the midbrain, including the lateral lemniscus and inferior colliculus. The additional wave patterns are anatomically undermined. The first two wave responses arise ipsilateral to the stimulus, while wave III and later represent bilateral auditory stimuli.

Testing reveals the absolute latencies of all of the waves, interpeak latency intervals, and the amplitudes of the waves. The altered latency of evoked waves from a stimulus indicates audiological disorders. The fifth peak is the most prominent, and the threshold of this wave is found to correlate well with behavioral hearing thresholds. Latencies of waves I to V at various stimulus intensities and interwave latencies (i.e., I–V, I–II, II–V) are used to assess the auditory functioning of the brainstem. This can provide important information regarding possible sites of lesion.

Altered wave patterns and peak latencies indicate retrocochlear lesions. For example, a tumor implicating CN VIII will either abolish wave pattern I and II or produce a prolonged interpeak latency between waves I

and III. Prolonged interpeak latencies and abnormal waveforms are commonly seen in multiple sclerosis, a demyelinating condition. However, if all wave patterns except the first are absent or abnormal, a structural brainstem abnormality is likely to be the cause.

DICHOTIC LISTENING

Commonly used for assessing cerebral dominance, dichotic listening is a noninvasive neuropsychological tool that uses auditory stimuli. It involves presenting simultaneous but slightly different auditory stimuli to both ears. The attention factors are minimized by requiring subjects to attend to both ears simultaneously and report the stimuli they perceive. When the linguistic material presented in both ears is largely similar and spoken in the same voice, attending to the stimuli from both ears poses processing difficulties. Even though an equal number of words is presented, subjects do not demonstrate a twofold gain, which would account for each item presented to both ears. Instead, the total stimuli reported from both ears range from 125 to 150%. Loss of information has been invariably greater for stimuli presented to the left and supposedly nondominant ear by 20 to 25%. This results in a natural right-ear advantage. This left-ear-specific loss of linguistic information and right-ear superiority were investigated in the pioneering work of Kimura in the 1960s. She attributed the right-ear advantage to its direct anatomical projections to the left hemisphere, which is dominant for language and speech (Fig. 20-12). The indirect anatomical projection to the language cortex accounts for the left-ear-specific information loss. The neurolinguistic implications of these findings are that right-ear performance can serve as an index for determining degrees of language lateralization. Strong support for the stronger contralateral auditory projections in dichotic listening came when the dichotic test results were validated by the observation of the left language lateralization by hemispheric infusion of sodium amobarbital.

LUMBAR PUNCTURE

The lumbar puncture (spinal tap) is used for diagnosing various infections and hemorrhages of the CNS that are not observable through CT. Chemical analysis of CSF also helps in the differential diagnosis of **multiple sclerosis**, **neurosyphilis**, **Guillain-Barré syndrome**, **carcinomatous meningitis**, and **neuropathies**. Lumbar puncture is contraindicated in cases of increased intracranial pressure because of the possibility of a brainstem herniation.

In lumbar puncture, a needle is inserted into the lumbar subarachnoid space while the patient leans forward (recumbent position) or lies on his or her side. The puncture is usually made between the third and fourth lumbar vertebrae because spinal penetration at this

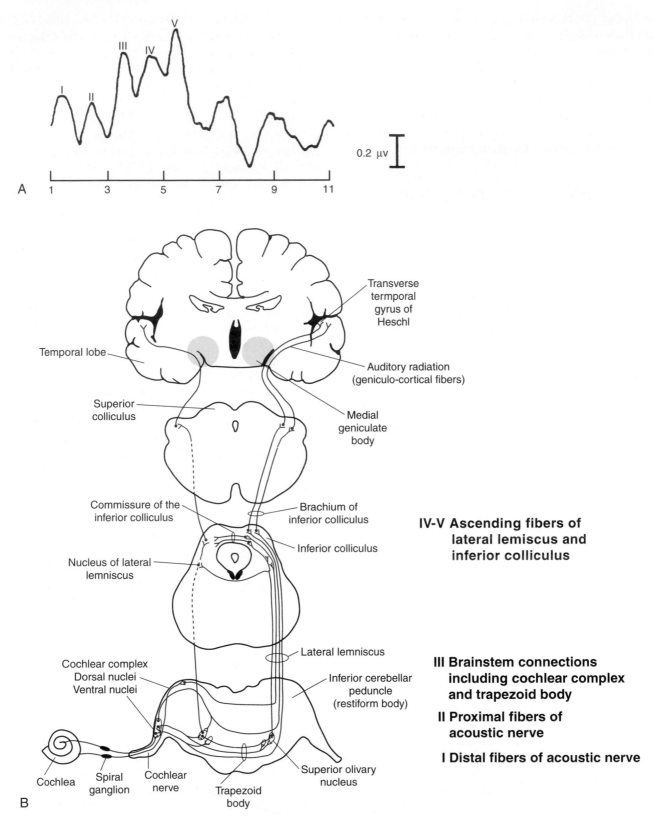

Figure 20-11. **A.** Normal brainstem auditory evoked responses within 10 msec from onset of clicks. **B.** Anatomical levels (Roman numerals) of auditory pathway have been implicated with brainstem response wave patterns.

point does not cause any injury to nerve fibers. Once the CSF starts flowing, the needle hub is attached to a manometer. The normal pressure in an adult is 80 to 150 mm H_2O, which may rise to 200 mm H_2O with the person seated. Increased intracranial pressure occurs in response to increased amounts of CSF, brain swelling, and brain tumor. A pressure level higher than normal suggests a pathological process. Ventricular pressure can also be measured by other invasive methods, such as inserting a catheter into the lateral ventricles.

NEUROSURGICAL PROCEDURES

Craniotomy, or Cortical Mapping

Craniotomy, a neurosurgical procedure, is undertaken to remove diseased brain tissue. Cortical stimulation brain mapping is used to avoid damaging sensorimotor and speech–language areas during cortical resections for seizures, tumors, and aneurysms.

Focal external electric stimulation is based on early observations by Fritsch and Hitzig (1870) and Bartholow (1874), who found that electric current externally applied to the exposed brain altered sensorimotor functions in animals and humans. After the safety and reliability of focal stimulation were established, stimulation mapping became a standard part of surgical treat-

ment for medically intractable epilepsy and was used to map the somatosensory cortex and to chart the human brain for memory and language at the Montreal Neurological Institute (Penfield and Roberts, 1959). Completed under local anesthesia while the patients remained awake, focal stimulation was used first to determine the stimulation threshold that produced after-discharges and second to determine whether the diseased part of the brain was critical for language and sensorimotor functions. Since many language functions take place around the diseased part of the brain, mapping of language in and around the area of pathology helps neurosurgeons determine whether it is safe to remove the diseased cortical tissues without any unacceptable loss primarily of higher mental functions (speech, language, and memory) and secondarily of sensorimotor functions. This mapping also helps determine the size and extent of the tissue that can be safely resected. As a rule of thumb, no tissue resection is undertaken from the somatosensory area in the frontoparietotemporal cortex unless there is preexisting hemiplegia or the diseased tissue is not involved with language.

In the post-Penfield era this technique has been extensively used to treat patients with epilepsy and in surgical management of other conditions, such as tumors and arteriovenous malformations. The focal stimulation acts like a reversible lesion of the brain ranging from 4 to 8 seconds; its interruption lasts only the duration of the applied current. Furthermore, the stimulation-induced interruption provides the most precise details about functional localization, since the lesion is only 0.5 to 3 mm in diameter. Also, it is not known to leave any lingering effect and/or postoperative aphasia. Carefully controlled stimulation parameters pose no safety concern to patients, cause no injury to the examined brain tissue, and produce no evidence of acute inflammation to the mapped region of the brain. Multiple samples of a single behavior from a single site allow for the necessary

Table 20-3. Five Peaks of Waves of Auditory Brainstem Response and Their Probable Site of Origin

Wave Number	Probable Site of Wave Pattern
I	Distal fibers of cranial nerve VIII
II	Proximal fibers of cranial nerve VIII
III	Brainstem connections including cochlear complex and trapezoid body
IV–V	Ascending fibers of the lateral lemniscus and inferior colliculus

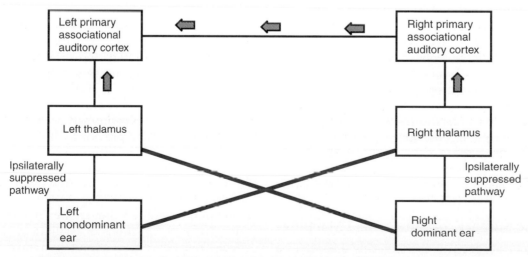

Figure 20-12. Anatomical model of ear projections to auditory cortex in a dichotic listening task.

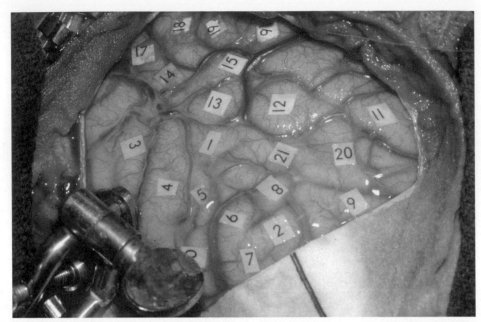

Figure 20-13. Exposed brain during electrocorticography. Numbered tickets mark sites that were functionally mapped during intraoperative neurolinguistic testing. Many of the numbered sites were implicated with language and memory functions.

statistical analysis and can help to determine whether the evoked linguistic errors are significant.

Interpretation of the physiological effects of focal stimulation is based on the interference it produces during ongoing activity. For example, if stimulation at a cortical site disrupts ongoing naming or speaking, the cortical area in question is considered to be functional for the task (Fig. 20-13). If the stimulation does not block or alter the naming or speaking process, the stimulated area is not considered to be involved in the ongoing activity. While evoking distant effects of the applied stimulation remains a possibility, the low current levels (below sensorimotor threshold) rule out any distant propagation of the current. The short duration of the applied current trains to the brain, however, is the only limitation of the technique. This operation is performed under local anesthesia to maintain a conscious patient who can participate in neurolinguistic testing. The patient answers questions while the cortex is stimulated with a bipolar electrode for a brief period. Stimulated areas that disrupt speech and/or produce motor movements are avoided during the resection of the lesion. This procedure of focal electric stimulation has been extensively used for mapping the language cortex in humans (Penfield and Roberts, 1959; Ojemann and Whitaker, 1978; Ojemann, 1983, 1992; Andy and Bhatnagar, 1983; Bhatnagar et al. 2000).

Stereotactic Surgery, or Subcortical Mapping

Stereotactic surgery involves placing a lesion or a stimulus electrode at a precise subcortical location to manage involuntary movements and intractable pain. The subcortical brain structures are mapped by electrical stimulation for guidance while the patient is under local anesthesia. Mapping optimizes the beneficial results from the involvement of normal structures. Two examples of stereotactic surgery are: (*a*) A lesion in the subthalamus or the ventrolateral nucleus of the thalamus is used to treat parkinsonian tremor., (*b*) A lesion in the globus pallidus is used in treatment of a parkinsonian tremor and rigidity.

Investigators have recently examined the subcortical participation in speech, language, and verbal memory by stimulating discrete subcortical areas through depth electrodes. Ojemann (1983) found that application of stimulation parameters, below threshold for induced language disturbance during a left thalamotomy, facilitated verbal recall. He attributed this facilitatory effect on the registration and recall of verbal stimuli to the thalamic evoked **alerting response mechanism** to verbal stimuli. Bhatnagar and colleagues (1989) noted a similar facilitatory effect on verbal memory from stimulation of the left centrum medianum, a neurolinguistically unexplored and previously unimplicated intralaminar thalamic nucleus with rich cortical and subcortical projections. Recently, Bhatnagar and colleagues (1990) have also found a similar, though quantitatively different, facilitatory effect on verbal memory from the stimulation of the right centromedianus nucleus of the thalamus. These observations of facilitatory neurolinguistic effects from subcortical stimulation have opened a new avenue of research.

Cordotomy

Cordotomy, a procedure used relatively infrequently, involves sectioning the lateral spinothalamic tract to relieve chronic pain; it is performed when medication proves ineffective. The operation is performed under local anesthesia so that the patient can tell the surgeon when the pain is relieved and in which part of the body it is no longer felt. The ventrolateral spinothalamic tract of the cord is sectioned on the side opposite to the painful body part (see Chapter 7 for the pathway mediating pain and temperature). The sectioning is performed three segments above the top segment level of pain. The spinal cord attachments of the dentate ligament are used as a reference point for sectioning the cord. They mark the plane between the overlying pyramidal tract and the underlying spinothalamic pain-conducting tract to be sectioned. The level of the sectioning is usually in the thoracic spinal cord for pain below the dermatomal nipple line. The cervical spinal cord is sectioned to eliminate pain in the upper extremities, shoulders, and neck.

Internal Carotid–External Carotid Anastomosis

A decrease in blood supply to the cortex and subcortical structures occurs when a blood vessel is occluded by a thrombosis, caused by either an embolus or local sclerotic plaque. As the blood supply is impeded, brain tissue distal to the thrombus loses function. Restoration of blood supply is performed by anastomosing the distal segment of the occluded artery to the superficial temporal artery. This surgery is performed through a craniotomy. At present, the benefits of this procedure are doubtful. It is used only with selected patients.

Carotid Endarterectomy

Occlusive sclerotic plaques are usually found at the region of common carotid bifurcation. Carotid endarterectomy is most frequently performed for occlusions of the common and/or internal carotid arteries. Carotid clamps are used for temporary occlusion of the vessel above and below the level of the thrombus. The thrombotic plaque is removed surgically through an incision overlying the thrombosed arterial site. The sclerotic plaque, which lines the inside of the vessel and occludes it, is removed by scraping it away from the inner vessel wall. The incision in the vessel wall is sutured after the plaque is removed; the temporary blood vessel clamps are released, and blood flow is reestablished.

Aneurysm Clipping

An aneurysm is a bulging defect of the blood vessel wall that looks like a protruding nipple or balloon attached to the vessel. Aneurysms that hemorrhage or cause neurological deficits and seizures require immediate attention. The medical management of an aneurysm involves lowering blood pressure to prevent bleeding; clipping is used to obliterate the neck or the attachment of the aneurysm to the blood vessels, thus disabling it. Aneurysms are also treated without opening the skull through coiling, which involves placing a platinum coil in the aneurysm. This coil causes a blood clot to form, sealing off the aneurysm.

GENETIC INHERITANCE

The way in which we pass our attributes to our children is the subject of genetics. What we know about inheritance and genetic transmission can be traced to the late-19th-century work of Gregor Mendel, who observed several patterns of inherited traits by examining the mating of different-colored flowers in and pea plants.

Genes regulates the formation, distribution, and cellular growth in an embryo. This genetic blueprint is received from both parents at the time of conception. After passing through mitotic and meiotic divisions, each parental germ cell (oogonia and spermatogonia) contains 22 somatic chromosomes and one sex chromosome (see Chapter 5). At conception, cells from the two parents combine their genetic code to form a zygote that contains 44 (22 + 22) autosomal chromosomes and X and Y sex chromosomes. The genes consist of 6 billion to 7 billion base pairs of DNA arranged linearly in 23 pairs of chromosomes. Each coiled chromosome contains tens of thousands of genes. One or more pairs of genes received from the parents regulate most physical traits, such as height, hair color, body shape, aptitude, and others.

Among these thousands of genes, everyone carries a few dysfunctional genes. Some diseases are caused by one faulty gene (**dominant inheritance**), and some morbid conditions occur when a defective gene comes from both parents (**recessive inheritance**). There is no immunity against genetic illness, and large numbers of serious disorders are associated with chromosome abnormalities. Chromosomal errors occur primarily during the formation of germ cells, when meiotic processes reduce chromosomes to the haploid number 23 and a gamete cell ends up with an extra chromosome resulting in trisomy. Most trisomies cause severe developmental deficits. **Down's syndrome** is the most common type of trisomy. Incidentally, most severe genetic malformations result in spontaneous abortions. Errors of genetic inheritance also have implications for altered physiological functions, such as metabolic, endocrine, and neurological diseases.

Tracing the distribution of genes in the extended family is an important concept in understanding inheritance. Researchers use standard symbols to construct pedigrees, charts used in genetics to analyze inheritance and to show ancestral history (Fig. 20-14).

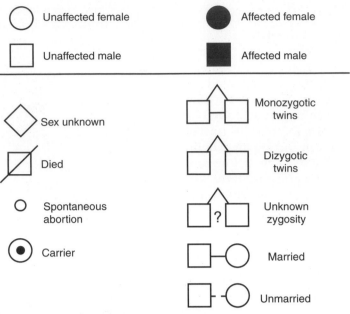

Figure 20-14. Pedigree chart.

Gregor Mendel related his observations to the mathematical probability of inheritance. Most mathematical patterns of gene expression are calculated on the basis of gene penetration. However, if the gene is not fully penetrated, the genetic traits may not follow the exact mathematical pattern. There are three common modes of genetic inheritance: dominant, recessive, and X-linked.

Dominant Inheritance

Even a single faulty gene can pass on a dominant autosomal genetic disease (Fig. 20-15). A child receives this kind of disease if he or she has one parent with the disorder. The defective gene dominates the gene from the other parent with which it is paired. In these cases, there is a 50% probability for each child to inherit the disease. At the same time there is a 50% chance that the child will not receive the faulty gene. Diseases inherited through dominant genes exhibit various degrees of symptoms, with severity ranging from mild to moderate degrees, most appearing late in life. There are more than 2000 known dominant autosomal disorders, but the most pertinent to students in communicative disorders is Huntington's chorea, a progressive degenerative disease.

Recessive Inheritance

Recessive inheritance requires that both parents carry the faulty gene and transmit that gene to the child (Fig. 20-16). If one parent alone is a carrier of the dysfunctional gene, this gene is not likely to be harmful because it is dominated by the normal gene that is received

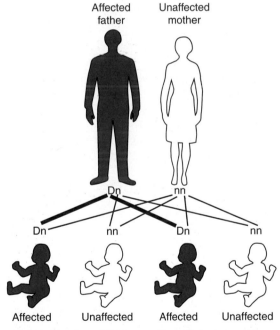

Figure 20-15. Dominant inheritance. One affected parent has a single faulty gene (D) that dominates its normal counterpart (n). Each child's chances of inheriting D or n from affected parent are 50%.

from the other parent. With so many genes passing from parents, it is quite rare for both parents to be affected with the same faulty gene; consequently, there is a low probability of this type of transmission. However, if a child receives a faulty gene from both parents, he or she is at risk for major birth defects. In such cases, each child has a 25% chance of inheriting the disease, a 25% chance of not inheriting the disease, and a 50% chance of re-

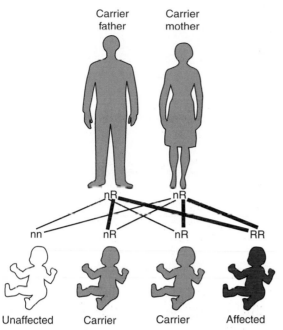

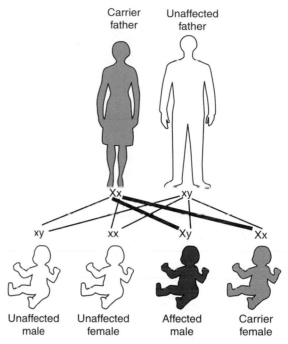

Figure 20-16. Recessive inheritance. Both parents, usually unaffected, carry a normal gene (n) that takes precedence over its faulty recessive counterpart (R). Each child's odds are (a) 25% risk of inheriting a double dose of mutant R genes that may cause a serious birth defect; (b) 25% chance of inheriting two n genes, being unaffected noncarrier; and (c) 50% chance of being an unaffected carrier.

Figure 20-17. Most common X-linked inheritance. Female chromosomes of unaffected mother carry one faulty gene (X) and one normal gene (x). Father has normal male X and Y chromosome complement. Each male child's odds are (a) 50% risk of inheriting faulty X and disorder; (b) 50% chance of inheriting normal X and Y chromosomes. Each female child's odds are (a) 50% risk of inheriting one faulty X gene, to be a carrier like mother; (b) 50% chance of inheriting no faulty gene.

ceiving the faulty gene from one parent, which would make the child a carrier of the dysfunctional gene. The child's probability of getting the autosomal recessive disorder is very high if the parents have common ancestors or are close relatives. Some well-known recessive disorders are cystic fibrosis and Tay-Sachs disease.

X-Linked Inheritance

Males and females carry different sex chromosomes, males have XY and females have XX. Consequently, a female may have a homogeneous gene on both X chromosomes, whereas a male cannot because he carries only one X chromosome. A fertilization of X (female) and X (male) results in a female child, whereas a fertilization of X (female) and Y (male) results in a male child.

X-linked inheritance involves genes situated in the X chromosomes. Generally, a mother carries a faulty gene in one of the X chromosomes (Fig. 20-17). In this case, a defective X chromosome appearing in a male child must have come from the mother because the father can only pass on a Y chromosome to the son.

If a girl receives a faulty X chromosome, it is dominated by the normal pair from the father. Overall, for each male child, this results in a 50% risk of inheriting the faulty gene and accompanying disorder, and for each female, it results in a 50% risk of inheriting the faulty gene (X) and not exhibiting the disease but becoming a carrier like the mother. Obiviously, no male-

to-male transmission of a faulty X gene occurs. Commonly known X-linked diseases are color blindness, hemophilia (blood clotting disorder), and Duchenne's muscular dystrophy.

SPECIFIC NEUROLOGICAL DISORDERS

Neurology is a highly clinical field that depends on careful observations of symptoms. It requires a solid knowledge of neuroanatomy to appraise symptoms clinically. Any alteration in neuronal functioning results in specific sensorimotor disturbances. Some of these disorders have been examined in the clinical information section in each chapter, but the disorders and medical concepts not previously covered are briefly discussed now.

Seizures and Epilepsy

Seizures are sensory, motor, cognitive, and affective disorders that result from abnormal electrical discharges in the brain (Fig. 20-18). Epilepsy refers to recurring seizures. Approximately 70 to 75% of seizures occur before age 20. More than 30% of them occur before age 4 or 5; they are mostly associated with high fever and may not be recurrent. The causative factors in 50% of seizure disorders are metabolic abnormalities, tumors, infarcts, infections, and physiological disturbances.

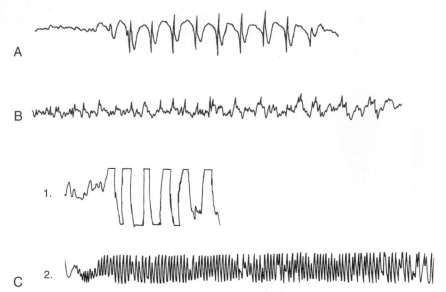

Figure 20-18. Electroencephalographic samples of high amplitude discharges and repeated spikes representing abnormal electrical activities in different types of seizures. **A.** Petite mal (absence) epilepsy in a 15-year-old boy. **B.** Psychomotor epilepsy. **C.** Grand mal (tonic–clonic) epilepsy with two frequency patterns.

Table 20-4. Classification of Seizures

Partial Seizures		Generalized	
Focal	Complex	Petit Mal	Grand Mal
Rhythmic spike and/or slow-wave focal discharges with sensorimotor, visceral and/or emotional symptoms	Abnormal electrical activity in amygdala, hippocampus, septum, mesodiencephalon, and association cortices with complex sensorimotor, visceral, emotional symptoms	Symmetrical 3-Hz spike and wave with brief episodes of automatisms	High-voltage spike and wave activities with varied frequencies and duration, usually associated with loss of consciousness and tonic-clonic movements

Among the remaining 50% of patients, no specific cause can be detected. Some factors that cause seizure disorders are **perinatal insult, trauma, anoxia, tumor,** and **metabolic disorders**.

In a normal brain, electrical activity is remarkably stable, and nerve membrane polarization and depolarization are delicately balanced. However, in epilepsy the brain's electrical activity becomes unstable. It is characterized by a prolonged high-frequency neuronal discharge, which represents rapid and excessive depolarization of membrane potentials (Fig. 20-18). The seizures occur when electrical activity in one or more brain structures rises above a critical threshold. Epileptic discharge can recruit neighboring and functionally related neuronal elements, and thus it replicates itself while spreading from one area to another. During the course of frequently recurring epileptic discharges, some neurons remain quiescent for varying periods, representing excessive depolarization (fatigue) or hyperpolarization (inhibition).

Epileptic seizures are commonly divided into two types: **partial** and **generalized**. Partial seizures are further divided into **partial focal (simple)** and **partial complex,** and generalized seizures may be either **petit mal (absence)** or **grand mal (tonic-clonic) seizures** (Table 20-4).

PARTIAL/FOCAL, OR SIMPLE, EPILEPSY

Partial/focal (elementary) epilepsy is usually caused by a single cortical or subcortical lesion. Symptoms are characterized by sudden onset of sensory and/or motor behaviors confined to a single body part such as the leg, arm, or face, depending on the lesion site. For example, a lesion in the motor cortex may generate jerking of the arm. Involvement of the sensory cortex causes altered sensory perception, such as numbness or tingling. Spread of the abnormal discharge activity to adjacent cortical areas recruits other body parts into the seizure. The progressive recruitment of other body parts is called the jacksonian march after the English neurologist who first described it. For example, a jacksonian seizure may start in the foot and spread to the lower leg, thigh, abdomen, shoulder, and arm. A jacksonian sensory spread may start as a tingling sensation in the thumb that spreads to the fingers, forearm, upper arm, and shoulder. An aura is a focal seizure characterized by a specific sensory experience that precedes the full-blown seizure. Auras are warnings of impending seizures. Patients generally remember the aura but do not remember the automatic behavior during the temporal lobe seizure that emanates from the amygdala and hippocampus. In some cases of focal epilepsy, medication may be effective. However, focal epilepsy usually responds best to localized surgical removal of the lesion and the surrounding seizing brain tissue.

PARTIAL COMPLEX, OR PSYCHOMOTOR, SEIZURES

Partial complex (psychomotor) seizures are due to congenital and postnatal lesions of the medial temporal lobe structures consisting of the amygdala, hippocampus, and overlying temporal cortex. These types of seizures, occurring most frequently in adults and older age groups, are characterized by recurring episodes of automatic, irrational behavior of which there usually is no memory. The individual is cognizant of neither the actions nor the consequences of them. In addition, the patient may have episodes of aggressive behavior. There are also notable cognitive deficits characterized by inattentiveness, unclear thinking, compulsive thoughts, sensory illusions, and apathy. These types of automatic behavior occur in complex partial seizures because the discharge spreads to the cortical association areas and thereby impairs the mechanisms of thought. The automatic actions represent programmed behaviors that are released from inhibition because they no longer are under direct control of the prefrontal associational cortex. In contrast, the premotor and primary sensorimotor cortices are spared. The emotional components of the automatism related to mood, sexuality, and aggression are generated in the hypothalamus and integrated with the cortically programmed behaviors at the level of the diencephalon and brainstem.

PETIT MAL, OR ABSENCE, SEIZURES

Petit mal (absence) seizures occur in children aged 3 to 12, and they usually disappear after the third decade of life. These seizures involve a brief loss of awareness and are often associated with staring, chewing, blinking, and occasional myoclonic jerks. A dominant familial predisposition is evident. The electrical discharge is primarily thought to involve a reverberating circuit between the cortex, thalamus, and brainstem reticular formation. The EEG brain wave pattern consists of a slow wave with spikes appearing at three per second. Drug therapy may control this type of seizure.

GRAND MAL, OR TONIC-CLONIC, SEIZURES

Grand mal (tonic-clonic) seizures usually involve the cortex, basal ganglia, diencephalon, and brainstem reticular formation. Symptoms of grand mal seizures include loss of consciousness followed by tonic convulsions consisting of repeated hyperextension of the body

Table 20-5. General Symptoms Associated with Tonic-Clonic Phases of Grand Mal Seizures

Tonic Phase	Clonic Phase
Unconsciousness	Alternate muscle relaxation
Falling to ground	Tongue biting
Spasticity in muscles	Salivation
Transient interruption of breathing	Turning blue

(tonic-clonic convulsions) and breath-holding spells resulting in cyanosis and tongue biting (Table 20-5). The average length of a tonic-clonic seizure is approximately 1 to 3 minutes. At the end of the seizure, the patient remains tired and listless for approximately an hour. During the seizure the EEG reveals high-frequency spikes.

A hereditary predisposition is thought to be the underlying substrate for grand mal epilepsy. The precipitating factors consist of strong emotional stimuli, hyperventilation, drugs, fever, infections, and physical stimuli such as loud noises and flashing lights. A grand mal seizure may last for several minutes before it stops completely. It is thought that two factors bring about the termination of these seizures: fatigue of the firing neurons and neuronal inhibition.

ANTIEPILEPTIC DRUGS

Diphenylhydantoin (phenytoin, or **Dilantin**), **phenobarbital**, and **carbamazepine** (**Tegretol**) are the three frequently used antiepileptic drugs. With these therapeutic drugs, there usually is a marked reduction of paroxysmal discharge, and consequently the seizures are controlled. Drug combinations are often used, especially in complex syndromes made up of two or more seizure types. If drug therapy is inadequate and if it is feasible, the discharging brain tissue is surgically removed.

Sleep and Altered Consciousness

As a diagnostic tool of cortical activity, the EEG is used to differentiate between altered states of consciousness such as **stupor**, **coma**, and **brain death**. It is also used to measure brain activity during **sleep**, which is another state of mind. The cerebral cortex, which is active during periods of wakefulness, controls sensorimotor activity through a stream of impulses that diminish during sleep. The cortical activity in the awakened state is regulated by the projections of the **reticular activating system** (**RAS**), which is responsible for cortical activation and arousal, and levels of consciousness. The RAS itself can be activated by any internal or external stimulus. Reduced activation of the RAS lowers consciousness and responsiveness (see Chapter 16).

Stupor is a level of significantly altered consciousness. Persons in stupor are minimally conscious and can be brought to a higher level of consciousness only through a strong stimulus, such as pain. Even after consciousness is regained, the individual may not fully participate in any activity and may lapse back into stupor. Coma, a deeper state of impaired consciousness, is a profoundly decreased level of wakefulness in which the patient remains unresponsive to painful stimuli and cannot be awakened. There is general amnesia for the duration of the coma in patients who recover. In case of brain death, the cerebral cortex is completely nonfunctional, while the brainstem reflexes—breathing and heartbeat control— may be preserved. Keeping such a person alive has become a bioethical issue and has been debated extensively.

Sleep, an active state of mind though different from wakefulness, is characterized by diminished responsiveness and is an important physiological state for replenishing body energy. Deprivation of sleep has been found to affect the quality of cortical functions and has been associated with difficulty in reasoning, attending, self-monitoring, and maintaining concentration. Sleep-deprived individuals are irritable and fatigued.

Normal sleep consists of two categories: **rapid eye movement (REM)** and **non–rapid eye movement (NREM)**. NREM sleep further consists of four (1–4) stages (Fig. 20-19). The EEG correlates of sleep are measured by the increased degree of the dominance of two slow waves, **theta** and **delta**, which become more and more synchronized as one enters the cycle of sleep.

One enters the REM and NREM stages many times during the sleep cycle. In the REM stage, the representative EEG pattern remains desynchronized, similar to the one seen in the awake stage (Fig. 20-20). It is characterized by mixed electric wave frequencies with θ- and decreased α-activity (1–2 cycles per second lower than waking). However, there is substantial inhibition of sensory systems and the motor neurons in the spinal cord and brainstem. This immobilizes skeletal muscles except for the muscles of eye and diaphragm. On one hand, the dominance of the parasympathetic system during REM slows down important body systems by lowering respiration, blood pressure, heartbeat, and body temperature. On the other hand, it increases gastric mobility.

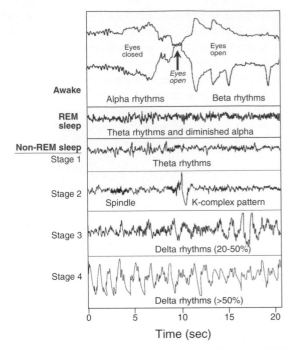

Figure 20-20. EEG rhythms during the stages of REM and NREM sleep.

Disconnected from the external stimuli during this stage, the CNS becomes sensitive to internally generated signals, as seen by the imagery experiences of dreams, which are accompanied by rapid movements of the eyes. Events like dreams, nightmare, erection, and bed wetting, of which individuals may not retain any memory, are known to occur at this stage.

The rest of sleep time is spent in NREM sleep, which is marked by a greater synchronization of electroencephalographic rhythms. In NREM sleep, muscle tension is significantly reduced, and movement, though possible, is minimal. This movement is usually limited to the movements that change body position, if needed. The energy consumption of the body remains low because of the dominance of the parasympathetic system. In terms of electrical functioning, the slow EEG rhythms with large amplitude represent the synchronized neuronal activity at this stage. During NREM sleep, a person progresses from stage 1 to stage 4; each of the stages is identified by a distinctive EEG pattern (Fig. 20-20). For example, stage 1, also called quiet wakefulness, is characterized by low-amplitude θ-EEG activity replacing the high-frequency α-wave pattern. The individual is fully relaxed, with eyes closed and fleeting thoughts. In terms of EEG activity, this stage is hard to distinguish from the REM stage. NREM stage 2 is marked by the emergence of short sharp bursts of α-waves, known as high-amplitude sleep spindles (12- to 14-Hz wave pattern) and K complexes in the presence of background θ-activity; the person at this stage is hard to awaken. NREM stage 3 is somewhat similar to stage 2, with 20 to 50% δ-activity

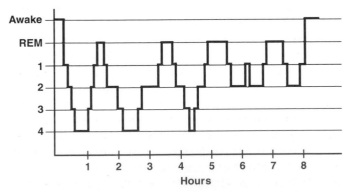

Figure 20-19. Time spent and stages of REM sleep.

and the sleeper in a state of extreme relaxation. Representing the deepest level of sleep, stage 4 is dominated by greater than 50% δ-electrical waves. The person at this stage is relaxed and difficult to awaken. Sleepwalking, sleep talking, and sleep terror are known to occur during δ-sleep, which includes stages 3 and 4. After progressing through these stages, one may reverse to different stages until reaching NREM stage 1 or REM level, completing the sleeping cycle. In a typical 7- to 8-hour sleep period, an individual alternates from NREM to REM stage about every 70 to 120 minutes. This cycle repeats about 3 to 5 times during the entire sleep period.

There are many sleep-related problems, such as disorders of initiating and maintaining sleep during normal sleeping periods, excessive daytime sleepiness, disorders of the sleep cycle, and dysfunctions associated with various stages of sleep. **Insomnia** (inability to initiate and maintain sleep during normal hours) is a common problem and is usually associated with such conditions as stress or emotional changes in life, most of which are temporary. **Hypersomnia**, or sleeping during normal waking hours, is caused by dysfunction of sleep. **Narcolepsy** is a common type of hypersomnia. In narcolepsy, which is inherited as an autosomal recessive trait, a person exhibits uncontrollable napping during the day. Other symptoms are cataplexy (brief loss of muscle tone with sudden emotional bursts), vivid hallucinations, and sleep paralysis, in which the patient appears awake but cannot move the limbs. One of the causes of hypersomnia is **obstructive sleep apnea**, in which excessive relaxation of the pharyngeal muscle closes the upper airway during sleep. In apnea, the person may stop breathing and awake in panic.

Toxic Encephalopathies

Encephalopathy refers to CNS dysfunctions that primarily result from impaired cellular metabolism. As discussed in Chapter 17, the metabolic functioning of the CNS depends on a consistent supply of oxygen and glucose supplied by blood. Any condition that interrupts this supply of glucose and oxygen to the brain can cause toxic or metabolic encephalopathy. The factors affecting brain metabolism can be intrinsic or extrinsic. Degenerative brain changes in Parkinson's, Huntington's, and Alzheimer's diseases are intrinsic factors, whereas externally introduced toxic agents and coagents are extrinsic factors.

The onset of toxic encephalopathy is usually gradual. Early signs include slowed cognitive processing, confusion, memory loss, impaired ability to communicate, difficulty finding words, depression, withdrawal, and indifference. In its advanced stages, these symptoms become more pronounced and include hallucinations, agitation, communicative breakdown, inattention, seizures, and coma.

Various conditions can alter the brain's metabolism and cause toxic encephalopathy. Persistent anoxia can severely affect the brain's oxygen supply. Both vascular and pulmonary diseases can contribute to anoxia. Lasting anoxia to the medulla depresses respiration and can be fatal. A depleted supply of glucose, as seen in **hypoglycemia**, and excessive concentration of blood sugar directly affect brain functioning. Also, **blood lead levels** greater than 40 mg per 100 mL cause lead poisoning, a condition common in children who live in old buildings with chipping lead paint. Manifestations of lead poisoning consist of hyperactivity, behavioral problems, psychomotor (lethargy) retardation, mental retardation, epilepsy, and neuropathy. Liver diseases and renal failure are the other causes of metabolic disturbances that can affect cognitive and sensorimotor functions and personality. Malnutrition and alcohol dependency are two of the most common causes of **thiamine deficiency** and can be seen in **Wernicke's** and **Korsakoff's encephalopathy**. However, in many instances, encephalopathic manifestations are reversible if they are treated early.

Myopathies

Myopathy is a collective term referring to a group of diverse muscle diseases caused by tissue degeneration, toxicity, and inflammatory changes. The primary complaint is muscle weakness, although muscles appear normal on clinical examination. Problems with speech and swallowing can also be found. There are various types of muscular abnormalities: **Muscular dystrophy** is a hereditary myopathy marked by progressive weakness and atrophy. **Duchenne's dystrophy** is an X-linked myopathy transmitted to male children from their mothers, who never manifest the condition. **Ocular** and **facial dystrophies** affect extrinsic ocular and facial muscles, causing dysarthria and severe problems with ocular movements.

Peripheral Neuropathies

Neuropathy is a disease of the peripheral nerves, interrupting the transmission of impulses from motor neurons to muscles. It can be inherited, idiopathic, or caused by trauma, toxicity, infection, or neoplastic growth. Neuropathy can involve a single peripheral nerve (mononeuropathy) or several peripheral nerves (polyneuropathy). Neuropathy may affect only sensory or motor functions or may involve both; the symptom profile may be acute, chronic, or relapsing. Common peripheral mononeuropathies include neuropathy at the wrist (carpal tunnel syndrome), elbow, or knee. Carpal tunnel syndrome results from the entrapment of the median nerve at the wrist level and is seen in people whose work activity regularly requires wrist movement. Elbow neuropathy involves the ulnar nerve, which is susceptible to damage at the elbow. Initial symptoms of ulnar neuropathy are numbness and tingling at the area of nerve distribution. The nerve involved in knee neuropathy is the peroneal. It is especially susceptible to damage as it passes laterally around the fibula. Sitting with the legs crossed is often a cause of this neuropathy, and foot drop as well as sensory and motor disturbances characterize it.

Cranial neuropathies usually involve muscles of the eye, jaw, or face. Lesions of the fibers supplying the ocular nerves can affect movements of the eye and the parasympathetic functions of the iris. Lesions of the trigeminal nerve result in sensory symptoms in the face and motor problems for the mastication muscles. Damage to the facial nucleus and its nerve results in facial paralysis (Bell's palsy) and visceral and parasympathetic disturbances.

Neoplastic Growth

Neoplasms (tumors) are abnormal tissue growth that is generally but not always slow and insidious. Because of the brain's ability to reorganize, tumors present very slow and subtle clinical signs. Neoplastic growth in the brain primarily increases intracranial pressure, which slowly irritates and damages the surrounding brain tissues. Some common clinical signs of brain tumors are double vision, headache, altered cognitive ability, nausea, and seizures. Most brain tumors originate from glia cells (gliomas). **Astrocytomas**, **ependymomas**, and **oligodendrogliomas** are common types of brain tumors; other brain tumors are the **meningiomas**, which arise from the dura mater, and **acoustic neuromas**, which arise from the Schwann cell sheath of the nerve.

Cerebral Infections

Various bacteria, viruses, and other organisms can cause infection in the CNS. Generally, infections' effect on the brain is diffuse, and they most commonly affect the meninges (meningitis) and the cerebral cortex (encephalopathy). Infections can also be local, such as cerebral abscess, which occur in different parts of the brain. Some common infections include **viral infections**, **herpes simplex**, *Escherichia coli*, **brain abscess**, **subdural empyema**, and **syphilis**.

SUMMARY

This chapter describes a few commonly used diagnostic techniques. Some prevalent neurological diseases and medical technical concepts are included. These topics directly apply to the management of neurology patients who are commonly seen by practicing audiologists, speech–language pathologists and professionals in behavior sciences, primarily in medical settings. Imag-

ing techniques are discussed to familiarize students with the procedures, principles, and purposes underlying different neurodiagnostic techniques. The chapter also addresses the importance of sodium Amytal for assessment of cerebral dominance, usually before craniotomy. A discussion of electroencephalography and electromyography explains how these tests are used to measure functioning of the brain cells and muscle fibers. The ways to record evoked potentials to specific and controlled sensory stimulation and their interpretation are also described. Finally, various neurological techniques and neurosurgical procedures, along with their neurolinguistic implications, are examined. Modes of genetic inheritance and a brief account of common neurological diseases are presented.

Technical Terms

angiogram	myopathy
computed tomography (CT)	neuropathy
cordotomy	paroxysmal discharge
craniotomy	positron emission
dichotic listening	tomography (PET)
dominant inheritance	recessive inheritance
electroencephalography	regional cerebral blood flow
encephalopathy	single proton emission
epilepsy	computed tomography
magnetic resonance	(SPECT)
imaging (MRI)	X-linked inheritance

Review Questions

1. Define the following terms:

angiogram	myopathy
computed tomography (CT)	neuropathy
cordotomy	paroxysmal discharge
craniotomy	positron emission
dichotic listening	tomography (PET)
dominant inheritance	recessive inheritance
electroencephalography	regional cerebral blood flow
encephalopathy	single photon emission
epilepsy	tomography (SPECT)
magnetic resonance imaging (MRI)	X-linked inheritance

2. Describe the techniques, purposes, and clinical significance of angiography, CT, SPECT, MRI, and PET.
3. Describe sodium Amytal infusion and its neurolinguistic significance.
4. Describe the diagnostic importance of EEG and discuss major types of brain waves.
5. Explain the pathophysiology of seizure disorders.
6. Describe clinical symptoms of partial and generalized seizures.
7. Discuss the spinal tap procedure.
8. Explain the diagnostic importance of electromyography.
9. Describe how do neuropathic and/or myopathic conditions affect electromyographic tracing.
10. Describe nerve conduction and its clinical implications.
11. Discuss the clinical significance of EMG.

12. Describe the evoked potential technique and clinical implications of the brainstem auditory evoked responses.
13. Describe the dichotic listening paradigm and its neurolinguistic implications.
14. Describe the neurosurgical procedures used for surgical ablation, lesion placement, anastomosing the internal carotid and external arteries, and removing fatty material from carotid arteries.
15. Discuss the physiology of sleep and its common disorders.
16. Describe the pathophysiology of myopathy and neuropathy.

17. Discuss the dominant, recessive, and X-linked modes of genetic inheritance, citing the risk probability associated with each of these transmission modes with a labeled diagram.
18. Explain why a father cannot pass an X-linked disorder to a male child.
19. Discuss common diseases and pathological conditions that are transmitted through dominant and recessive genes.
20. Describe encephalopathy, myopathy, peripheral neuropathy, neoplastic growth, and cerebral infections.

Appendices

APPENDIX A. COMMON ABBREVIATIONS

a or **aa**   of each, arteries
ab   abortion
ABG   arterial blood gas
abd/Abd   abdomen, abductor
abn   abnormal
ABR   auditory brainstem response, absolute bed rest
a.c./ac   before a meal
ACTH   adrenocorticotrophic hormone
ad/AD   right ear, to, up to, Alzheimer's disease
ADHD   attention deficit hyperactivity disorder
ADL   activities of daily living
ad lib.   freely, at pleasure, as desired
adm   admission
AFP   α-fetoprotein
alc   alcohol
ALS   amyotrophic lateral sclerosis, acute lateral sclerosis, advanced life support
AMA   against medical advice, American Medical Association
amb   ambulatory
AMI   acute myocardial infarction
amt   amount
angio   angiogram
A-P   anteroposterior
aq/AQ   aqueous, water
ARDS   adult respiratory distress syndrome
ARF   acute renal failure
as/AS   left ear
ASA   aspirin (acetylsalicylic acid), atrial septal aneurysm
ASAP   as soon as possible
as tol   as tolerated
au/AU   both ears, allergenic (allergy) units
AV   arteriovenous, atrioventricular
b.i.d./BID   twice daily
BK   below knee; bullous keratopathy
BM   bowel movement
BP   blood pressure
BR   bedrest
BS   bowel sounds, blood sugar, barium swallow

Bx   biopsy
c̄   with
C   Celsius, Calorie (kilocalorie)
Ca   calcium, cathode
CA   cancer, carcinoma, cardiac arrest
CAB   coronary artery bypass
cal   calorie(s)
cap.   capsule
CAT   computed axial tomography
cath   catheter, catheterization
CBC   complete blood count
CBR   complete bed rest
CC/C.C.   chief complaint
CCU   coronary care unit, critical care unit
CHF   congestive heart failure
CHI   closed head injury
CHO   carbohydrate
chol   cholesterol
circ   circumcision, circulation
Cl   chloride
cl liq   clear liquid
cm   centimeter
c/o   complaint of
CO   carbon monoxide, cardiac output
CPR   cardiopulmonary resuscitation
CSF   cerebrospinal fluid
CT   computed tomography, carpal tunnel, chemotherapy
CVA   cerebrovascular accident
CVP   central venous pressure
Cx   cervix, cancel
CXR   chest x-ray
/d   per day
DAT   diet as tolerated, dementia of the Alzheimer type
d/c   discharge, discontinue
del   delivery, delivered
disch.   discharge
DOA   dead on arrival
DPT   diphtheria-pertussis-tetanus (immunization)
DRG   diagnosis-related groups
DTR   deep tendon reflexes
DW   distilled water, daily weight
Dx   diagnosis
E   enema, edema, eye

EBL   estimated blood loss
ECG   electrocardiogram
ECT   electroconvulsive therapy
EDC   estimated date of confinement
EEG   electroencephalogram
EENT   eyes, ears, nose, and throat
EKG   see ECG
EMG   electromyogram
ENG   electronystagmography
ENT   ear, nose, throat
ER   emergency room
ESR   erythrocyte sedimentation rate
exam.   examination
ext/EXT   extract, external, extremity
F   Fahrenheit
FBS   fasting blood sugar
Fe   iron
FH   family history
FHT   fetal heart tone
FSH   follicle-stimulating hormone
FTA   blood test for syphilis
Fx   fracture
g/gm   gram
GB   gallbladder, Guillain-Barré (syndrome)
GI   gastrointestinal
GTT   glucose tolerance test, drops
gyn/GYN   gynecology
h/hr   hour
H   hypodermic, heart, head, height, Hydrogen
HA   headache, hearing aid, heart attack
Hb/Hgb/Hg   hemoglobin
HBP   high blood pressure
Hg   mercury
H/O   history of
H₂O   water
H₂O₂   hydrogen peroxide
HOB   head of bed
H&P   history and physical
hs/HS   hour of sleep (bedtime)
HT   height, hypertension, hearing test, heart transplant
Hx   history, hospitalization
IBS   irritable bowel syndrome
ICU   intensive care unit

IM   intramuscular, infectious mononucleosis
inj.   injection
IPPB   intermittent positive pressure breathing
IUD   intrauterine device
i.v./IV   intravenous, invasive
IVC   intravenous cholangiogram, inferior vena cava, inspiratory vital capacity
K   potassium
KCl   potassium chloride
kg   kilogram
KO   keep open
KUB   kidney, ureter, bladder
KVO   keep vein open
L/l   liter
lab.   laboratory
lac   laceration
lap   laparotomy, laparoscopy
lat   lateral
LE   lower extremities, left ear, left eye
lg   large
LLL   left lower lobe
LLQ   left lower quadrant
LMP/lmp   last menstrual period
LP   lumbar puncture, low protein
LPN   licensed practical nurse
lt   left, light
LUL   left upper lobe
LUQ   left upper quadrant
MCA   middle cerebral artery, middle cerebral aneurysm, motorcycle accident
μg   microgram
mg   milligram
MI   myocardial infarction
mL/ml   milliliter
mm   millimeter
MRI   magnetic resonance imaging
MS   multiple sclerosis, mitral stenosis
Na   sodium
NA   not applicable, not admitted
NaCl   sodium chloride
NAS   no added salt, neonatal abstinence syndrome
NB   newborn, needle biopsy
neg   negative
NG   nasogastric
NICU   neurological intensive care unit, neonatal intensive care unit, neurosurgical intensive care unit
noc./noct   night/nocturnal
n.p.o.   nothing by mouth
N&V   nausea and vomiting
NVS   neurological vital signs

O₂   oxygen
OB   obstetrics
OD   right eye, overdose, optic disc
oint   ointment
OM   otitis media, osteomyelitis
OOB   out of bed
OP   outpatient, operation, oropharynx, osteoporosis
Ophth   ophthalmic
OR   operating room
ortho   orthopedics
OS/O.S.   left eye, oral surgery
OT   occupational therapy
OU   both eyes
oz   ounce
p̄   after (post)
PA   physician assistant, posterior-anterior
p.c./pc   after meals
PCA   posterior cerebral artery, posterior communicating artery
PCU   primary care unit, progressive care unit
PCV   packed cell volume
PDR   Physician's Desk Reference
Peds.   pediatrics
PEEP   positive end-expiratory pressure
PERRLA   pupils equal, regular, reactive to light and accommodation
PET   positron emission tomography
PICU   pediatric intensive care unit
PKU   phenylketonuria
pm/PM   between noon and midnight
PO   by mouth (per os), postoperative
post op   postoperative
PP   postpartum, postprandial (after meals), pulse pressure
PPD   purified protein derivative, postpartum day
p.r.   through rectum
PR   pulse rate, premature
PRBC   packed red blood cells
pre-op   preoperative, before surgery
PRN/prn   whenever necessary
pt   patient, pint
PT   physical therapy, preterm
PTA   prior to admission, pure-tone average, physical therapy assistant
q   every
qam   every morning
qd   every day
qhr   every hour
qid   four times a day
qn   every night

qod   every other day
qoh   every other hour
qt   quart
R   rectal, respiration
RBC   red blood cells, red blood count
REM   rapid eye movement
resp.   respirations
RLL   right lower lobe
RLQ   right lower quadrant
RN   registered nurse
R/O   rule out
ROM   range of motion, right otitis media
RR   recovery room, respiratory rate
rt   right
RT   respiratory/radiation/recreational therapy
RUL   right upper lobe
RUQ   right upper quadrant
Rx   therapy, prescription, treatment
s̄   without
sc/SC   subcutaneous(ly)
SLP   speech–language pathologist
SOB   shortness of breath
SOM   serous otitis media
s/p   status post
ss   a half
stat.   immediately
supp   suppository
surg   surgical
Sx   symptoms, surgery
Sz/sz   seizure
T/temp.   temperature
tab   tablet
TAT   tetanus antitoxin, till all taken
TB   tuberculosis
TCT   thrombin clotting time
TIA   transient ischemic attack
t.i.d.   three times a day
TO   telephone order
TPN   total parenteral nutrition
trach.   tracheostomy, tracheal
TWE   tap water enema
Tx   treatment, traction, transplant
U   unit (Note: It is best to spell out to minimize confusion)
UA   urinalysis
UGI   upper gastrointestinal
UTI   urinary tract infection
vag   vaginal
VER   visual evoked response
VS   vital signs
WA   while awake
WBC   white blood cells, white blood count
WC   wheelchair, whooping cough
wt.   weight

APPENDIX B. MEDICAL TERMINOLOGY

Common Prefixes and Suffixes

PREFIXES

a-, ab- (L.)   from or away from, as in abduct

a-, an- (G.)   absence or negation, as in agenesis or anopsia

ad- (L.)   to or toward, as in afferent (*d* changes to *f* if it precedes *f*)

amb-, ambi-, ambo- (L.)   both, both sides, about, around, as in ambidextrous

bi-, bis- (L.)   two or double, as in bilateral

contra- (L.)   against or opposite, as in contralateral

de- (L.)   from, down, away, as in decerebration

di- (G.)   double, as in diplopia

dia- (G.)   through, between, across, as in diagnosis

dis-, di- (L.)   away from, apart, in different directions, as in dislocation

dys- (G.)   bad or difficult, as in dysphagia

endo-, ento- (G.)   within or inside, as in endocardium

epi- (G.)   upon, on, above, as in epidermis

exo-, ecto- (G.)   outside or without, as in ectoderm

extra-, exter-, extro- (L.)   outside, in addition to, beyond, as in exteroceptor

hemi- (G.)   half, as in hemiplegia

homo- (G.)   likeness, steady, same, as in homonymous

hyper- (G.)   above, beyond, excessive, over, as in hypertension

hypo- (G.)   less than, below, under, beneath, as in hypotension

infra- (L.)   below or beneath, as in infraorbital

inter- (L.)   in the midst or between, as in interhemispheric

intra- (L.)   inside or within, as in intrahemispheric

ipsi- (L.)   same, as in ipsilateral

mal- (L.)   abnormal or bad, as in malocclusion

mes-, meso- (G.)   middle, as in mesoderm

meta- (G.)   transformation, after, beyond, changed to, as in metabolism

neo- (G.)   new, as in neocortex

para- (G.)   beside, alongside of, resembling, as in paralgesia

peri- (G.)   about or around, as in perisylvian

poly- (G.)   much or many, as in polyneural

pre- (L.), **pro-** (G.)   before or in front of, as in prophase

pros- (G.)   before, toward, facing, as in prosencephalon

retro- (L.)   behind or back, as in retrograde

sub- (L.)   in small quantity or beneath, as in subdural or subarachnoid

supra- (L.)   above, beyond, on the upper side, as in supratentorial

syn-, sym- (G.)   joined or together, as in synapse or sympathy (*syn-* appears as *sym-* before the letters *b, p, ph,* and *m*)

tact- (L.)   touch, as in tactile

trans-, tra- (L.)   across or through, as in transection

SUFFIXES

-al (G.)   relating to, characteristic of, similar to, as in bacterial

-algia, -algesia (G.)   suffering or pain, as in neuralgia

-ate (G.)   to cause, as in dehydrate

-culus (L.)   a little one, as in fasciculus

-cyst (G.)   sac with membranous lining, as in blastocyst

-eal (L.)   pertaining to, characteristic of, similar to, as in pharyngeal

-ectomy (G.)   excision of, removal of, cutting away, as in lobectomy

-emia (G.)   referring to blood, as in anemia

-genic, -genesis (G.)   produced from or pertaining to origin, as in epileptogenic

-gram (G.)   tracing or record, as in audiogram

-graph (G.)   writing or recording, as in electroencephalograph

-ia, -y (G.)   condition of or an abnormal state of, as in dementia

-ial (L.)   of, like, suitable for, as in branchial

-iasis (G.)   diseased or pathological state or condition, as in psoriasis

-ic, -ac, -tic (G.)   relating to or similar to, as in syphilitic

-ile (L.)   capable of, tending to, like, as in contractile

-illa (L.)   a little one, as in fibrilla

-in, -ine (G.)   chemical substance, as in chlorine

-ine (L.)   pertaining to, characteristic of, similar to, as in feminine

-ist, -ast (G.)   suffix of agency denoting one who does something, as in otologist

-itis (G.)   inflammation, as in meningitis

-ity, -ety, -ty (L.)   the state of, as in morbidity

-ium (G.)   part, area, lining, as in pericardium

-ize (G.)   to do or to treat by special method, as in anesthetize

-logia, -ology (G.)   study or science of, as in audiology

-oma (G.)   tumor, as in meningioma

-opia (G.)   vision, as in hyperopia

-or (L.)   one who or that which does a specified action, as in tensor

-osis (G.)   act or process of, status, state of disease, as in osteosis

-path, -pathic, -pathy (G.)   suffering or disease, as in neuropathy

-rrhea (G.)   watery secretion, flow, discharge, as in rhinorrhea

-sis, -sia (G.)   process, action, pathological state, condition, as in parablepsia

-te, -t (G.)   suffix of agency denoting person or thing that does something, as in gamete

-ter (G.)   the means of or the place for, as in ureter

-tomy (G.)   excision (cutting) or surgically placed lesion, as in thalamotomy

-ure (L.)   noun suffix denoting an act, a process, or the result of an act, as in fracture

Common Latin and Greek Lexical Roots

Acoustic

akoustikos (G.) = hearing; ic = suff.

Pertaining to sound or the sense of hearing.

Acrocephalia

akron (G.) = extremity; kephale (G.) = head; ia = suff.

Pointed condition of the top of the cranium.

Acromastitis

akron (G.) = extremity; mastos (G.) = breast; itis = suff.

Inflammation of the nipple.

Acupuncture

acus (L.) = needle; punctura (L.) = puncture; e = suff.

Puncture with needles for therapeutic purposes.

Adenoid

aden (G.) = gland; eidos (G.) = form, shape.

Having the appearance of a gland.

Adiadochokinesia

a = negative; diadochos (G.) = succeeding; kinesis (G.) = movement; ia = suff.

Impaired ability to perform alternating movements.

Agnosia

a = negative; gnosis (G.) = knowledge; ia = suff.

Impaired ability to relate meaning/interpretation to an object or form while basic sensory modality is intact.

Agraphia

a = negative; graphein (G.) = to write; ia = suff.

A writing disorder acquired after a brain lesion.

Alexia

a = negative; lexis (G.) = word; ia = suff.

Impaired ability to comprehend written words.

Ambidextrous

ambi (L.) = on both sides; dexter (L.) = right; ous = suff.

Referring to a person able to use both hands equally well.

Amygdala

amygdalum (L.), derived from amygdale (G.) = almond.

An almond-shaped limbic nucleus.

Anadipsia

ana (G.) = intensive; dipsa (G.) = thirst; ia = suff.

Intense thirst.

Anesthesia

an (G.) = not; aisthesis (G.) = sensation; ia = suff.

Partial or total loss of sensation.

Angiography

angeion (G.) = vessel; graphein (G.) = to write; y = suff.

A radiographic study of blood vessels.

Annulose

annulus (L.) = ring, ose = suff.

Having or characterized by a ring or rings.

Anopsia

an = negative; opsis (G.) = vision; ia = suff.

An impairment of vision.

Ansa peduncularis

ansa (L.) = handle; pedunculus (L.) = a little foot; aris (L.) = adjectival suff.

Fibers passing from the thalamus through the thalamic radiation.

Antithrombin

anti (G.) = against, opposing; thrombos (G.) = clot; in = suff.

A substance that inhibits coagulation of the blood. (The Greek word *thrombus* denotes a blood clot obstructing a blood vessel or a cavity of the heart.)

Aphasia

a = negative; phasis (G.) = speech; ia = suff.

An acquired language disorder.

Apraxia

a = negative; praxis from prattein (G.) = to act; ia = suff.

A disorder in the ability to execute skilled movements voluntarily.

Aqueduct

aqua (L.) = water; ductus (L.) = duct.

Canal or passage, as in the cerebral aqueduct.

Arachnoid

arachne (G.) = spider's web; eidos (G.) = form.

A meningeal layer resembling a spider web.

Arthritis

arthron (G.) = joint; itis = suff.

Inflammation of a joint accompanied by pain, swelling, and changes in structure.

Astereognosis

a = negative; stereos (G.) = solid; gnosis (G.) = knowledge.

Impaired ability to recognize objects by feel or tactile manipulation.

Astrocyte

astron (G.) = star; kytos (G.) = hollow (cell); e = suff.

A supporting cell.

Asynergy

a = negative; syn (G.) = with; ergon (G.) = work; y = suff.

Absence of synergic muscle movements.

Ataxia

a = negative; taxis (G.) = order; ia = suff.

Absence of muscle coordination.

Athetosis

a = negative; thetos (G.) = placed; osis = suff.

An involuntary motor movement.

Autonomic

autos (G.) = self; nomos (G.) = law; ic = suff.

Self-controlling.

Autotoxin

autos (G.) = self; toxikon (G.) = poison; in = suff.

Poison generated within the body it affects.

Binocular

bis, bin (L.) = two; oculus (L.) = eye; ar = suff.

Pertaining to both eyes.

Brachycardia

brachys (G.) = short; kardia (G.) = heart.

Slow heart action.

Brachiocephalic

brachium (L.) = arm; kephale (G.) = head; ic = suff.

Pertaining to the arm and the head.

Brachium

brachium (L.), derived from brachion (G.) = arm.

Armlike long fiber bundles in the central nervous system.

Bradykinesia

bradys (G.) = slow; kinesis (G.) = movement; ia = suff.

Slow movement.

Buccal
bucca (L.) = mouth; al = suff.
Pertaining to cheek or mouth, as in buccal cavity.

Calciferous
calx (L.) = lime; ferre (L.) = to carry; ous = suff.
Containing calcium, lime , or chalk.

Cardiology
kardia (G.) = heart; logos (G.) = word, reason; y = suff.
Study of the heart.

Carpoptosis
karpos (G.) = wrist; ptosis (G.) = a falling.
Wrist drop.

Cephalad
kephale (G.) = head; ad = suff.
Toward the head.

Cerebellum
cerebellum (L.) = a diminutive form of cerebrum.
A part of the brain containing small sulci and gyri (folia).

Cerumen
cera (L.) = wax; men = suff.
A substance secreted by glands at the outer third of the ear canal.

Chiragra
cheir (G.) = hand; agra (G.) = seizure.
Pain in the hand.

Chondrogenesis
chondros (G.) = cartilage; genesis (G.) = generation, birth.
Formation of cartilage.

Chondroplasty
chondros (G.) = cartilage; plassein (G.) = to mold; y = suff.
Surgical repair of cartilage.

Chorea
chorea (L.), derived from choros (G.) = dance.
Dancelike involuntary muscle movements.

Chromatolysis
chroma/chromatos (G.) = color; lysis (G.) = dissolution.
Dissolution of cellular microstructures in reaction to an injury.

Clonus
klonus (G.) = turmoil.
Spasmodic contraction and relaxation.

Commissure
commissura (L.) = a joining together.
Transverse band of nerve fibers passing over the midline in the central nervous system.

Craniomalacia
kranion (G.) = skull; malakia (G.) = softening.
Softening of the skull bones.

Cryesthesia
krymos (G.) = cold; aisthesis (G.) = sensation; ia = suff.
Sensitivity to cold.

Cuneate, Cuneiform
cuneus (L.) = wedge; forma (L.) = shape.
Wedge-shaped.

Cynantrophy
kyon (G.) = dog; anthropos (G.) = man; y = suff.
Insanity in which the patient behaves like a dog.

Cysticotomy
kystis (G.) = bladder, sac; tome (G.) = incision; y = suff.
Surgical incision of cystic bile duct.

Cystitis
kystis (G.) = bladder, sac; itis = suff.
Inflammation of bladder.

Dactylomegaly
daktylos (G.) = finger; megalos (G.) = great; y = suff.
Abnormal size of fingers and/or toes.

Dehydrate
de (L.) = from; hydor (G.) = water; ate = suff.
Deprive of, lose, or become free of water.

Dendrite
dendron (G.) = tree; ite = suff.
Receptive endings of nerve cells.

Dermatome
derma (G.) = skin; tome (G.) = cutting.
A skin area innervated by nerves originating from a single spinal segment.

Diaphragm
diaphragma (G.) = a partition.
A thin membrane, such as one used in dialysis; a musculomembranous wall separating the abdomen from the thoracic cavity.

Diencephalon
dia (G.) = through; enkephalos (G.) = brain.
A subcortical structure consisting of thalamus and hypothalamus.

Digital
digitus (L.) = finger; al = suff.
Referring to a finger or a toe.

Dilatant
dilatare (L.) = to enlarge; ant = suff.
Anything that causes dilation.

Dilation
dilatare (L.) = to enlarge; ion = suff.
Expansion of an organ.

Dormant
dormio (L.) = sleep; ant = suff.
Sleeping; inactive.

Dura
durus (L.) = hard.
Outermost meningeal layer.

Dysmetria
dys (G.) = bad; metron (G.) = measure; ia = suff.
Impaired control of range and strength of muscle.

Dysphonia
dys (G.) = bad; phone (G.) = voice; ia = suff.
Difficulty in speaking.

Electroencephalogram
elektron (G.) = relationship to electricity; enkephalos (G.) = brain; gramma (G.) = something written.
A tracing on an electroencephalograph, which is an instrument that records the electrical activity of the brain.

Encephalomeningitis
enkephalos (G.) = brain; meninx/meningos (G.) = membrane; itis = suff.
Inflammation of the brain and its membranes.

Esotropia
es (G.) = into; tropos (G.) = a turn; ia = suff.
A turning of the eye inward.

Falx
falx (L.) = sickle.
A sickle-shaped dural extension separating cerebral (falx cerebri) and cerebellar (falx cerebelli) hemispheres.

Fasciculus
diminutive of fascis (L.) = bundle.
A bundle of fibers carrying functionally similar information.

Femoral
femoralis (L.) = pertaining to femur.
Pertaining to the femur (thigh).

Foramen
foramen (L.) = a passage or opening.
A passage or opening as between two.

Fornical
fornix (L.) = arch; al = suff.
Pertaining to or resembling fornix, an arch-shaped fiber tract connecting hippocampus and mamillary bodies.

Fovea
fovea (L.) = a pit or depression.
Depressed area in center of macula lutea.

Gametogenesis
gamein (G.) – to marry; genesis (G.) = generation, birth.
Formation of gametes—oogenesis or spermatogenesis.

Genial
geneion (G.) = chin; al = suff.
Pertaining to the chin.

Geriatrics
geras (G.) = old age; iatrike (G.) = medical treatment; ics = suff.
Study and treatment of physical and mental products of old age.

Glia
glia (G.) = glue.
Support of central nervous system.

Globus pallidus
globus (L.) = a ball; pallidus (L.) = white or lightly colored.
A basal ganglia structure located between internal capsule and putamen.

Glossolalia
glossa (G.) = tongue; lalia (G.) = babble.
Repetition of senseless remarks unrelated to the subject at hand.

Glossopathy
glossa (G.) = tongue; pathos (G.) = disease; y = suff.
Disease of the tongue.

Gonarthrotomy
gona (G.) = knee; arthron (G.) = joint; tome (G.) = incision; y = suff.
Incision of the knee joint.

Haploid
haploos (G.) = simple; eidos (G.) = form, shape.
Possessing half the diploid or normal number of chromosomes found in somatic or body cells.

Helicotrema
helix (G.) = coil; trema (G.) = hole.
Opening at the tip of the cochlear canal where the scala tympani and the scala vestibuli come together.

Hemialgia
hemi (G.) = half; algos (G.) = pain; ia = suff.
Pain in half of the body.

Hemianesthesia
hemi (G.) = half; an (G.) = not; aisthesis = sensation; ia = suff.
Loss of sensation in half of the body.

Hemiasthenia
hemi (G.) = half; asthenia (G.) = weakness.
Weakness in half of the body.

Hemiballismus
hemi (G.) = half; ballismos (G.) = dancing.
Flinging, involuntary movements.

Hemiparesis
hemi (G.) = half; paresis (G.) = paralysis.
Paralysis of half of the body.

Hemiplegia
hemi (G.) = half; plege (G.) = a stroke; ia = suff.
Paralysis of half of the body.

Hemorrhage
haima (G.) = blood; rhegnynai (G.) = to burst forth; e = suff.
Abnormal discharge of blood externally or internally.

Hepatology
hepatikos (G.) = liver; logos (G.) = word, reason; y = suff.
The study of the liver.

Heterophasia
heteros (G.) = other; phasis (G.) = speech; ia = suff.
Use of meaningless words instead of those intended.

Hippocampal
hippokampos (G.) = sea horse; al = suff.
Pertaining to the hippocampus.

Hydrocephalus
hydro (G.) = water; kephale (G.) = head.
Excessive production/retention of cerebrospinal fluid in ventricles.

Hyperosmia
hyper (G.) = excessive; osme (G.) = smell; ia = suff.
Abnormal sensitivity to odors.

Hypertrophy
hyper (G.) = excessive; trophe (G.) = nourishment; y = suff.
Increase in size of an organ or structure owing to growth rather than tumor formation.

Hypnolepsy
hypnos (G.) – sleep; lepsis (G.) = seizure; y = suff.
Irresistible sleepiness; narcolepsy.

Hypoglycemia
hypo (G.) = under; glykys (G.) = sweet; haima (G.) = blood; ia = suff.
Deficiency of sugar in the blood.

Hysterectomy
hystera (G.) = womb; ektome (G.) = excision; y = suff.
Excision of the uterus.

Idiopathy
idios (G.) = own; pathos (G.) = disease; y = suff.
A primary disease without apparent external cause.

Incision
incisio (L.) = to cut; ion = suff.
A cut made with a knife.

Insular
insula (L.) = island; ar = suff.
Pertaining to any insula, especially the central lobe (isle of Reil) of the cerebral hemispheres.

Kinesthesia
kinesis (G.) = movement; aisthesis (G.) = sensation; ia = suff.
A sensation associated with limb movement.

Lability
labi (L.) = to slip; ilis = adj. element; ity = suff.
State of being unstable or changeable.

Lacrimal
lacrima (L.) = tear; al = suff.
Pertaining to tears.

Laloplegia
lalia (G.) = babble; plege (G.) = stroke; ia = suff.
Paralysis of speech muscles without affecting action of the tongue.

Lemniscus
limniskos (G.) = ribbon.
A bundle of nerve fibers in central nervous system.

Lepidoma
lepis (G.) = scale; oma (G.) = tumor.
A tumor derived from lepidic tissue; rind tumor.

Leptomeninges
leptos (G.) = thin, slim; meninx/meningos (G.) = membrane.
Pia mater and arachnoid as distinct from dura mater because of their thinner structure.

Leptorrhine
leptos (G.) = thin, slim; rhis (G.) = nose; ine = suff.
Having a very thin or slender nose.

Logagnosia
logos (G.) = word; a (G.) = not; gnosis (G.) = knowledge; ia = suff.
Word blindness.

Macrocephaly
makros (G.) = large; kephale (G.) = head; y = suff.
Abnormal largeness of the head.

Macrophthalmia
makros (G.) = large; ophthalmos (G.) = eye; ia = suff.
Abnormally large eyeballs.

Macula
macula (L.) = a spot.
A small circular region in the retina.

Malar
mala (L.) = cheek; ar = suff.
Pertaining to the cheekbone.

Mammilla
mamma (L.) = breast; illa (L.) = a little one.
Nipple.

Mamillary
mammilla (L.) = nipple; y = suff.
Nipple-shaped mamillary bodies of hypothalamus.

Mania
mania (G.) = madness.
Madness, characterized by excessive excitement.

Mesencephalon
mesos (G.) = middle; enkephalos (G.) = brain.
Midbrain, which lies between diencephalon and pons.

Metencephalon
meta (G.) = after; enkephalos (G.) = brain.
Brain region, which develops into pons and cerebellum.

Microglia
mikros (G.) = small; glia (G.) = glue.
A supporting (glia) cell in brain.

Microtia
mikros (G.) = small; ous/otos (G.) = ear; ia = suff.
Unusually small size of the auricle or external ear.

Monophyletic
monos (G.) = single; phyle (G.) = tribe; tic = suff.
Originating from a single source.

Myasthenia
mys (G.) = muscle; asthenia (G.) = weakness.
Muscular weakness.

Myelatelia
myelos (G.) = marrow, spinal cord; ateleia (G.) = imperfection.
Defective development of the spinal cord.

Myelencephalon
myelos (G.) = marrow; enkephalos (G.) = brain.
Brain region that develops into medulla.

Myometer
mys (G.) = muscle; metron (G.) = measure; ter = suff.
Device for measurement of muscular contractions.

Nephrohypertrophy
nephros (G.) = kidney; hyper (G.) = excessive; trophe (G.) = nourishment; y = suff.
Overgrowth or dilation of the kidneys.

Neocerebellum
neos (G.) = new; cerebellum (L.) = diminutive of cerebrum.
Newest part of cerebellum.

Neocortex
neos (G.) = new; cortex (L.) = bark.
Most recent six-layered cellular growth in brain.

Neurilemma
neuron (G.) = nerve; lemma (G.) = husk.
Thin, membranous sheath enveloping a nerve fiber.

Neurohistology
neuron (G.) = nerve; histos (G.) = tissue; logos (G.) = study; y = suff.
The study of nervous tissue.

Neurotology
neuron (G.) = nerve; ous/otos (G.) = ear; logos (G.) = word, reason; y = suff.
The study of the inner ear and its neural connections.

Nocturnal
nocturnus (L.) = at night; al = suff.
Pertaining to or occurring in the night.

Nocuous
nocuus (L.) = noxious, harmful.
Being noxious or harmful.

Nyctalgia
nyx (G.) = night; algos (G.) = pain; ia = suff.
Pain during the night.

Nystagmus
nystagmos (G.) = a nodding.
Involuntary rhythmic oscillation of eyes.

Oligodendrocyte
oligos (G.) = few; dendron (G.) = tree; kytus (G.) = hollow (cell); e = suff.
Supporting cell.

Oligodontia
oligos (G.) = little; odont (G.) = tooth; ia = suff.
A hereditary developmental anomaly characterized by fewer teeth than normal.

Ontogeny
on (G.) = being; gennan (G.) = to produce; y = suff.
History of the development of an individual; ontogenesis.

Oogenesis

oon (G.) = egg; genesis (G.) = birth, generation.
Formation and development of the ovum.

Ophthalmology

ophthalmos (G.) = eye; logos (G.) = word, reason; y = suff.
The study of the eye.

Ossicle

ossiculum (L.) = little bone; e = suff.
Any small bone, as one of the three bones of the ear.

Osteonecrosis

osteo (G.) = bone; nekrosis (G.) = state of death.
Death of bone tissue.

Osteoradionecrosis

osteon (G.) = bone; radiatio (L.) = radiation; nekrosis (G.) = state of death.
Death of a bone following irradiation.

Osteosclerosis

osteon (G.) = bone; skleros (G.) = hard; osis = suff.
An abnormal increase in thickening and density of bone.

Paleencephalon

palaios (G.) = old; enkephalos (G.) = brain.
Phylogenetically older portion of the brain.

Pallium

pallium (L.) = cloak.
The cerebral cortex with its adjacent white substance.

Palpebrate

palpebra (L.) = eyelid; ate = suff.
Concerning an eyelid.

Papilloma

papilla (L.) = nipple; oma (G.) = tumor.
Any benign epithelial tumor.

Paraplegia

para (G.) = beside; plege (G.) = a stroke; ia = suff.
Paralysis of both legs.

Pathophysiology

pathos (G.) = disease; physis (G.) = nature; logos (G.) = word, reason; y = suff.
The study of how normal physiological processes are altered by disease.

Pediatrician

pais (G.) = child; iatrikos (G.) = healing; ian = suff.
A specialist in the treatment of children's diseases.

Pericranium

peri (G.) = around; kranium (G.) = skull.
Fibrous membrane around cranium periosteum of skull.

Perispondylitis

peri (G.) = around; spondylos (G.) = vertebra; itis = suff.
Inflammation of the parts around a vertebra.

Phagocyte

phagein (G.) = to eat; kytos (G.) = cell; e = suff.
A scavenger cell, such as microglia, having the ability to ingest and destroy particular substances, such as bacteria.

Pia mater

pia mater (L.) = tender mother.
Innermost layer of meninges.

Platypelvic

platys (G.) = broad; pelvis (L.) = a basin; ic = suff.
Having a broad pelvis.

Pneumatology

pneuma, pneumatos (G.) = air, breath; logos (G.) = word, reason; y = suff.
Science of gases and air, their chemical properties, and use in treatment.

Pneumohemorrhagica

pneuma, pneumatos (G.) = air, breath; haima (G.) = blood; rhegnynai (G.) = to burst forth; ica = suff.
Hemorrhage into pulmonary air cells.

Potency

potentia (L.) = power; y = suff.
Strength of a medicine.

Presbyacusia

presbys (G.) = old; akousis (G.) = hearing; ia = suff.
Decreased hearing sensitivity due to advancing age.

Presbyatrics

presbys (G.) = old; iatrikos (G.) = healing; ics = suff.
Science of old age and its treatment.

Presbyophrenia

presbys (G.) = old; phren (G.) = mind; ia = suff.
Senile psychotic syndrome.

Presbyopia

presbys (G.) = old; ops (G.) = eye; ia = suff.
Decreased visual sensitivity due to advancing age.

Proprioception

proprius (L.) = one's own; capio (L.) = to take; ion = suff.
The awareness of posture, movement, and changes in equilibrium and the knowledge of position, weight, and resistance of objects in relation to the body.

Prosencephalon

pros (G.) = at; enkephalos (G.) = brain.
Front end of neural tube, which develops into forebrain (telencephalon and diencephalon).

Protrusion

protrudere (L.) = to project; ion = suff.
Condition of being forward or projecting.

Ptosis

ptosis (G.) = a dropping.
Dropping or drooping of an organ or part.

Pulvinar

pulvinus (L.) = cushioned seat; ar = suff.
A prominent and cushion-like part of the thalamus comprising a portion of the posterior nuclei.

Quadriplegia

quadri (L.) = four; plege (G.) = stroke; ia = suff.
Paralysis of four extremities (both arms and legs).

Rachitomy

rhachis (G.) = spine; tome (G.) = incision; y = suff.
Surgical cutting of the vertebral column.

Renipuncture

ren (L.) = kidney; punctura (L.) = a piercing; e = suff.
Surgical puncture of the capsule of the kidney.

Resonance

resonantia (L.) = resound; ce = suff.
Quality or act of resounding.

Restiform

restis (L.) = rope; forma (L.) = form.
Rope-shaped fasciculus, inferior cerebellar peduncle, containing afferent fibers to cerebellum.

Retrouterine

retro (L.) = behind; uterus (L.) = womb; ine = suff.
Behind the uterus.

Retroversion

retro (L.) = back; versio (L.) = a turning; ion = suff.
A turning or state of being turned back.

Rhombencephalon

rhombos (G.) = a lozenge-shaped figure; enkephalos (G.) = brain.
Brain vesicle that develops into metencephalon (pons and cerebellum) and myelencephalon (medulla).

Rostrum

rostrum (L.) = beak.
Rostral part of corpus callosum.

Sclerosis

skleros (G.) = hard or stiff; osis (G.) = abnormal process or state.
A hardening of an organ, e.g., arteriosclerosis.

Senescence

senescens (L.) = growing old; ce = suff.
The process of growing old or the period of old age.

Senility

senilis (L.) = old; ty = suff.
The state of being old; weakness of old age either mentally or physically.

Sensiblity

sensibilitas (L.) = to feel or perceive stimuli; y = suff.
The capacity to receive and respond to stimuli.

Sinistrogyration

sinister (L.) = left; gyros (G.) = circle; ion = suff.
Inclination to the left.

Somatic

somatikos (G.) = bodily.
Related to the body.

Somesthetic

soma (G.) = body; aisthesis (G.) = sensation; ic = suff.
General somesthetic sensations are pain, temperature, and touch.

Sphygmophone

sphygmos (G.) = pulse; phone (G.) = voice.
Instrument for hearing the pulse beat.

Striatum

striatum (L.) = having been grooved.
The corpus striatum, a structure in the brain consisting of two basal ganglia and the fibers of the internal capsule which separate them.

Subaural

sub (L.) = under, below; auris (L.) = ear; al = suff.
Pertaining to the area below the ear.

Symbiosis

syn (G.) = together; bios (G.) = life; is = suff.
Condition in which two organisms live together for mutual benefit.

Symphysis

symphysis (G.) = growing together.
A line of fusion between two bones that are separate in early development.

Synapse

synaptein (G.) = to join; se = suff.
Junction between two neurons.

Syringomyelia

syrinx/syringos (G.) = pipe, tube; myelos (G.) = marrow; ia = suff.
A cavity formation in spinal gray.

Tachycardia

tachys (G.) = swift; kardia (G.) = heart.
An abnormal rapidity of heart action.

Tectum

tectum (L.) = roof.
Superior colliculi located dorsal to cerebral aqueduct in midbrain.

Telencephalic

telos (G.) = end; enkephalos (G.) = brain; ic = suff.
Pertaining to the telencephalon or endbrain.

Telencephalon

telos (G.) = end; enkephalos (G.) = brain.
Brain region that develops into neocortex, basal ganglia, and limbic system.

Temporal

tempus/temporis (L.) = period of time; al = suff.
Pertaining to or limited in time.

Teratogenesis

teratos (G.) = monster; genesis (G.) = birth, generation.
Development of abnormal structures in an embryo; development of a severely deformed fetus.

Tetraplegia

tetra (G.) = four; plege (G.) = stroke; ia = suff.
Paralysis of both arms and legs; quadriplegia.

Thalamic

thalamos (G.) = inner chamber; ic = suff.
Pertaining to the thalamus.

Thermanalgesia

therme (G.) = heat; an (G.) = not; algesis (G.) = sense of pain; ia = suff.
Inability to experience reaction to heat because of cerebral lesion.

Torticollis

tortus (L.) = twisted; collum (L.) = neck.
Deformity characterized by a twisted neck; wryneck.

Toxigenic

toxikon (G.) = poison; gennan (G.) = to produce; ic = suff.
Producing toxins or poisons.

Ultrasonic

ultra (L.) = beyond; sonus (L.) = sound; ic = suff.
Pertaining to sounds of frequencies above approximately 20,000 cycles per second.

Unicellular

unus (L.) = one; cellula (L.) = a little box; ar = suff.
Having only one cell.

Vasodilation

vas (L.) = vessel; dilatare (L.) = to enlarge; ion = suff.
Dilation of a blood vessel.

Venom

venenum (L.) = poison.
A poison excreted by some animals, such, as insects or snakes, and transmitted by bites and stings.

Vertigo

vertigo (L.) = a turning round.
Sensation either of moving around in space or of having objects move about the person.

Visceromegaly

viscera (L.) = body organs; megalos (G.) = great; y = suff.

Generalized enlargement of the abdominal visceral organs.

Vision

visio (L.) = a seeing; ion = suff.

Act of viewing external objects.

Glossary

Abdominal reflex—contraction of the abdominal wall on stroking the overlying skin; absence of this reflex is associated with pyramidal tract lesions (upper motor neuron).

Abduction—movement of limb away from the central body axis.

Abembryonic (vegetal pole)—pertaining to a region opposite to the implanting embryo.

Abscess—local accumulation of pus from liquified tissue resulting in displacement of tissues.

Absolute refractive period—time immediately following the action potential in which no other action potential can be initiated.

Acalculia—impaired ability, acquired after brain damage, to perform simple arithmetic calculation.

Accommodation—changes that the lens undergoes to keep a moving object in focus.

Acetylcholine—neurotransmitter commonly released by neurons in the central and peripheral nervous systems; neurons that release acetylcholine are called cholinergic neurons.

Acetylcholinesterase—enzyme that breaks acetylcholine into acetic acid and choline.

Acquired immunodeficiency syndrome—viral disease in which a virus attacks body's own immune system.

Achromatic—without color.

Action potential—electrical impulse representing a transient fluctuation in membrane potentials; propagated along axonal process.

Adaptation—diminished sensitivity of a receptor to continued stimulation.

Adduction—movement of limb toward the midline or central body axis.

Adenohypophysis—anterior lobe of the pituitary gland.

Adipsia—condition in which one does not feel thirsty.

Adrenal cortex—outer portion of the adrenal gland, which releases cortisol on stimulation by pituitary gland.

Adrenaline—catecholamine neurotransmitter also called epinephrine; synthesized from norepinephrine.

Adrenergic—relating to nerve cells that synthesize epinephrine or norepinephrine.

Afferent—axonal fibers that conduct impulses toward the central nervous system or nerve cell body.

Agnosia—acquired impairment in recognizing objects while the modalities of sensation are normally functioning.

Agraphia—impaired ability, acquired after brain damage, to express through writing.

Akinesia—slow initiation or loss of movements.

Alar lamina— alar plate zone of the embryonic neural tube dorsal to the sulcus limitans; dorsal gray columns of spinal cord and sensory centers of the brain develop from this region.

Albinism—genetic condition involving partial or total lack of pigments in skin, hair, and eyes.

Alexia—impaired ability, acquired after brain damage, to comprehend written information.

Alkalosis—condition resulting from an increased acid (Ph) in body fluid.

Allantois—one of the fetal membranes related to urinary bladder development; not functionally important in human development.

Allelic gene—genes at corresponding positions (loci) in a chromosome pair.

α-Motor neuron—fast-conducting motor neurons (alpha) in the spinal cord that supply extrafusal fibers of skeletal muscles.

α-Wave (α-rhythm)—brain wave with a frequency between 8 Hz and 13 Hz; occurs when subject is relaxed with eyes closed.

Alternating hemiplegia—clinical condition resulting from a lesion in the brainstem; involves cranial nerve impairments on side ipsilateral to lesion with hemiplegia and sensory loss on opposite side.

Alzheimer's disease—chronic degenerative condition in brain characterized by irreversible loss of memory, language, and cognition.

Amnesia—impaired ability to remember; forgetting information preceding cortical injury is retrograde amnesia; inability to learn newer information after injury is anterograde amnesia.

Amnion—fetal membrane that encloses the embryo and fetus; later the amniotic cavity is the sole cavity for the pregnant uterus.

Amygdaloid nucleus—temporal limbic structure that regulates emotional and autonomic responses.

Amyotrophic—pertaining to muscular atrophy, as in amyotrophic lateral sclerosis.

Amyotrophic lateral sclerosis (ALS, Lou Gehrig's dis-

ease)—progressive degenerative condition of spinal and cortical motor neurons characterized by muscular weakness and atrophy.

Anabolism—building of energy and cellular metabolic substances needed for the body.

Analgesia—absence of normal pain sensation; drugs that relieve pain are analgesic agents.

Anaphase—third stage in cell division.

Anastomosis—site of communication between two blood vessels.

Anencephaly—birth defect in which the forebrain and/or midbrain is small or missing; caused by defective fusion of neural tube during embryological development.

Anesthesia—loss of pain sensation.

Aneurysm—local balloonlike dilation of a blood vessel caused by a weakened arterial wall or genetic defect.

Angiography—modified x-ray technique that involves injection of radiopaque substance for examining blood vessels.

Anlagen—see *Primordium*.

Annulospiral nerve endings—specialized receptors that mediate muscle stretch.

Anomia—impaired ability to name objects.

Anorexia nervosa—psychological disease in which a patient is fatally weakened by loss of appetite.

Anosmia—partly or fully impaired ability to smell.

Anosognosia—failure to recognize one's own disease.

Anterior medullary velum—cerebellar structure that forms roof of the fourth ventricle.

Anterograde reaction—see *Wallerian degeneration*.

Antibody—defensive substance produced internally in response to a specific antigen in the body.

Antigen—foreign substance in the body that triggers a response from the immune system.

Aphagia—impaired ability to swallow.

Aphasia—impaired ability to process language, resulting from brain damage.

Apneustic area—pontine respiratory center that stimulates the medullary inspiratory center.

Apraxia—impaired ability to execute skilled motor acts, not caused by muscle paralysis or incoordination, sensory deficits, or incomprehension.

Aqueduct—canal within brainstem that connects the third and fourth ventricles.

Aqueous humor—watery substance similar to cerebrospinal fluid that is continuously produced and drained in the posterior chamber of the eye.

Arachnoid trabecula—fibrous tissue that crosses the space between the arachnoid and pia mater.

Arachnoid villi (granulations)—wormlike tufted structures that drain cerebrospinal fluid from subarachnoid space into the superior sagittal sinus.

Archicerebellum—oldest part of the cerebellum; includes flocculus and nodulus and is related to equilibrium.

Arteriosclerosis—narrowing of arterial lumen due to accumulation of lipids, fatty substances, and cholesterol along intimal walls of blood vessels; one cause of hypertension.

Arteriovenous malformation—congenital condition in which tangled and twisted arteries and veins are interconnected in a localized area.

Artery—vessel carrying blood from the heart to body parts.

Asphyxia—condition resulting from insufficient intake of oxygen.

Asthenia—muscle weakness caused by cerebellar dysfunctioning.

Astigmatism—focusing disorder in which vertical and horizontal rays focus at two different points on the retina; results from irregular lens and/or cornea curvature.

Astrocytes—neuroglia cells that support nerve cells and contribute to blood-brain barrier.

Asynergia—impaired ability to perform coordinated movements sequentially.

Ataxia—lack of coordination in sequential muscular activities, resulting from cerebellar pathology.

Atheroma—thickening of arterial walls occurring in atherosclerosis.

Atherosclerosis—see *Arteriosclerosis*.

Athetosis—involuntary slow, writhing movements of limbs.

Attenuation reflex—contraction of middle ear muscles resulting in a decreased auditory sensitivity.

Atonia—lack of muscle tone.

Atrophy—wasting away of a muscle, organ, or other tissue.

Atrophy of denervation (fiber wasting)—severely reduced muscle mass with loss of muscle fibers, resulting from prolonged loss (6 months or more) of lower motor neuron innervation of these fibers.

Atrophy of disuse—reduction in muscle mass without loss of muscle fibers (cells) caused by decreased contractile activity.

Audiogram—graphic representation of hearing thresholds at various frequencies.

Audiometry—assessment of hearing sensitivity for a range of pure tones using the decibel (dB) scale.

Auditory association cortex—brain region located around the primary auditory cortex, responsible for the elaboration of auditory information.

Autoimmunity—condition in which antibodies are produced and attack the body's own normal tissues.

Autonomic ganglia—group of nuclei in peripheral nervous system that mediate impulses from the central nervous system to various visceral organs, muscle tissues, and glands.

Autonomic nervous system—division of the peripheral nervous system with sympathetic and parasympathetic fibers; works subconsciously and innervates blood vessels, internal organs, and glands.

Autoregulation—cerebral mechanism for controlling blood flow to the brain.

Autosomal—related to chromosomes other than sex chromosomes.

Autosomal dominance—mode of genetic expression in which each offspring has a 50% probability of inheriting a condition.

Axial muscles—muscles that regulate movements of the body and trunk.

Axon—neuronal process capable of conducting neuronal impulses to other cell bodies.

Axon collateral (terminal bouton, presynaptic terminal)—end region of axon.

Axonal hillock—site where the axon joins the cell.

Axonal reaction—chromatolytic changes in the soma following damage to an axon.

Babinski reflex—dorsal flexion of great toe and fanning of other toes when sole of foot is stroked; presence of this reflex in adults indicates pyramidal tract (upper motor neuron) pathology; named after French neurologist Joseph Babinski.

Ballism—violent flinging movements usually involving one side of the body; associated with a lesion of the subthalamic nucleus.

Basal ganglia—group of subcortical nuclei (caudate, globus pallidus, and putamen) within white matter in each cerebral hemisphere; important in regulation of movement.

Basal lamina—basal plate zone of the embryonic neural tube ventral to the sulcus limitans; ventral gray columns of the spinal cord and motor centers of the brain develop from this region, also called the basal plate.

Basis pedunculi (pes peduncle, crus cerebri)—includes descending motor fibers in midbrain on each side.

Bell's palsy—facial paralysis caused by facial nerve pathologies; paralyzed muscles are pulled toward unaffected side.

Bilaminar embryo—human embryo in second week.

Binocular vision—visual field area simultaneously processed in both eyes.

Biopsy—removal of tissue from the living body, usually for microscopic examination.

Bitemporal hemianopia—loss of temporal visual fields for both eyes.

Blast—immature cell.

Blastocyst—stage in the first week of human development.

Blastomere—cell resulting from cleavage of a fertilized ovum.

Blind spot—small area in retina through which the optic nerve exits the eyeball; with no photoreceptors present, this area does not respond to light.

Blood-brain barrier—physiological barrier unique to brain arteries that prevents release of noxious substances in blood from entering the brain.

Blood pressure—force exerted by blood pumped against arterial walls.

Blood urea nitrogen—examination of the nitrogen from urea in the blood for determining the adequacy of kidney function.

Brachial plexus—network of nerve fibers supplying arm, forearm, and hand.

Brachium—armlike fiber bundle; brachium of inferior colliculus represents auditory fiber bundle that connects inferior colliculus to medial geniculate body of thalamus; brachium of superior colliculus mediates visual information from lateral geniculate body of thalamus to pretectal region in midbrain.

Brachium conjunctivum—see *Superior cerebellar peduncle.*

Brachium pontis—see *Middle cerebellar peduncle.*

Bradykinesia—slow motor movements.

Brainstem—stem part of the brain that consists of midbrain, pons, and medulla.

Brain waves—cellular electrical activity recorded from brain surface.

Branchial arches—five pairs of arched embryological structures that develop into laryngeal, pharyngeal, and facial muscles.

Broca's aphasia—type of aphasia associated with a lesion in the premotor cortex and characterized by impaired verbal output.

Brodmann areas—mapped areas of the brain representing various cytoarchitectonic structures.

Calvarium—superior portion of the cranium; has a domelike appearance.

Canal of Schlemm—circular venous sinus canal that drains the aqueous humor from anterior chamber of the eyeball.

Capillary—terminal branch of artery that carries blood to tissues.

Cardiac muscle—heart muscle.

Carotid vascular system—system formed by the internal carotid artery that supplies blood to the brain; divided into middle and anterior cerebral arteries.

Catabolism—metabolic breakdown of complex substances into simpler substances such as food digestion and oxidation of nutrient molecules for energy.

Catecholamine—group of neurotransmitters including epinephrine, norepinephrine, and dopamine; cells that produce these neurotransmitters are catecholaminergic.

Cauda equina—nerve fibers that extend beyond spinal cord.

Caudal—toward back of brain or tail of the spinal cord.

Caudate nucleus—basal ganglia nucleus with motor functions.

Central gray—reticular core around the cerebral aqueduct.

Central sulcus—obliquely descending sulcus on lateral surface of brain that forms the boundary between the frontal and parietal lobes.

Cerebellar cortex—cellular layer of the cerebellum.

Cerebellar peduncles—three pairs of fiber tracts that connect the cerebellum with the brainstem.

Cerebellum—rhombencephalon derivative; important motor control center.

Cerebral aqueduct (iter)—narrow ventricular passage in midbrain that connects the third and fourth ventricles.

Cerebral cortex—sheet of gray matter that consists of six layers of cells and covers the cerebral hemisphere.

Cerebral hemisphere—two major parts of the cerebrum connected by the corpus callosum.

Cerebrospinal fluid—clear fluid produced in ventricular cavity; protects the brain by forming a cushion in the subarachnoid space around the central nervous system.

Cerebrovascular accident (CVA, stroke)—interruption of blood supply to brain tissue.

Cerebrum—two cerebral hemispheres connected by the corpus callosum.

Chemotherapy—chemical treatment of a disease.

Cholesterol—fatlike substance found in animal fat, bile, blood, and other body parts.

Cholinergic—pertaining to cells that secrete acetylcholine.

Chordotomy—surgical sectioning of tract in the spinal cord.

Chorea—rhythmic, graceful, involuntary movements, predominantly of distal extremities and muscles of the face, tongue, and pharynx; striatum is the suspected site of lesion.

Chorion—fetal membrane enclosing the embryo; it forms part of the placenta and is highly active and functional.

Choroid plexus—pia capillary network invaginated in the ventricles that produces cerebrospinal fluid.

Chromatolysis—swelling and dissolution of cellular organelles, specifically Nissl bodies, in response to injury.

Chromosomes—strands of condensed chromatin (DNA) within nucleus; associated with RNA and histones.

Ciliary muscle—eye muscle that regulates lens thickness in visual accommodation; its contraction reduces tension on suspensory ligaments, inducing a spherical shape of the lens for near vision.

Cingulate gyrus—limbic–cortical structure midsagittal above the corpus callosum; has emotional, somatic, and autonomic functions.

Circadian rhythm—any rhythm with a period of one day.

Circle of Willis—arterial circle at the base of the brain that connects carotid and vertebrobasilar system; the major anastomotic point in the brain.

Claustrum—subcortical gray structure; concerned with unconscious motor activity.

Cleavage—progressive mitotic division of the fertilized ovum.

Climbing fibers—cerebellar afferent fibers (olivocerebellar projections) that directly activate Purkinje cells.

Coagulation—blood clot formation.

Cochlea—fluid-filled spiral structure that contains the organ of Corti, the sensory end organ of hearing.

Coelom—body cavity containing visceral organs: heart, lungs, intestines, testes, etc.

Cogwheel rigidity—condition of rhythmic interruption of resistance in a hypertonic muscle during passive manipulation.

Colic—painful spasmodic movement in any hollow internal tube, occurs mostly in the abdomen.

Collateral circulation—alternative blood flow via an anastomosis to an area that has lost its blood supply; also called ventricular trigone.

Collateral trigone—region from which the lateral ventricles diverge into temporal and occipital horns.

Color blindness—X-linked genetic condition in which perception of one or more colors is impaired.

Commissural fibers—association fibers that travel across the midline and connect both cerebral hemispheres.

Computed tomography (CT)—X-ray technique that provides cross-sectional images of the brain and body.

Conceptus—developing human along with its membranes; any developmental stage from zygote through birth.

Concussion—brain injury associated with brief loss of consciousness in absence of any visible structural damage.

Conduction aphasia—type of aphasia associated with arcuate fasciculus lesion and characterized by disproportionately impaired verbal repetition with nearly normal comprehension and speaking.

Conductive hearing loss—hearing loss resulting from an interrupted transmission of sound through the outer or middle ear to the cochlea.

Cones—retinal cells responsible for the highest level of visual acuity and color discrimination.

Conjugate—simultaneous movement of both eyes in the same direction, important for focusing and reading.

Connecting stalk—forerunner of the umbilical cord; formed of extraembryonic mesoderm.

Contralateral—side opposite the midline.

Contusion—brain injury characterized by a bruise under the unbroken skin.

Conus medullaris—terminal point of the spinal cord.

Convex—elevated, as the surface of a lens.

Convolution—rounded elevation forming the surface of the cerebral hemispheres, also called gyrus (pl. gyri).

Cornea—outermost layer of the eye.

Coronal—vertical section dividing the brain into front and back.

Corona radiata—sensorimotor fibers above the internal capsule.

Corpora quadrigemina—tectal structure; four egg-shaped structures (inferior and superior colliculi) in the dorsal midbrain that serve as reflex centers for vision and audition.

Corpus callosum—massive bundle of axonal fibers that interconnects the cortex of the two cerebral hemispheres.

Corpus striatum—see *Striatum*.

Cortex—collection of nerve cells that forms the external surface of the brain.

Corticobulbar tract—pyramidal tract fibers that descend from the cortex to the brainstem and activate motor nuclei of cranial nerves.

Corticospinal tract—pyramidal tract fibers that descend from the cortex to the spinal cord and activate spinal motor neurons.

Cortisol—steroid hormone released by the adrenal cortex that inhibits the immune system and mobilizes energy.

Cranial nerves—12 pairs of nerves in the peripheral nervous system that innervate buccofacial muscles and mediate sensations of vision, smell, and touch from face, head and neck.

Craniotomy—surgical procedure used to open the skull for brain operations.

Cranium bifidum— embryological malformation marked by absence of cranial bone fusion leading to herniation of meninges and cortex.

Cremasteric reflex—retraction of the testicle on stroking the skin of the inner thigh; absence of this reflex indicates a pyramidal tract lesion (upper motor neuron).

Cristae—vestibular sensory hair cells embedded in a gelatinous mass that project into the ampulla of each of the three semicircular canals.

Crossed extension reflex—withdrawal of a limb to painful stimuli with the extension of opposite side lower extremities.

CT scan—see *Computed tomography*.

Cuneus—occipital lobe region on midsagittal surface.

Cupula—gelatinous mass that contains hairs (cilia) of sensory hair cells and forms a cone that projects into the endolymph of semicircular canal.

Cutaneous—general sensation from skin.

Cytoarchitectonism—related to structure, organization, and arrangement of nerve cells in the brain.

Cytoarchitectural map—map of brain areas based on their cellular composition.

Cytological—related to cells.

Cytoplasm—substances within cellular plasma but external to nucleus.

Cytotrophoblast—cellular layer developing from trophoblast; forms components of fetal membranes, such as amnion, chorion, and placenta.

Dark adaptation—process of retina becoming sensitive to dim light.

Decerebrate rigidity—sustained contractions of extensor muscles that result from lesions in the brainstem reticular formation above the vestibular nucleus.

Decibel—unit of sound intensity.

Decussation—crossing over of fibers; e.g., crossing of pyramidal tract and dorsal column lemniscal fibers in the medulla.

Deep cerebellar nuclei—nuclei embedded within the cerebellar medullary region, e.g., dentate, emboliform, globose, and fastigial nuclei.

Dementia—acquired progressive impairment of intellectual functions caused by brain damage.

Dendrites—cellular processes that receive impulses from other cells.

Denticulate ligaments—fibrous ligaments attaching the spinal cord to surrounding dura mater.

Depolarization—changes in membrane potentials in which the cellular interior changes from negative (resting potential) to positive.

Dermatome—body region that receives its sensory and motor innervation from a single spinal nerve.

Diabetes insipidus—excessive thirst and urination caused by inadequate secretion of antidiuretic hormone.

Diabetes mellitus—disease in which glucose is not adequately oxidized in the body tissue because of insufficient insulin.

Diadochokinesia—ability to make rapid alternating movements of limbs; requires coordinated activity of pairs of muscles.

Dichotic listening—neuropsychological testing tool that involves simultaneous presentation of auditory stimuli to both ears.

Diencephalon—inner part of the brain that lies between the cerebral hemispheres and midbrain; includes the thalamus and hypothalamus.

Diffusion—temperature-based movement of molecules from a region of high concentration to an area of low concentration, resulting in a balanced distribution.

Diopter—unit used for measuring the refractive power of the eye, which is reciprocally connected to the focal distance.

Diplopia—pathological condition of double vision in which a single object is seen as two objects.

Disjunction—separation of bivalent chromosomes during anaphase.

Diuresis—excessive secretion and passage of urine; commonly seen in diabetes mellitus.

Diurnal—occurring every day.

DNA (deoxyribonucleic acid)—double-stranded molecular structure containing genetic information.

Dominant inheritance—denoting a nonfunctional allele possessed by one of the parents, which dominates the contrasting allele (the recessive) from the other parent.

Dopamine—neurotransmitter commonly released by brainstem neurons; deficiency of it causes Parkinson's disease.

Dorsal—toward superior surface of brain.

Dorsal horn—region of the spinal cord containing sensory cell bodies.

Duchenne's muscular dystrophy—disease of muscular atrophy transmitted through X-linked inheritance.

Dura mater—outermost layer of the three meninges.

Dysarthria—disorders of motor speech that result from central or peripheral disturbances of muscular control.

Dysdiadochokinesia—impaired ability to undertake rapidly alternating movements.

Dysphagia—difficulty in swallowing.

Ectoderm—outermost of the three primary germ layers.

Edinger-Westphal nucleus—visceral nucleus of the oculomotor nerve that regulates pupil constriction and lens accommodation.

Efferent—axonal fibers that mediate nerve impulses away from the central nervous system and cell body.

Electroencephalography—technique for recording electrical activity of the brain.

Embolism—blocking of an artery by a piece of clot (sclerotic tissue) that has detached from an atherosclerotic plaque.

Embryoblast—inner cell mass that gives rise to embryo proper.

Embryonic (animal) pole—region of blastocyst with inner cell mass; opposite pole is abembryonic (vegetal) pole.

Emmetropia—normal vision in which light rays converge on the retina.

Encapsulated endings—ovoid fluid-filled receptors with multiple layers; highly sensitive to deformation.

Encephalopathy—dysfunction of the central nervous system because of a degenerative disease of the brain.

Endoderm—innermost of the three primary germ layers.

Endolymph—fluid that fills the semicircular canals, utricle, and saccule.

Endoneurium—layer of connective tissue that wraps axons of peripheral nerves

Endorphin—one of the peptides in the brain that is concerned with pain; acts similar to morphine.

Endothelial cells—layer of cells lining the blood vessels.

Ependymal cells—layer of cells that lines the interior surface of the ventricular cavity.

Epiblast—embryonic germ layer on the dorsal aspect of the bilaminar disk that gives rise to ectoderm, neuroectoderm, and mesoderm.

Epicritic—fine discriminative touch; includes two-point touch, stereognosis, and graphesthesia.

Epilepsy—sensory, motor, cognitive, and affective disorders that result from abnormal electric discharges in brain.

Epinephrine (adrenaline)—important reticular formation catecholamine neurotransmitter synthesized from norepinephrine.

Epineurium—connective tissue sheath that surrounds a peripheral nerve.

Epithalamus—part of the thalamus.

Equilibrium—state of body balance in space; dynamic equilibrium maintains balance when moving; static equilibrium maintains balance in relatively stationary (nonmovement) states.

Estrogen—female sex hormones that promote development of sex characteristics.

Eustachian tube—tube that connects the middle ear with the nasopharynx; equalizes air pressure on both sides of tympanic membrane (eardrum).

Excitatory postsynaptic potential—impulses that activate the postsynaptic cell to generate an action potential.

Expanded tip endings—receptors with expanded tips; slow-transmitting and moderately adapting mechanoreceptors.

Extension—movement that straightens a limb.

Extensor—muscle that causes extension when it contracts.

Extraembryonic—prefix indicating derivation from a trophoblast.

Extrafusal fibers—contractile portion of muscle fibers that forms the bulk of a muscle.

Falx cerebelli—triangular vertical extension from tentorial cerebelli that separates the two cerebellar hemispheres.

Falx cerebri—large, sickle-shaped extension of dura between two hemispheres.

Far point—point from which light rays originate.

Fasciculation—Involuntary contractions of groups (fasciculi) of muscle fibers.

Fasciculus cuneatus—sensory fibers carrying sensations of fine discriminative touch from the upper half of the body.

Fasciculus gracilis—sensory fibers carrying sensations of fine discriminative touch from the lower half of the body.

Fibrillation—spontaneous twitch of individual muscle fibers.

Filum terminale—fibrous extension of the spinal cord attached to coccyx

Fissure—groove region bordering the gyri on the brain surface, also called sulcus (pl. sulci).

Flaccid—weak, having less than normal tone (muscle).

Flaccid dysarthria—motor speech disorder associated with degeneration of lower motor neurons.

Flexion—movement that bends a limb.

Flexor—muscle that causes flexion when it contracts.

Focal length—distance between the lens and point where light rays converge to form a focused image.

Focal point—point at which light rays converge for focusing.

Foramen—opening.

Foramen magnum—opening through which the medulla exits from the base of the skull.

Forebrain—brain region derived from the rostral embryonic brain and includes the telencephalon and diencephalon.

Fornix—bundle of fibers that mediates two-way connections among hypothalamus, septum, and hippocampus and is important in visceral functions.

Fovea—dipped area in the macula lutea; site of central fixation responsible for sharp vision.

Free nerve endings—small and slowly conducting mechanoreceptors; associated with pain and temperature.

Frequency—rate of complete cycles of vibrations, expressed in Hertz.

GABA—major inhibitory neurotransmitter of the brain synthesized from glutamate; its deficiency in the striatum is implicated with Huntington's chorea.

GABA-ergic neurons—inhibitory neurotransmitter neurons in basal ganglia.

Gametes—male and female sex cells.

Gametogenesis—process through which male and female sex cells develop.

γ-Motor neurons—slow-conducting, small spinal motor neurons (gamma) that supply intrafusal muscle fibers.

Ganglia—group of nerve cell bodies in the peripheral nervous system.

Gene expression—process that converts gene coded information into the operating of a cell and structure.

Gene mutation—any spontaneous heritable changes in the sequencing of DNA elements.

General functions—touch, pain, and temperature information, processed by general receptors.

Generalized seizure—extensive and synchronized electrical activity in nerve cells that spreads to the entire brain.

Gene—unit of heredity located at a fixed position on a particular chromosome.

Genome—complete DNA sequence containing entire genetic information of an individual or a species.

Glia cells—secondary cells (astroglia, microglia, and oligodendroglia) in the nervous system that serve as supportive connective tissue.

Globus pallidus—part of the basal ganglia that is involved with motor activity.

Golgi tendon organ—receptor in muscle tendons that is sensitive to tension in muscles.

Gonadotropic hormones—hormones secreted in the anterior pituitary gland (adenohypophysis) that regulate sex gland cells.

Graphesthesia—discriminative sensory ability to recognize the outline of letters, words, or symbols written on the surface of skin.

Gray matter—term used for the collection of cell bodies in the central nervous system.

Gyrus—bump formation that lies between two sulci.

Helicotrema—end region of the cochlea that connects the scala vestibuli to the scala tympani.

Hemianesthesia—loss of sensation on one side of the body.

Hemianopsia—loss of vision in half of the visual field.

Hemiballism—violent flinging movements on one side of the body.

Hemiparesis—paralysis of one side of body.

Hemophilia—X-linked disorder of blood clotting.

Hemorrhage—discharging of blood from a ruptured artery.

Heredity—passage of parental characteristics to offspring via genes.

Heschl's gyri—short, oblique convolutions in the lateral sulcus that form the primary auditory cortex.

Hippocampus (hippocampal formation)—limbic structure bordering the lateral ventricle inferior horns; thought to be related to memory functions.

Histology—microscopic study of tissue structures.

Homeostatic—related to maintenance of the bodily environment.

Homonymous hemianopia—loss of vision in same visual fields for both eyes.

Homunculus—representation of the body in the sensorimotor cortex.

Hormones—chemical substances that originate in an organ and regulate important body activities.

Huntington's chorea—progressive condition of dominant inheritance characterized by involuntary movements, cognitive deficits, and dysarthric speech.

Hydrocephalus—accumulation of cerebrospinal fluid in brain ventricles secondary to its impaired absorption.

Hypalgesia—increased threshold for pain resulting in decreased sensitivity to pain.

Hyperalgesia—decreased threshold for pain marked by increased response to painful stimuli.

Hyperopia—visual refraction error in which light rays focus behind the retina (farsightedness).

Hyperparathyroidism—increased level of parathyroid secretion.

Hyperplasia—increase in cell number.

Hyperthermia—unusually high fever.

Hypertrophy—increase in size of cells or organs.

Hypoblast—embryonic germ layer on ventral aspect of the bilaminar disk that gives rise to endoderm.

Hyponatremia—low level of serum sodium.

Hyporeflexia—diminished or reduced reflexive movements that usually result from pathology in the lower motor neurons.

Hypothalamus—diencephalic structure beneath the thalamus that secretes hormones and regulates feeding, fighting, and sexual behavior.

Hypotonia—reduced tone and lessened resistance to passive movement in muscle.

Hypoxemia—low oxygen level in arterial blood.

Hypoxia—below-normal level of oxygen in body tissues.

Ideomotor apraxia—inability to carry on skilled purposeful movements because of a disconnection between motor and ideational centers.

Idiopathic—describing a disease without an apparent cause.

Immunity—body's natural power to resist the attack of disease or harmful agents.

Impulse—action potential.

Incus—middle ear bone.

Inertia—tendency of matter to resist change in motion (if matter is at rest, it remains at rest; if moving, it continues to move until acted on by an external force).

Infarct—area of damaged tissue caused by insufficient or blocked blood supply.

Inferior cerebellar peduncle—restiform body; one of the fiber bundles connecting the cerebellum with the brainstem; mediates spinal inputs to the cerebellar hemispheres.

Inferior colliculus—midbrain structure affecting auditory reflexes and transmission of auditory signals to the medial geniculate body of the thalamus.

Inferior mesenteric ganglia—prevertebral sympathetic nucleus.

Inflammation—edematous response by tissue to an injury.

Infundibular stem—stalk of the pituitary gland.

Inhibitory postsynaptic potentials—impulses that inhibit the capacity of a postsynaptic cell to generate an action potential.

Insomnia—inability to sleep.

Insula (isle of Reil)—triangular cortical brain area buried within the lateral sulcus.

Intensity—amplitude of sound waves that determines loudness; refers to strength of molecular movement.

Interhemispheric—relating to a structure common to both cerebral hemispheres or a structure between them.

Internal arcuate fibers—crossing fibers of dorsal lemniscal system at the medulla.

Internal capsule—collection of ascending and descending fibers at the diencephalic level.

Interneurons—associational neurons that interconnect other nerve cells within the central nervous system; their function is either to facilitate or to inhibit signals.

Intracranial pressure—pressure within the cranium or skull.

Intrafusal fibers—specialized muscle fibers that run parallel to extrafusal fibers and contain muscle spindles, the muscle stretch receptors.

Intrahemispheric—related to structures within one hemisphere.

Ion—particle formed when an electrolyte goes into solution.

Ionic equilibria—electrical potential difference that regulates the ionic concentration gradient across the cell membrane.

Ion selectivity—membrane permeability to selected ions.

Ipsilateral—related to the same side in contrast to the opposite side.

Iris—colored contractile membrane that covers the anterior chamber and regulates pupil size.

Ischemia—reduced supply of blood.

Iter—see *Cerebral aqueduct.*

Karyotype—presentation of an individual's chromosomes arranged in a standard format according to their shapes and sizes.

Kinesthesia—ability to detect the range and direction of limb movements.

Klüver-Bucy syndrome—behavioral syndrome that results from bilateral ablation of the amygdala and surrounding temporal tissues; characterized by indiscriminate eating, oral exploration, fearlessness, loss of aggression, psychic blindness, and inappropriate hypersexuality.

Korsakoff's syndrome—neurological syndrome of confusion, confabulation, social apathy, and amnesia secondary to chronic alcoholism.

Labyrinth—system of intercommunicating bony canals and cavities that constitute the inner ear and have a membranous lining; lining forms specialized sensory organs that project into the endolymph of the canals.

Lacrimal gland—gland in the orbit responsible for secretion of tears.

Lamina terminalis (lamina terminalis hypothalami)—thin plate derived from telencephalon; rostral end of former neural tube; later in development, it forms the anterior wall of the third ventricle of the cerebrum.

Lateral geniculate body—thalamic nucleus responsible for transmission of visual information to cortex.

Lateral lemniscus—fibers projecting auditory impulses between superior olivary nucleus and inferior colliculus.

Lateral ventricle—ventricular cavity in the cerebral hemisphere.

Lemniscus—collection of nerve fibers carrying similar information.

Leukemia—malignant blood disease marked by abnormal white blood cells.

Light adaptation—physiological process through which retinal cells gradually become less sensitive to bright light.

Light reflex—constriction of the pupil in response to light.

Limbic lobe—phylogenetically, an old part of the brain that regulates reproductive behavior, instinctual reflexes, and vegetative activities.

Locus ceruleus—important reticular formation nucleus in the brainstem that produces norepinephrine and widely projects to various brain areas.

Logarithm—exponent that indicates the power to which a number is raised to produce another number.

Lower motor neurons—motor nuclei through which the central nervous system sends impulses to muscles and glands; muscles deprived of efferent impulses atrophy.

Lumbar puncture—diagnostic procedure in which a needle is inserted in lower lumbar section of vertebral canal to drain a small amount of cerebrospinal fluid.

Luminosity curve—visual representation of spectral sensitivity of photoreceptors to light rays of various wavelengths.

Macrophage—phagocytic cell that digests and removes cellular debris in the brain.

Macula—specialized sensory structure in the vestibular apparatus that contributes to the maintenance of static equilibrium.

Macula lutea—yellowish area in the posterior retina that predominantly contains cones and corresponds to the central visual field.

Magnetic resonance imaging (MRI)—imaging technique with magnetic tracer to provide clear tissue resolution.

Malleus—middle ear ossicle attached to the tympanic membrane.

Mechanoreceptors—sensory receptor responsible for selective stimuli.

Medial forebrain bundle—important limbic fiber bundle that interconnects forebrain, limbic structures, hypothalamus, and the midbrain tegmentum and connects to dopaminergic, noradrenergic, and serotonic neurons.

Medial geniculate body—thalamic nucleus responsible for transmitting auditory information to the cortex.

Medial lemniscus—sensory fiber tract formed in medulla by crossed sensory fibers; carries discriminative touch and proprioception.

Medial longitudinal fasciculus—brainstem fiber bundle that runs on each side of the midline in the brainstem beneath the fourth ventricle and interconnects ocular cranial nerve nuclei with vestibular projections.

Meiosis—cell division during the formation of sex cells in which the number of chromosomes is halved.

Membrane potential—electric voltage across a cell membrane.

Memory—ability to retain learned information.

Ménière's disease—chronic condition of the membranous labyrinth edema characterized by progressive hearing loss, vertigo, and tinnitus.

Meninges—three protective membranes (dura, arachnoid, and pia) that cover the central nervous system.

Meningitis—bacterial or viral infection of the central nervous system that causes inflammation in meningeal membranes.

Mesoderm—middle of the three primary germ layers.

Metabolism—cellular biochemical activities that include analytical (catabolic) and synthetic (anabolic) reactions that generate energy.

Metaphase—stage in mitotic cellular division.

Metastasis—spread of disease from one part of the body to another, as with migration of cancerous cells.

Microcephaly—embryological malformation in which the brain and skull cap are small in comparison to the face size.

Microfilaments—as protein actin, contributors to the cellular skeleton.

Microglia—scavenger glia cells that remove cellular debris.

Microtubules—represented as straight protein tubulin, contributors to the cellular skeleton; responsible for axoplasmic transport.

Micturition—urination.

Midbrain—part of the brainstem between the pons and diencephalon; also called mesencephalon.

Middle cerebellar peduncle (brachium pontis)—bundle of fibers that connects the cerebellum with basilar pons.

Middle ear—air-filled cavity containing three bones.

Miosis—condition of contracted pupillary aperture.

Mitosis—cell division in which the daughter cell receives identical number and kind of chromosomes.

Modiolus—conical bony structure that wraps the cochlea around it.

Monoamines—subgroup of small molecular neurotransmitters derived from amino acids.

Monocular vision—visual field processed by only one eye.

Morula—tiny sphere of blastomeres.

Mossy fibers—afferent fibers that include all sensory projections to the cerebellum, except for olivocerebellar fibers.

Motor cortex—cortical region consisting of Brodmann area 4; involved with control and regulation of voluntary movements.

Motor end plate—postsynaptic membrane at the neuromuscular junction.

Motor neuron—neuron in the anterior horn of the spinal cord that controls muscle cells and causes muscle contraction.

Motor unit—neuronal unit that consists of motor neurons, their axonal processes, myoneural junctions, and innervated muscles.

Multipolar cells—neurons containing three or more neurites.

Muscle spindles—receptors in muscles; sensitive to changes in length of muscles.

Mutation—spontaneous changes in gene or chromosomal structure.

Myalgia—pain in muscles.

Myasthenia gravis—autoimmune neuromuscular disorder that results from growth of antibodies to acetylcholine receptors.

Mydriasis—dilation of the pupil.

Myelin—sheath of lipid and cell membrane wrapped around an axon.

Myoneural junction—synapse between a lower motor neuron axon terminal and a skeletal muscle fiber.

Myopathy—disease of muscles.

Myopia—nearsightedness; refraction error in which light rays converge in front of the retina.

Myosin—thin filament protein of muscle fibers that contributes to the contraction of muscle fibers by chemical interactions.

Myotatic reflex—reflexive muscle contraction in response to muscle stretch.

Necrosis—island of dead tissue surrounded by normal tissue.

Neocerebellum—phylogenetically, new part of the cerebellum that includes the posterior lobe; concerned with skilled movements.

Neocortex—six-layer cerebral cortex found in mammals only.

Neologisms—unrecognizable word formations.

Nerve cell—specialized cell of nervous system that conducts electrical impulses.

Neural crest—segmental neuroectodermal tissue that separates from the neural tube dorsally before it closes; develops into elements of the peripheral nervous system and other specialized structures.

Neuralgia—pain extending along the course of a nerve.

Neural plate—thickened midline plate of neuroectoderm that develops into the neural tube, giving rise to the central nervous system.

Neural tube—embryological structure that results from fusion of neural folds and develops into the brain and spinal cord.

Neuraxis—brain and spinal axis.

Neurilemma—outermost covering of axons formed by Schwann cells; in the peripheral nervous system.

Neurite—thin tube-shaped process extending from a neuronal cell; further divided into an axon and dendrite.

Neuritis—inflammation of a nerve or nerves.

Neuroblast—immature cell prior to cell division.

Neurofibrillary tangles—age-induced twisting of fibers in the soma of nerve cells, often associated with Alzheimer's disease and Down's syndrome.

Neurofilaments—important components of the cellular skeleton; serve as channels for intracellular communication.

Neuroleptic—tranquilizer; a class of drugs used for treating psychoses.

Neuromuscular junction—myoneural junction; the space between neuron and muscle.

Neuron—nerve cell with a cell body and its processes that participate in impulse transmission.

Neuropathy—nerve disease.

Neuropharmacology—the study of drug effects on the nervous system.

Night blindness (nyctalopia)—inability to see at night after a normal period of dark adaptation.

Nissl body—endoplasmic structure in neuronal cell body that participates in protein synthesis.

Nociceptor—receptor sensitive to harmful stimuli, such as pain.

Node of Ranvier—intervening space between two internodes (segments) of myelin.

Nondisjunction—failure of two homologous chromosomes or two chromatids to dissociate during meiosis; results in one cell having an extra chromosome and the other cell missing one.

Non-REM (non–rapid eye movement, NREM) sleep—stage of sleep characterized by slow and large waves; marked with some muscle tone and paucity of dreams.

Nonspecific nuclei—group of thalamic nuclei that receive inputs from diffuse sources and project to diffuse cortical areas, e.g., intralaminar nuclei that mediate reticular projections to the cortex and influence synchronization of brain electrical activity.

Noradrenergic synapses—nerve endings where norepinephrine is released.

Norepinephrine—catcholamine neurotransmitter also called noradrenalin; released by neurons primarily in the pons and medulla; cells that produce norepinephrine are called noradrenergic cells.

Notochord—primitive solid skeletal structure derived from specialized mesodermal cells; retained in intervertebral disk as the nucleus pulposus; ventral to neural tube.

Nucleolus—structure in the nucleus of a cell body; contains RNA needed for protein synthesis.

Nucleus—controlling center of a nerve cell.

Nucleus pulposus—adult remnant of notochord in intervertebral disk.

Nystagmus—oscillatory movement of eyeballs composed of slow and fast components; identified according to direction of fast component.

Occipital lobe—region of the cerebrum.

Octonia—gelatinous mass that incorporates sensory hair cells covered by a thin layer of densely packed calcium carbonate crystals.

Olfaction—sense of smell.

Olfactory bulb—bulb-shaped brain structure that receives input from olfactory receptor neurons.

Olfactory cortex—region of the cerebral cortex connected to the olfactory bulb; includes the uncus, amygdaloid nucleus, and anterior region of the parahippocampal gyrus.

Olfactory epithelium—cellular sheet that lines the nasal passages and contains olfactory receptor neurons.

Oligodendroglia—glial cell that produces the myelin sheath around axons in the central nervous system.

Oogenesis—development of a female sex cell (ovum).

Oogonia—primordial cell from which an oocyte is derived.

Ophthalmoplegia—paralysis of extrinsic or intrinsic eye muscles.

Opsin—protein found in rhodopsin of rods.

Optic chiasm—structure where the right and left optic

nerves converge and part of the fibers from each nerve decussate to form the optic tracts.

Optic disk (papilla)—area through which the optic nerve exits and arteries enter the eyeball.

Optic nerve—bundle of ganglion cell reception that passes from the eye to the optic chiasm.

Optic radiation—collection of axons coursing from the lateral geniculate body to the visual cortex.

Optic tectum—structure used to describe the superior colliculus.

Optic tract—collection of retinal ganglion cell axons stretching from the optic chiasm to the brainstem.

Organ of Corti—auditory receptor organ that contains hair cells and supporting cells.

Osmotic pressure—pressure exerted by active elements in a solution.

Ossicles—three small bones in the middle ear: malleus, incus, and stapes.

Otitis media—inflammation of the middle ear resulting in conductive hearing loss.

Oval window—hole in the bony cochlea at which movement of the ossicles is transferred to movement of the fluids in the cochlea.

Oxidation—chemical dissolution of nutrients for energy.

Oxytocin (Pitocin)—peptide hormone released from the posterior pituitary; stimulates uterine contractions in pregnant uterus to induce delivery and ejection of milk from mammary glands.

Pacinian corpuscle—mechanoreceptor in the skin sensitive to vibrations.

Paleocerebellum—anterior lobe of the cerebellum, primarily concerned with equilibrium and locomotion.

Papez circuit—neuronal circuit connecting the hypothalamus and cortex; serves pain and emotion.

Papilla— see *Optic disk*.

Parahippocampus—memory-related cortical region in medial surface of temporal lobe.

Paralysis—loss of under voluntary control on muscles; spastic paralysis is associated with upper motor neuron syndrome; flaccid paralysis is associated with lower motor neurons.

Paraphasia—inappropriate selection of words and phonemes.

Parasympathetic system—division of the autonomic nervous system with nuclei in craniosacral region; concerned with conservation of body energy.

Parenchyma—functionally specialized cells of an organ.

Paresthesia—abnormal sensation, such as numbness, crawling, twisting, and itching.

Parkinson's disease—movement disorder of the basal ganglia characterized by resting tremor, muscular rigidity, and paucity of movements.

Paroxysmal discharge—periodic abnormal electrical discharge.

Peduncle—bundle of fibers that connects the cerebellum and brainstem.

Periaqueductal gray matter—region surrounding the cerebral aqueduct in the midbrain.

Perilymph—fluid in the scala vestibuli and tympani.

Peripheral nervous system—part of the nervous system that includes all cranial and spinal nerves.

Peristalsis—wavelike contracting movements in a hollow structure that propels the content.

Peritoneal cavity—potential abdominal space between layers of parietal and visceral peritoneum.

Periventricular zone—hypothalamic region that medial to the third ventricle.

Permeability—property of brain vessels that restricts the passage of fluids and substances.

PET—see *Positron emission tomography*.

pH—indicator of acidity and alkalinity in a solution.

Phagocyte—macrophagic microglia cells that ingest cellular debris.

Phantom pain—sensation of pain apparently originating from an amputated limb.

Photopsin—visual pigment found in retinal cones.

Photoreceptors—specialized retinal cells that transfer light energy into action potentials.

Pia mater—inner most layer of the three meninges.

Pineal gland—thalamic gland organ; important in diurnal rhythm.

Pituitary gland—hypothalamic structure of hormone synthesis in the central nervous system; divided into a large anterior lobe (adenohypophysis) and a small posterior lobe (neurohypophysis).

Planum temporale—area of the superior temporal lobe found to be larger in the left temporal lobe.

Plasticity—brain's ability to reorganize and modify functions and adapt to internal and external changes.

Poikilothermy—condition in which the temperature of an organism is similar to the temperature of the environment.

Polar bodies—products of cell division during maturation of the ovum that consists of almost all nuclear materials; do not develop further and are lost.

Polarization—electrical resting state of a cell characterized by polarity of ions inside and outside the cell.

Poliomyelitis—acute viral disease of lower motor neurons in the spinal cord and brainstem.

Polydipsia—condition characterized by excessive fluid intake.

Polyuria—condition characterized by excessive discharge of urine.

Pontine nuclei—clusters of nuclei that mediate cortical projections to the cerebellar cortex.

Portal system—two sets of capillaries supplying blood to the anterior pituitary gland (adenohypophysis).

Positron emission tomography (PET)—dynamic imaging technique that measures cellular metabolism using radioactive substances.

Postcentral gyrus (somesthetic cortex, primary sensory cortex)—cortical area behind the central sulcus that integrates sensory inputs from the body and provides sensory awareness.

Posterior—tail or caudal direction.

Preganglionic and postganglionic neurons—autonomic nervous system projections that travel indirectly via small autonomic ganglia. A preganglionic neuron has its cell body in the brainstem and spinal cord, and it projects out of the central nervous system to a postganglionic neuron.

Precentral gyrus—primary motor cortex rostral to the central sulcus.

Prechordal plate—region of tall hypoblastic cells anterior to the notochord; with ectoderm, it forms the oropharyngeal membrane.

Precuneus—parietal lobe region in the midsagittal surface.

Prefrontal cortex—rostral region of the frontal cortex with connections to the dorsomedial thalamus.

Premotor cortex—area anterior to the motor cortex that programs and regulates skilled movements.

Preoptic area—anterior portion of hypothalamus above optic chiasm.

Primary auditory cortex—Brodmann area 41; cortical area on the superior temporal gyrus.

Primitive streak—thickened region of epiblastic cells in the dorsal caudal midline of the embryo in the third week; epiblastic cells transform into mesoderm–mesenchymal cells through this region.

Primordium—earliest identifiable rudiment of tissue seen during development.

Principal (inferior) olivary nucleus—nucleus that projects spinal and reticular information to the cerebellum.

Pronation—movement that turns the palm downward.

Prophase—first stage in cell division.

Proprioception—internal awareness of position, posture, and movement.

Protopathic—primitive sensory system that includes pain, temperature, and crude touch.

Protraction—movement that projects a limb or organ forward.

Pseudobulbar palsy—pathological condition involving bilateral supranuclear paralysis of the cranial nerve nuclei; has significant implications for spastic dysarthria.

Psychosis—severe form of mental disorder characterized by disorganization of thinking, personality, and behavior.

Pterygopalatine ganglion—parasympathetic postganglion of the facial nerve.

Pupil—opening through which light enters the eye and strikes the retina.

Pupillary light reflex—change in diameter of the pupils in response to projected light; mediated by visceral fibers of the oculomotor cranial nerve from the brainstem to the iris.

Purkinje cells—large cerebellar nerve cells.

Putamen—anatomical structure of the basal ganglia.

Pyramidal decussation—crossing of motor fibers that takes place in the most caudal medulla.

Pyramidal tract—tract that carries motor fibers to the brainstem and spinal cord.

Quadriplegia—paralysis of all four limbs.

Raphe nucleus—collection of reticular cells along the midline in the brainstem; diffusely project to all levels of the brain.

Rapid eye movement (REM) sleep—sleep stage characterized by high frequency, low-amplitude electroencephalographic waves, vivid dreams, and rapid eye movements.

Recessive inheritance—genetic mode of inheritance in which both parents transmit the same nonworking gene.

Reciprocal inhibition—neuronal arrangement in the nervous system in which activation of nerve cells for agonistic muscles simultaneously inhibits motor nerve cells of antagonistic muscles; ensures that when one muscle is contracting, its paired muscle is relaxing.

Red nucleus—midbrain cell cluster that relays cerebellar outputs to the motor cortex and spinal cord.

Referred pain—internal organ pain sensed in other body parts or areas.

Reflex—stereotyped involuntary motor response to a stimulus.

Refraction—bending of light rays as they travel from one medium to another.

Regional cerebral blood flow—neuroradiological technique that measures blood flow to functionally active brain areas by monitoring a radioactive tracer.

Reissner's membrane—cochlear membrane that separates the scala media from the scala vestibuli.

Restiform body—see *Inferior cerebellar peduncle*.

Resting membrane potential—membrane potential of −70 mV; at this stage, the nerve cell is not generating action potentials.

Reticular formation—diffuse core of brainstem nuclei with extensive projections that integrates the entire nervous system and is involved with cortical arousal and muscle tone.

Retina—neural layer of the eye that contains photoreceptor cells.

Retinal (visual yellow)—light-absorbing molecule of rhodopsin in rods, an aldehyde of vitamin A.

Retinotectal potentials—axons that leave the retina and synapse upon the superior colliculus.

Retraction—movement that pulls back a limb or organ.

Retrograde reaction—see *Axonal reaction*.

Rhodopsin—visual purple pigment found in rod cells.

Rigidity—stiff state of muscle; clasp knife is a transient state of increased resistance of extensors to passive muscle movement, which melts away; cogwheel is a quality of jerky resistance felt during passive muscle movement.

Rods—retinal photoreceptors responsible for night vision.

Rostral—toward the front of the head.

Rubrospinal tract—group of axons involved with motor movements; descends from the red nucleus and terminates on the motor neurons in the spinal cord.

Sagittal—vertical section dividing the brain into left and right halves.

Saltatory conduction—propagation of an action potential along a myelinated axon.

Scala media—cochlear region lying between the scala vestibuli and scala tympani.

Scala tympani—perilymph-filled lowermost compartment of the cochlea; connected to the scala vestibuli through helicotrema.

Scala vestibuli—perilymph-filled uppermost compartment of the cochlea; connected to the scala tympani through the helicotrema.

Schwann cells—glial cells that form myelin around axons in the peripheral nervous system.

Sclera—outer (white) layer of the eye ball.

Sclerosis—hardening of a structure.

Scotopic vision—night vision mediated by rod cells.

Semicircular canals—three circular canals containing sensory organs, suspended in endolymph for reflex control of dynamic equilibrium.

Semiovale center—mass of white matter below the cerebral cortex.

Sensorineural loss—deafness resulting from a dysfunctioning organ of Corti or cochlear nerve.

Sensory receptors—nerve endings that respond to environmental changes by producing action potentials.

Septum pellucidum—thin membrane above septal nuclei; anteriorly divides the lateral ventricles.

Serotonergic—cells that produce serotonin neurotransmitter.

Serotonin—important central nervous system neurotransmitter that plays a role in sleep and wakefulness.

Single photon emission tomography (SPECT)—dynamic imaging technique that measures cerebral blood flow using a radioactive substance.

Sinus—hollow channel covered with dura in the brain; receives deoxygenated blood.

Skeletal muscle—muscle that contains striated fibers; move bones around a joint.

Soma—cell body; central region of the neuron.

Somatic—relating to structures derived from a series of mesodermal somites, including skeletal muscles.

Somite—segmental blocklike mass of mesoderm on either side of the notochord; gives rise to muscles, vertebral bodies, and skin.

Somatostatin—chemical capable of inhibiting the release of somatotropin, a protein hormone, by the anterior lobe of the pituitary gland.

Spastic hemiplegia—paralysis of one side of the body after a lesion in the pyramidal tract.

Special functions—vision- and audition-related information, mediated by specialized receptors.

Specific nuclei—group of thalamic nuclei that project definitive information to functionally committed specific cortical areas; e.g., lateral geniculate body is concerned with vision and projects to primary visual cortex.

SPECT—see *Single photon emission tomography*.

Spermatogenesis—development of a male sex cell (spermatozoon).

Spermatogonia—male germ cell or gamete, undifferentiated and arising from the seminiferous tubule, dividing into two primary spermatocytes.

Spina bifida—embryonic malformation marked by the opened vertebral column; has several subtypes, for which see text.

Spinal anesthesia—injection of liquid anesthetic into the lumbar spinal subarachnoid space that causes a temporary loss of sensation in the lower body extending up to the level of injection.

Spinal nerve—nerve of the spinal cord that innervates the body.

Spinocerebellar tract—fiber bundle that mediates unconscious proprioception to the cerebellum.

Spinothalamic—axonal pathways that conduct sensory impulses from the spinal cord to the thalamus.

Spinothalamic pathway—ascending bundle of fibers that mediates pain, touch and temperature sensation.

Stapes—middle ear ossicle that is attached to the oval window.

Static labyrinth—maintenance of a balanced position of the head and body in space against gravity during rest and during straight-line head movements.

Stenosis—narrowing of arteries.

Stereognosis—identification of objects by tactual sensation of shape, texture, and size.

Stereotaxic/stereotactic—a precise method of destroying or manipulating deep-seated brain structures, located by use of three-dimensional; a common treatment method in neurosurgery.

Strabismus—optic disorder in which the eyes are not directed at the same object.

Stretch reflex—muscular contraction elicited by a passive muscle stretch.

Striate cortex—primary visual cortex; Brodmann area 17.

Striatum—collective word for the basal ganglia nuclei of the putamen and caudate nucleus.

Subarachnoid space—space filled with cerebrospinal fluid; between the pia mater and arachnoid membrane.

Subcallosal gyrus—limbic structure.

Subdural space—potential space between the dura mater and arachnoid membrane.

Substantia gelatinosa—neurons in the dorsal spinal column that receive nociceptive information.

Substantia nigra—midbrain structure related to motor functions.

Subthalamic nucleus—subthalamic structure with motor functions.

Subthalamus—subthalamic nucleus, zona incerta, and fields of H.

Superior cerebellar peduncle—branchium conjunctivum; one of the fiber bundles that connects the cerebellum with brainstem.

Superior colliculus—midbrain structure related to visual reflexes, such as ocular accommodation and coordinated head and eye movements.

Superior olivary nucleus—nucleus in the medullary tegmentum that is the first to receive projections from both cochleae.

Supination—movement that causes the palm to turn upward.

Supraoptic nucleus—hypothalamic nucleus.

Sympathetic chain—series of interconnected ganglia adjacent to the vertebral column.

Sympathetic system—one division of the autonomic nervous system with axonal projections from the thoracic and lumbar spinal regions; concerned with expenditure of body energy with regulation of bodily responses in flight or fight situation.

Synapse—point of junction between two neurons.

Syncytiotrophoblast—syncytial layer without cell boundaries differentiated from the trophoblast; enters into the formation of the placenta and its membrane.

Tactile—related to the sense of touch.

Tardive dyskinesia—involuntary slow and stereotyped movements of facial muscles; a side effect of psychotropic drugs, such as haloperidol.

Tay-Sachs disease—disorder of autosomal recessive inheritance resulting in fatal brain damage with deterioration of mental and physical functions, convulsions, and enlarged head; common in Eastern European Jews.

Tectorial membrane—membrane that hangs over the hair cells in the cochlea.

Tectospinal tract—tract that originates from nuclei in the superior colliculi and terminates on spinal motor neurons; regulates head and neck movements.

Tectum—area dorsal to the cerebral aqueduct in the midbrain; reflex center for vision and audition.

Tegmentum—area in the brainstem ventricular floor that contains sensorimotor nuclei and cranial nerves.

Telophase—final stage in the development of a nucleus.

Tendon—nerve fiber that attaches a muscle to bone.

Teratogen—fetotoxic drug that causes development of abnormal structures in an embryo, resulting in a deformed fetus.

Teratogenesis—abnormal development of an embryo that results in a deformed fetus.

Terminal bouton—end region of the axon that makes synaptic contact.

Testosterone—male sex hormone produced by the testicle; promotes the development of sperm and sexual characteristics.

Thalamus—major diencephalic structure on either side of the third ventricle; important in sensorimotor integration and projection to the cortex.

Third ventricle—cerebrospinal fluid–filled space in the diencephalon.

Thrombosis—formation of a local clot that blocks the lumen of a blood vessel.

Thymus—lymphoid structure that functions as an endocrine gland.

Thyrotropin—thyroid trophic hormone secreted by adenohypophysis.

Tonotopic—systemic organization of frequency distribution in the auditory cortex.

Tract—bundle of nerve fibers in the central nervous system.

Trapezoid body—transverse crossing fibers of the auditory pathway in the pons.

Tremor—rhythmic pill-rolling movements of fingers at rest, along with akinesia and rigidity that characterize Parkinson's disease; intention tremor occurs during movement and results from cerebellar pathology.

Trigeminal nerve—nerve responsible for sensation from the face, head, and mouth; its motor fibers regulate the muscles of mastication.

Trilaminar embryo—human embryo in the third week.

Trisomy—abnormal addition of a third chromosome of one type to a diploid set.

Trophoblast—outer cell mass differentiating into cytotrophoblast and syncytiotrophoblast.

Uncus—structure of the limbic system that contributes to the sense of smell.

Unipolar neuron—neuron with a single process (neurite).

Upper motor neurons—cell bodies in the motor cortex and their descending axonal processes that synapse on cranial and spinal motor neurons; with lesions in motor cortex, lower motor neurons become free of inhibitory and facilitatory forebrain inputs, which results in impaired volitional muscle control, spastic paralysis, and hyperreflexia.

Vasoconstriction—decreased diameter of a blood vessel.

Vasodilation—increased diameter of a blood vessel resulting in greater blood flow.

Vasomotor center—neural network in the medulla that controls arterial blood pressure and pulse rate.

Vasopressin—hypothalamic antidiuretic hormone transported to the posterior lobe of the pituitary gland.

Vein—vessel that transports circulated blood from body to heart.

Venous sinus system—veins and sinuses responsible for draining blood and cerebrospinal fluid; veins collect blood from the brain and empty it into sinuses or dilated channels.

Ventral—location below the point of reference or the bottom of a brain structure.

Ventral horn—ventral region of the spinal cord that houses motor neurons.

Ventral root—bundle of fibers that exits from the spinal ventral horns.

Ventricles—interconnected brain cavities in which cerebrospinal fluid is produced.

Vermis—midline structure of the cerebellum.

Vertebra—segment of spinal bone.

Vertex—highest point of dorsal surface of head.

Vertigo—sensation that one's body or outer world is rotating in space.

Vesicle (brain)—subdivision of embryonic neural tube, each with a wall of neuroectoderm and a cavity.

Vestibular apparatus—part of the inner ear responsible for detecting head motion.

Vestibule—cavernous part of the inner ear consisting of the utricle and saccule, which contain sensory organs needed to facilitate reflex control of static equilibrium.

Vestibulospinal tract—fibers that descend from vestibular nuclei to spinal motor neurons and regulate posture.

Viscera—internal organs of the ventral body cavity.

Visceral—vital organs of the body that have nonstriated muscles and are innervated by the autonomic nervous system; visceral activity relates to functions of respiration, phonation, and digestion.

Visceral functions—activities of the muscles of respiration, digestion, swallowing, phonation, and speech.

Visceral muscles—muscles of the heart, spleen, great vessels and digestive, respiratory, urogenital, endocrine, and speech systems.

Viscerosomatic—related to the viscera and body.

Visual acuity—assessment of the ability to resolve details of distant objects; tested with Snellen's chart.

Visual field—area seen by both eyes when looking straight ahead.

Vitreous humor—jellylike substance in the posterior cavity of the eye; prevents eyeball from collapsing and contributes to intraocular pressure.

Wada test—procedure in which the cerebral cortex is transiently anesthetized for assessing its functions.

Wallerian degeneration—structural changes in distal portion of an axon after it is sectioned and disconnected from the cell body.

Watershed—tertiary brain area peripheral to primary distribution areas for anterior, posterior, and middle cerebral arteries; derives its blood via the branches of the three cortical arteries.

White matter—collective term for axonal bundles in the central nervous system.

Withdrawal reflex—withdrawal of limb because of painful stimuli.

X-linked inheritance—genetic inheritance mode where diseases are transmitted by a gene or genes on the X (sex) chromosome.

Yolk sac (primary)—transient membranous structure of the embryo that disappears completely.

Yolk sac (secondary)—specialized structure that separates from the embryo early in development and may persist through birth; its proximal stalk gives rise to ileal (Meckel's) diverticulum.

Young-Helmholtz trichromic theory—theory that relates the color perception on the activation of three types of cones.

Zone of Lissauer—outermost region of the spinal dorsal horn that receives fibers carrying pain and temperature from the body.

Zygote—fertilized ovum (first stage in human development).

References

LISTED REFERENCES

Alexander MP, and Benson DF. The aphasias and related disturbances. In Joynt RJ, Ed. Clinical Neurology, vol. 1. Philadelphia: Lippincott, 1998:1–58.

Alexander MP, Naeser MA, and Palumbo CL. Correlations of subcortical CT lesion sites and aphasia profiles. Brain 1987;110:961–991.

Andy OJ, and Bhatnagar SC. Inhibitory effects of thalamic stimulation on acquired stuttering: physiological evidence from four neurosurgical subjects. Brain Lang 1992;42:385–401.

Andy OJ, and Bhatnagar SC. Thalamic-induced stuttering (surgical observations). J Speech Hear Res 1991;34:796–800.

Benson DF. The third alexia. Arch Neurol 1977;34:327–331.

Benson DR, Sheremata WA, Bouchard R, Segarra JM, Price D, and Geschwind N. Conduction aphasia: a clinicopathological study. Arch Neurol 1973;28:339–346.

Bhatnagar SC, and Andy OJ. Alleviation of acquired stuttering from thalamic stimulation. J Neurol Neurosurg Psychiatry 1989; 52:1182–1184.

Bhatnagar SC, Andy OJ, Korabic EW, Saxena VK, Hellman RS, Collier BD, and Krohn L. The effect of thalamic stimulation in processing of verbal stimuli in dichotic listening tasks: a case study. Brain Lang 1989;36:236–251.

Bhatnagar SC, Andy OJ, Korabic EW, and Tikofsky RS. The effect of bilateral thalamic stimulation in verbal recall. J Neurolinguistics 1990a;5:407–425.

Bhatnagar SC, Andy OJ, Korabic EW, and Tikofsky RS. Effects of bilateral thalamic stimulation on dichotic verbal processing. J Neurolinguistics 1990b;5:407–425.

Bhatnagar SC, Mandybur GT, Buckingham HW, and Andy OJ. Language representation in the human brain: evidence from cortical mapping. Brain Lang 2000;74:238–259.

Blumer D, and Benson BF. Personality changes with frontal and temporal lesions. In Benson DF, and Blumer D, Eds. Psychiatric Aspects of Neurologic Disease. New York: Grune & Stratton, 1975: 151–170.

Damasio H. Neuroanatomical Correlates of the Aphasias. In Sarno MT, Ed. Acquired Aphasia, 3rd ed. San Diego: Academic, 1998:43–70.

Darley FL, Aronson AE, and Brown JR. Motor Speech Disorders. Philadelphia: Saunders, 1975.

DeRenzi E, Motti F, and Nichelli P. Imitating gestures: a quantitative approach to ideomotor apraxia. Arch Neurol 1980;37:6–10.

Evans DA, Funkenstein HH, Albert MS, Scherr PA, Cook NR, Crown MJ, Hebert LE, Hennekens CH, and Taylor JO. Clinically diagnosed Alzheimer's disease: an epidemiologic study in a community population of older persons. JAMA 1989;262:2551–2556.

Gado M, Hanaway J, and Frank R. Functional anatomy of the cerebral cortex by computed tomography. J Comput Assist Tomogr 1979;3:1–19.

Gerstmann J. Zur Symptomatologie der Hirnlasionen im Bergangsgebiet der unteren Parietal und mittleren Occipitalwindung (das Syndrom: Fingeragnosie, Rechts-Links Stцrung, Agraphie, Akalkulie). Nervenartzt 1930:691–695. Translated in Rittenberg DA, and Hochberg FH, Eds. Neurological Classics in Modern Translation. New York: Hafner Press, 1977:150–154.

Geschwind N. The apraxias: neural mechanisms of disorders of learned movement. Am Sci 1975;63:188–195.

Geschwind N, and Levitsky W. Human brain: left-right asymmetries in temporal speech region. Science 1968;161:186–187.

Geschwind N, Quadfasel F, and Segarra J. Isolation of the speech area. Neuropsychologia 1968;6:327–340.

Goldman-Rakic PS. The prefrontal landscape: implications of functional architecture for understanding human mentation and the central executive. Philos Trans R Soc Lond B Biol Sci 1996;351:1445–1453.

Kirshner HS. Apraxia of speech: a linguistic enigma. A neurologist's perspective. Semin Speech Lang 1992;13:14–24.

Kirshner HS, Casey PF, Henson J, and Heinrich JJ. Behavioral features and lesion localization in Wernicke's aphasia. Aphasiology 1989;3:169–176.

Kirshner HS, Tanridag O, Thurman L, and Whetsell WO Jr. Progressive aphasia without dementia: two cases with focal spongiform degeneration. Ann Neurol 1987;22:527–532.

Langman J, Shimada M, and Rodier P. Floxuridine and its influence on postnatal cerebellar development. Pediatr Res 1972;6:758–764.

Lassen NA, Ingvar DH, and Skinhoj E. Brain function and blood flow. Sci Am 1978;239:62–71.

Lavine RA. Neurophysiology: The Fundamentals. Lexington: D.C. Heath & Co., 1983.

Lecours AR. Myelogenetic correlates of development of speech and language. In Lenneberg EH, and Lenneberg E, Eds. Foundation of Language Development, vol. 1. New York: Academic, 1975: 121–135.

Lenneberg EH. Biological Foundations of Language. New York: Wiley, 1967.

Mazziotta JC, Phelps ME, Carson RE, and Kuhl DE. Tomographic mapping of human cerebral metabolism: sensory deprivation. Ann Neurol 1982;12:435–444.

Mazziotta JC, Phelps ME, Miller J, and Kuhl DE. Tomographic mapping of human cerebral metabolism: normal unstimulated state. Neurology 1981;31:503–506.

Mesulam M-M. Slowly progressive aphasia without generalized dementia. Ann Neurol 1982;11:592–598.

Metter EJ. Neuroanatomy and physiology of aphasia: evidence from positron emission tomography. Aphasiology 1987;1:3–33.

Metter EJ, and Hanson WR. Brain imaging as related to speech and language. In Darby J, Ed. Speech Evaluation in Neurology. New York: Grune & Stratton, 1985:123–160.

Metter EJ, Jackson C, Kempler D, Hanson WR, Mazziotta JC, and Phelps ME. Glucose metabolic asymmetries in chronic Wernicke's, Broca's and conduction aphasias. Neurology 1986;36(suppl 1):317.

Mohr JP, Pessin MS, Finklestein S, Funkenstein HH, Duncan GW, and Davis KR. Broca aphasia: pathologic and clinical. Neurology 1978;28:311–324.

Naeser MA, Alexander MP, Helm-Estabrooks N, Levine HL, Laughlin SA, and Geschwind N. Aphasia with predominantly subcortical lesion sites—description of three capsular/putaminal aphasia syndromes. Arch Neurol 1982;39:2–14.

Naeser MA, and Hayward RW. Lesion localization in aphasia with cranial computed tomography and the Boston diagnostic aphasia examination. Neurology 1987;28:545–551.

Naeser MA, Hayward RW, Laughlin SA, Becker JMT, Jernigan TL, and Zatc LM. Quantitative CT scan studies in aphasia. Part II. Comparison of the right and left hemisphere. Brain Lang 1981;12: 165–189.

Naeser MA, Palumbo CL, Helm-Estabrooks N, Stiassny-Eder D, and Albert M. Severe nonfluency in aphasia. Role of the medial subcallosal fasciculus and other white matter pathways in recovery of spontaneous speech. Brain 1989;112:1–38.

Neary D, and Snowden J. Fronto-temporal dementia: nosology, neuropsychology, and neuropathology. Brain and Cognition 1996;31:176–187.

Ochipa C, Rothi LJG, and Heilman KM. Ideational apraxia: a deficit in tool selection and use. Ann Neurol 1989;25:190–193.

Ojemann GA. Brain organization for language from the perspective of electrical stimulation mapping. Behav Brain Res 1983;6:189–230.

Ojemann G, Ojemann J, Lettich E, and Berger M. Cortical language localization in left, dominant hemisphere. An electrical stimulation mapping investigation in 117 patients. J Neurosurg 1989; 71:316–326.

Penfield W, and Rasmussen T. The Cerebral Cortex of Man: A Clinical Study of Localization of Function. New York: Macmillan, 1950.

Penfield W, and Roberts L. Speech and Brain Mechanisms. Princeton: Princeton University, 1959.

Shallice T, and Warrington EK. Auditory-verbal short-term memory impairment and conduction aphasia. Brain Lang 1977;4:479–491.

Tikofsky RS, and Hellman R. Brain single photon emission computed tomography, newer activation and intervention studies. Semin Nucl Med 1991;21:42–57.

Wada, J. and Rasmussen, T. Intracarotid injection of sodium amytal for the lateralization of cerebral dominance. Journal of Neurosurgery 1960;17:266–282.

Yakovlev PI, and Lecours AR. The myelogenetic cycles of regional maturation of the brain. In Minkowski A, Ed. Regional Development of the Brain in Early Life. Oxford: Blackwell, 1967:3–70.

SUGGESTED REFERENCES

Adams RD, Victor M, and Ropper AH. Principles of Neurology, 6th ed. New York: McGraw-Hill, 1997.

Andreasen NC. Brain Imaging: Applications in Psychiatry. Washington, D.C.: American Psychiatric Press, 1989.

Angevine JB, and Cotman CW. Principles of Neuroanatomy. New York: Oxford University, 1981.

Arey LB. Developmental Anatomy, 7th ed. Philadelphia: Saunders, 1974.

Bear MF, Connors BW, and Paradiso MA. Neuroscience: Exploring the Brain, 2nd ed. Baltimore: Lippincott-Williams & Wilkins, 2001.

Brodal P. The Central Nervous System: Structure and Function, 2nd ed. New York: Oxford University Press, 1997.

Brodmann K. Vergleichende Lokalisation lehre der Grosshirnrinde in ihren Prinzipien dargestellt auf Grunddes Zellenbaues. Leipzig: Barth, 1909.

Brooks VB. The Neural Basis of Motor Control. New York: Oxford University Press, 1986.

Brown AG. Nerve Cells and Nervous Systems: An Introduction to Neuroscience. New York: Springer-Verlag, 1994.

Carpenter MB. Core Text of Neuroanatomy, 4th ed. Baltimore: Williams & Wilkins, 1991.

Crafts RC. A Textbook of Human Anatomy, 2nd ed. New York: John Wiley & Sons, 1979.

Crosby EC, Humphrey T, and Lauer EW. Correlative Anatomy of the Nervous System. New York: Macmillan, 1962.

DeArmond SJ, Fusco MM, and Dewey MM. Structure of the Human Brain: A Photographic Atlas, 3rd ed. New York: Oxford University Press, 1989.

Garoutte B. A Survey of Functional Neuroanatomy, 3rd ed. Millbrae CA: Mill Valley Medical Publishers, 1994.

Gelb DJ. Introduction to Clinical Neurology. Boston: Butterworth-Heinemann, 1995.

Gilman S, and Newman SW. Manter and Gatz's Essentials of Clinical Neuroanatomy and Neurophysiology, 9th ed. Philadelphia: Davis, 1996.

Gluhbegovic N, and Williams TH. The Human Brain: A Photographic Guide. Haggertown MD: Harper & Row, 1980.

Guyton AC. Textbook of Medical Physiology, 9th ed. Philadelphia: Saunders, 1998.

Guyton AC. Basic Neuroscience: Anatomy and Physiology, 2nd ed. Philadelphia: Saunders, 1991.

Haines DE, Ed. Fundamental Neuroscience, 2nd ed. New York: Churchill Livingstone, 2000.

Haines DE. Neuroanatomy: An Atlas of Structures, Sections, and Systems, 5th ed. Baltimore: Lippincott-Williams & Wilkins, 2000.

Hamilton WJ, and Mossman HW. Hamilton, Boyd, and Mossman's Human Embryology: Prenatal Development of Form and Function, 4th ed. Cambridge: Heffer, 1972.

Heimer L. The Human Brain and Spinal Cord: Functional Neuroanatomy and Dissection Guide, 2nd ed. New York: Springer-Verlag, 1994.

Kandel ER, Schwartz JH, and Jessell TM, Eds. Essentials of Neural Science and Behavior. Norwalk CT: Appleton & Lange, 1996.

Kandel ER, Schwartz JH, and Jessell TM. Principles of Neural Science, 4th ed. New York: McGraw-Hill, 2000.

Kaufman DM. Clinical Neurology for Psychiatrists, 4th ed. Philadelphia: Saunders, 1995.

Kelly DE. Bailey's Textbook of Microscopic Anatomy, 1st ed. Baltimore: Williams & Wilkins, 1984.

Kiernan JA. The Human Nervous System: An Anatomical Viewpoint, 7th ed. Philadelphia: Lippincott-Williams & Wilkins, 1998.

Kingsley RE. Concise Text of Neuroscience, 2nd ed. Philadelphia: Lippincott-Williams & Wilkins, 1999.

Kirshner HS. Behavioral Neurology: A Practical Approach. New York: Churchill Livingstone, 1985.

Kirshner HS, Ed. Handbook of Neurological Speech and Language Disorders. New York: Marcel Dekker, 1994.

Marcus E, Jacobson S, and Curtis B. An Introduction to the Neurosciences, 2nd ed. Baltimore: Williams & Wilkins, 1996.

Marieb EN. Essentials of Human Anatomy and Physiology, 6th ed. Menlo Park CA: Benjamin-Cummings, 2000.

Martini FH. Fundamentals of Anatomy and Physiology, 4th ed. Englewood Cliffs NJ: Prentice Hall, 1997.

Menkes JH. Textbook of Child Neurology, 5th ed. Baltimore: Williams & Wilkins, 1995.

Mesulam MM, Ed. Principles of Behavioral Neurology. Philadelphia: Davis, 1985.

Moore KL, and Persaud TVN. The Developing Human: Clinically Oriented Embryology, 6th ed. Philadelphia: Saunders, 1998.

Nauta WJH, and Feirtag M. Fundamental Neuroanatomy. New York: Freeman, 1986.

Netter F. The CIBA Collection of Medical Illustrations. Nervous System: Anatomy and Physiology, vol. 1 part I. West Caldwell NJ: Ciba-Geigy, 1983.

Nolte J. The Human Brain: An Introduction to Its Functional Anatomy, 4th ed. St. Louis: Mosby–Year Book, 1998.

Pansky B, Allen DJ, and Budd GC. Review of Neuroscience, 2nd ed. New York: McGraw-Hill Health Professions Division, 1991.

Parent A. Carpenter's Human Neuroanatomy, 9th ed. Baltimore: Williams & Wilkins, 1996.

Sadler TW, and Baik, S. Langman's Medical Embryology, 8th ed. Baltimore: Lippincott Williams & Wilkins, 2000.

Solomon EP, and Phillips GA. Understanding Human Anatomy and Physiology. Philadelphia: Saunders, 1987.

Tortora GJ, and Grabowski, SR. Principles of Anatomy and Physiology, 9th ed. Reading MA: Addison-Wesley Educational, 2000.

Von Bekesy G. Experiments in Hearing. Woodbury NY: Acoustical Society of America, 1989.

Weiner HL, Levitt LP, and Rae-Grant A. Neurology, 6th ed. Baltimore: Williams & Wilkins, 1999.

Weinreb EL. Anatomy and Physiology. Reading MA: Addison-Wesley Longman, 1982.

Werner JK. Neuroscience: A Clinical Perspective. Philadelphia: Saunders, 1980.

Wiederholt WC. Neurology for Non-Neurologists, 3rd ed. Philadelphia: Saunders, 1995.

Wilkinson IM. Essential Neurology, 3rd ed. Malden MA: Blackwell Science, 1999.

Williams PL, and Warwick R. Functional Neuroanatomy of Man. Philadelphia: Saunders, 1975.

Williams PL, and Bannister LH, Eds. Gray's Anatomy: The Anatomical Basis of Medicine and Surgery, 3rd ed. New York: Churchill Livingstone, 1995.

Figure and Table Credits

FIGURES

Figure 1.4. Based on Williams PL, Ed. Gray's Anatomy, 38th ed. Edinburgh: Churchill Livingstone, 1995.

Figure 1.7. From Carpenter MB. Core Text of Neuroanatomy, 4th ed. Baltimore: Williams & Wilkins, 1991.

Figure 2.1B. Modified from Guyton AC. Organ Physiology: Structure and Function of the Nervous System. Philadelphia: Saunders, 1976.

Figure 2.3. From Haines DE. Neuroanatomy: an Atlas of Structures, Sections, and Systems, 5th ed. Baltimore: Lippincott-Williams & Wilkins, 2000.

Figure 2.5. From Haines DE. Neuroanatomy: an Atlas of Structures, Sections, and Systems, 5th ed. Baltimore: Lippincott-Williams & Wilkins, 2000.

Figure 2.6. Based on Parent A. Carpenter's Human Neuroanatomy, 9th ed. Baltimore: Williams & Wilkins, 1996.

Figure 2.7. From Haines DE. Neuroanatomy: an Atlas of Structures, Sections, and Systems, 5th ed. Baltimore: Lippincott-Williams & Wilkins, 2000.

Figure 2.8. From Haines DE. Neuroanatomy: an Atlas of Structures, Sections, and Systems, 5th ed. Baltimore: Lippincott-Williams & Wilkins, 2000.

Figure 2.9. From Parent A. Carpenter's Human Neuroanatomy, 9th ed. Baltimore: Williams & Wilkins, 1996.

Figure 2.10. From Haines DE. Neuroanatomy: an Atlas of Structures, Sections, and Systems, 5th ed. Baltimore: Lippincott-Williams & Wilkins, 2000.

Figure 2.11. From Haines DE. Neuroanatomy: an Atlas of Structures, Sections, and Systems, 5th ed. Baltimore: Lippincott-Williams & Wilkins, 2000.

Figure 2.12. Modified from Carpenter MB. Core Text of Neuroanatomy, 4th ed. Baltimore: Williams & Wilkins, 1991.

Figure 2.13. Modified from Carpenter MB. Core Text of Neuroanatomy, 4th ed. Baltimore: Williams & Wilkins, 1991.

Figure 2.15. From Haines DE. Neuroanatomy: an Atlas of Structures, Sections, and Systems, 5th ed. Baltimore: Lippincott-Williams & Wilkins, 2000.

Figure 2.16. From Haines DE. Neuroanatomy: an Atlas of Structures, Sections, and Systems, 5th ed. Baltimore: Lippincott-Williams & Wilkins, 2000.

Figure 2.17. From Parent A. Carpenter's Human Neuroanatomy, 9th ed. Baltimore: Williams & Wilkins, 1996.

Figure 2.18. From Parent A. Carpenter's Human Neuroanatomy, 9th ed. Baltimore: Williams & Wilkins, 1996.

Figure 2.19. Modified from Carpenter MB. Core Text of Neuroanatomy, 4th ed. Baltimore: Williams & Wilkins, 1991.

Figure 2.20. From Parent A. Carpenter's Human Neuroanatomy, 9th ed. Baltimore: Williams & Wilkins, 1996.

Figure 2.21. From Parent A. Carpenter's Human Neuroanatomy, 9th ed. Baltimore: Williams & Wilkins, 1996.

Figure 2.24B. Modified from Haines DE. Neuroanatomy: an Atlas of Structures, Sections, and Systems, 5th ed. Baltimore: Lippincott-Williams & Wilkins, 2000.

Figure 2.27, A and B. From Haines DE. Neuroanatomy: an Atlas of Structures, Sections, and Systems, 5th ed. Baltimore: Lippincott-Williams & Wilkins, 2000.

Figure 2.28. Modified from Mettler FA. Mettler's Neuroanatomy, 2nd ed. St. Louis: Mosby, 1948.

Figure 2.29. From Haines DE. Neuroanatomy: an Atlas of Structures, Sections, and Systems, 5th ed. Baltimore: Lippincott-Williams & Wilkins, 2000.

Figure 2.31. Modified from Carpenter MB. Core Text of Neuroanatomy, 4th ed. Baltimore: Williams & Wilkins, 1991.

Figure 2.32. Modified from Carpenter MB. Core Text of Neuroanatomy, 4th ed. Baltimore: Williams & Wilkins, 1991.

Figure 2.34. Modified from Parent A. Carpenter's Human Neuroanatomy, 9th ed. Baltimore: Williams & Wilkins, 1996.

Figure 2.36. Modified from Carpenter MB. Core Text of Neuroanatomy, 4th ed. Baltimore: Williams & Wilkins, 1991.

Figure 2.38. Modified from Carpenter MB. Core Text of Neuroanatomy, 4th ed. Baltimore: Williams & Wilkins, 1991.

Figure 2.39. Modified from Heimer L. The Human Brain and Spinal Cord: Functional Neuroanatomy and Dissection Guide. New York: Springer-Verlag, 1983.

Figure 2.40. A. From Mettler FA. Mettler's Neuroanatomy, 2nd ed. St. Louis: Mosby, 1948. B. Haines DE. Neuroanatomy: an Atlas of Structures, Sections, and Systems, 5th ed. Baltimore: Lippincott-Williams & Wilkins, 2000.

Figure 2.41. From Carpenter MB. Core Text of Neuroanatomy, 4th ed. Baltimore: Williams & Wilkins, 1991

Figure 2.42. From Parent A. Carpenter's Human Neuroanatomy, 9th ed. Baltimore: Williams & Wilkins, 1996.

Figure 2.43. From Mettler FA. Mettler's Neuroanatomy, 2nd ed. St. Louis: Mosby, 1948.

Figure 2.44. From Mettler FA. Mettler's Neuroanatomy, 2nd ed. St. Louis: Mosby, 1948.

Figure 2.45. A. Based on Heimer L. The Human Brain and Spinal Cord: Functional Neuroanatomy and Dissection Guide. New York: Springer-Verlag, 1983. B. Based on House EL, and Pansky B. A Functional Approach to Neuroanatomy. New York: McGraw-Hill, 1967.

Figure 2.46A. From Parent A. Carpenter's Human Neuroanatomy, 9th ed. Baltimore: Williams & Wilkins, 1996.

Figure 2.47. From Carpenter MB. Core Text of Neuroanatomy, 4th ed. Baltimore: Williams & Wilkins, 1991.

Figure 2.48. From Carpenter MB. Core Text of Neuroanatomy, 4th ed. Baltimore: Williams & Wilkins, 1991.

Figure 2.49. Modified from Kiernan JA. The Human Nervous System: An Anatomical Viewpoint, 7th ed. Philadelphia: Lippincott-Williams & Wilkins, 1998.

Figure 2.50. From Parent A. Carpenter's Human Neuroanatomy, 9th ed. Baltimore: Williams & Wilkins, 1996.

Figure 3.2. From Haines DE. Neuroanatomy: an Atlas of Structures, Sections, and Systems, 5th ed. Baltimore: Lippincott-Williams & Wilkins, 2000.

Figure 3.3. From Haines DE. Neuroanatomy: an Atlas of Structures, Sections, and Systems, 5th ed. Baltimore: Lippincott-Williams & Wilkins, 2000.

Figure 3.4. From Haines DE. Neuroanatomy: an Atlas of Structures, Sections, and Systems, 5th ed. Baltimore: Lippincott-Williams & Wilkins, 2000.

Figure 3.5. From Haines DE. Neuroanatomy: an Atlas of Structures, Sections, and Systems, 5th ed. Baltimore: Lippincott-Williams & Wilkins, 2000.

Figure 3.6. Modified from Haines DE. Neuroanatomy: an Atlas of Structures, Sections, and Systems, 5th ed. Baltimore: Lippincott-Williams & Wilkins, 2000.

Figure 3.7. From Haines DE. Neuroanatomy: an Atlas of Structures, Sections, and Systems, 5th ed. Baltimore: Lippincott-Williams & Wilkins, 2000.

Figure 3.9. From Haines DE. Neuroanatomy: an Atlas of Structures, Sections, and Systems, 5th ed. Baltimore: Lippincott-Williams & Wilkins, 2000.

Figure 3.10. From Haines DE. Neuroanatomy: an Atlas of Structures, Sections, and Systems, 5th ed. Baltimore: Lippincott-Williams & Wilkins, 2000.

Figure 3.11. From Haines DE. Neuroanatomy: an Atlas of Structures, Sections, and Systems, 5th ed. Baltimore: Lippincott-Williams & Wilkins, 2000.

Figure 3.12. From Haines DE. Neuroanatomy: an Atlas of Structures, Sections, and Systems, 5th ed. Baltimore: Lippincott-Williams & Wilkins, 2000.

Figure 3.13. From Haines DE. Neuroanatomy: an Atlas of Structures, Sections, and Systems, 5th ed. Baltimore: Lippincott-Williams & Wilkins, 2000.

Figure 3.14. From Haines DE. Neuroanatomy: an Atlas of Structures, Sections, and Systems, 5th ed. Baltimore: Lippincott-Williams & Wilkins, 2000.

Figure 3.15. From Haines DE. Neuroanatomy: an Atlas of Structures, Sections, and Systems, 5th ed. Baltimore: Lippincott-Williams & Wilkins, 2000.

Figure 3.16. From Haines DE. Neuroanatomy: an Atlas of Structures, Sections, and Systems, 5th ed. Baltimore: Lippincott-Williams & Wilkins, 2000.

Figure 3.17. From Haines DE. Neuroanatomy: an Atlas of Structures, Sections, and Systems, 5th ed. Baltimore: Lippincott-Williams & Wilkins, 2000.

Figure 3.18. From Haines DE. Neuroanatomy: an Atlas of Structures, Sections, and Systems, 5th ed. Baltimore: Lippincott-Williams & Wilkins, 2000.

Figure 3.19. From Haines DE. Neuroanatomy: an Atlas of Structures, Sections, and Systems, 5th ed. Baltimore: Lippincott-Williams & Wilkins, 2000.

Figure 3.20. Modified from Haines DE. Neuroanatomy: an Atlas of Structures, Sections, and Systems, 5th ed. Baltimore: Lippincott-Williams & Wilkins, 2000.

Figure 3.21. From Haines DE. Neuroanatomy: an Atlas of Structures, Sections, and Systems, 5th ed. Baltimore: Lippincott-Williams & Wilkins, 2000.

Figure 3.22. From Haines DE. Neuroanatomy: an Atlas of Structures, Sections, and Systems, 5th ed. Baltimore: Lippincott-Williams & Wilkins, 2000.

Figure 3.23. From Haines DE. Neuroanatomy: an Atlas of Structures, Sections, and Systems, 5th ed. Baltimore: Lippincott-Williams & Wilkins, 2000.

Figure 3.24. From Haines DE. Neuroanatomy: an Atlas of Structures, Sections, and Systems, 5th ed. Baltimore: Lippincott-Williams & Wilkins, 2000.

Figure 3.25. From Haines DE. Neuroanatomy: an Atlas of Structures, Sections, and Systems, 5th ed. Baltimore: Lippincott-Williams & Wilkins, 2000.

Figure 3.26. Courtesy of Duane E. Haines, Department of Anatomy, University of Mississippi Medical Center.

Figure 4.1. Redrawn from DuPraw EJ. DNA and Chromosomes. New York: Holt, Rinehart & Winston, 1970.

Figure 4.2. From Sadler TW. Langman's Medical Embryology, 8th ed. Philadelphia: Lippincott-Williams & Wilkins, 2000.

Figure 4.3. From Sadler TW. Langman's Medical Embryology, 8th ed. Philadelphia: Lippincott-Williams & Wilkins, 2000.

Figure 4.4. From Sadler TW. Langman's Medical Embryology, 8th ed. Philadelphia: Lippincott-Williams & Wilkins, 2000.

Figure 4.5. From Sadler TW. Langman's Medical Embryology, 8th ed. Philadelphia: Lippincott-Williams & Wilkins, 2000.

Figure 4.6. From Sadler TW. Langman's Medical Embryology, 8th ed. Philadelphia: Lippincott-Williams & Wilkins, 2000.

Figure 4.7. From Sadler TW. Langman's Medical Embryology, 8th ed. Philadelphia: Lippincott-Williams & Wilkins, 2000.

Figure 4.8. From Sadler TW. Langman's Medical Embryology, 8th ed. Philadelphia: Lippincott-Williams & Wilkins, 2000.

Figure 4.9. From Sadler TW. Langman's Medical Embryology, 8th ed. Philadelphia: Lippincott-Williams & Wilkins, 2000.

Figure 4.10. From Sadler TW. Langman's Medical Embryology, 8th ed. Philadelphia: Lippincott-Williams & Wilkins, 2000.

Figure 4.11. From Sadler TW. Langman's Medical Embryology, 8th ed. Philadelphia: Lippincott-Williams & Wilkins, 2000.

Figure 5.1B. Modified from Kiernan JA. The Human Nervous System: An Anatomical Viewpoint, 7th ed. Philadelphia: Lippincott-Williams & Wilkins, 1998.

Figure 5.5. Based on Marieb EN. Essentials of Human Anatomy and Physiology, 4th ed. Menlo Park CA: Benjamin-Cummings, 1994.

Figure 5.8. Modified from Gilman S, and Newman SW. Manter and Gatz's Essentials of Clinical Neuroanatomy and Neurophysiology, 9th ed. Philadelphia: Davis, 1996.

Figure 5.9. Courtesy of Dr. Leighton Mark, Department of Neuroradiology, Medical College of Wisconsin.

Figure 6.1AB. Modified from Parent A. Carpenter's Human Neuroanatomy, 9th ed. Baltimore: Williams & Wilkins, 1996.

Figure 7.4B. Modified from Parent A. Carpenter's Human Neuroanatomy, 9th ed. Baltimore: Williams & Wilkins, 1996.

Figure 7.5B. Modified from Parent A. Carpenter's Human Neuroanatomy, 9th ed. Baltimore: Williams & Wilkins, 1996.

Figure 7.6. Modified from Parent A. Carpenter's Human Neuroanatomy 9th ed. Baltimore: Williams & Wilkins, 1996.

Figure 7.7B. Modified from Parent A. Carpenter's Human Neuroanatomy, 9th ed. Baltimore: Williams & Wilkins, 1996.

Figure 7.8. Modified from Parent A. Carpenter's Human Neuroanatomy, 9th ed. Baltimore: Williams & Wilkins, 1996.

Figure 7.9B. Modified from Crosby E, Humphrey T, and Lauer E. Correlative Anatomy of the Nervous System. New York: Macmillan, 1962.

Figure 7.10. Modified from Carpenter MB. Core Text of Neuroanatomy, 4th ed. Baltimore: Williams & Wilkins, 1991.

Figure 8.1. Based on Carpenter MB. Core Text of Neuroanatomy, 4th ed. Baltimore: Williams & Wilkins, 1991.

Figure 8.2AB. Redrawn from Lavine RA. Neurophysiology, the Fundamentals. Lexington MA: Heath, 1983.

Figure 8.5. Modified from Lavine RA. Neurophysiology, the Fundamentals. Lexington MA: Heath, 1983.

Figure 8.6. Based on Eyzaguiuirre C, and Fiddone S. Physiology of the Nervous System. Chicago: Yearbook, 1975.

Figure 8.9. Modified from Carpenter MB. Core Text of Neuroanatomy, 4th ed. Baltimore: Williams & Wilkins, 1991.

Figure 8.14. Modified from Carpenter MB. Core Text of Neuroanatomy, 4th ed. Baltimore: Williams & Wilkins, 1991.

Figure 9.2. Redrawn from Lavine RA. Neurophysiology: the Fundamentals. Lexington MA: Collamore Press, 1983.

Figure 9.3. From Parent A. Carpenter's Human Neuroanatomy, 9th ed. Baltimore: Williams & Wilkins, 1996.

Figure 9.4. From Parent A. Carpenter's Human Neuroanatomy, 9th ed. Baltimore: Williams & Wilkins, 1996.

Figure 9.6. Modified from Parent A. Carpenter's Human Neuroanatomy, 9th ed. Baltimore: Williams & Wilkins, 1996.

Figure 9.7. Modified from Carpenter MB. Core Text of Neuroanatomy, 4th ed. Baltimore: Williams & Wilkins, 1991.

Figure 9.9. Modified from Carpenter MB. Core Text of Neuroanatomy, 4th ed. Baltimore: Williams & Wilkins, 1991.

Figure 9.10. From Haines DE. Neuroanatomy: an Atlas of Structures, Sections, and Systems, 5th ed. Baltimore: Lippincott-Williams & Wilkins, 2000.

Figure 10.2B. Based on Kandel ER, Schwartz JH, and Jessell TM. Principles of Neural Science, 4th ed. New York: McGraw-Hill, 2000.

Figure 10.3C. Modified from Curtis BA, Jacobson S, and Marcus EM. An Introduction to the Neurosciences. Philadelphia: Saunders, 1972.

Figure 10.4. Modified from Carpenter MB. Core Text of Neuroanatomy, 4th ed. Baltimore: Williams & Wilkins, 1991.

Figure 10.5. Based on House EL, and Pansky B. A Functional Approach to Neuroanatomy. New York: McGraw-Hill, 1967.

Figure 10.6. Based on House EL, and Pansky B. A Functional Approach to Neuroanatomy. New York: McGraw-Hill, 1967.

Figure 11.2. Modified from Parent A. Carpenter's Human Neuroanatomy, 9th ed. Baltimore: Williams & Wilkins, 1996.

Figure 11.4. Modified from Parent A. Carpenter's Human Neuroanatomy, 9th ed. Baltimore: Williams & Wilkins, 1996.

Figure 11.6. Modified from Parent A. Carpenter's Human Neuroanatomy, 9th ed. Baltimore: Williams & Wilkins, 1996.

Figure 11.7. Modified from Carpenter MB. Core Text of Neuroanatomy, 4th ed. Baltimore: Williams & Wilkins, 1991.

Figure 11.8. Modified from Carpenter MB. Core Text of Neuroanatomy, 4th ed. Baltimore: William & Wilkins, 1991.

Figure 11.10, A and B. Based on Gardener E. Fundamentals of Neurology. Philadelphia: Saunders, 1975.

Figure 11.12. Modified from Carpenter MB. Core Text of Neuroanatomy, 4th ed. Baltimore: Williams & Wilkins, 1991.

Figure 12.1AB. Modified from Carpenter MB. Core Text of Neuroanatomy, 4th ed. Baltimore: Williams & Wilkins, 1991.

Figure 12.2. A. From Parent A. Carpenter's Human Neuroanatomy, 9th ed. Baltimore: Williams & Wilkins, 1996. **B.** From Mettler FA. Mettler's Neuroanatomy, 2nd ed. St. Louis: Mosby, 1948.

Figure 12.3. From Parent A. Carpenter's Human Neuroanatomy, 9th ed. Baltimore: Williams & Wilkins, 1996.

Figure 12.4. From Parent A. Carpenter's Human Neuroanatomy, 9th ed. Baltimore: Williams & Wilkins, 1996.

Figure 12.5. A. Modified from Carpenter MB. Core Text of Neuroanatomy, 4th ed. Baltimore: Williams & Wilkins, 1991. **B.** Based on Guyton AC. Textbook of Medical Physiology, 7th ed. Philadelphia: Saunders, 1986.

Figure 13.1B. Modified from Carpenter MB. Core Text of Neuroanatomy, 4th ed. Baltimore: Williams & Wilkins, 1991.

Figure 13.4. Modified from Parent A. Carpenter's Human Neuroanatomy, 9th ed. Baltimore: Williams & Wilkins, 1996.

Figure 13.5. Modified from Parent A. Carpenter's Human Neuroanatomy, 9th ed. Baltimore: Williams & Wilkins, 1996.

Figure 13.6. Modified from Parent A. Carpenter's Human Neuroanatomy, 9th ed. Baltimore: Williams & Wilkins, 1996.

Figure 14.1. A. Modified from Parent A. Carpenter's Human Neuroanatomy, 9th ed. Baltimore: Williams & Wilkins, 1996.

Figure 14.2. Modified from Parent A. Carpenter's Human Neuroanatomy, 9th ed. Baltimore: Williams & Wilkins, 1996.

Figure 14.7. From Haines DE. Neuroanatomy: an Atlas of Structures, Sections, and Systems, 5th ed. Baltimore: Lippincott-Williams & Wilkins, 2000.

Figure 15.1. From Mettler FA. Mettler's Neuroanatomy, 2nd ed. St. Louis: Mosby, 1948.

Figure 15.2. Modified from Moore KL, and Persaud TVN. The Developing Human: Clinically Oriented Embryology, 6th ed. Philadelphia: Saunders, 1998.

Figure 15.3, A and B. From Parent A. Carpenter's Human Neuroanatomy, 9th ed. Baltimore: Williams & Wilkins, 1996.

Figure 15.7. From Carpenter MB. Core Text of Neuroanatomy, 4th ed. Baltimore: Williams & Wilkins, 1991.

Figure 15.8. From Carpenter MB. Core Text of Neuroanatomy, 4th ed. Baltimore: Williams & Wilkins, 1991.

Figure 15.9. Redrawn from Carpenter MB. Core Text of Neuroanatomy, 4th ed. Baltimore: Williams & Wilkins, 1991.

Figure 15.10. Modified from Carpenter MB. Core Text of Neuroanatomy, 4th ed. Baltimore: Williams & Wilkins, 1991.

Figures 15.11, 15.14, 15.15, 15.18, 15.19, 15.22-15.26, 15.28-15.32. Based on information illustrated in House EL, and Pansky B. A Functional Approach to Neuroanatomy. New York: McGraw-Hill, 1967.

Figure 15.12. Modified from Carpenter MB. Core Text of Neuroanatomy, 4th ed. Baltimore: Williams & Wilkins, 1991.

Figure 15.13. Redrawn from Kaufman DM. Clinical Neurology for Psychiatrists, 3rd ed. Philadelphia: Saunders, 1990.

Figure 15.16. Redrawn from Kaufman DM. Clinical Neurology for Psychiatrists, 3rd ed. Philadelphia: Saunders, 1990.

Figure 15.17. Modified from Carpenter MB. Core Text of Neuroanatomy, 4th ed. Baltimore: Williams & Wilkins, 1991.

Figure 15.21. Modified from Carpenter MB. Core Text of Neuroanatomy, 4th ed. Baltimore: Williams & Wilkins, 1991.

Figure 15.29. Redrawn from Van Allen MW, and Rodnitzky RL. Pictorial Manual of Neurologic Tests, 2nd ed. Chicago: Yearbook, 1981.

Figure 16.6. From Carpenter MB. Core Text of Neuroanatomy, 4th ed. Baltimore: Williams & Wilkins, 1991.

Figure 16.7. From Carpenter MB. Core Text of Neuroanatomy, 4th ed. Baltimore: Williams & Wilkins, 1991.

Figure 16.8. From Carpenter MB. Core Text of Neuroanatomy, 4th ed. Baltimore: Williams & Wilkins, 1991.

Figure 16.9. From Carpenter MB. Core Text of Neuroanatomy, 4th ed. Baltimore: Williams & Wilkins, 1991.

Figure 16.10. From Carpenter MB. Core Text of Neuroanatomy, 4th ed. Baltimore: Williams & Wilkins, 1991.

Figure 17.2. From Carpenter MB. Core Text of Neuroanatomy, 4th ed. Baltimore: Williams & Wilkins, 1991.

Figure 17.3A. From Carpenter MB. Core Text of Neuroanatomy, 4th ed. Baltimore: Williams & Wilkins, 1991.

Figure 17.4A. From Carpenter MB. Core Text of Neuroanatomy, 4th ed. Baltimore: Williams & Wilkins, 1991.

Figures 17.8, 9AB, 17.10AB. Courtesy of Dr. Leighton Mark, Department of Neuroradiology, Medical College of Wisconsin.

Figure 17.11. From Parent A. Carpenter's Human Neuroanatomy, 9th ed. Baltimore: Williams & Wilkins, 1996.

Figure 17.12, A. and B. From Carpenter MB. Core Text of Neuroanatomy, 4th ed. Baltimore: Williams & Wilkins, 1991.

Figure 18.2A. From Parent A. Carpenter's Human Neuroanatomy, 9th ed. Baltimore: Williams & Wilkins, 1996.

Figure 20.1-20.2. Courtesy of Dr. Varun K. Saxena, Center for Neurological Disorders, Milwaukee, Wisconsin.

Figure 20.4AB. Courtesy of Dr. Leighton Mark, Department of Neuroradiology, Medical College of Wisconsin.

Figure 20.6. Courtesy of Dr. John Mazziotta, Reed Institute, UCLA Medical Center, Los Angeles, California.

Figure 20.7AB. Courtesy of Dr. Howard S. Kirshner, Vanderbilt Medical Center, Nashville, Tennessee.

Figure 20.11B. Modified from Carpenter MB. Core Text of Neuroanatomy, 4th ed. Baltimore: Williams & Wilkins, 1991.

Figure 20.12. Modified from Bhatnagar SC, Andy OJ, Korabic EW, and Tikofsky RS. Effects of bilateral thalamic stimulation on dichotic verbal processing. J Neurolinguistics 1990;4:407-425.

Figure 20.15. Modified from Genetic Counseling. White Plains NY: March of Dimes Birth Defects Foundation Booklet 9-0022, Jul 1984.

Figure 20.16. Modified from Genetic Counseling. White Plains NY: March of Dimes Birth Defects Foundation Booklet 9-0022, Jul 1984.

Figure 20.17. Modified from Genetic Counseling. White Plains NY: March of Dimes Birth Defects Foundation Booklet 9-0022, Jul 1984.

TABLES

Table 4.1. Modified from Arey LB. Developmental Anatomy. Philadelphia: Saunders, 1966.

Table 4.2. Modified from Moore KL, and Persaud TVN. The Developing Human, Clinically Oriented Embryology, 5th ed. Philadelphia: Saunders, 1993.

Table 4.3. Modified from Menkes JH. Textbook of Child Neurology, 5th ed. Baltimore: Williams & Wilkins, 1990:210.

Index

Page numbers in *italics* denote figures; those followed by a "t" denote tables.